# Laryngeal Manifestations
# of Systemic Diseases

# Laryngeal Manifestations of Systemic Diseases

Abdul-Latif Hamdan, MD, EMBA, MPH, FACS
Robert Thayer Sataloff, MD, DMA, FACS
Mary J. Hawkshaw, BSN, RN, CORLN

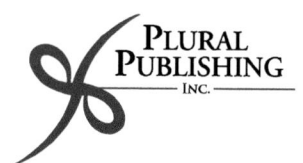

PLURAL
PUBLISHING
INC.

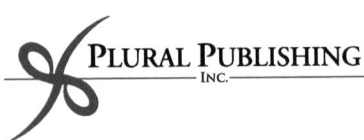

5521 Ruffin Road
San Diego, CA 92123

e-mail: information@pluralpublishing.com
Website: http://www.pluralpublishing.com

NOTICE TO THE READER
Care has been taken to confirm the accuracy of the indications, procedures, drug dosages, and diagnosis and remediation protocols presented in this book and to ensure that they conform to the practices of the general medical and health services communities. However, the authors, editors, and publisher are not responsible for errors or omissions or for any consequences from application of the information in this book and make no warranty, expressed or implied, with respect to the currency, completeness, or accuracy of the contents of the publication. The diagnostic and remediation protocols and the medications described do not necessarily have specific approval by the Food and Drug administration for use in the disorders and/or diseases and dosages for which they are recommended. Application of this information in a particular situation remains the professional responsibility of the practitioner. Because standards of practice and usage change, it is the responsibility of the practitioner to keep abreast of revised recommendations, dosages, and procedures.

**Library of Congress Cataloging-in-Publication Data:**

Names: Hamdan, A. L. (Abdul Latif), editor. | Sataloff, Robert Thayer, editor. | Hawkshaw, Mary, editor. | Based on (work): Sataloff, Robert Thayer. Professional voice. Fourth edition.
Title: Laryngeal manifestations of systemic diseases / [edited by] Abdul-Latif Hamdan, Robert Thayer Sataloff, Mary J. Hawkshaw.
Description: San Diego, CA : Plural Publishing, [2019] | "Some of the material in this book was derived from Sataloff, RT. Professional Voice: The Science and Art of Clinical Care, Fourth Edition. San Diego, California: Plural Publishing, Inc.; 2017 . . . much of the material in Laryngeal Manifestations of Systemic Disease is new, reworked, and/or expanded"—Pref. | Includes bibliographical references and index.
Identifiers: LCCN 2018028889 | ISBN 9781635501292 (alk. paper) | ISBN 1635501296 (alk. paper)
Subjects: | MESH: Voice Disorders—physiopathology | Voice—physiology | Larynx—pathology
Classification: LCC RF510 | NLM WV 500 | DDC 616.85/506—dc23
LC record available at https://lccn.loc.gov/2018028889

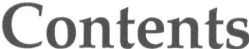

# Contents

# Preface

Voice conveys much more than intellectual messages. Most people recognize vocal expression of emotion. For example, when we answer a phone call from a parent, we need to hear no more than the word "hello" to know whether the call brings good news or bad. Similarly, voice change may offer the first indication of various systemic disorders. *Laryngeal Manifestations of Systemic Disease* summarizes the vocal changes that occur with disorders throughout the body. It is common for dysphonia to be the first manifestation of systemic disease. So, familiarity with laryngeal manifestation of systemic disease is important not only for otolaryngologists and phoniatrists, but also for family practitioners, internists, medical students, physician assistants, nurse practitioners, nurse clinicians, speech-language pathologists, singing voice specialists, acting voice specialists, voice teachers, and others entrusted with the care, education, and health of the human voice. This book is intended for all such professionals, and for patients, particularly professional voice users, who want to know as much as possible about their instrument and conditions that might affect it adversely.

*Laryngeal Manifestations of Systemic Disease* synthesizes current knowledge about voice modifications associated with various disorders.

After providing basic introductory information in the initial chapters, the chapters in this book review pathophysiology of systemic diseases and their effects on phonation, with summaries of current literature; and we have attempted to assist clinicians by including intriguing cases and images. Some of the material in this book was derived from R.T. Sataloff *Professional Voice: The Science and Art of Clinical Care, Fourth Edition* (2017), San Diego, California: Plural Publishing, Inc., with the permission of Plural Publishing, Inc. However, although that publication is recent, much of the material in *Laryngeal Manifestations of Systemic Disease* is new, reworked, and/or expanded.

Chapter 1, Clinical Anatomy and Physiology of the Voice, contains a great deal of information about laryngeal anatomy, neuroanatomy, respiratory function and other topics that, to the best of our knowledge, has not been synthesized in similar detail in a single source elsewhere, except in Sataloff's *Professional Voice: The Science and Art of Clinical Care, Fourth Edition*, from which this chapter has been republished. Chapter 2 on Genetics of the Voice reviews what is known about the genetics of voice from a clinical perspective. Genetic considerations are increasingly important to understanding and treating systemic disease. In Chapter 3 on the Impact of Aging on the Voice, we summarize vocal changes associated with the aging process, a common and expected cause of voice modification. Chapter 4, Common Medical Diagnoses and Treatments in Patients with Voice Disorders: An Introduction and Overview, provides insights on a great many maladies that may alter the voice, some of which are covered in much greater details in subsequent chapters. Chapter 5 on Sleep, Body Fatigue, and Voice reviews the importance of sleep and general well-being to vocal health, and dysphonic changes that might be expected with deficiencies in either. Laryngeal Manifestations of Neurologic Disorders are discussed in Chapter 6. In this chapter, various neurological conditions are summarized including tremor, multiple sclerosis, myasthenia gravis, dystonia, and others. Understanding the pathophysiology of their effects on voice should be of value to anyone caring for the many patients with such maladies. In addition to covering various aspects of psychological assessment and treatment, Chapter 7 on Psychological Aspects of Voice Disorders integrates information on the role of psychological professionals and others involved in management of emotional and psychological challenges in voice patients. Chapter 8, Impact of the Auditory System on Voice, reviews dysphonia associated with hearing function and dysfunction. Laryngeal Manifestations of Respiratory Disorders, Chapter 9, reviews the many effects of respiratory dysfunction upon phonation. Since "support," or the power source of the voice, depends upon efficient pulmonary function and aerobic conditioning, respiratory disorders commonly are associated with dysphonia. Allergies often cause dysphonia, and basic, clinically practical information on this topic is presented in Chapter 10. In Chapter 11 on Laryngeal Manifestations of Gastrointestinal Disorders, the impact of gastroenterological dysfunction upon phonation is reviewed in detail, with special attention to laryngopharyngeal reflux. This chapter includes approximately 600 references in a comprehensive update of this important topic and it is republished from the fourth edition of Sataloff's book on Professional Voice. Laryngeal Manifestations of Autoimmune Disorders, Chapter 12, reviews many of the autoimmune diseases that may affect the voice including rheumatoid arthritis, systemic lupus erythematosus, and others. Chapter 13, Laryngeal Manifestations of Endocrine Disorders, provides an overview of endocrinologic dysfunction. The voice is extremely sensitive to even slight changes in the hormonal environment, and good laryngologists commonly diagnose endocrinologic disorders based on a presenting complaint of dysphonia. Chapter 14 on Bodily Injuries and Their Effects on the Voice, presents the consequences of trauma upon phonation. Any injury that causes pain (back, neck, extremity, shoulder, or elsewhere) that alters posture or muscle function and balance may affect the voice. Chapter 15 on Medications and the Voice reviews the voice effects associated with many medications commonly prescribed for disorders throughout the body. Not only systemic disease but also its treatment may be responsible for a voice complaint.

We hope that this book will prove useful for our readers and will help make all of us better holistic diagnosticians. When a patient presents with a voice complaint and we diagnose a previously unrecognized systemic disease, we may not only improve the voice, but we also may save a life.

—Abdul-Latif Hamdan, MD, EMBA, MPH, FACS,
American University of Beirut Medical Center

—Robert T. Sataloff, MD, DMA, FACS,
Drexel University College of Medicine

—Mary J. Hawkshaw, RN, BSN, CORLN,
Drexel University College of Medicine

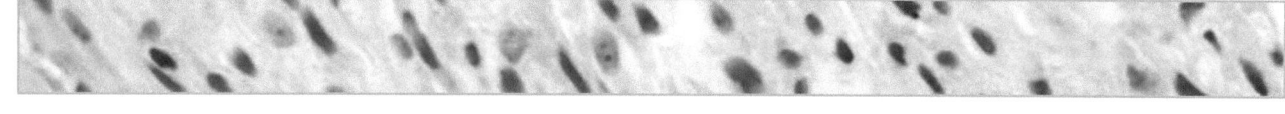

# Contributors

**Joseph Anticaglia, MD**
Ear, Nose, and Throat Associates of New York
Flushing, New York
*Chapter 15*

**Donald O. Castell, MD**
Professor of Medicine
Director of Esophageal Disorders Program
Department of Gastroenterology and Hepatology
Charleston, South Carolina
*Chapter 11*

**John R. Cohn, MD, FCCP**
Professor of Medicine and Pediatrics
Thomas Jefferson University
Philadelphia, Pennsylvania
*Chapter 10*

**Abdul-Latif Hamdan, MD, EMBA, MPH, FACS**
Professor of Otolaryngology, Head and Neck
    Surgery
Head, Division of Laryngology
Director of "Hamdan Voice Unit"
American University of Beirut Medical Center
Beirut, Lebanon
*Chapters 3, 5, 6, 9, 12, 13*

**Mary J. Hawkshaw, RN, BSN, CORLN**
Research Professor
Department of Otolaryngology-Head and Neck
    Surgery
Drexel University College of Medicine
Philadelphia, Pennsylvania
*Chapters 2, 3, 4, 5, 6, 9, 10, 11, 12, 13, 15*

**Reinhardt J. Heuer, PhD**
Professor Emeritus
Department of Communication Sciences and
    Disorders
Temple University
Adjunct Professor
Department of Otolaryngology-Head and Neck
    Surgery
Drexel University College of Medicine
Philadelphia, Pennsylvania
*Chapter 7*

**Philip O. Katz, MD**
Professor
Department of Medicine
Division of Gastroenterology
Weill Cornell Medical Center
New York, New York
*Chapter 11*

**Kirsten Meenan, BS**
Drexel University College of Medicine
Philadelphia, Pennsylvania
*Chapter 15*

**Patricia A. Padams, RN, BSN, CEN**
Nurse Manager and Clinical Research Coordinator
(In association with John R. Cohn, MD)
Thomas Jefferson University
Philadelphia, Pennsylvania
*Chapter 10*

**Jonathan J. Romak, MD**
Instructor
Department of Otolaryngology-Head and Neck
    Surgery
Drexel University College of Medicine
Philadelphia, Pennsylvania
*Chapter 15*

**Deborah Caputo Rosen, RN, PhD**
President
Caputo Rosen Consulting
Philadelphia, Pennsylvania
*Chapter 7*

**David A. Sasso, MD, MPH**
Assistant Clinical Professor
Child Study Center
Yale School of Medicine
New Haven, Connecticut
*Chapter 7*

**Dahlia M. Sataloff, MD**
Chairman, Department of Surgery
Pennsylvania Hospital
Professor of Clinical Surgery
University of Pennsylvania

Perelman School of Medicine
Philadelphia, Pennsylvania
*Chapter 11*

**Johnathan B. Sataloff, BS, BA**
Harvard Medical School
Harvard University
Boston, MA
*Chapter 4*

**Robert Thayer Sataloff, MD, DMA, FACS**
Professor and Chairman
Department of Otolaryngology-Head and Neck
  Surgery
Senior Associate Dean for Clinical Academic
  Specialties
Drexel University College of Medicine
Chairman, The Voice Foundation
Chairman, American Institute for Voice and Ear
  Research

Faculty, Academy of Vocal Arts
Philadelphia, Pennsylvania
*Chapters 1, 2, 3, 4, 5, 6, 7, 8, 9, 10, 11, 12, 13, 14, 15*

**Morgan A. Selleck, MD**
Resident
Department of Otolaryngology-Head and Neck
  Surgery
Chapel Hill School of Medicine
University of North Carolina
Chapel Hill, North Carolina
*Chapter 8*

**Michelle White, BA**
Drexel University College of Medicine
Philadelphia, Pennsylvania
*Chapter 15*

# Clinical Anatomy and Physiology of the Voice

*Robert Thayer Sataloff*

## Anatomy

The anatomy of the voice is not limited to the region between the suprasternal notch and the hyoid bone. Practically all body systems affect the voice. The larynx receives the greatest attention because it is the most sensitive and expressive component of the vocal mechanism, but anatomic interactions throughout the patient's body must be considered in treating voice disorders. It is helpful to think of the larynx as composed of 4 anatomic units—skeleton, mucosa, intrinsic muscles, and extrinsic muscles—as well as vascular, neurological, and other related structures. The glottis is the space between the vocal folds. The term *vocal cords* was abandoned in favor of the term *vocal folds* more than 3 decades ago. Vocal folds is a more accurate description of the structure, as described below (although not quite so accurate as the German term "vocal lips"). Moreover, the word "cord" often makes people think of a string-like structure, and vocal fold motion is not similar to a vibrating string.

### Laryngeal Skeleton: Cartilages, Ligaments, and Membranes

The most important parts of the laryngeal skeleton are the thyroid cartilage, the cricoid cartilage, and the 2 arytenoid cartilages (Figure 1–1). The laryngeal cartilages are connected by soft attachments that allow changes in their relative angles and distances, thereby permitting alterations in the shape and tension of the tissues extended between them. The intrinsic muscles of the larynx are connected to these cartilages.

For example, one of the intrinsic muscles, the thyro-arytenoid (TA), extends on each side from the arytenoid cartilage to the inside of the thyroid cartilage just below and behind the thyroid prominence. The medial belly of the TA is also known as the vocalis muscle, and it forms the body of the vocal fold.

The pyramidal, paired arytenoid cartilages sit atop the superior edge of the cricoid cartilage. They each include a muscular process, a vocal process and an apex, a body, and a complex, concave articular surface. They are hyaline cartilages, except for the vocal process, and the apices in some cases, which are composed of fibroelastic cartilage. The hyaline portions generally begin to ossify at around 30 years of age.[2] Clinically, arytenoid asymmetry is common. Hamdan et al. studied 110 singers (male-to-female ratio of 2:1) and found no correlation between arytenoid asymmetry and vocal symptoms.[3] In a later study, they also found no correlation between arytenoid asymmetry and posture, neck tension, or glottal attack.[4] Bonilha et al also found that arytenoid asymmetry was common, but there were no statistically significant differences in prevalence of arytenoid asymmetries comparing subjects with normal voices and those with dysphonia.[5]

Ossification of the thyroid cartilage begins earlier, usually at around 20 years of age, and usually begins posteriorly and inferiorly.[2] The 2 thyroid laminae join in the midline, forming an angle of approximately 120° in women and approximately 90° in men. The thyroid prominence is also more noticeable in men and is commonly known as the "Adam's apple." Just above the thyroid prominence, the thyroid laminae form a "V," the thyroid notch. Posteriorly, the

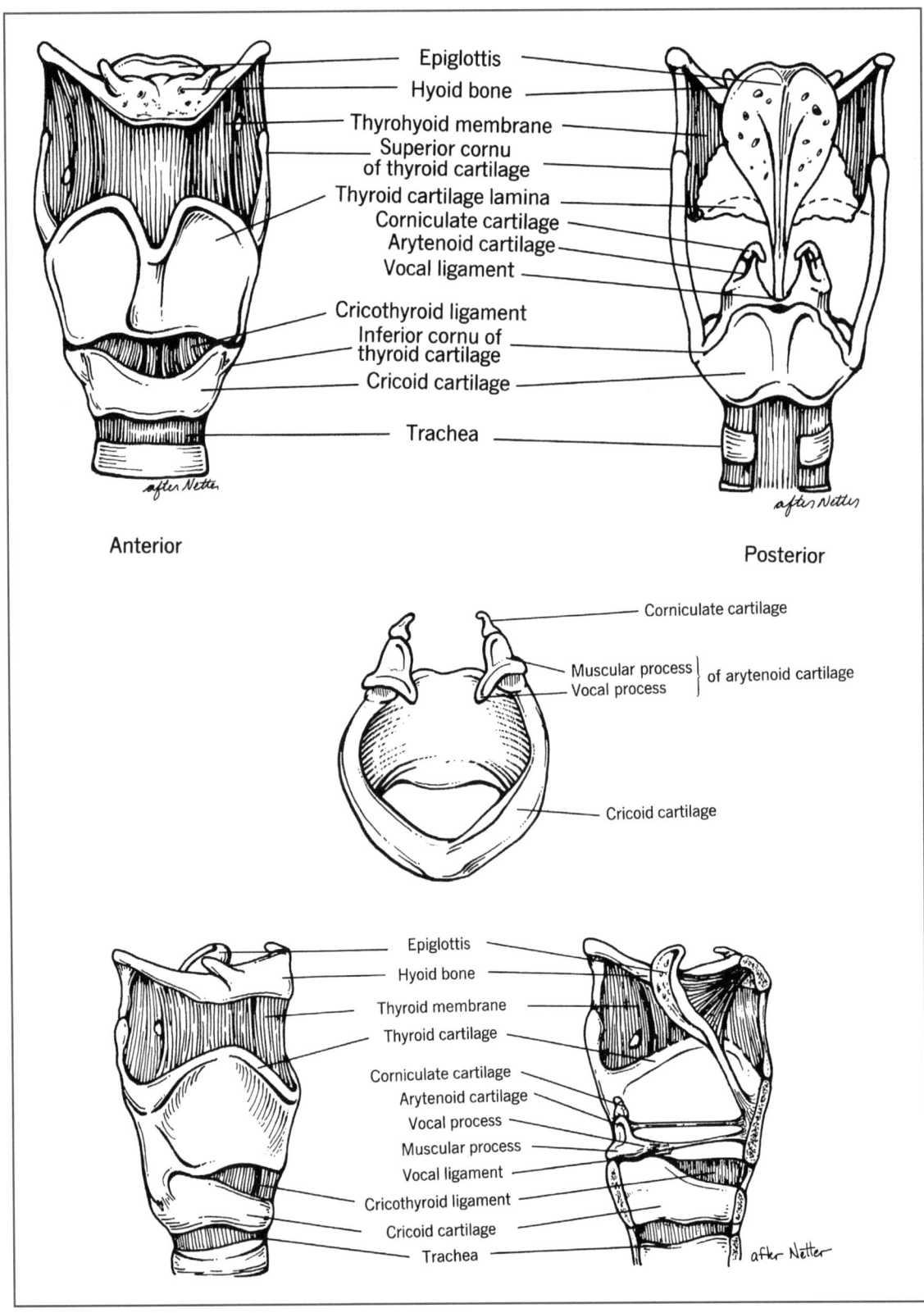

Epiglottis
Hyoid bone
Thyrohyoid membrane
Superior cornu of thyroid cartilage
Thyroid cartilage lamina
Corniculate cartilage
Arytenoid cartilage
Vocal ligament
Cricothyroid ligament
Inferior cornu of thyroid cartilage
Cricoid cartilage
Trachea

after Netter

Anterior

after Netter

Posterior

Corniculate cartilage
Muscular process
Vocal process
of arytenoid cartilage
Cricoid cartilage

Epiglottis
Hyoid bone
Thyroid membrane
Thyroid cartilage
Corniculate cartilage
Arytenoid cartilage
Vocal process
Muscular process
Vocal ligament
Cricothyroid ligament
Cricoid cartilage
Trachea

after Netter

**A**

**Figure 1–1. A.** Cartilages of the larynx. *(continues)*

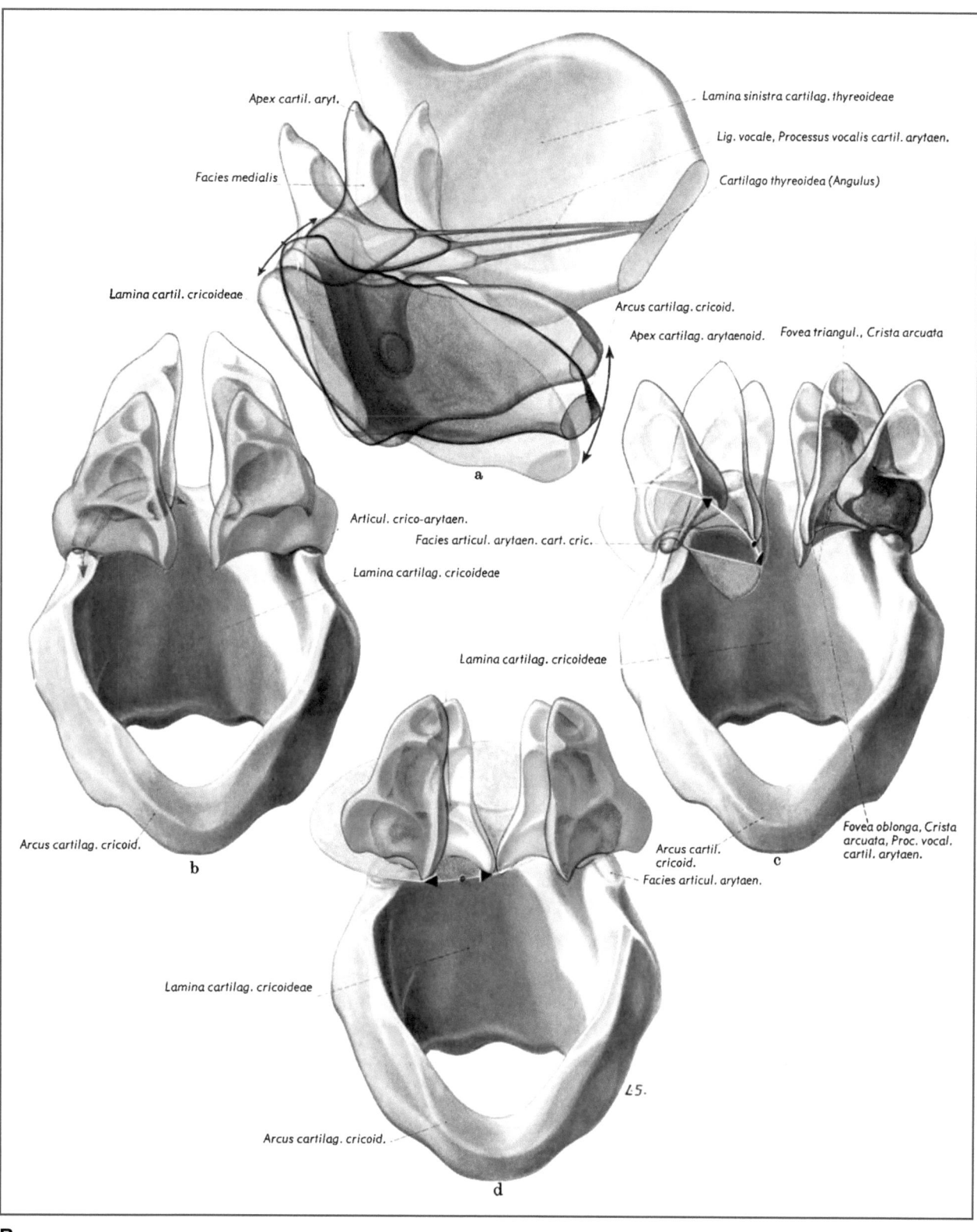

B

**Figure 1–1.** *(continued)* **B.** Schematic representation of position changes of laryngeal cartilages illustrating the most extreme positions achieved by each. (Reproduced with permission from Pernkopf.[1])

laminae extend to form superior and inferior cornua (horns). The superior cornu connects to the hyoid bone via the thyrohyoid ligament. The inferior cornu is connected to the cricoid cartilage by a synovial cricothyroid joint. The joint is encased in a capsular ligament, which is strengthened posteriorly by a fibrous band. Movement of the paired cricothyroid joints is diarthrodial. The primary movement is rotary, with the cricoid rotating around a transverse axis passing through both joints. Gliding in various directions also occurs to a limited extent. This joint tends to move anteromedially during vocal fold adduction and posterolaterally during vocal fold abduction and permits the anterior aspects of the cricoid and thyroid cartilages to be brought more closely together to increase vocal fold length (and frequency of phonation, or pitch) in response to cricothyroid (CT) muscle contraction.

The perichondrium of the thyroid cartilage is thinner internally than externally. Externally, in the midline, there is a tiny landmark that can be helpful in identifying the position of the anterior commissure.[6] This small, diamond-shaped surface depression is associated with a slightly lighter color compared to the adjacent thyroid cartilage. It is found in the anterior midline, approximately halfway between the thyroid notch and the inferior border of the thyroid cartilage, and a small, unnamed artery travels through this tiny depression, as described by Adams et al.[6] The landmark is referred to sometimes as Montgomery's aperture. At a corresponding location on the inner surface, there is a small protrusion that is devoid of perichondrium. This is the point of attachment of Broyles ligament and the anterior commissure tendon. The rest of the thyroid cartilage is covered with fairly thick perichondrium, and the smooth, concave inner surface is covered by a mucosal membrane. Broyles ligament is formed by the vocal ligament (which is also the upper border of the conus elasticus), the internal perichondrium of the thyroid cartilage, and the thyroepiglottic ligament.

The oblique line is another important external landmark of the thyroid cartilage. It runs anteroinferiorly from a superior thyroid tubercle located just inferior to the superior cornu, and it extends to the inferior thyroid tubercle located at the lower border of the thyroid lamina. The oblique line is actually a ridge to which the thyrohyoid, sternothyroid, and inferior pharyngeal constrictor muscles attach. Fibers from the palatopharyngeus and stylopharyngeus muscles attach to the posterior border of the thyroid cartilage.

The signet ring–shaped cricoid cartilage is the only circumferential cartilaginous structure in the airway. Its posterior lamina may rise to a height of approximately 30 millimeters (mm), and its anterior arch may be only a few millimeters in height. Not only is the anterior aspect of the arch thin, but it also ossifies later than the posterior aspect of the cricoid cartilage, which begins to ossify in the early to mid-20s. Because the anterior portion of the arch is both thin and tends to ossify later, it is particularly prone to fracture during surgical manipulation. This should be remembered in procedures such as cricothyroid approximation; traction should always be centered laterally on the cricoid arch, rather than near the midline. The cricoid and thyroid cartilages are joined through the cricothyroid joints. These synovial joints vary among individuals. They have been divided into 3 groups.[7] In group 1, the rotation axis of the cricothyroid joint is located in the lower third of the joint (13 of 24 specimens studied); in group 2, it is located in the middle third of the joint (5/23); and in group 3 the effective axis of rotation is located in the lower third of the cricoid cartilage. Elongations of the vocal fold were 12% in group 1, 8% in group 2, and 3% in group 3. These differences may be important for patients undergoing cricothyroid approximation surgery, but more research is needed to confirm these findings and investigate their clinical implications. The cricoid is connected to the thyroid cartilage not only through the cricothyroid joints, but also through the cricothyroid membrane and its midline thickening known as the cricothyroid ligament.

Internal dimensions of the cricoid cartilage and trachea vary substantially. Such information is important with regard to tracheal intubation, dilatation, stenting, endoscopy, anastomosis, and transplantation. The luminal cross sections vary between and among men and women. The smallest dimension occurs in the frontal plane.[8] In women, this measures approximately 11.6 mm, with a range of 8.9 to 17 mm. In men, it is about 15 mm, with a range of 11 to 21.5 mm. The distance between the cricoarytenoid joint facets varies from person to person, as well, as does the angle between longitudinal axes of the cricoarytenoid joint facets (42°–74° in women, 37°–75° in men).[8] Morphometric characteristics of the larynx have also been studied by Jotz et al.[9] They examined larynges of 50 male and 50 female fresh cadavers of humans older than 40 years. All laryngeal measurements were greater in men than in women except for the thyroid angle that was greater in women. There was no significant difference in morphological comparison between men and women among various age groups.

The cross section of the trachea is also highly variable, with a frontal diameter reported as narrow as 9.9 mm in women and 12 mm in men.[8] The marked variation in size and shape highlights the difficulty in creating a standardized rigid stent. It should also be noted that the diameter of the cricoid ring in some women is too narrow to permit the atraumatic passage of an endotracheal tube with a 7-mm internal diameter. Anatomic variation also must be taken into consideration during laryngotracheal replacement or transplantation.

In addition to the cricoid, thyroid, and paired arytenoid cartilages, there are numerous other components of the laryngeal skeleton and the related structures. The superior aspect of the laryngeal skeleton is the hyoid bone, which is usually ossified by age 2. The hyoid bone attaches to the mylohyoid, geniohyoid, and hyoglossus muscles superiorly and inferiorly connects to the thyroid cartilage via the thyrohyoid membrane. This U-shaped bone has an inferiorly located lesser cornu and a superiorly located greater cornu on each side.

The epiglottis is a fibroelastic cartilage that is shaped like a leaf and narrows inferiorly where it becomes the petiole. The petiole attaches to the inner surface of the thyroid cartilage immediately below the thyroid notch by the thyroepiglottic ligament. The superior aspect of the epiglottis faces the base of the tongue anteriorly and the laryngeal inlet posteriorly. The hyoepiglottic ligament connects the posterior surface of the hyoid bone to the lingual surface of the epiglottis. On its laryngeal surface, the epiglottis contains a protuberance that sometimes obscures view of the anterior commissure. This is the epiglottic tubercle. Perichondrium is less densely adherent to the epiglottic cartilage on the lingual surface than on the laryngeal surface, explaining why epiglottic edema tends to be more prominent in the vallecula than in the laryngeal inlet. However, edema on the lingual surface can push the epiglottis posteriorly, resulting in airway obstruction. The preepiglottic space is formed by the mucosa of the vallecula superiorly, the thyroid cartilage and thyrohyoid membrane anteriorly, and the epiglottis posteriorly and inferiorly. Blood vessels and lymphatic channels course through this space.

There are several cartilages of less functional importance located above the thyroid cartilage. The cartilages of Santorini, or corniculate cartilages, are fibroelastic and are found above the arytenoid cartilages. They help improve the rigidity of the aryepiglottic folds. Like the epiglottis and many other elastic cartilages, they do not ossify. The cuneiform cartilages (cartilages of Wrisberg) also do not ossify, even though they consist of hyaline cartilage. They are located in the aryepiglottic folds and also improve rigidity, helping to direct swallowing toward the piriform sinuses. The triticeal cartilages are located laterally within the thyrohyoid ligaments. These structures are hyaline cartilages and often do ossify

(as may the lateral thyrohyoid ligaments themselves). They may easily be mistaken on x-rays for foreign bodies. The lateral thyrohyoid ligaments are actually thickenings of the thyrohyoid membrane. There is also more central thickening called the medial thyrohyoid ligament. The laryngeal vessels and the internal branches of the superior laryngeal nerves enter the thyrohyoid membrane posterior to the lateral thyrohyoid ligaments. The thyrohyoid ligaments and membranes are among the structures that suspend the larynx directly or indirectly from the skull base. The other structures that do so include the stylohyoid ligaments, the thyrohyoid ligaments and membrane, the thyroepiglottic ligaments, the cricothyroid ligaments and membrane, the cricoarytenoid ligaments, and the cricotracheal ligament and membrane.

The arytenoid cartilages are capable of complex motion. Previously, it was believed that the arytenoids rock, glide, and rotate. More accurately, the cartilages are brought together in the midline and revolve over the cricoid. It appears as if individuals use different strategies for approximating the arytenoids, and these strategies may influence a person's susceptibility to laryngeal trauma that can cause vocal process ulcers and laryngeal granulomas.

The larynx contains 2 important, large, paired "membranes," the triangular membranes and the quadrangular membranes (Figure 1–2). The paired triangular membranes form the conus elasticus. Each triangular membrane is attached to the cricoid and thyroid cartilages anteriorly (the base of the triangular membrane), to the cricoid cartilage inferiorly, and to the vocal process of the arytenoid cartilage posteriorly (the apex of the triangular membrane). The superior edge of each fibroelastic triangular membrane is the vocal ligament, forming the intermediate and deep layers of lamina propria of the vocal folds, as discussed below. These structures extend anteriorly to form a portion of Broyles ligament. More anteriorly, a portion of the conus elasticus constitutes the cricothyroid ligament.

Like the upper border of the triangular membrane, the upper and lower borders of the quadrangular membrane are free edges. The upper border of each quadrangular membrane is the aryepiglottic fold, bilaterally. The lower border extends from the inferior aspect of the epiglottis to the vocal process of the arytenoid cartilages and forms part of the vestibular (or ventricular) fold, or false vocal fold. Superior and inferior thickenings in the quadrangular membrane form the aryepiglottic ligament and the vestibular ligament, respectively. The quadrangular membrane is shorter in vertical height posteriorly than anteriorly. Lateral to these structures is a region called the paraglottic space. It is bounded laterally by the thyroid

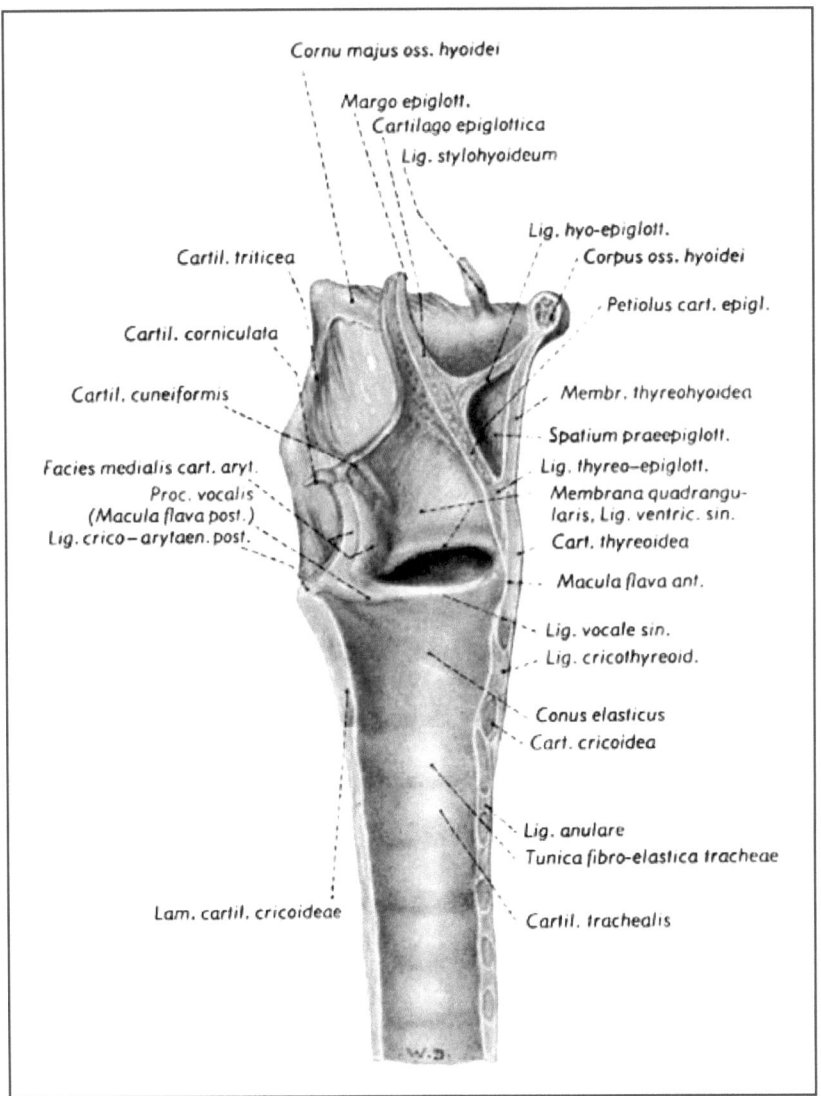

Cornu majus oss. hyoidei

Margo epiglott.
Cartilago epiglottica
Lig. stylohyoideum

Lig. hyo-epiglott.
Corpus oss. hyoidei

Cartil. triticea

Petiolus cart. epigl.

Cartil. corniculata

Cartil. cuneiformis

Membr. thyreohyoidea
Spatium praeepiglott.
Lig. thyreo-epiglott.
Membrana quadrangu-
laris, Lig. ventric. sin.
Cart. thyreoidea
Macula flava ant.

Facies medialis cart. aryt.
Proc. vocalis
(Macula flava post.)
Lig. crico-arytaen. post.

Lig. vocale sin.
Lig. cricothyreoid.

Conus elasticus
Cart. cricoidea

Lig. anulare
Tunica fibro-elastica tracheae

Lam. cartil. cricoideae

Cartil. trachealis

**Figure 1–2.** Internal view of the larynx illustrating the position of the quadrangular and triangular membranes. (Reproduced with permission from Pernkopf.[1])

lamina and medially by the supraglottic mucosa covering the vestibular fold from the ventricle to the aryepiglottic fold. There is a thin, elastic membrane that is contiguous above with the quadrangular membrane and below with the conus elasticus, forming an intermediate segment of elastic tissue that encloses the laryngeal ventricle. The paraglottic space is contiguous with the space between the cricoid and thyroid cartilages. The laryngeal inlet lies between the aryepiglottic folds.

The region formed by the paired ventricular and aryepiglottic folds is designated as "supraglottis." A pouch of mucosa between the under surface of the false vocal folds and the upper surface of the true vocal folds is called the ventricle of Morgagni, or the

laryngeal ventricle. The superior aspect of the laryngeal ventricle is known as the saccule of Hilton. The supraglottis extends from the tip of the epiglottis to the junction between the floor and lateral wall of the laryngeal ventricle. Hence, most clinicians define the floor of the ventricle as part of the glottic larynx. A detailed understanding of the supraglottic larynx is becoming more important clinically because of advances in transoral robotic surgery (TORS), as illustrated by Goyal et al who described anatomic variations in the superior laryngeal neurovascular bundle and differences in anatomic perspective using a robot.[10] The glottic larynx also includes the true vocal folds, anterior commissure, and interarytenoid region at the level of the vocal folds posteriorly (commonly, and incorrectly, referred to as the posterior commissure). The subglottis begins at the junction of squamous and respiratory epithelium under the vibratory margin of the vocal folds, about 5 mm below the beginning of the vibratory margin. The subglottis ends at the inferior border of the cricoid cartilage.

### Larynx: Mucosa

With the exception of the vocal folds, the epithelial lining of most of the vocal tract is pseudostratified, ciliated columnar epithelium, typical respiratory epithelium involved in handling mucous secretions. The vibratory margin of the vocal fold is covered with nonkeratinizing, stratified squamous epithelium, better suited than respiratory epithelium to withstand the trauma of vocal fold contact. Vocal fold

lubrication is created by cells in several areas. The saccule, the posterior surface of the epiglottis, and the aryepiglottic folds contain seromucinous, tubuloalveolar glands that secrete serous and/or mucinous lubricant. There are also goblet cells within the respiratory epithelium that secrete mucus. These are especially common in the area of the false vocal folds. The goblet cells and glands also secrete glycoproteins, lysozymes, and other materials essential to healthy vocal fold function. The laryngeal mucosa also contains immunologically active Langerhans cells.[11] In most people, secretory glands are not located near the vibratory margin.

The vibratory margin of the vocal folds is much more complicated than simply mucosa overlying muscle. It consists of 5 layers (Figure 1–3).[15] The thin, lubricated epithelium covering the vocal folds forms the area of contact between the vibrating vocal

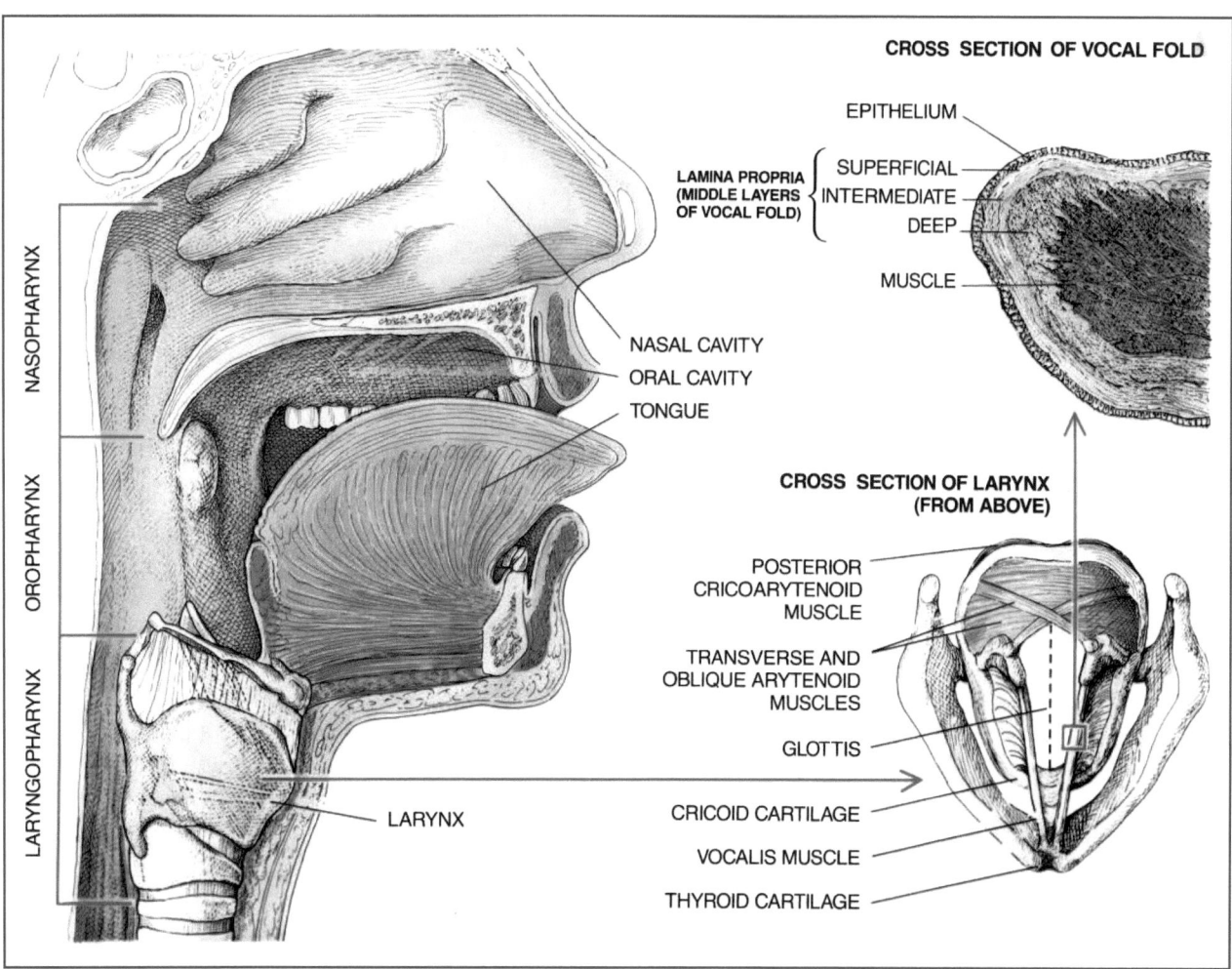

**A**

**Figure 1–3. A.** An overview of the larynx and vocal tract, showing the vocal folds, and the region from which the vocal fold was sampled to obtain the cross section showing the layered structure. (Reprinted with permission from Sataloff.[12]) *(continues)*

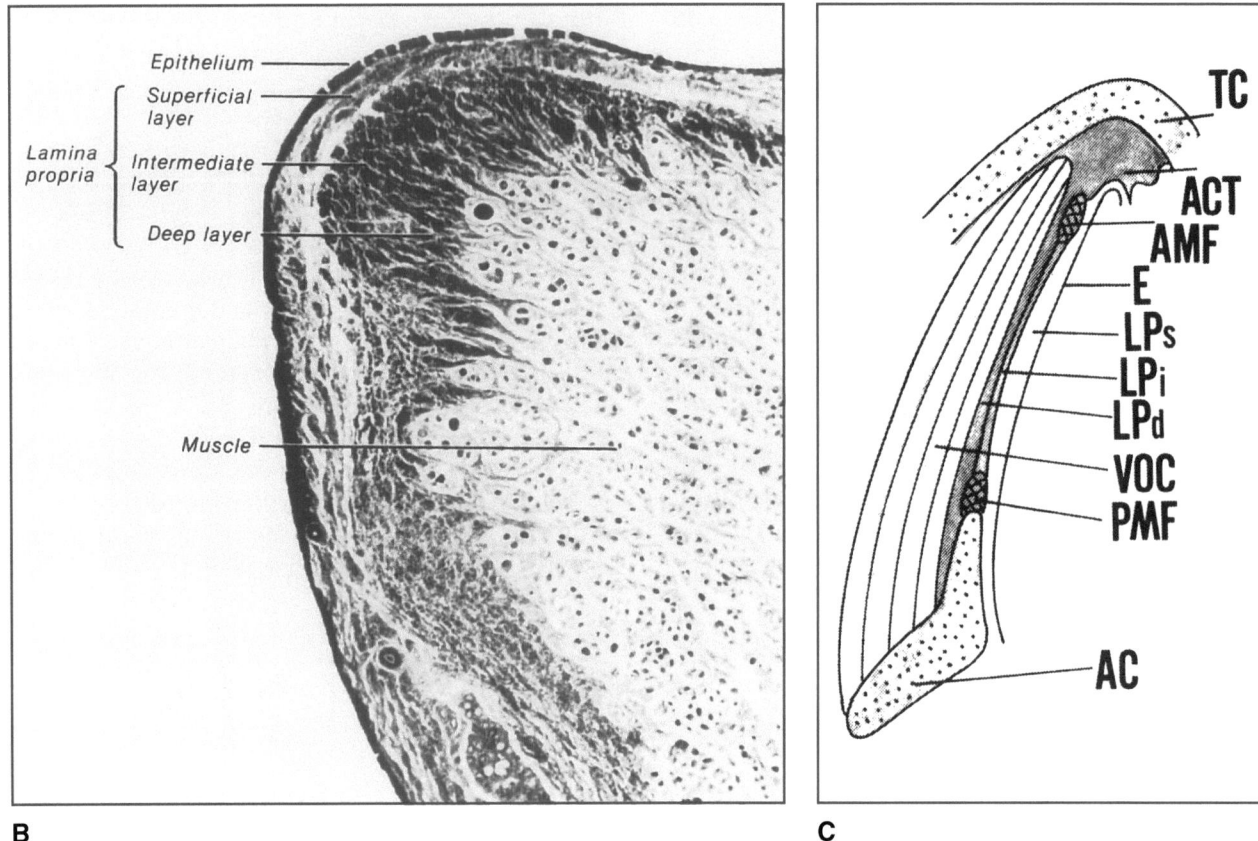

B                                                                C

**Figure 1–3.** *(continued)* **B.** The structure of the vocal fold. (Reprinted with permission from Hirano.[13(p5)]) **C.** Schematic representation of a horizontal section of the vocal fold. TC, thyroid cartilage; ACT, anterior commissure tendon; AMF, anterior macula flava; PMF, posterior macula flava; AC, arytenoid cartilage; E, epithelium; LP, lamina propria; s, superficial layer; i, intermediate layer; d, deep layer; VOC, vocalis muscle. (Reproduced with permission from Gray et al.[14])

folds and acts somewhat like a capsule, helping to maintain vocal fold shape. The superficial layer of the lamina propria, also known as Reinke space, is composed of loose fibrous components and matrix and lies immediately below the epithelial layer. It contains very few fibroblasts and consists of a network of mucopolysaccharides, hyaluronic acid, and decorin that provide for the flexibility required of the vocal fold cover layer.[16–19] In normal vocal folds the superficial lamina propria also contains fibronectin. Fibronectin is also thought to be deposited as a response to tissue injury.[20] The superficial lamina propria also contains elastin precursors (elaunin and oxytalin), but relatively few mature elastin or collagen fibers. Ordinarily, it has few or no lymphatics, secretory glands, or capillaries. Myofibroblasts and macrophages were found in the superficial lamina propria in about one-third of laryngeal specimens studied by Catten et al[19] and were more common in women than in men. The third layer of the vocal folds is the intermediate layer of the lamina propria.

Mature elastin fibers make up most of the intermediate layer. They are arranged longitudinally. This layer also contains large quantities of hyaluronic acid, a relatively inflexible space filler that is hydrophilic and is believed to act as a shock absorber.[17] Fibromodulin also is present in the intermediate layer.[18] The deep layer of the lamina propria, the fourth layer, is composed primarily of longitudinally arranged collagenous fibers and is rich in fibroblasts. De Melo et al analyzed the distribution of collagen in the lamina propria.[21] They described a layer of thick collagen type 1 immediately below the epithelium, and a second, more dense layer superficial to the thyroarytenoid muscle and penetrating between muscle fibers. A layer of collagen type 3 was located between the 2 collagen type 1 layers. The collagen fibers formed an intertwined "wicker basket" network within the lamina propria which helps explain how the vocal fold is able to stretch, despite containing nonstretchable fibers. Interestingly, the authors also noted segmental areas of disarray in the intertwining collagen layers in older patients, suggesting that the variation in histoarchitecture might be related to voice changes common among elderly patients. Prades et al reported similar findings and noted that the mean thickness of the superficial layer of lamina propria is about 13% of the total lamina propria.[22] The intermediate layer constitutes about 51%, and the deep layer makes up about 36% of the lamina propria. The TA or vocalis muscle constitutes the body of the vocal fold and is the fifth layer, as well as one of the intrinsic laryngeal muscles. The region that consists of the intermediate and deep layers of the lamina propria is called the vocal ligament and lies immediately below Reinke space. It is important to note that this layered structure of the vocal folds is not present at birth, but rather begins developing at around the age of 7 or 8 years and is not completed until the end of adolescence.[23,24] There are other differences between the pediatric and adult larynx that are not reviewed in this chapter, but many are discussed elsewhere in this book in connection with relevant clinical entities. A great deal more information is available about the ultrastructure of human vocal folds and may be found in other literature.[25]

Although variations along the length of the membranous vocal fold are important in only a few situations, the surgeon, in particular, should be aware that they exist. The mucosa (epithelium and lamina propria, together) of the normal adult male has been described as being approximately 1.1-mm thick. The superficial layer is about 0.3 mm, the vocal ligament is about 0.8 mm,[26] and the epithelium is about 5–25 cells (about 50 microns) in thickness.[27] However, particularly interesting research by Friedrich et al shows additional interesting complexity and variation in the anatomy of the vocal fold.[28] Friedrich et al divided the vocal fold into 5 histological and functional portions. Three of the portions included the musculomembranous vocal fold, and the other 2 regions were divisions of the posterior glottic region and included the region of the vocal process of the arytenoids, which constitutes the cartilaginous portion of the vocal folds and the lateral wall of the posterior glottis. They also found significant differences between men and women in terms of not only absolute measurements, but also relative dimensions of various portions of the vocal fold. In particular, the middle portion of the musculomembranous vocal fold was twice as long in men (8.5 mm) as in women (4.6 mm), accounting for 37% of total glottic length in men and only 29% in women. The authors speculate that this difference in the length of the vibrating portions of the vocal folds may explain why the fundamental frequency ratio between men and women is approximately 1:2, while

the overall laryngeal dimensions are only 1:1.5. In addition to variations in length, Friedrich et al also found that the thickness of the lamina propria varied depending on location along the length of the vocal fold and on gender (Figure 1–4). Friedrich's elegant research should be interpreted in the historical context of earlier observations, some of which appear to provide data that are contradictory to his. Actually, the methods of observation and intent of the studies differed; most of the findings in the various studies are reconcilable.

The vocal folds join anteriorly. The area of union is known as the anterior commissure. A "commissure" is a point of coming together. Hence, the term *posterior commissure* has been discouraged, because the vocal folds do not come together in posterior larynx. However, this terminology has been challenged by Tucker and Tucker,[29] who argue that histologic data showing the posterior union the cricoid cartilage justify the use of the term *posterior commissure*. Their view has not been accepted widely, and most laryngologists still agree with Hirano et al[30] and refer to "the posterior glottis" or "the posterior larynx," rather than the posterior commissure. In 1986, Hirano et al[30] studied the posterior glottis in 20 specimens obtained from autopsy, photographing the larynges from above and below in neutral, adducted, and abducted conditions. They also studied the histology of the posterior glottis in the same 3 conditions. Hirano et al defined the posterior glottis as consisting of 3 portions: the posterior wall of the glottis, the lateral wall of the posterior glottis, and the cartilaginous portion of the vocal fold. They noted that the posterior larynx closes at the supraglottis during vocal fold adduction, rather than at the glottis, thus producing a conical space that can be seen only from below. Using this methodology, they calculated that the posterior glottis accounted for 35%–45% of the entire glottic length, and 50%–65% of the entire glottic area. The mucosa covering the posterior glottis consisted of ciliated epithelium, and the lamina propria consisted of only 2 layers. The superficial layer was looser in structure, and the deep layer was composed of dense elastic and collagenous fibers with numerous mucosecretory glands. Many of the fibers in the deep layer ran vertically in the region of the posterior wall of the glottis, but the fibers on the lateral wall were found to run obliquely. This study provided useful, interesting anatomic information. However, in interpreting its physiological significance, it should be remembered that abduction and adduction were accomplished by threads attached to the muscular processes of the arytenoid cartilages; the results may or may not be identical to the complex motions that occur during phonation in a living human.[30]

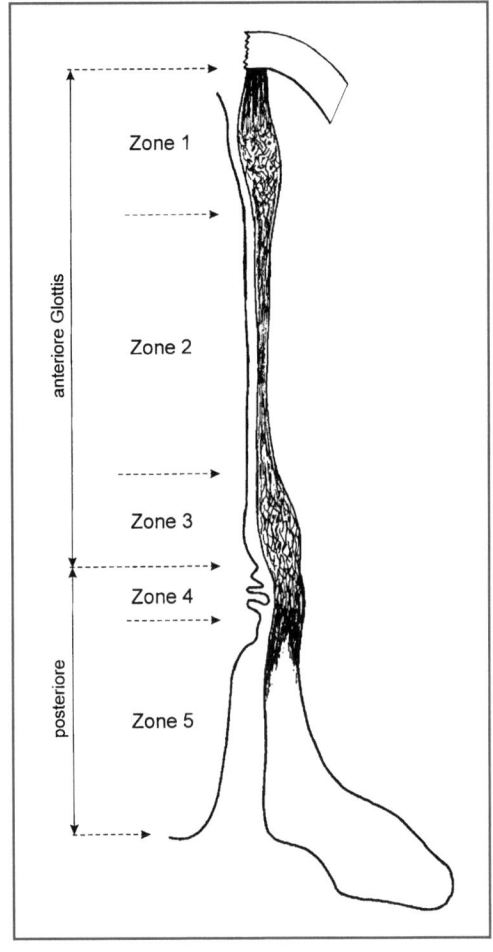

**A**

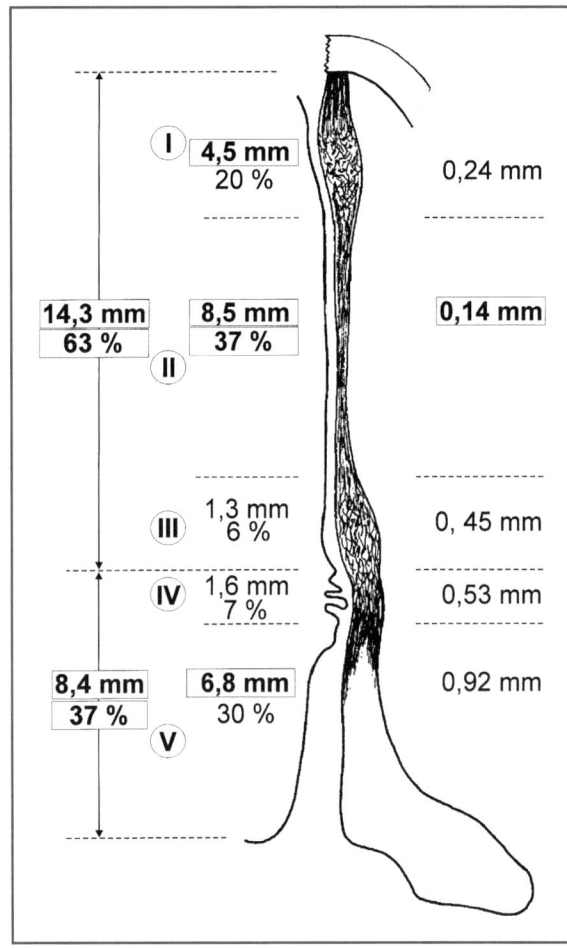

**B**

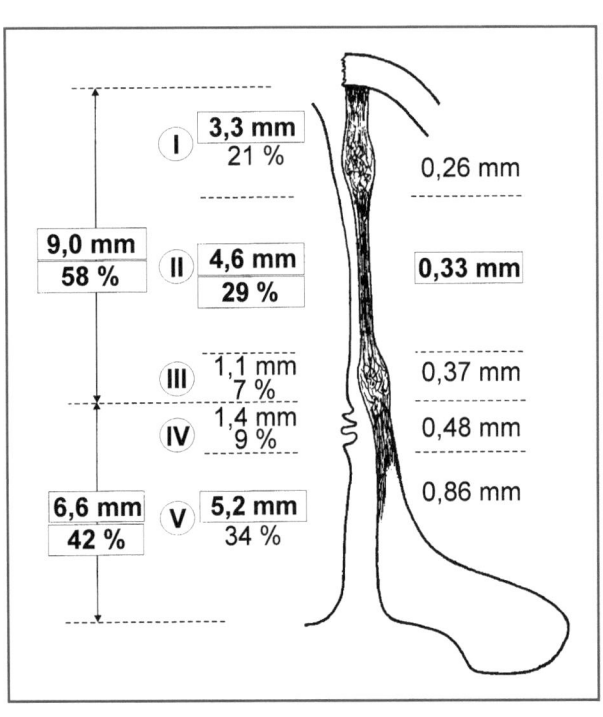

**C**

Figure 1–4. **A.** Vocal fold divided into zones. **B.** Proportions of the vocal fold constituted by each zone in men. **C.** Thickness of the lamina propria in millimeters in women. Note that the European numbering system is used in which 0.45 mm is written as 0,45 mm. (Courtesy of Gerhardt Friederich, MD.)

It has long been recognized that particularly striking variations occur at the anterior and posterior portions of the musculomembranous vocal fold, the region between the vocal process and attachment of the vocal fold to the thyroid cartilage.[31] Anteriorly, the intermediate layer of the lamina propria becomes thick, forming an oval mass called the anterior macula flava. This structure is composed of stroma, fibroblasts, and elastic fibers. Anteriorly, the anterior macula flava inserts into the anterior commissure tendon (Broyles ligament). The anterior commissure tendon is a mass of collagenous fibers, which is connected to the midpoint of the thyroid cartilage anteriorly, the anterior macula flava posteriorly, and the deep layer of the lamina propria laterally. As Hirano has pointed out, this arrangement allows the stiffness to change gradually from the pliable musculomembranous vocal fold to the stiffer thyroid cartilage.[31] Sato et al have described stellate cells in the macula flava that are related to fibroblasts, but which appear to constantly synthesize extracellular matrices that are required for normal human vocal fold mucosal function.[32–34] Changes in extracellular matrices alter vocal fold function, particularly viscoelasticity, and these changes are associated with some aspects of vocal aging. Aging changes in the vocal fold stellate cells in the macula flava may be responsible for some of the age-related extracellular matrices alterations.[35–38] Sato also demonstrated that stellate cells of the macula flava were more sensitive to radiation-induced change than many of the other components of vocal folds.[39] These findings suggest that radiation may damage the ability of stellate cells to generate precursors of collagenous and elastic fibers, indicating that radiation causes changes not only in fiberblasts and other components of the lamina propria, but also in the ability of the stellate cells in the macula flava to maintain normal vocal fold homeostasis. Fuja et al cultured vocal fold stellate cells and demonstrated induced deactivation.[40] Their data suggest that the stellate cells are a potential target for research on the physical elastic properties of vocal fold mucosa during normal phonation, aging, scar, fibrosis, and other conditions.

A similar gradual change in stiffness occurs posteriorly where the intermediate layer of the lamina propria also thickens to form the posterior macula flava, another oval mass that is structurally similar to the anterior macula flava. The posterior macula flava attaches to the vocal process of the arytenoid cartilage through a transitional structure that consists of chondrocytes, fibroblasts, and intermediate cells.[41] Thus, the stiffness progresses from the flexible musculomembranous vocal fold to the slightly stiffer macula flava, to the stiffer transitional structure, to the elastic cartilage of the vocal process, and to the hyalin cartilage of the arytenoid body. It is believed that this gradual change in stiffness serves as a cushion that may protect the vocal folds from mechanical damage caused by contact or vibrations.[41] It may also act as a controlled damper that smooths mechanical changes during vocal fold movements. This arrangement seems particularly well suited to vibration, as are other aspects of the vocal fold architecture. For example, blood vessels in the vocal folds begin posteriorly and anteriorly and run parallel to the vibratory margin, with very few vessels entering the mucosa perpendicular to the free edge of the vibratory margin or from the underlying muscle. Even the elastic and collagenous fibers of the lamina propria run approximately parallel to the vibratory margin, allowing them to compress against each other or pull apart from each other flexibly and parallel with the forces of the mucosal wave. The more one studies the vocal fold, the more one appreciates the beauty of its engineering.

Functionally, the 5 layers have different mechanical properties and are analogous to ball bearings of different sizes that allow the smooth shearing action necessary for proper vocal fold vibration. The posterior two-fifths (approximately) of the vocal folds are cartilaginous, and the anterior three-fifths are musculomembranous (from the vocal process forward) in adults. Under normal circumstances, most of the vibratory function critical to voice quality occurs in the musculomembranous portion.

Mechanically, the vocal fold structures act more like 3 layers consisting of the cover (epithelium and superficial layer of the lamina propria), transition (intermediate and deep layers of the lamina propria), and the body (the vocalis muscles). Understanding this anatomy is important because different pathologic entities occur in different layers and require different approaches to treatment. For example, fibroblasts are responsible for scar formation. Therefore, lesions that occur superficially in the vocal folds (eg, nodules, cysts, and most polyps) should permit treatment without disturbance of the intermediate and deep layers, where fibroblast proliferation, or scar formation, occurs.

In addition to the 5 layers of the vocal fold, there is a complex basement membrane connecting the epithelium to the superficial layer of the lamina propria.[42] The basement membrane is a multilayered, chemically complex structure. It gives rise to type VII collagen loops that encircle type III collagen fibers in the superficial layer of the lamina propria (Figure 1–5). Current research has changed substantially

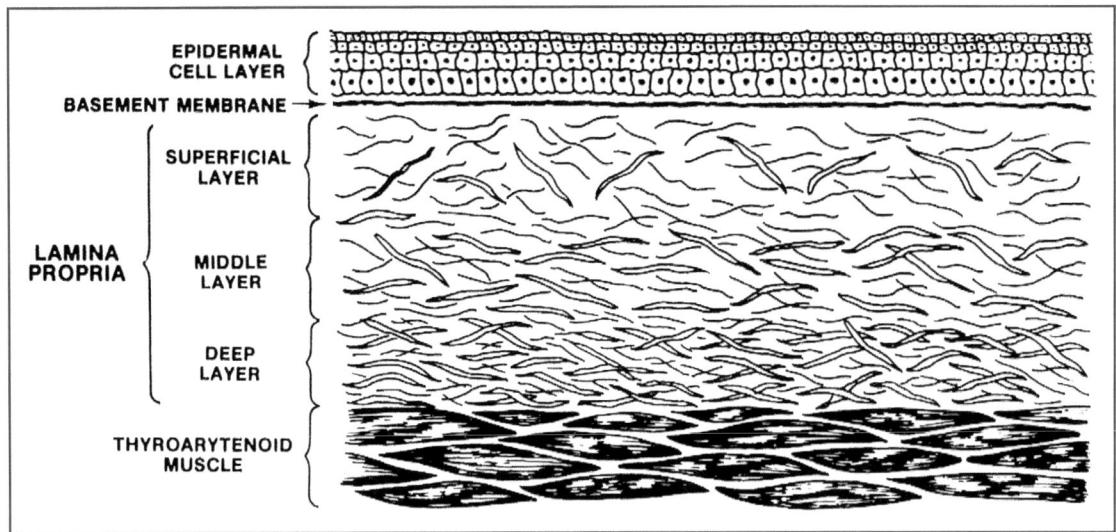

**A**

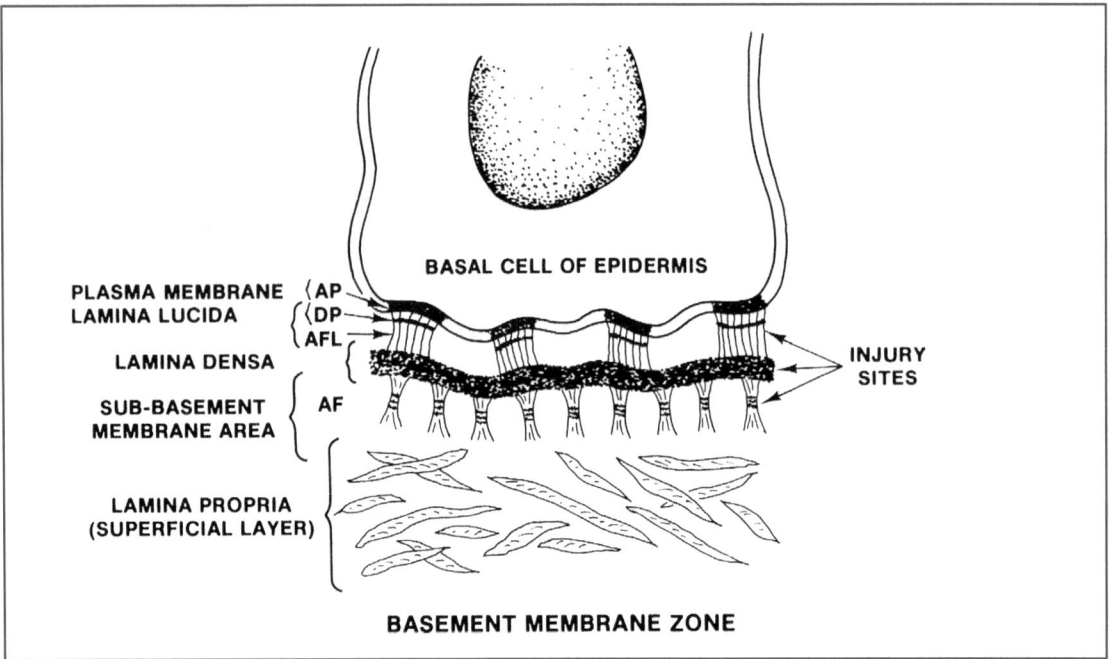

**B**

**Figure 1–5. A.** Structure of the vocal fold (not drawn to scale). The basement membrane lies between the epithelium and the superficial layer of the lamina propria. (Reproduced with permission from Gray,[42]) **B.** Basement membrane zone. Basal cells are connected to the lamina densa by attachment plax (AP) in the plasma membrane of the epidermis. Anchoring filaments (AFL) extend from the attachment plax through the subbasal densa plate (DP) and attach to the lamina densa (dark single-layer, electron-dense band just beneath the basal cell layer.) The subbasement membrane zone consists of anchoring fibers (AFs) that attach to the lamina densa and extend into the superficial layer of the lamina propria. Type VII collagen fibers attach to the network of the lamina propria by looping around type III collagen fibers. (Reproduced with permission from Gray.[42]) *(continues)*

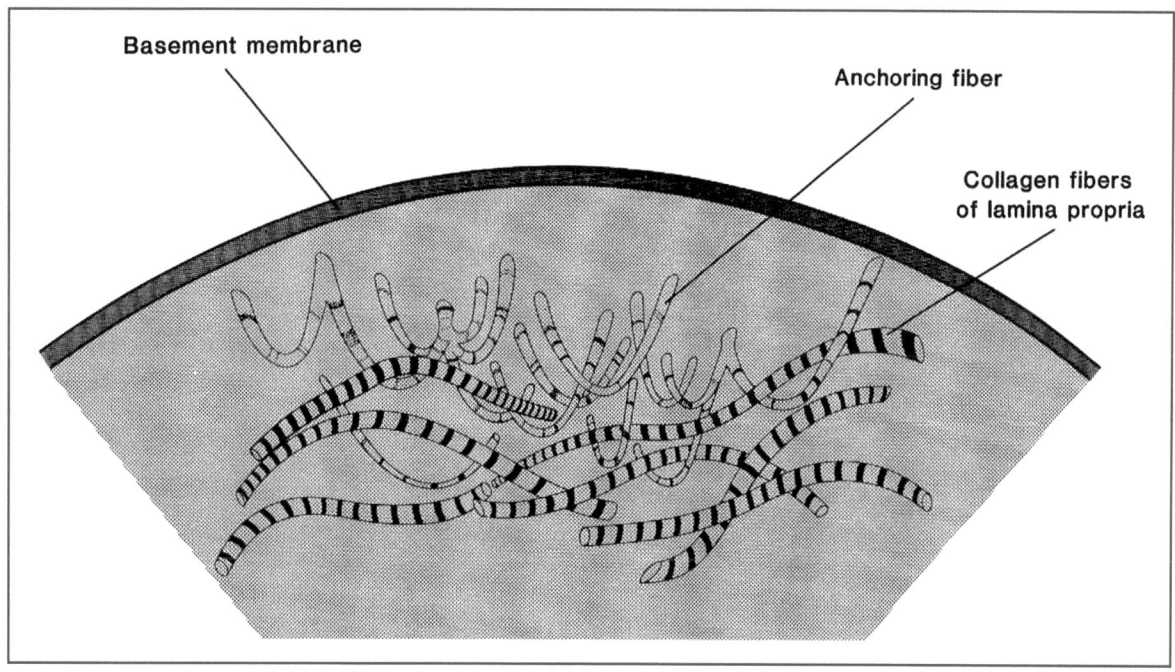

**C**

**Figure 1–5.** *(continued)* **C.** Type VII collagen anchoring fibers pass from the basement membrane, reinserting into it. Through the anchoring fiber loops pass type III collagen fibers of the superficial layer of lamina propria. (Courtesy of Steven Gray, MD.)

our understanding of vocal fold composition and function. For example, in his description of the basement membrane zone, Gray described a chain link–fence arrangement of anchoring fibers, which he believes permits tissue compression and bending.[16] The density of the anchoring fibers is greatest in the area of greatest vibration and shearing stresses, in the middle of the musculomembranous portion of the vocal folds. Knowledge of the basement membrane has already been important in changing surgical techniques, as discussed later in this book. It also appears important in other matters, such as the ability to heal following trauma, the development of certain kinds of vocal fold pathology, and in histopathologic differential diagnosis.

The vocal folds may be thought of as the oscillators of the vocal mechanism.[43] Above the true vocal folds are tissues known as the "false vocal folds." Unlike the true vocal folds, they do not make contact during normal speaking or singing. However, they may produce voice during certain abnormal circumstances. This phenomenon is called dysphonia plica ventricularis. Until recently, the importance of the false vocal folds during normal phonation was not appreciated. In general, they are considered to be used primarily for forceful laryngeal closure; they come

into play during pathological conditions. However, contrary to popular practice, surgeons should recognize that they cannot be removed without affecting phonation. The physics of airflow through the larynx is very complex, involving vortex formation and sophisticated turbulence patterns that are essential to normal phonation. The false vocal folds provide a downstream resistance, which is important in this process, and they probably play a role in vocal tract resonance, as well.

**Laryngeal: Blood Supply and Lymphatic Drainage**

The larynx receives its blood supply primarily from the inferior and superior laryngeal arteries and the cricothyroid artery. The superior laryngeal arteries arise from the superior thyroid arteries, which are branches of the external carotid arteries. The superior laryngeal arteries course with the superior laryngeal nerves, piercing the thyrohyoid membrane with the internal branch of the superior laryngeal nerve. The superior laryngeal arteries supply the structures related to the quadrangular membranes and piriform sinuses, primarily above the cricoid cartilage. These include the epiglottis, aryepiglottic fold, thyroarytenoid (TA) muscle, lateral cricoarytenoid (LCA) muscle, interarytenoid (IA) muscle, and vocal fold mucosa. There are anastomoses with the superior laryngeal artery on the contralateral side and with the inferior laryngeal artery. The cricothyroid (CT) artery also arises from the superior thyroid artery and supplies the CT muscle and membrane, some of the extrinsic laryngeal musculature, and portions of the subglottic pharynx (after penetrating the cricothyroid membrane). The inferior laryngeal arteries arise from the inferior thyroid arteries, branches of the thyrocervical trunk. On the left, the inferior thyroid artery may arise directly from the subclavian artery. The inferior laryngeal arteries travel with the recurrent laryngeal nerves to supply the posterior cricoarytenoid (PCA) muscle, and probably portions of the true vocal fold ventricles and false vocal folds, in some cases. The superior laryngeal veins join the internal jugular veins, and the inferior laryngeal veins empty into the thyrocervical trunks and from there communicate with the subclavian venous system.

The blood supply to the vocal fold mucosa deserves special attention. It is unusual in several ways. The vocal folds contain only small vessels including arterioles, venules, and capillaries. They run parallel to the vibratory margin of the vocal fold, entering from anterior or posterior, and they have frequent arteriovenous anastomoses.[44] This arrangement appears to optimize vessel patency and blood flow even in the presence of the substantial shearing forces encountered during high-pressure phonation. Although Franz and Aharinejad have suggested that there are venous connections between the mucosa and muscle,[44] other authors disagree.[45,46] There appear to be no direct communications between the microvasculature of the superficial lamina propria and the medial belly of the thyroarytenoid (vocalis) muscle. However, Franz and Aharinejad appear to have been correct in suggesting that the serpentine course of subepithelial vessels is engineered to accommodate safely the extreme changes in length and tension that may occur during phonation.[45] The appearance of blood vessels on the superior surfaces of vocal folds may vary in the presence of laryngeal pathology. For example, De Biase and Pontes[47] reviewed 280 videolaryngoscopic images divided into groups of 70 patients each with vocal nodules (VNs), polyps, minimal structural alterations (MSAs) or no abnormalities (control group). Visible superior surface vessels were found in 91.4% of the MSA group, 77.1% of patients with polyps, 44.7% of VN subjects, and 31.4% of controls. Longitudinal and transverse vessels were present in 74.3% and 37.1% (respectively) of the MSA group, 65.7% and 22.9% of subjects with pol-

yps, 34.3% and 12.9% of VN patients, and only 25.7% and 5.7% of controls. Tangled vessels were present in only the MSA subjects (8.6%). Abrupt changes in vessel caliber and sinuous vessels were found in the subjects with polyps (21.4% and 5.7%, respectively) and MSA subjects (61.4% and 27.1%).

The vessels along the vibratory margin have a different structure than those on the superior surface of the vocal fold or in the TA muscle.[24] For example, capillaries along the vibratory margin are lined by endothelial cells and encircled by pericytes with tight intercellular junctions. The endothelial cells have intermediate-thickness filaments near the cell nucleus and bundles of thick filaments adjacent to the luminal cell membrane.[46] These filaments, together with the lamellate structure of the basement membrane and its interspersed myocytes and pericytes, form a lattice that stabilizes the structure of the microvessels, helping them to tolerate the high shearing forces that can be generated during phonation.[46] This structure enhances mechanical support and helps explain the relative infrequency with which vocal fold hemorrhage occurs, even during forceful phonation. The other vessels of the vocal fold and laryngeal muscles are composed mainly of simple, endothelial-lined capillaries of the continuous (nonfenestrated) variety (the most common type of capillary).[48]

Lymphatic drainage from the larynx occurs through superficial and deep systems, although the deep system is most important. The superficial lymphatic system communicates bilaterally and provides only intramucosal drainage. Each deep system is submucosal and drains its lateral structures. Lymphatic drainage from the larynx courses superiorly and inferiorly. Supraglottic lymphatic vessels travel with the superior laryngeal and superior thyroid vessels to deep cervical lymph nodes (levels II and III) associated with the internal jugular veins. This drainage may be bilateral. There are also lymphatic vessels from the laryngeal ventricles that course through the cricothyroid membrane and thyroid gland en route to the prelaryngeal, prethyroid, supraclavicular, pretracheal, and paratracheal lymph nodes. Inferiorly, lymphatic vessels from the glottic and subglottic larynx form 2 posterolateral pedicles and a middle pedicle. The posterolateral pedicles travel unilaterally with the inferior thyroid artery to the deep lateral cervical (levels III and IV), subclavian, paratracheal, and tracheoesophageal lymph nodes. The middle pedicle courses through the cricothyroid membrane, communicating with pretracheal and delphian nodes, which drain into the deep cervical lymph nodes. There is scant lymphatic drainage from the true vocal folds.

**Larynx: Intrinsic Muscles**

The intrinsic muscles are responsible for abduction, adduction, and tension of the vocal folds (Figures 1–6 and 1–7). All but one of the muscles on each side of the larynx are innervated by the 2 recurrent (or inferior) laryngeal nerves, which are discussed in detail below. Because these nerves usually run long courses from the neck down into the chest and back up to the larynx (hence, the name "recurrent"), they are easily injured by trauma, neck surgery, and thoracic surgery. The left recurrent laryngeal nerve is more susceptible to injury during chest surgery because of its course around the aortic arch. The right recurrent laryngeal nerve, however, is more likely to have an oblique course laterally in the neck and thus may be at greater risk for injury in neck surgery. Such injuries may result in abductor and adductor paralysis of the vocal fold. The remaining muscle, the CT muscle, is innervated by the superior laryngeal nerve on each side, which is especially susceptible to viral and traumatic injury.

For some purposes, including electromyography and surgery, it is important to understand the function of individual laryngeal muscles in detail. The muscles of primary functional importance are those innervated by the recurrent laryngeal nerves including the thyroarytenoid (TA), posterior cricoarytenoid (PCA), lateral cricoarytenoid (LCA), and interarytenoid or arytenoideus (IA), and the superior laryngeal nerves including the cricothyroid (CT) (Figures 1–6, 1–7, and 1–8).

The TA muscle adducts, lowers, shortens, and thickens the vocal folds, thus rounding the vocal fold's edge. Thus, the cover (epithelium and superficial layer of lamina propria) and transition (intermediate and deep layers of lamina propria) are effectively made slacker, while the body is stiffened.

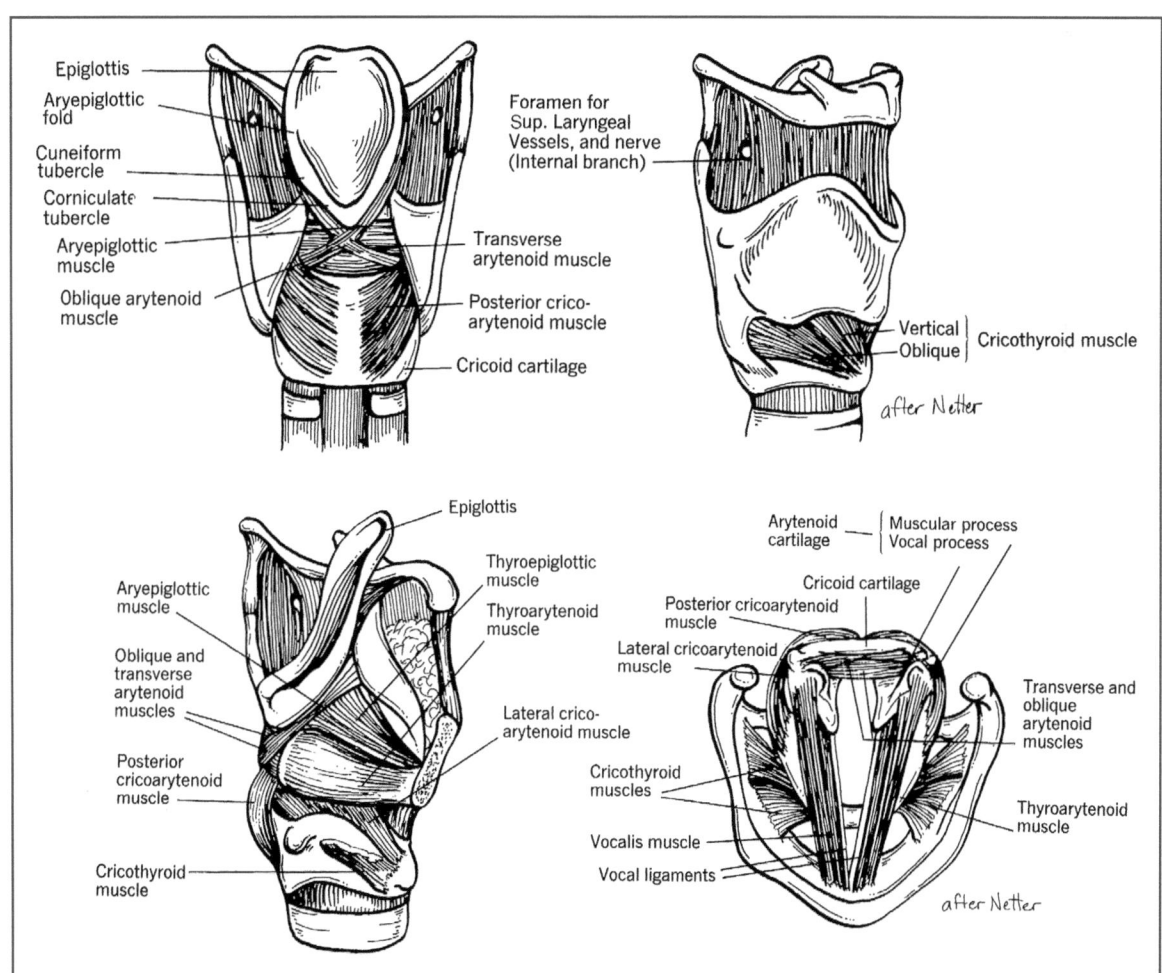

**Figure 1–6.** The intrinsic muscles of the larynx.

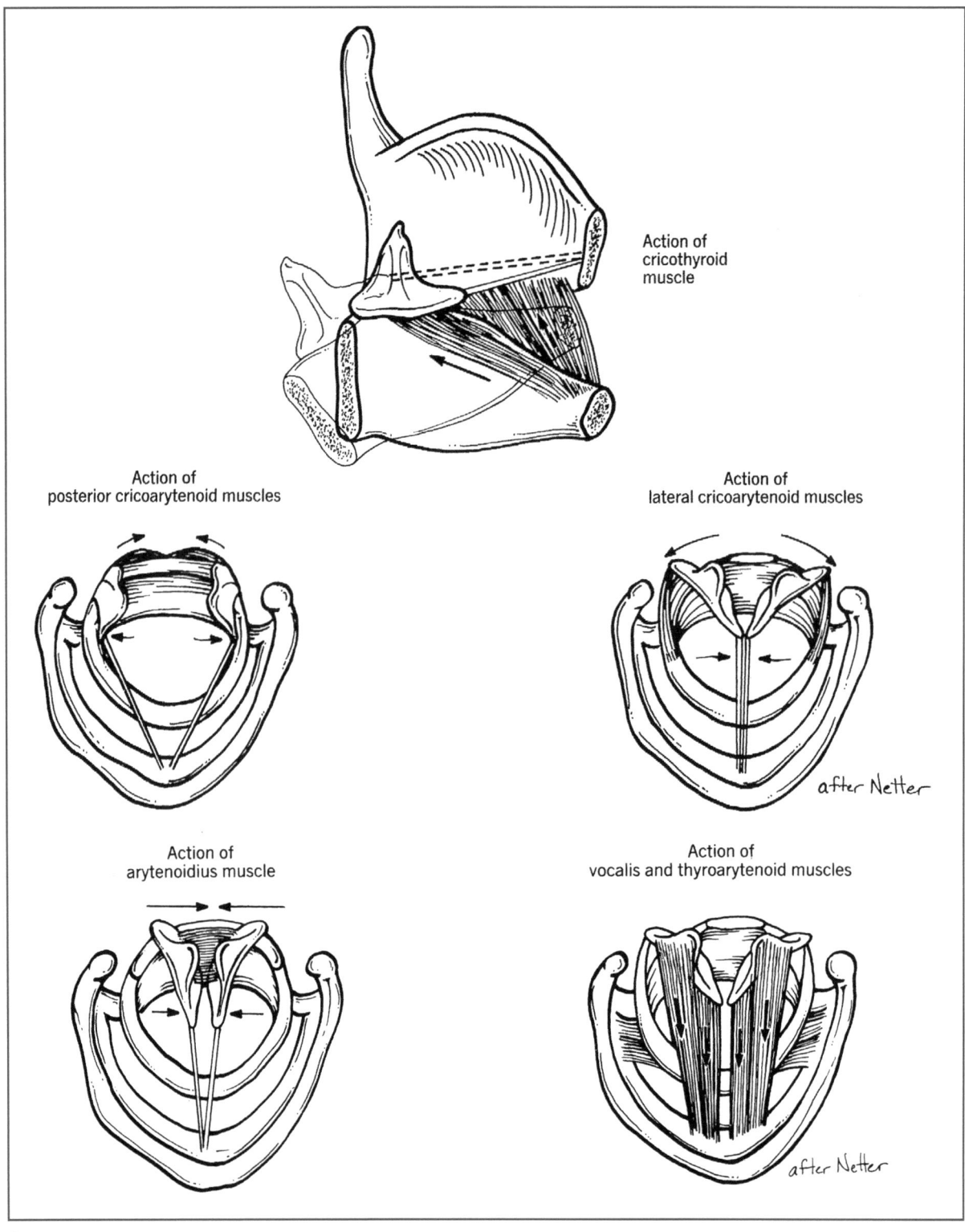

Action of
cricothyroid
muscle

Action of
posterior cricoarytenoid muscles

Action of
lateral cricoarytenoid muscles

after Netter

Action of
arytenoidius muscle

Action of
vocalis and thyroarytenoid muscles

after Netter

**A**

**Figure 1–7. A.** Action of the intrinsic muscles. In the bottom 4 figures, the directional arrows suggest muscle actions but may give a misleading impression of arytenoid motion. These drawings should not be misinterpreted as indicating that the arytenoid cartilage rotates around a vertical axis. The angle of the long axis of the cricoid facets does not permit some of the motion implied in this figure. However, the drawing still provides a useful conceptualization of the effect of individual intrinsic muscles, so long as the limitations are recognized. *(continues)*

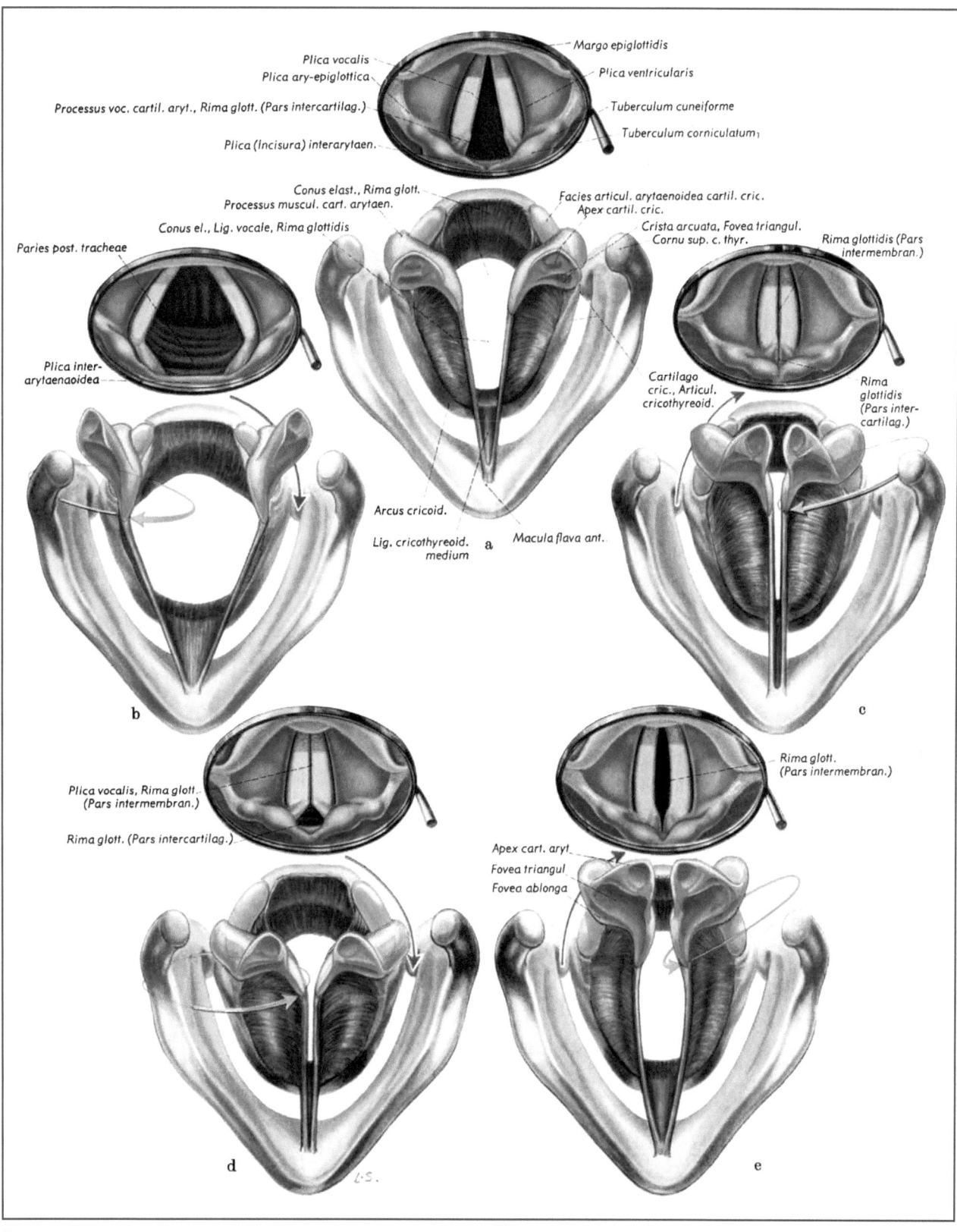

**B**

**Figure 1–7.** *(continued)* **B.** The shapes of the glottis as seen on mirror examination and on anatomic preparations during rest (a), inspiration (b), phonation (c), whispering (d), and falsetto singing (e). (Reproduced with permission from Pernkopf.[1])

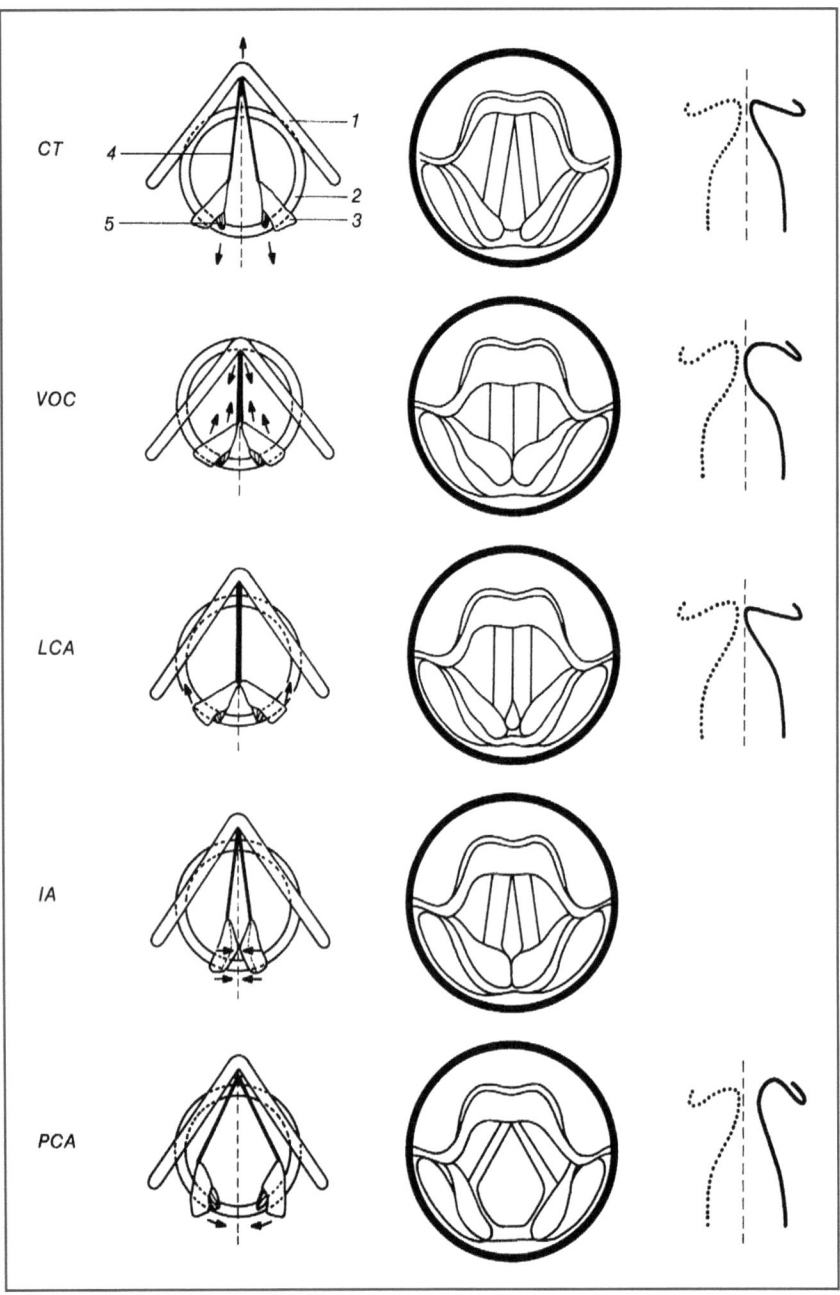

**A**

**Figure 1–8. A.** Schematic presentation of the function of the laryngeal muscles. The left column shows the location of the cartilages and the edge of the vocal folds when the laryngeal muscles are activated individually. The arrows indicate the direction of the force exerted. 1, thyroid cartilage; 2, cricoid cartilage; 3, arytenoid cartilage; 4, vocal ligament; 5, posterior cricoarytenoid ligament. The middle column shows the views from above. The right column illustrates contours of frontal sections at the middle of the musculomembranous portion of the vocal fold. The dotted line illustrates the vocal fold position when no muscle is activated. CT, cricothyroid; VOC, vocalis; LCA, lateral cricoarytenoid; IA, interarytenoid; PCA, posterior cricoarytenoid. (Reproduced with permission from Hirano M.[13(p8)]) *(continues)*

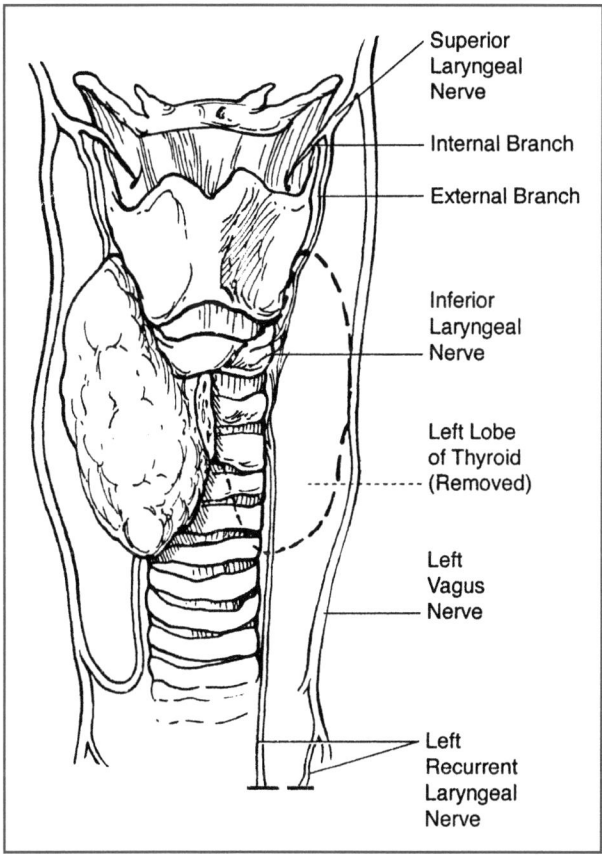

**B**

Figure 1–8. *(continued)* **B.** The superior and recurrent laryngeal nerve branch from the vagus nerve and enter the larynx.

Adduction from vocalis muscle (the medial belly of the TA) contraction is active, particularly in the musculomembranous segment of the vocal folds. Contraction of the vocalis muscle tends to lower vocal pitch. The thyroarytenoid originates anteriorly from the posterior (interior) surface of the thyroid cartilage and inserts into the lateral base of the arytenoid cartilage, from the vocal process to the muscular process. More specifically, the superior bundles of the muscle insert into the lateral and inferior aspects of the vocal process and run primarily in a horizontal direction. The anteroinferior bundles insert into the anterolateral aspect of the arytenoid cartilage from its tip to an area lateral to the vocal process. (These fibers are associated primarily with the lateral belly.) The most medial fibers run parallel to the vocal ligament and insert onto the medial aspect of the vocal process. There are also cranial fibers that extend into the aryepiglottic fold. Anteriorly, the vertical organi-

zation of the muscle results in a twisted configuration of muscle fibers when the vocal fold is adducted. The neuromuscular organization of the medial belly of the TA muscle is more complex than previously believed. Research by Sanders helped clarify these complexities. He has shown, for example, that muscle groups along the superior and inferior margin of the medial (contact) surface of the vocal folds function differently from one another.[49] The thyroarytenoid is the third largest intrinsic muscle of the larynx. The TA muscle is divided into 2 compartments. The medial compartment is also known as the vocalis muscle. It contains a high percentage of slow-twitch muscle fibers. The lateral compartment has predominantly fast-twitch muscle fibers. One may suspect that the medial compartment (vocalis) is specialized for phonation, whereas the lateral compartment (muscularis) is specialized for vocal fold adduction, but these suppositions are unproven. De Campos et al studied TA muscle in comparison with tongue, because the tongue muscle is considered the most complex structure in the body with regard to movements and muscle fiber orientation.[50] The authors speculated that TA complexities might be correlated with similar muscle structure. They found that both tongue and TA muscle showed the same percentage of transverse (about 72%), undefined (about 15%), and longitudinal (about 10%) fibers. In contrast to these similarities, they found no morphometric correlation comparing the structures of the recurrent laryngeal nerve and the hypoglossal nerve. Studies of TA muscle using myosin antibodies have shown that TA muscle contains unique extrafusal fibers containing tonic myosin, but no muscle spindles.[51] These findings suggest similarities between thyroarytenoid muscle function and extraocular muscles, both of which perform unloaded (non-weight-bearing) contractions without afferent information from native muscle spindles.

The LCA muscle is a small muscle that adducts, lowers, elongates, and thins the vocal fold. All layers are stiffened, and the vocal fold edge takes on a more angular or sharp contour in response to LCA muscle contraction. It originates on the superior lateral border of the cricoid cartilage and inserts into the anterior lateral surface of the muscular process of the arytenoid. It is an extremely important adductor and is especially important in the initial movement from abduction to adduction. The bilaterally innervated IA muscle (arytenoideus, or interarytenoid muscle, a medium-sized intrinsic muscle) primarily adducts the cartilaginous portion of the vocal folds. It is particularly important in providing medial compression to close the posterior glottis. It has relatively little effect on the stiffness of the musculo-membranous portion. The interarytenoid muscle is the only unpaired laryngeal muscle. It is innervated by the recurrent laryngeal nerve and receives fibers from the internal branch of the superior laryngeal nerve (although there is no evidence that the internal branch of the superior laryngeal nerve provides motor innervation to this muscle. The IA muscle consists of transverse and oblique fibers. The transverse fibers originate from the lateral margin of one arytenoid and insert into the lateral margin of the opposite arytenoid. The oblique fibers originate posteriorly and inferiorly from the base of the cricoid cartilage, but they extend around the apex of the arytenoid cartilage to continue as the aryepiglottic musculature.

The PCA muscle abducts, elevates, elongates, and thins the vocal fold by rocking the arytenoid cartilage posterolaterally. All layers are stiffened, and the edge of the vocal fold is rounded during PCA muscle contraction. It is the second largest intrinsic muscle. It originates over a broad area of the posterolateral portion of the cricoid lamina and inserts on the posterior surface of the muscular process of the arytenoid cartilage, forming a short tendon that covers the cranial aspect of the muscular process. Asanau et al studied the PCA.[52] They found 2 separate muscle bellies in all cases. They contained 1, 1-11A, and 11A fibers, but comparing the vertical and horizontal bellies of the PCA revealed differences in the fiber-type composition. They also noted regional differences in both bellies of the PCA. They suggested that the PCA should be considered as a combination of 2 functional subunits differing significantly in muscle fiber-type composition, rather than as a single muscle.

When the superior laryngeal nerves are stimulated, the CT muscles move the vocal folds into the paramedian position. They also lower, stretch, elongate, and thin the vocal folds, stiffening all layers and sharpening the vocal folds' contours. It is the largest intrinsic laryngeal muscle and is largely responsible for longitudinal tension, a very important factor in control of pitch. Contraction of the CT muscles tends to increase vocal pitch through their lengthening effect on the vocal folds. The CT muscle originates from the anterior and lateral portions of the arch of the cricoid cartilage and has 2 bellies. The oblique belly inserts into the posterior half of the thyroid lamina and the anterior portion of the inferior cornu of the thyroid cartilage. The vertical (erect) belly inserts into the inferior border of the anterior aspect of the thyroid lamina.

Intrinsic laryngeal muscles are skeletal muscles. Skeletal muscles are composed primarily of 3 types of fibers. Type I fibers are highly resistant to fatigue, contract slowly, and utilize aerobic (oxidative) metabolism. They have low glycogen levels, high levels of oxidative enzymes, and are relatively smaller in diameter. Fast-contracting type IIB fibers are subdivided into types IIA, IIB, and IIX. The myosin heavy-chain isoform in each fiber type is primarily responsible for determining contraction speed. Only type I, IIA, and IIX fibers are present in humans. Type IIA fibers use principally oxidative metabolism but contain both a high level of oxidative enzymes and glycogen. They contract rapidly but are also fatigue resistant. Type IIB fibers are found in small mammals and are the most fatigable but fastest-contracting fiber types. They also are the largest in diameter. They utilize anaerobic glycolysis primarily and contain a large amount of glycogen but relatively few oxidative enzymes. Human laryngeal muscles generally contain a mixture of type I, IIA, and IIX fibers, with the proportion of each varying from muscle to muscle. The fiber composition of laryngeal muscles differs from that of most larger skeletal muscles. Elsewhere, muscle fiber diameters are fairly constant, ranging between 60 and 80 microns. In laryngeal muscles, there is considerably more variability,[53,54] and fiber diameters vary between 10 and 100 microns, with an average diameter of 40–50 microns. The TA and lateral CT muscles are designed for rapid contraction. Laryngeal muscles have a higher proportion of type IIA fibers than most other muscles, which makes them particularly well suited to rapid contraction with fatigue resistance.[55] In addition, many laryngeal motor units have multiple neural innervations. There appear to be approximately 20–30 muscle fibers per motor unit in a human CT muscle,[56] suggesting that the motor unit size of this laryngeal muscle is similar to that of extraocular and facial muscles.[57] In the human TA muscle, 70%–80% of muscle fibers have 2 or more nerve endplates and some fibers have as many as 5 nerve endplates.[58] Only 50% of CT and LCA muscle fibers have multiple endplates, and multiple endplates are even less common in the PCA muscle (5%). It is still not known whether one muscle fiber can be part of more than one motor unit (receive endplates from different motor neurons), or whether all of the endplates on each muscle are associated with the same motor neuron.[55]

Recent research has provided additional interesting observations in laryngeal muscles. Wu et al found that human PCA and TA muscles express 3 types of myosin heavy-chain (MyHC) isoforms, including slow type I, fast type 2A, and fast type 2X.[59] Single-fiber analysis has demonstrated regional differences, and the common occurrence of hybrid fibers.[59] Recent research by Malmgren and coworkers has also demonstrated that laryngeal muscles remain capable of spontaneous regeneration over a lifetime and that the proportion of regenerating fibers (identified immunohistochemically by the presence of the developmental myosin isoforms) increases as the TA muscle ages.[60] Malmgren et al also speculate that the increase in regenerating fibers may be a compensatory response to an age-related increase in muscle fiber injury or death. These new findings are consistent with clinical observations that many "aging changes" of the voice can be reversed through voice therapy.[61]

**Larynx: Innervation**

The recurrent and superior laryngeal nerves are branches of the 10th cranial nerves, or the vagus nerves, which are the longest of the cranial nerves. The vagus nerves originate from 8 to 10 rootlets in a groove in the brainstem between the olive and inferior cerebellar peduncles, in close association with the origins of the 9th and 11th cranial nerves. The rootlets attach to the medulla oblongata in the brainstem, and course below the cerebellar flocculus, where they unite to form the 10th cranial nerve, which exits the cranium through the jugular foramen with the spinal accessory nerve, the glossopharyngeal nerve, and the jugular vein. The hypoglossal nerve exits the skull through the hypoglossal canal, which is adjacent to the jugular foramen and separated from it by a septum. The first ganglion of the vagus nerve is the jugular ganglion, which is located in the jugular foramen, and is known also as the superior ganglion of the vagus nerve. The nodose ganglion (inferior ganglion) is the second ganglion of the vagus nerve and is located in the neck, slightly inferior to the jugular foramen. The vagus nerve contains branchial motor fibers, somatic sensory fibers (from the posterior external auditory canal, from skin adjacent to the ear in some people, and from the tympanic membrane and pharynx), special sensory fibers (taste), visceral motor fibers, and visceral afferent fibers (from the upper respiratory tract, esophagus, stomach, pancreas, abdominal viscera, aortic bodies, aortic arch, and heart). Cells for the visceral, special sensory afferent, and somatic sensory afferent fibers originate in the jugular ganglion and the nodose ganglion. Visceral afferent fibers have cell bodies in the inferior vagal ganglion. Their axons ascend to the medulla oblongata, then descend in the tractus solitarius from which they enter the caudal aspect of the nucleus of the tractus solitarius, also called the nucleus solitarius. Sensory afferent fibers from the larynx and pharynx travel with the visceral afferent fibers via the recurrent and superior laryngeal nerves to their cell bodies in the inferior ganglion.

The nucleus ambiguus is the branchial motor nucleus for the external branch of the superior laryngeal nerve, the recurrent laryngeal nerve, and the pharyngeal nerve and its plexus. Bilateral corticobulbar fibers from the motor cortexes descend through the internal capsule to synapse with the nucleus ambiguus. This bilateral innervation is important in maintaining coordinated, voluntary control of the laryngeal muscles. The motor neurons of the CT muscle are situated rostrally in the nucleus ambiguus, just caudal to the nucleus of the facial nerve. More rostrally, the motor neurons of the TA, LCA, and PCA muscles are located in overlapping pools.[62,63] The LCA, TA, and IA motor neurons are located in close association to each other (partially overlapping) and are separate from the CT motor neurons, which are more rostrally co-located with pharyngeal and palatal motor neurons.[64] Davis and Nail[62] have shown that there are larger motor neurons associated with the TA and LCA muscles (fast-acting muscles used to constrict and protect the airway) than with the PCA and CT muscle (slower-acting muscles that dilate the airway for respiration). Many other neuromotor regions of importance to phonation are beyond the scope of this chapter (mouth, tongue, palate, pharynx, chest, abdomen) but should be considered part of the anatomy of the voice.

Premotor neurons, or interneurons, control motor neurons; motor neurons with multiple functions may be controlled by more than 1 premotor neuron. For example, for phonation, the premotor neuron controlling the TA muscle is associated with the nucleus retroambiguus, located caudally in the medulla. However, for swallowing functions, the TA muscle can be driven by premotor neurons elsewhere in the medulla and pons.[65]

The periaqueductal gray (PAG) matter is a central area of particular interest to voice specialists and has been studied elegantly by several investigators, especially Pamela Davis, PhD, in Sydney, Australia. The PAG is a region of gray matter, composed of neuronal cell bodies, surrounding the cerebral aqueduct. It is contiguous with gray matter surrounding the third ventricle in the hypothalamus and thalamus rostrally and with gray matter surrounding the pontine portion of the fourth ventricle caudally. Stimulation of the PAG, or of other regions that stimulate the PAG (such as the hypothalamus),[66] produces vocalization; destruction of the PAG produces mutism.[67–70] The neurons in the PAG form longitudinal columns and are essential to emotional expression.[71] The lateral column of neurons in the PAG is responsible for vocalization, increases in blood pressure and heart rate associated with the fight-or-flight response, alterations in bodily blood flow, and nonopioid analgesia.[72–75] PAG neurons control vocalization by anastomosing with cells in the nucleus retroambiguus, the origin of premotor neurons discussed above. In addition to stimulating motor neurons in the nucleus ambiguus associated with the larynx, the nucleus retroambiguus stimulates motor neurons associated with chewing; movements of the tongue, palate, face, and pharynx; and motor activity in the chest and abdomen.[62] The PAG region receives numerous connections from the cortex,[76] and it may be involved in emotional expression associated with the voice in speech and song. It clearly plays an important role in spontaneous emotional voicing in animals, newborns, and adult humans.[77] The PAG matter is also involved in muscle control during respiration,[72,78,79] a function linked closely with phonation. Interestingly, Davis and coworkers have shown that vocalization activated by the PAG is also associated with laryngeal and vagal afferent input, suggesting that the duration of vocalization is controlled, not just by stimulation of vocalization (including emotional content), but also by the amount of air available in the lungs.[80] Ambalavanar demonstrated that afferents from the internal branch of the superior laryngeal nerve travel to the portions of the PAG involved in vocalization, which may be the pathway associated with coordinating such reflex control.[81] Interestingly, the Lombard effect, which is so important to speakers and singers (the tendency to speak more loudly in the presence of background noise), is also represented in the PAG.[82]

Bandler et al have suggested that the PAG may not activate and deactivate laryngeal, respiratory, and orofacial motoneurons directly, but rather may establish "emotional and vocal readiness," with activation actually being dependent on higher brain structures.[75] They suggest that this may explain why damage to the PAG and/or the anterior cingulate cortex produces mutism, even when other components of the voluntary vocal motor system are intact, and why motor cortex injury does not cause mutism when the lateral PAG remains intact to produce emotional vocalization.

Broca area and the sensory-motor regions of the lateral cerebral cortex are involved in control for vocalization. In 1959, Penfield and Roberts published classic descriptions of the function of the primary motor cortex based on cortical stimulation performed in patients with epilepsy.[83] Vocalization was localized in the lowest portion of the cortical strip. Stimulation of this region produced activity not only in laryn-geal muscles, but also in those of the jaw, lips, and tongue. The premotor cortex (Brodmann area 6) is located close to the primary voice motor cortex, as is the supplementary motor region, which is involved in initiation of speech. Adjacent subcortical areas are also important for speech, but their functions are not understood completely. Most axons in the cerebral cortex cross the midline. So, functions such as motor control from the left hemisphere may affect primarily the right side of the body. However, some functions, including those controlled by cranial nerves (ie, facial and laryngeal muscle function), may be ipsilateral and/or contralateral.

Studies utilizing dynamic imaging techniques such as positron emission tomography (PET) have begun to improve our understanding of function in these areas of the brain. Perry et al used PET to study singing.[84] They found hyperperfusion during singing in various areas associated with the motor cortex, including the anterior cingulate cortex, precentral gyri, anterior insula, supplementary motor area, and the cerebellum. The central nervous system specializations that enable processing of acoustically complex voice signals are not understood fully, although it is likely that there are "voice cells" in the brain. Using functional magnetic resonance imaging (fMRI), in 2011 Perrodin et al identified "voice cells" analogous to "face cells" in the brains of monkeys.[85] Unlike face cells, they found that voice clusters contain moderate proportions of voice cells that exhibit high stimulus selectivity. Looking at a broader prospective of the brain's management of speech production, Simonyan and Horwitz published a review of laryngeal motor cortical control during speech and other laryngeal activities.[86] They suggested that the location of the laryngeal motor cortex is in the primary motor cortex and its direct connections with the brainstem laryngeal motor neurons in humans, as opposed to its location in the premotor cortex with only indirect connections to the laryngeal motor neurons in nonhuman primates. They suggested that this major evolutionary development in humans is associated with the human ability to speak and vocalize voluntarily. In addition to dynamic imaging (cerebral blood flow) fMRI studies, a variety of other methods can be used to study neurophysiology of brain function, including neuropsychological testing, dichotic listening, dichaptic touching, split-field tachistoscopic viewing, electroencephalography with evoked potential testing, and other techniques. Some of these approaches have been used to study cerebral dominance and its relationship to musical faculty. It is popularly believed that music and art are associated with the type of thinking performed primarily in the right brain of a right-handed individual, while language is represented primarily by processes in the left brain. At present, it is unclear whether these traditional models are valid; it seems probable that complex interactions involving numerous cortical and subcortical areas of both sides of the brain are involved in complicated activities such as emotional expression through speech or song. In a particularly interesting study, Kleber et al examined the brains of expert opera singers, conservatory-level voice students, and laymen during singing of an Italian aria, using fMRI.[87] The researchers were interested in evaluating effects of motor-skill training. Their experiments revealed that voice training is associated with increased functional activation bilaterally of the primary somatosensory cortex representing articulators in the larynx. There was additional activation in the right primary sensory motor cortex, the inferior parietal lobe, and the dorsolateral prefrontal cortex bilaterally. Expert singers also showed subcortical changes including increased activation in the basal ganglia, thalamus, and cerebellum. Increased vocal training also correlated with increased activity of a cortical network for enhanced kinesthetic motor control and sensory motor guidance, as well as increased involvement of motor memory areas at the cerebellar and subcortical levels. Further research into these observations should provide interesting information that might be applied to voice training, diagnosis, and rehabilitation. Although other areas of the brain are beyond the scope of this chapter, it should be noted that there are many brain activities of interest and importance to voice patients and clinicians. For example, hearing is essential to optimal voice and speech production, so understanding auditory brain function also is important for voice care, as is understanding areas involved in emotion and many other functions.

The superior laryngeal nerve branches off the vagus nerve high in the neck at the inferior end of the nodose ganglion. It travels between the internal and external carotid arteries, dividing into an internal and external branch near the posterior aspect of the hyoid bone. The external branch courses inferiorly with the superior thyroid artery and vein over the constrictor muscle and through the posterior cricothyroid membrane into the larynx (see Figure 8–8B). Chuang et al studied the anatomic positions of the external branch of the superior laryngeal nerve in Chinese adults. They noted that the inferior corner of the thyroid cartilage was a reliable landmark for identifying the external branch but that there were variations in the position of the nerve.[88] Using the Cernea classification,[89] after investigating 86 nerves in 43 cadavers they identified Cernea type 1 position

in 16.2% (nerve crossing the superior thyroid vessels more than 1 cm above the horizontal plane passing through the upper border of the superior pole of the thyroid gland), type 2a anatomy in 39.5% (nerve crossing the vessels less than 1 cm above the horizontal plane), and type 2b in 38.3% (nerve crossing the superior thyroid vessels below the horizontal plane). They concluded that 77.8% of the superior laryngeal nerve external branches studied were in positions of high risk for injury during thyroid surgery. These findings are similar to those of other authors.[90,91] The authors recommended identifying the nerve inferiorly at the inferior cornu of the thyroid cartilage and reported a nerve identification rate significantly better than that reported by authors who identify the nerve distally at the inferior constrictor-cricothyroid junction[92] but different from those of Cernea[89] and others.[93–95] While it is possible that there may be racial differences (the Chuang study was performed off Chinese adults), Furlan studied the question and found no statistically significant different between ethnic groups, but they reported variations in the external branches superior laryngeal nerve related to individual stature and thyroid volumes.[94] The external branch supplies the CT muscle. An extension of the external branch may also supply motor and sensory innervation to the vocal folds. Wu et al have identified this extension of the external branch of the superior laryngeal nerve as the human communicating nerve.[96] This neural connection was found in 12 (44%) of 27 specimens. When present, it exited the medial surface of the cricothyroid muscle and entered the lateral surface of the thyroarytenoid muscle. The communicating nerve was composed of an intramuscular branch, which combined with the recurrent laryngeal nerve or terminated within the thyroarytenoid muscle directly, and an extramuscular branch that passed through the thyroarytenoid muscle and terminated in the subglottic mucosa in the region of the cricoarytenoid joint. The communicating nerves contain an average of 2510 myelinated axons, of which 31% were motor neurons. Wu et al believe that when the communicating nerve is present, it supplies a second source of motor innervation to the thyroarytenoid muscle and extensive sensory innervation to the subglottic area and cricoarytenoid joint.

The internal branch of the superior laryngeal nerve is responsible primarily for sensation in the mucosa at and above the level of the vocal fold, but it may be responsible for some motor innervations of laryngeal muscles, as well. The internal branch of the superior laryngeal nerves is divided into 3 divisions.[97] The superior division supplies the mucosa on the laryngeal surface of the epiglottis. The middle division supplies portions of the true vocal folds, false vocal folds, and the aryepiglottic folds. The inferior division supplies the mucosa of the arytenoids, the portion of the subglottis not supplied by the recurrent laryngeal nerve, the upper esophageal sphincter, and the anterior wall of the hypopharynx. The internal branch of the superior laryngeal nerves also supplies the thyroepiglottic and cricoarytenoid joints.

Terminal sensory nuclei also are involved in reflex pathways associated with the reticular formation. The distributions of the sensory nerves within the larynx in humans remain somewhat speculative, being inferred primarily from research performed in cats.[98] Yoshida and coworkers found that the internal branch at the superior laryngeal nerve supplies the ipsilateral side of the epiglottis, aryepiglottic fold, arytenoid eminence, rostral aspect of the vocal fold, vestibule, and mucosa overlying the PCA muscle. The posterior branch of the recurrent laryngeal nerve divides into two branches, one of which goes to Galen anastomosis. The other sensory branch provides bilateral supply with ipsilateral dominance to the caudal aspect of the vocal fold and the subglottic region. Some fibers from the internal branch of the superior laryngeal nerve join with fibers from the posterior branch of the recurrent laryngeal nerve to share innervation of the posterior wall of the glottis and the medial aspect of the arytenoids bilaterally with ipsilateral predominance.[99] The cell bodies of the sensory fibers arise primarily in the nodose ganglion and project to the ipsilateral nucleus solitarius. Special sensory fibers for taste from the epiglottis and the larynx course with the vagus nerve to the tractus solitarius and its nucleus.

The recurrent laryngeal nerves branch off the vagus in the chest. On the left, the nerve usually loops around the aortic arch from anterior to posterior and passes lateral to the ligamentum arteriosum behind the arch to enter the tracheoesophageal groove. Occasionally, the nerve is not "recurrent" and does not loop around the aortic arch. Instead it branches directly off the vagus nerve in the neck and courses directly to the larynx. On the right, it usually loops around the brachiocephalic or subclavian artery. This anatomic relationship is usually, but not always, present; and nonrecurrent recurrent nerves occur, probably in less than 1% of people. Nonrecurrent right "recurrent" laryngeal nerves are seen most commonly when the right subclavian artery arises from the descending aorta. In such cases, the "recurrent" nerve arises in the neck and travels directly to the larynx. The recurrent nerves travel superiorly in the tracheoesophageal grooves, entering the larynx between the esophagus and tracheopharyngeus

muscle. As they course toward the larynx, the recurrent nerves give off branches to the heart, esophagus, trachea, pharynx, and larynx. The recurrent nerves run perpendicularly between the first 2 branches of the inferior thyroid artery and are attached closely to the posterior, medial aspect of the thyroid lobe. They enter the larynx coursing just below or under the inferior constrictor muscle and communicate with the ansa Galeni, a connection between the posterior branch of the recurrent laryngeal nerve and the internal branch of the superior laryngeal nerve, which is described in more detail in the next paragraph below. Interestingly, it has been found that the myelinated fibers in the left recurrent laryngeal nerve are larger in diameter than those on the right.[100] This led Malmgren and Gacek to speculate that differences in fiber size may allow the simultaneous activation of laryngeal muscles via faster transmission rates on the left, despite the fact that the right recurrent laryngeal nerve is shorter than the left[101] and thus should otherwise transmit faster causing signal activation sooner. More recently, Jotz et al reexamined the question of histological asymmetry of the RLN.[102] They found that the intraperineural area and perimeter of fibers of the right RLN were statistically larger than those of the left RLN. They speculated that the morphological differences were related to the different time of arrival of the stimulus to the laryngeal muscles.

Within the larynx, the recurrent laryngeal nerve crosses from posterior to anterior usually at a level slightly below the cricoarytenoid joint. Usually, the recurrent nerve passes approximately 4 to 5 mm posterior to the cricothyroid joint, but in up to about 15% of adults, the nerve may split around the joint, or it may pass anterior to it. These landmarks may be particularly important during surgical procedures in which identification of the cricothyroid joint is necessary. As the recurrent nerve enters the region of the cricothyroid joint, it divides into branches to each of the intrinsic muscles to which it provides motor innervation. It appears that the first branch usually goes to the PCA muscle. This posterior branch also innervates the IA muscles. An anterior branch courses toward the LCA muscle and supplies the TA muscle, as well. Detailed studies of the courses and variations on the terminal branches of the recurrent laryngeal nerves have not yet been published. Research is currently underway to address this deficiency in knowledge, which has become relevant clinically because of surgical procedures such as thyroarytenoid neurectomy. Consequently, the thyroarytenoid branch was studied first.[103] In this study, we determined that the median distance from the inferior tubercle of the thyroid cartilage to the thyroarytenoid branch of the recurrent laryngeal nerve was 3.75 mm. Fifty-four percent of the nerves traveled in a horizontal direction within the larynx, but vertical and oblique orientations were observed. The thyroarytenoid division of the recurrent laryngeal nerve branched in approximately 20% of specimens. From this study, we concluded that surgeons performing thyroarytenoid neurectomy can identify the likely position of the thyroarytenoid nerve by measuring approximately 4 mm from the inferior tubercle along a perpendicular line. In most specimens, the nerve was encountered within 1 to 4 mm from the inferior tubercle. In 2007, the author (RTS) and colleagues performed similar studies on the innervation of the posterior cricoarytenoid muscle, in an effort to explore the practicality of PCA nerve section for abductor spasmodic dysphonia.[104] Microscopic dissection allowed the identification and measurement of the branches from the recurrent laryngeal nerves (RLNs) to the PCA in the 43 human cadaver larynges. The cricothyroid (CT) joint was the primary landmark for measurement. All of the PCA muscles received innervation from the anterior division of the RLN. The number of direct branches from the RLN ranged from 1 to 5 (average 2.3). More than 70% of PCA muscles also received 1–3 branches off of the branch to the interarytenoid (IA) muscle. Less than half of PCA muscles received any kind of nerve branches from the posterior division of the RLN. Branches to the PCA most commonly departed the main RLN in its vertical segment, and all entered the muscle from its deep surface. Branches departed the RLN within an average of 9.5 mm from the CT joint; the branch to the IA occurred distal to this point. The innervation to the PCA is complex and redundant, and the segment of the RLN supplying those branches is difficult to expose safely. For these reasons, selective denervation or reinnervation procedures limited to the PCA nerve branches may be difficult technically. When needing only to denervate the PCA, this can be accomplished by removing a portion of the PCA and the underlying nerve supply, maximizing efforts to avoid injury to the branches to the IA muscle. In addition to motor innervation, the recurrent laryngeal nerves are also responsible for sensory innervation primarily below the level of the true vocal folds, and of the spindles of the intrinsic muscles,[105] although they may supply portions of the vocal folds as noted above. There are interconnections between the superior and recurrent laryngeal nerves, particularly in the region of the IA muscles. The IA muscles are also the only laryngeal muscles that receive bilateral innervation (both recurrent laryngeal nerves).

Sympathetic innervation of the larynx is from the superior cervical ganglion. Parasympathetic inner-

vation from the dorsal motor nucleus travels to the supraglottic larynx with the internal branch of the superior laryngeal nerves and to the subglottic larynx with the recurrent laryngeal nerves. The larynx also contains other important structures not discussed in detail in this chapter, including chemoreceptors, taste buds, and various mechanoreceptors, Meissner corpuscles, free nerve endings, and Merkel cells. The superior and recurrent laryngeal nerves are also connected through the ramus communicans, also called the ansa Galeni or nerve of Galen, which supplies motor innervation to the tracheal and the esophageal mucosa and the smooth muscle of the trachea. It also supplies the chemoreceptors and baroreceptors of the aortic arch. The laryngeal chemoreflex is an interesting phenomenon that produces cardiovascular changes and central apnea in response to chemical stimulation of the larynx.[106,107] The laryngeal chemoreflex may be triggered by stimuli such as gastric acid and can produce responses including laryngeal adduction, bronchoconstriction, hypotension, bradycardia, apnea, and possibly sudden infant death syndrome.[108] Like sudden infant death syndrome, the laryngeal chemoreflex is seen usually only in infants under the age of 1. It differs from the glottic closure reflex in response to swallowing and from laryngospasm, which involves glottic closure without central apnea or cardiovascular changes. There is also a laryngeal reflex that results in glottic closure in response to gentle supraglottic tactile stimulation.

The larynx also contains low-threshold, rapidly adapting proprioceptors and low-threshold slowly adapting proprioceptors. The low-threshold, rapidly adapting proprioceptors are found in laryngeal joint capsules and control laryngeal muscle tone during joint movement (such as during singing or speech). Low-threshold, slowly adapting proprioceptors are found in the laryngeal muscles and help to fine-tune laryngeal muscle tone during activities such as phonation. The laryngeal proprioceptors are associated with 2 interesting polysynaptic reflex arcs that were identified in 1966.[109] When stimulated, the facilitatory reflex arc increases the rate of motor unit firing in the TA and CT muscles. When the inhibitory reflex arch is stimulated, motor unit firing is decreased in the TA, CT, and sternothyroid muscles. Proprioceptors are probably also important in control of laryngeal muscle tone during respiration.[110]

**Larynx: Extrinsic Muscles**

Extrinsic laryngeal musculature maintains the position of the larynx in the neck. This group of muscles includes primarily the strap muscles. Because raising or lowering the larynx may alter the tension or angle between laryngeal cartilages, thereby changing the resting lengths of the intrinsic muscles, the extrinsic muscles are critical in maintaining a stable laryngeal skeleton that permits effective movement of the delicate intrinsic musculature. In the Western classically trained singer, the extrinsic muscles maintain the larynx in a relatively constant vertical position throughout the pitch range. Such training of the intrinsic musculature results in vibratory symmetry of the vocal folds, producing regular periodicity of vocal fold vibration. This contributes to what the listener perceives as a "trained" voice.

The extrinsic muscles may be divided into those below the hyoid bone (infrahyoid muscles) and those above the hyoid bone (suprahyoid muscles). The infrahyoid muscles include the thyrohyoid, sternothyroid, sternohyoid, and omohyoid muscles (Figure 1–9). As a group, the infrahyoid muscles are laryngeal depressors. The thyrohyoid muscle originates obliquely from the thyroid lamina and inserts into the lower border of the greater cornu of the hyoid bone. Contraction brings the thyroid cartilage and the hyoid bone closer together, especially anteriorly. The sternothyroid muscle originates from the first costal cartilage and the posterior aspect of the manubrium of the sternum, and it inserts obliquely on the thyroid cartilage. Contraction lowers the thyroid cartilage. The sternohyoid muscle originates from the clavicle and posterior surface of the manubrium of the sternum, inserting into the lower edge of the body of the hyoid bone. Contraction lowers the hyoid bone. The inferior belly of the omohyoid originates from the upper surface of the scapula and inserts into the intermediate tendon of the omohyoid muscle low in the lateral neck. The superior belly originates from the intermediate tendon and inserts into the greater cornu of the hyoid bone. The omohyoid muscle pulls the hyoid bone down, lowering it.

The suprahyoid muscles include the digastric, mylohyoid, geniohyoid, and stylohyoid muscles. As a group, the suprahyoid muscles are laryngeal "elevators." The posterior belly of the digastric muscle originates from the mastoid process of the temporal bone and inserts into the intermediate tendon of the digastric, which connects to the hyoid bone. The anterior belly originates from the inferior aspect of the mandible near the symphysis and inserts into the digastric intermediate tendon. The anterior belly pulls the hyoid bone anteriorly and raises it. The posterior belly pulls the hyoid bone posteriorly and also raises it. The mylohyoid muscle originates from the inner aspect of the body of the mandible (mylohyoid

line) and inserts into a midline raphe on the hyoid, connecting with fibers from the opposite side. It raises the hyoid bone and pulls it anteriorly. The geniohyoid muscle originates from the spine at the mental symphysis of the mandible and inserts on the anterior surface of the body of the hyoid bone. It raises the hyoid bone and pulls it anteriorly. The stylohyoid muscle originates from the styloid process and inserts into the body of the hyoid bone. It raises the hyoid bone and pulls it posteriorly. Coordinated interaction among the extrinsic laryngeal muscles is needed to control the vertical position of the larynx, as well as other positions such as laryngeal tilt.

### The Supraglottic Vocal Tract

The supraglottic larynx, tongue, lips, palate, pharynx, nasal cavity (see Figure 1–3A), oral cavity, and possibly the sinuses shape the sound quality produced by the vocal folds by acting as resonators. Minor alterations in the configuration of these structures may produce substantial changes in voice quality. The hypernasal speech typically associated with a cleft palate and/or the hyponasal speech characteristic of severe adenoid hypertrophy are obvious. However, mild edema from an upper respiratory tract infection, pharyngeal scarring, or changes in muscle tension produce less obvious sound alterations. These are immediately recognizable to a trained vocalist or astute critic, but they often elude the laryngologist.

### The Tracheobronchial Tree, Lungs, Thorax, Abdomen, and Back

The lungs supply a constant stream of air that passes between the vocal folds and provides power for voice production, which is especially important in singing (Figure 1–10). Singers often are thought of as having "big chests." Actually, the primary respiratory difference between trained and untrained singers is not increased total lung capacity, as popularly assumed. Rather, the trained singer learns to use a higher proportion of the air in his or her lungs, thereby decreasing his or her residual volume and increasing respiratory efficiency.[111]

The abdominal musculature is the so-called "support" of the singing voice, although singers generally refer to their support mechanism as their "diaphragm." The function of the diaphragm muscle in singing is complex, and somewhat variable from singer to singer (or actor to actor). The diaphragm primarily generates inspiratory force. Although the abdomen can also perform this function in some situations,[112] it is primarily an expiratory-force generator.

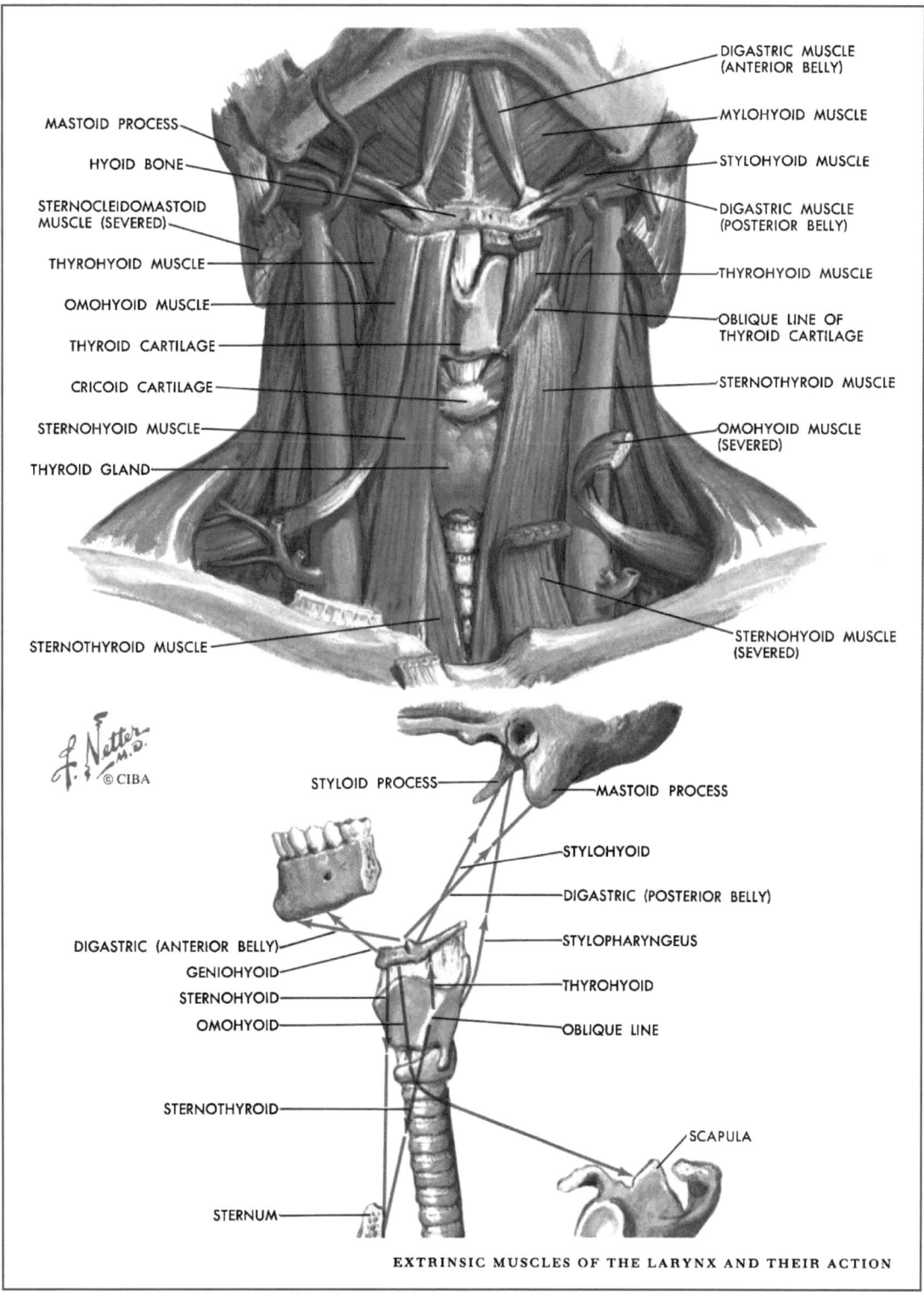

**Figure 1–9.** Extrinsic muscles of the larynx and their actions. (From *The Larynx. Clinical Symposia.* New Jersey: CIBA Pharmaceutical Company; 1964;16[3]: Plate 4. Copyright 1964. Icon Learning Systems, LLC, a subsidiary of MediMedia USA Inc. Reprinted with permission from Icon Learning Systems, LLC, illustrated by Frank H. Netter, MD. All rights reserved.)

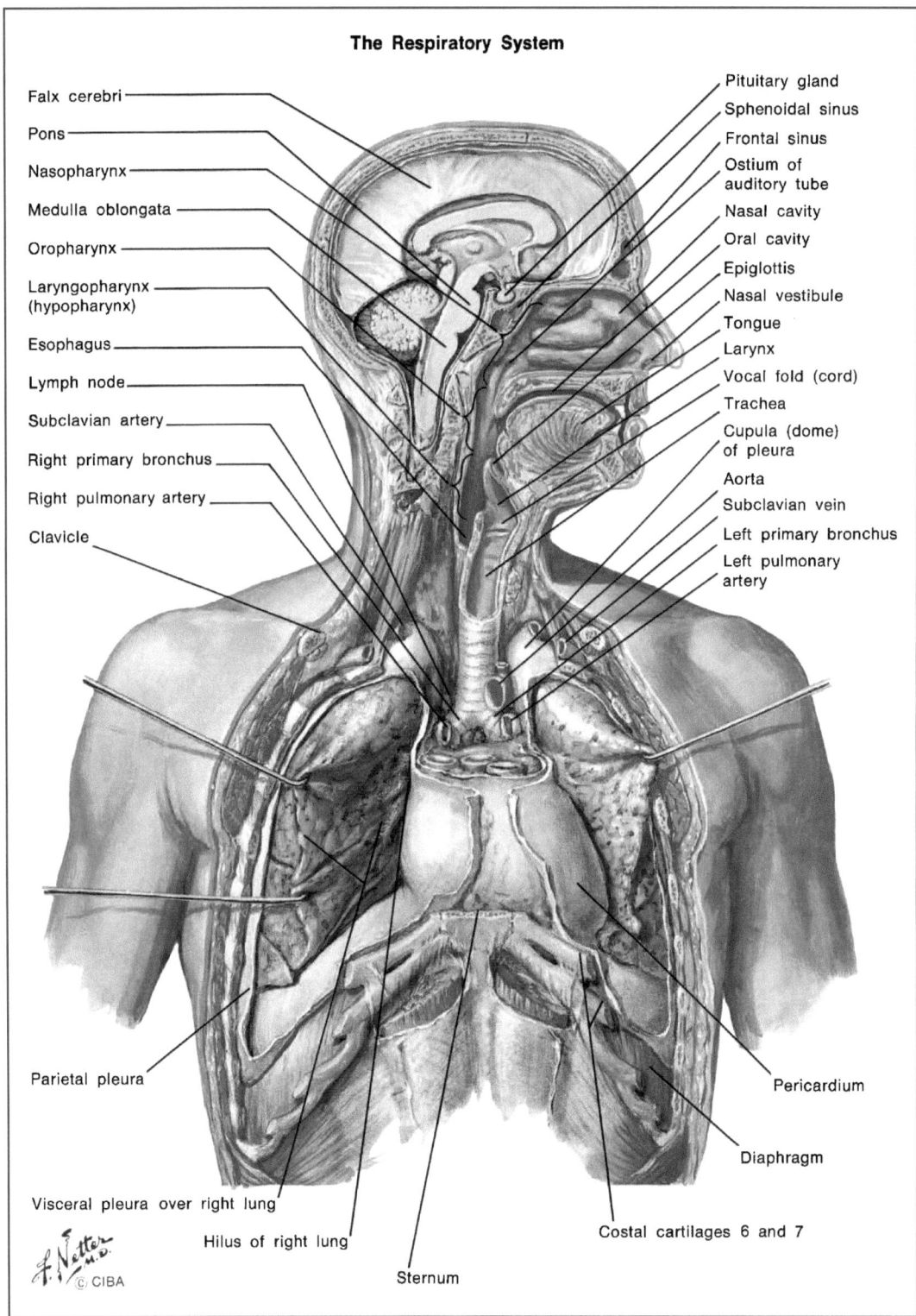

**The Respiratory System**

Falx cerebri

Pons

Nasopharynx

Medulla oblongata

Oropharynx

Laryngopharynx (hypopharynx)

Esophagus

Lymph node

Subclavian artery

Right primary bronchus

Right pulmonary artery

Clavicle

Pituitary gland

Sphenoidal sinus

Frontal sinus

Ostium of auditory tube

Nasal cavity

Oral cavity

Epiglottis

Nasal vestibule

Tongue

Larynx

Vocal fold (cord)

Trachea

Cupula (dome) of pleura

Aorta

Subclavian vein

Left primary bronchus

Left pulmonary artery

Parietal pleura

Pericardium

Diaphragm

Visceral pleura over right lung

Hilus of right lung

Costal cartilages 6 and 7

Sternum

**Figure 1–10.** The respiratory system, showing the relationship of supraglottic structures. The line marking the vocal fold actually stops on the false vocal fold. The level of the true vocal fold is slightly lower. The diaphragm is also visible in relation to the lungs, ribs, and abdomen muscles. (From The Development of the Lower Respiratory System. *Clinical Symposia.* New Jersey: CIBA Pharmaceutical Company; 1975;27[4]: Plate 1. Copyright 1964. Icon Learning Systems, LLC, a subsidiary of MediMedia USA Inc. Reprinted with permission from Icon Learning Systems, LLC, illustrated by Frank H. Netter, MD. All rights reserved.)

Interestingly, the diaphragm is coactivated by some performers during singing and appears to play an important part in the fine regulation of singing.[113] Actually, the anatomy and physiology of support for phonation are quite complicated and not understood completely. Both the lungs and rib cage generate passive expiratory forces under many common circumstances; however, passive inspiratory forces also occur. The active respiratory muscles working in concert with passive forces include the intercostal, abdominal, back, and diaphragm muscles. The principal muscles of inspiration are the diaphragm and external intercostal muscles. Accessory muscles of inspiration include the pectoralis major; pectoralis minor; serratus anterior; subclavius; sternocleidomastoid; anterior, medial, and posterior scalenus, serratus posterior and superior; latissimus dorsi; and levatores costarum muscles. During quiet respiration, expiration is largely passive. Many of the muscle used for active expiration (forcing air out of the lungs) are also employed in "support" for singing and acting voice tasks, including abdominal, back, and chest muscles.

Muscles of active expiration either raise the intra-abdominal pressure forcing the diaphragm upward or decrease the diameter of the ribs or sternum to decrease the volume dimension of the thorax, or both. They include the internal intercostals, which stiffen the rib interspaces and pull the ribs down; the transversus thoracis, the subcostal muscles, and the serratus posterior inferior muscles, all of which pull the ribs down; and the quadratus lumborum, which depresses the lowest rib. In addition, the latissimus dorsi, which may also act as a muscle of inspiration, is capable of compressing the lower portion of the rib cage and can act as a muscle of expiration as well. The above muscles all participate in active expiration and support. However, the primary muscles of active expiration are the abdominal muscles. They include the external oblique, internal oblique, rectus abdominus, and transversus abdominus muscles. The external oblique is a flat broad muscle located on the side and front of the lower chest and abdomen. Upon contraction, it pulls the lower ribs down and raises the abdominal pressure by displacing abdominal contents inward. It should be noted that this muscle is strengthened by leg lifting and lowering and other exercises but is not developed effectively by traditional trunk curls or sit-ups. Appropriate strengthening exercises of the external oblique muscles are often neglected in voice training. The internal oblique is a flat muscle in the side and front walls of the abdomen. It lies deep to the external oblique. When contracted, the internal oblique drives the abdominal wall inward and lowers the lower ribs. The rectus abdominis runs parallel to the midline of the abdomen, originating from the xiphoid process of the sternum and the fifth, sixth, and seventh costal (rib) cartilages. It inserts into the pubic bone. It is encased in the fibrous abdominal aponeurosis. Contraction of the rectus abdominis also forces the abdominal contents inward and lowers the sternum and ribs. The transversus abdominis is a broad muscle located under the internal oblique on the side and front of the abdomen. Its fibers run horizontally around the abdomen. Contraction of the transverse abdominis compresses the abdominal contents, elevating intraabdominal pressure. Back (especially lower back) and other muscles (eg, iliocostalis dorsi, iliocostalis lumborum, longissimus dorsi) are also extremely important to power source "support" function, and especially to support for projected speech and singing.

The abdominal and back musculatures receive considerable attention in vocal training. The purpose of support is to maintain an efficient, constant power source and inspiratory-expiratory mechanism. There is disagreement among voice teachers as to the best model for teaching support technique. Some experts describe positioning the abdominal musculature under the rib cage; others advocate distension of the abdomen. Either method may result in vocal problems if used incorrectly, but distending the abdomen (the inverse pressure approach) is especially dangerous, because it tends to focus the singer's muscular effort in a downward and outward direction, which is ineffective. Thus, the singer may exert considerable effort, believing he or she is practicing good support technique, without obtaining the desired effect. Proper abdominal muscle training is essential to good singing and speaking, and the physician must consider abdominal function when evaluating vocal dysfunction.

### The Musculoskeletal System

Musculoskeletal conditioning and position throughout the body (posture) affect the vocal mechanism and may produce tension or impairment of function, resulting in voice dysfunction or injury. Stance deviation, such as from standing to supine, produces obvious changes in respiratory function. However, lesser changes, such as distributing one's weight over the calcaneus rather than forward over the metatarsal heads (a more athletic position), alter the configuration of the abdominal and back muscle function enough to influence the voice. Tensing arm and shoulder muscles promote cervical muscle strain, which can adversely affect laryngeal function. Careful control of muscle tension is fundamental to good vocal technique. In fact, some teaching methods use musculoskeletal conditioning and relaxation as the primary focus of voice training.

### The Psychoneurological System

The psychological constitution of the singer or professional voice user impacts directly on the vocal mechanism. Psychological phenomena are reflected through the autonomic nervous system, which controls mucosal secretions and other functions critical to voice production. The nervous system is also important for its mediation of fine muscle control. This fact is worthy of emphasis, because minimal voice disturbances may occasionally be the first sign of serious neurologic disease.

## Physiology

The physiology of voice production is exceedingly complex and will be summarized only briefly in this chapter. Greater detail may be found elsewhere in this book. For more information, the reader is advised to consult subsequent chapters and other literature, including publications listed in the bibliographies of other chapters and in the Suggested Readings list near the end of this book. Respiratory physiology is included in some detail below.

### Overview of Phonatory Physiology

Volitional voice production begins in the cerebral cortex. Complex interactions among the centers for speech, musical, and artistic expression establish the commands for vocalization. The "idea" of the planned vocalization is conveyed to the precentral gyrus in the motor cortex, which transmits another set of instructions to motor nuclei in the brainstem and spinal cord (Figure 1–11). These areas transmit the complicated messages necessary for coordinated activity of the laryngeal, thoracic, and abdominal musculature and of the vocal tract articulators and resonators. Additional refinement of motor activity is provided by the extrapyramidal (cerebral cortex, cerebellum, and basal ganglion) and the autonomic nervous systems. These impulses combine to produce a sound that is transmitted not only to the ears of listeners but also to those of the speaker or singer. Auditory feedback is transmitted from the ear to the cerebral cortex via the brainstem, and adjustments are made to permit the vocalist to match the sound produced with the intended sound. There is also tactile feedback from the throat and other muscles involved in phonation that undoubtedly help in fine-tuning vocal output, although the mechanism and role of tactile feedback are not fully understood. In many trained singers, the ability to use tactile feedback effectively is cultivated as a result of frequent interference with auditory feedback by ancillary noise in the concert environment (eg, an orchestra or band).

The voice requires interactions among the power source, the oscillator, and the resonator. The power source compresses air and forces it toward the larynx. The vocal folds close and open, permitting small bursts of air to escape between them. Numerous factors affect the sound produced at the glottal level, as discussed in greater detail in a subsequent chapter. Several of these factors include the pressure that builds up below the vocal folds (subglottal pressure), the amount of resistance to opening the glottis (glottal impedance), volume velocity of airflow at the glottis, and supraglottal pressure. The vocal folds do not vibrate like the strings on a violin. Rather, they separate and collide somewhat like buzzing lips. The number of times they do so in any given second (ie, their frequency) determines the number of air puffs that escape. The frequency of glottal closing and opening is a factor in pitch determination. Other factors affect loudness, such as subglottal pressure, glottal resistance, and amplitude of vocal fold displacement from the midline during each vibratory cycle. The sound created at the vocal fold level is a buzz, similar to the sound produced when blowing between 2 blades of grass. This sound contains a complete set of harmonic partials and is responsible in part for the acoustic characteristics of the voice. However, complex and sophisticated interactions in the supraglottic vocal tract may accentuate or attenuate harmonic partials, acting as resonators (Figure 1–12). This portion of the vocal tract is largely responsible for the beauty and variety of the sound produced.

Interactions among the various components of the vocal tract ultimately are responsible for all the vocal characteristics produced. Many aspects of the voice still lack complete understanding and classification. Vocal range is reasonably well understood, and broad categories of voice classifications are generally accepted (Figure 1–13). Other characteristics, such as vocal register, are controversial. Registers are expressed as quality changes within an individual voice. From low to high, they may include vocal fry, chest, middle, head voice, falsetto, and whistle,

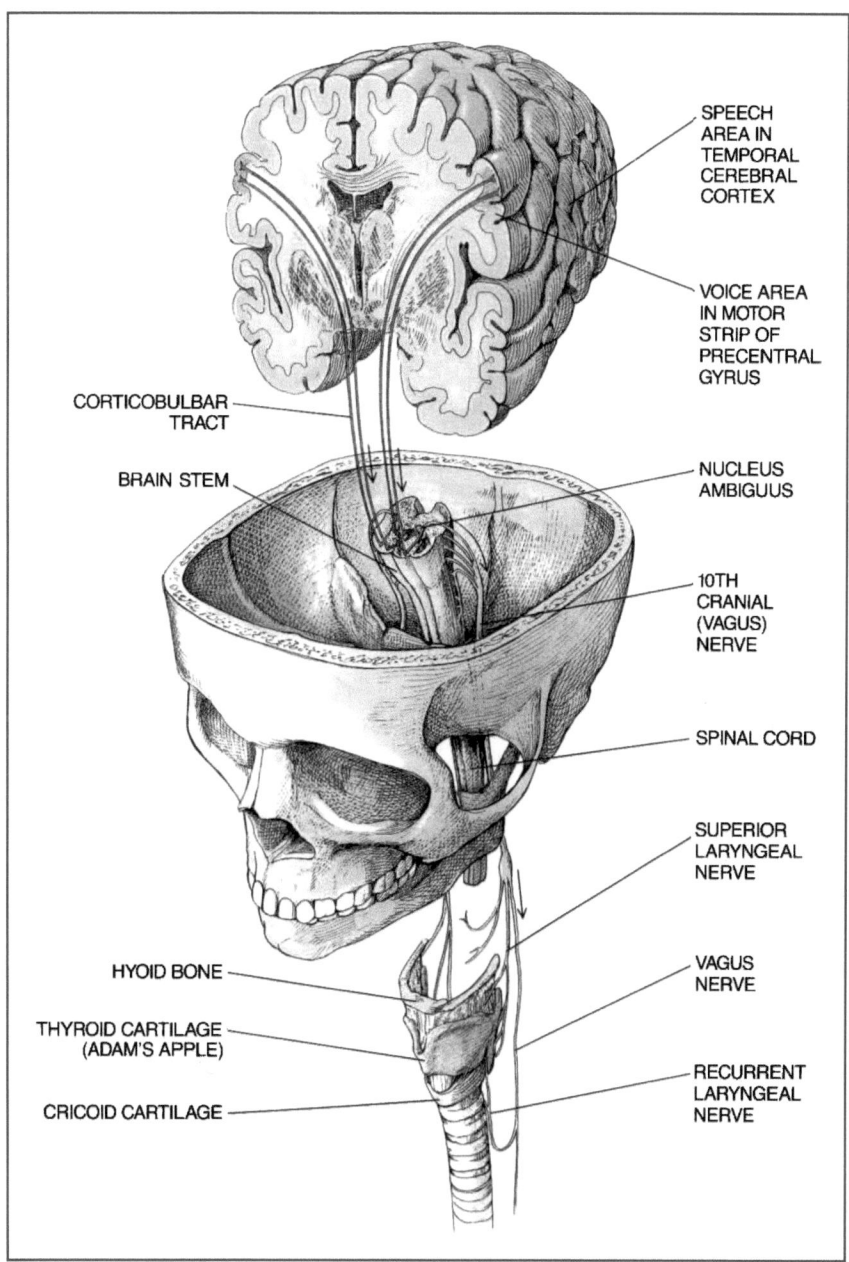

**Figure 1–11.** How the voice is produced. The production of speech or song, or even just a vocal sound, entails a complex orchestration of mental and physical actions. The idea for making a sound originates in the cerebral cortex of the brain—for example, in the speech area. The movement of the larynx is controlled from the voice area and is transmitted to the larynx by various nerves. As a result, the vocal folds vibrate, generating a buzzing sound. It is the resonation of that sound throughout the area of the vocal tract above the glottis—an area that includes the pharynx, tongue, palate, oral cavity, and nose—that gives the sound the qualities perceived by a listener. Auditory feedback and tactile feedback enable the speaker or singer to achieve fine-tuning of the vocal output. (Reproduced with permission from Sataloff.[12])

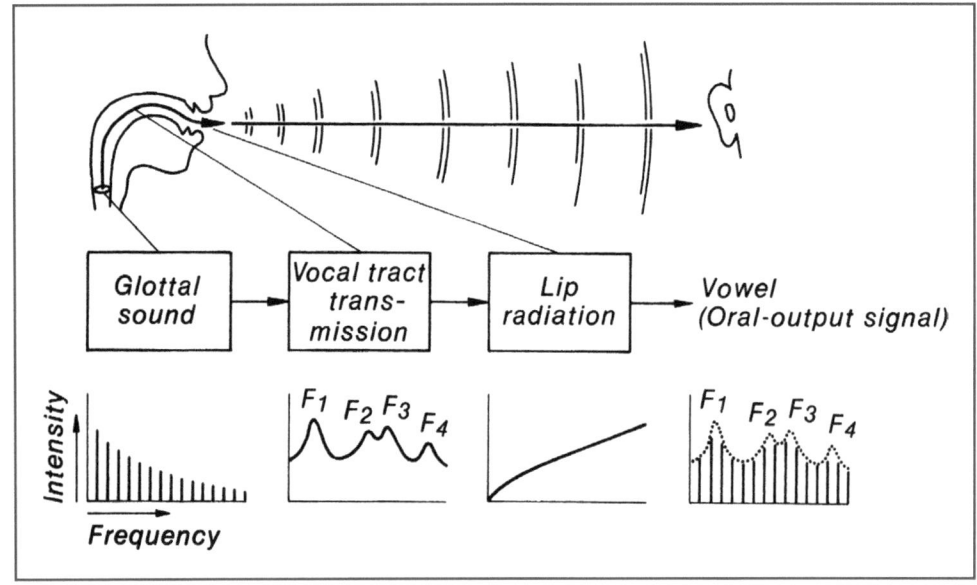

**Figure 1–12.** Some of the factors determining the spectrum of a vowel. (Reproduced with permission from Hirano.[13(p67)])

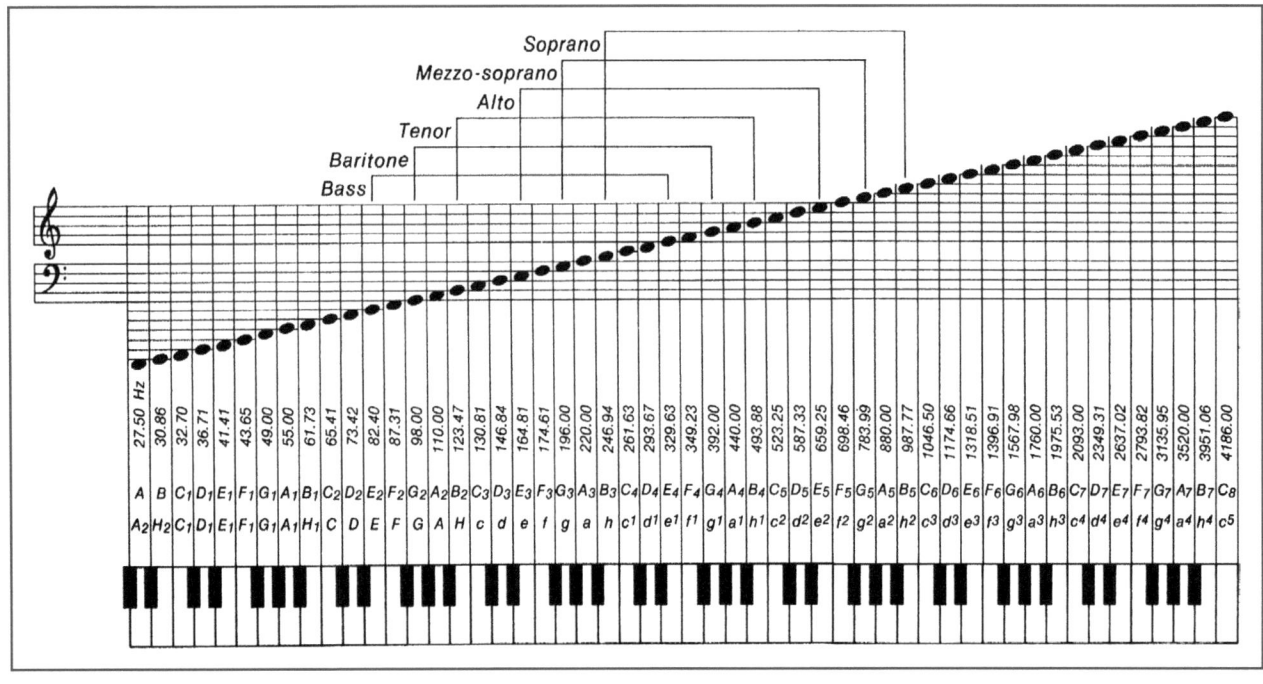

**Figure 1–13.** Correlation between a piano keyboard, pitch names (the lower in capital letters is used in music and voice research, and in this book), frequency, musical notation, and usual voice range. (Reproduced with permission from Hirano.[13(p89)])

although not everyone agrees that all categories exist. The term *modal register*, used most frequently in speech terms, refers to the voice quality generally used by healthy speakers, as opposed to a low, gravelly vocal fry, or high falsetto.

Vibrato is a rhythmic variation in frequency and intensity. Its exact source remains uncertain, and its desirable characteristics depend on voice range and the type of music sung. It appears most likely that the frequency (pitch) modulations are controlled primarily by intrinsic laryngeal muscles, especially the cricothyroid and adductor muscles. However, extrinsic laryngeal muscles and muscles of the supraglottic vocal tract may also play a role. Intensity (loudness) variations may be caused by variations in subglottal pressure, glottal adjustments that affect subglottal pressure, secondary effects of the frequency variation because of changes in the distance between the fundamental frequency and closest formant, or rhythmic changes in vocal tract shape that cause fluctuations in formant frequencies. When evaluating vibrato, it is helpful to consider the waveform of the vibrato signal, its regularity, extent, and rate. The waveform is usually fairly sinusoidal, but considerable variation may occur. The regularity, or similarity of each vibrato event compared to previous and subsequent vibrato events, is greater in trained singers than in untrained voice users. This regularity appears to be one of the characteristics perceived as a "trained sound." Vibratory extent refers to deviation from the standard frequency (not intensity variation) and can be less than ±0.1 semitone in some styles of solo and choral singing, such as some Renaissance music. For most well-trained Western operatic singing, the usual vibrato extent at comfortable loudness is ±0.5 to 1 semitone for singers in most voice classifications. Vibrato rate (the number of modulations per second) is generally 5–7. Rate may also vary greatly from singer to singer and in the same singer. Vibrato rate can increase with increased emotional content of the material, and rate tends to decrease with older age (although the age at which this change occurs is highly variable). When variations from the central frequency become too wide, a "wobble" in the voice is perceived; this is generally referred to as tremolo. It is not generally considered a good musical sound, and it is unclear whether it is produced by the same mechanisms responsible for normal vibrato. Ongoing research should answer many of the remaining questions.

## Respiration

Basic functions of the nose, larynx, and elemental concepts of inspiration and expiration are discussed elsewhere in this book. However, a brief review of selected aspects of pulmonary function is included here to assist readers in understanding the processes that underlie "support," as well as in understanding pulmonary disorders and their assessment.

Starting from the mouth, the respiratory system consists of progressively smaller airway structures. The trachea branches at the carina into mainstem bronchi, which then branch into progressively smaller bronchial passages and terminate in alveoli. Gas exchange (oxygen and carbon dioxide, primarily) between the lungs and the bloodstream occurs at the alveolar level. Air moves in and out of the alveoli in order to permit this exchange of gases. Air is forced out of the alveoli to create the airstream through which phonation is produced. Hence, ultimately alveolar pressure is the primary power source for phonation and is responsible for the creation of the subglottal pressure involved in vocal fold opening and closing. Alveolar pressure is actually greater than subglottal pressure during phonation and expiration, because some pressure is lost due to airway resistance between alveoli and the larynx. As the air passes the alveoli, it enters first the bronchioles, which are small, collapsible airways surrounded by smooth muscle but devoid of cartilage. From the bronchioles, air passes to progressively larger components of the bronchial tree and eventually to the trachea. These structures are supported by cartilage and are not fully collapsible, but they are compressible and respond to changes in external pressure during expiration and inspiration. During expiration, the pressure in the respiratory system is greatest in the alveolus (alveolar pressure) and least at the opening of the mouth where pressure is theoretically equal to atmospheric pressure. Thus, theoretically, all pressure is dissipated between the alveolus and the mouth during expiration due to airway resistance between these structures. Expiration pressure is the total of the elastic recoil combined with active forces created by muscular compression of the airway. The active pressure is distributed throughout all the components of the airway, although it may exert greater effect on the alveoli and bronchioles because they are fully collapsible. When the airway is opened, the air pressure in the alveoli (alveolar pressure) is equal to the atmospheric pressure in the room. In order to fill the alveoli, the alveolar pressure must be decreased to less than atmosphere pressure, creating a vacuum, which sucks air into the lungs. In order to breathe out, alveolar pressure must be greater than atmospheric pressure. As discussed above, there are passive and active forces operative during the inspiratory/expiratory process.

To clarify the mechanisms involved, the alveoli may be thought of as tiny balloons. If a balloon is filled with air, and the filling spout is opened, the elastic properties of the balloon will allow most of the air to rush out. This is analogous to passive expiration, which relies on the elastic properties of the respiratory system. Alternatively, we may wrap our hands around the balloon and squeeze the air out.

This may allow us to get the air out faster and more forcefully, and it will allow us to get more of the air out of the balloon than is expelled through the passive process alone. This is analogous to active expiration, which involves the abdominal, chest, and back muscles. If we partially pinch the filling spout of the balloon, air comes out more slowly because the outflow tract is partially blocked. The air also tends to whistle as it exits the balloon. This is analogous to obstructive pulmonary disease, and its commonly associated wheeze. If we try to blow up the balloon while our hands are wrapped around it, the balloon is more difficult to inflate and cannot be inflated fully, because it is restricted physically by our hands. This is somewhat analogous to restrictive lung disease. Under these circumstances, it may also take more pressure to fill the balloon, because the filling process must overcome the restricting forces. Under any of these circumstances, the more we fill the alveolar "balloon," the greater the pressure, as long as the balloon is not ruptured. When the pressure is greater, the increased elastic recoil results in more rapid and forceful air escape when the air is released. The pressure inside the balloon can be increased even above its maximal elastic recoil level simply by squeezing the outside of the balloon. This analogy is helpful in understanding the forces involved in breathing (especially expiration) and in generating support for phonation.

Although inspiration is extremely important, this discussion will concentrate primarily on expiration, which is linked so closely to "support" for speech and singing. The elastic component of expiratory pressure (specifically, alveolar pressure) depends on lung volume and the elastic forces exerted by the chest and the lungs. The lung is never totally deflated. At rest, it is inflated to about 40% of total lung capacity (TLC). The amount of air in the lungs at rest is the functional residual capacity (FRC). At FRC, the thorax is at a volume much less than its rest (or a neutral) posture, which is actually closer to 75% of TLC. Hence, at FRC the thorax has a passive tendency to expand, as happens during inspiration. Conversely, at FRC the lung is greater than its neutral position and would collapse if it were not acted upon by other forces. The collapsing elastic forces of the lung are balanced by the expanding elastic forces of the thorax. The lung and thorax interact closely, and their relative positions of contact vary constantly. This is facilitated by the anatomy of the boundary zone. The inner surface of the thorax is covered by a membrane called the parietal pleura, and the lung is covered by a similar membrane called the visceral pleura. A thin layer of pleural fluid exists between them. Hydrostatic forces

hold these surfaces together while allowing them to slide freely. Under pathologic circumstances (eg, following surgery or radiation) these surfaces may stick together, impairing lung function and affecting support for phonation adversely.

Thoracic and lung elastic behavior can be measured. The basic principle for doing so involves applying pressure and noting the volume changes caused by the pressure. This creates a pressure/volume (P/V) curve. The slope with the P/V curve for the thorax reflects its compliance (cCW), and the slope of the P/V curve for the lung represents its compliance (CL). When pressure is applied to the entire system, a difference P/V curve is created and its slope reflects the compliance of the entire respiratory system (CRS). Starting from FRC, if air is expelled the volume of the system is dropped below FRC, and an expanding force is created. It is increased as the volume decreases. Conversely, during inspiration above FRC, collapsing forces increase with increasing volume.

To phonate, we inspire, increasing volumes well above FRC. If we wish simply to expire, we relax and the passive elastic recoil forces air out of the alveoli, because inflating them has created an alveolar pressure that is greater than atmospheric pressure (and is predictable using the pressure-volume curve). The deeper the inspiration, the greater is the elastic recoil, hence the greater the expiratory air pressure. Inspiration from FRC is an active process, primarily. Thoracic muscles elevate the ribs and increase the diameter of the thorax. The external intercostal muscles are important to this process. Inspiration also involves contraction of the diaphragm muscle, which flattens and also increases thoracic volume, and accessory muscles discussed above.

Expiration is created by forces that decrease thoracic volume. If the entire thoracic and pulmonary complex is thought of as a balloon, this process is easy to understand. If one wishes to increase the pressure in a balloon to force the air out, one simply squeezes the balloon. When the container (balloon or thorax) containing a volume of gas (air) is decreased, the pressure in the gas increases. Expiration is achieved by muscles that pull the ribs down or compress the abdominal contents and push them up, making the volume of the thorax smaller. The principal muscles involved are the internal intercostal muscles, which decrease intercostal space and pull the ribs down, abdominal, back, and other muscles, as reviewed earlier in this chapter.

For projected phonations such as singing or acting, support involves (essentially, is) active expiration. After inspiration, elastic recoil and external forces created by expiratory muscles determine alveolar pressure, which is substantially greater than atmospheric pressure. The combination of passive (elastic) and active (muscular) forces pushes air out against airway resistance. As the pressure decreases on the path from alveolar (maximal to mouth atmospheric) pressure, there is a point at which the pressure inside the airway equals the active expiratory pressure (without the elastic recoil component), which is called the *equal pressure point* (EPP). As expiration continues toward the mouth, pressure drops below the EPP. As airway pressure diminishes below the active expiratory pressure, the airways begin to collapse. This physiologic collapse of the airways increases airway resistance by decreasing the diameter of the airways. The greater the active expiratory forces, the greater is the airway compression after the EPP has been passed. Expiratory pressure and airway compression are important to the control of expiratory airflow rate and are influenced by EPP.

Under normal circumstances, the EPP is reached in the cartilaginous airways, which do not collapse completely ordinarily, even during very forceful expiration or phonation. This is part of the physiological mechanism that allows us to continue to sing even as we are running out of air. However, under pathologic circumstance, the location of the EPP may be shifted. Asthma is the classic example. During bronchospasm or bronchoconstriction, the diameter of the bronchioles is narrowed by smooth muscle contraction, and airway resistance in the bronchioles is increased. Hence, as the air moves from the alveoli into the bronchioles, airway pressure diminishes much more quickly than normal, and EPP may be reached closer to the alveoli and bronchioles, in smaller airways that collapse more easily and more completely. In severe circumstances, the distal airways may collapse fully causing hyperinflation of the lungs and trapping air in the alveoli. Expiratory airflow rate is lowered substantially by the increased resistance in the distal airways, resulting in a lower-than-normal subglottic pressure. This can have profoundly adverse effects on phonation.

Other lung dysfunction also can impair subglottal pressure even if airway resistance is normal. The classic example is emphysema, which occurs commonly in smokers. This condition results in damage to the alveoli. Consequently, because elastic recoil pressures are lower, alveolar pressure is decreased compared to normal. Even if the active expiratory forces are normal, if passive (elastic) expiratory forces are decreased, the normal airway resistance acting against diminished alveolar pressure will shift the EPP distally toward or into collapsible airways. Even

when active expiratory efforts are increased under these circumstances, they do not help because they collapse the distal airways trapping air in the alveoli, and diminishing subglottal pressure.

Although this overview is oversimplified and highlights only some of the more important components of lower respiratory physiology, it is important for laryngologists to bear these principles in mind in order to understand the importance of diagnosis and treatment of respiratory dysfunction in voice professionals. In patients with Olympic voice demands, even slight changes from optimal physiology may have profound consequences on phonatory function, and they are responsible commonly for compensatory efforts that are diagnosed (correctly) as hyperfunctional voice use (muscle tension dysphonia). If we treat voice hyperfunction as if it were the primary problem, failing to recognize that it is secondary to an underlying, organic, pulmonary disorder, then treatment will not be successful in the long term, and preventable voice dysfunction and vocal fold injury may ensue.

## Other Considerations

In addition to the obvious clinical implications of a thorough understanding of laryngeal anatomy, newer technology offers interesting potential for study and teaching of laryngeal anatomy. For example, Hunter and Titze[114] presented an elegant report on more than 1500 measurements from 37 subjects. They suggested that, using a database of individual subject laryngeal dimensions, it should be possible to design a laryngeal model that could be changed from one subject to the next, predicting subject-specific laryngeal function. They also speculated that such work could lead to computer modeling of patient-specific laryngeal disorders and prediction of therapeutic outcomes. Although this elegant research was published more than a decade ago, its potential has not been realized, yet.

Newer technologies also have been applied to teaching laryngeal anatomy. The time-honored method of teaching human anatomy is through cadaver dissection; however, this traditional method has fallen out of favor in contemporary medical school curricula in the United States,[115] United Kingdom,[116] Australia,[117] and Holland.[118] Computer-aided instruction has risen in popularity, and the Association of American Medical Colleges (AAMC) recognizes the ubiquitous nature of these new educational technologies as being mainstream and integral to the medical school curriculum.[119] Hu et al has created a 3-dimensional, educational computer model of the larynx to teach laryngeal anatomy to medical students and residents.[120] Cadaveric necks were imaged with computed tomography and magnetic resonance imaging, and segmentation software was used to render the 3-dimensional images. This computer program has been received warmly by students.[120] Prospective randomized controlled trials have shown that this computer program is as efficacious as standard written lecture notes in teaching laryngeal anatomy.[121–123]

## Conclusion

This chapter and those that follow provide only enough information on the terminology, components, and workings of the voice to permit an understanding of practical, everyday clinical problems and their solutions. The otolaryngologist, speech-language pathologist, singing or acting teacher, singer, actor, or other voice professional would benefit greatly from more extensive study of voice science.

**Acknowledgment.** The author is grateful to Mary Hawkshaw for her assistance in reviewing this chapter.

## References

1. Pernkopf E. *Atlas of Topographical and Applied Human Anatomy*. Munich, Germany: Urban & Schwarzenberg; 1963.
2. Hatley W, Samuel E, Evison G. The pattern of ossification in the laryngeal cartilages: a radiological study. *Br J Radiol*. 1965;38:585–591.
3. Hamdan AL, Husseini ST, Halawi A, Sibai A. Arytenoid asymmetry in relation to vocal symptoms in singers. *J Voice*. 2011;25(2):241–244.
4. Husseini ST, Ashkar J, Halawi A, Sibai A, Hamdan AL. Arytenoid asymmetry in relation to posture, neck tension and glottal attack in singers. *J Voice*. 2011;63(5):264–268.
5. Bonilha HS, O'Sields M, Gerlach TT, Deliyski DD. Arytenoid adduction asymmetries in persons with and without voice disorders. *Logoped Phoniatr Vocol*. 2009;34(3):128–134.
6. Adams J, Gross N, Riddle S, Andersen P, Cohen JI. An external landmark for the anterior commissure. *Laryngoscope*. 1999;109:1134–1136.
7. Storck C, Gehrer R, Fischer C, et al. The role of the cricothyroid joint anatomy in cricothyroid approximation surgery. *J Voice*. 2011;25(5):632–637.
8. Randestad Å, Lindholm CE, Fabian P. Dimensions of the cricoid cartilage and the trachea. *Laryngoscope*. 2000;110:1957–1961.
9. Jotz GP, Stefani MA, Pereira da Costa Filho O, Malysz T, Soster PR, Leão HZ. A morphometric study of the larynx. *J Voice*. 2014;28(6):668–672.
10. Goyal N, Yoo F, Setabutr D, Goldenberg D. Surgical anatomy of the supraglottic larynx using the da Vinci robot. *Head Neck*. 2014;36(8):1126–1131.
11. Thompson AC, Griffin NR. Langerhan cells in normal and pathological vocal cord mucosa. *Acta Otolaryngol* (Stockh). 1995;115:830–832.
12. Sataloff RT. The human voice. *Sci Am*. 1992;267:108–115.
13. Hirano M. *Clinical Examination of Voice*. New York, NY: Springer-Verlag; 1981.
14. Gray S, Hirano M, Sato K. Molecular and cellular structure of vocal fold tissue. In: Titze IR, ed. *Vocal Fold Physiology*. San Diego, CA: Singular Publishing Group; 1993:4.
15. Hirano M. Structure and vibratory pattern of the vocal folds. In: Sawashima M, Cooper FS, eds. *Dynamic Aspects of the Speech Production*. Tokyo, Japan: University of Tokyo Press; 1977:13–27.
16. Gray SD, Pignatari SS, Harding P. Morphologic ultrastructure of anchoring fibers in normal vocal fold basement zone. *J Voice*. 1994;8:48–52.
17. Hammond TH, Zhou R, Hammond EH, Pawlak A, Gray SD. The intermediate layer: a morphologic study of the elastin and hyaluronic acid constituents of normal vocal folds. *J Voice*. 1997;11:59–66.
18. Hammond TH, Gray SD, Butler J, Zhou R, Hamond E. Age and gender-related elastin distribution changes in human vocal folds. *Otolaryngol Head Neck Surg*. 1998;119:314–322.
19. Catten M, Gray SD, Hammond TH, Zhou R, Hammond E. Analysis of cellular location and concentration in vocal fold lamina propria. *Otolaryngol Head Neck Surg*. 1998;118:663–667.
20. Gray SD, Hammond E, Hanson DF. Benign pathologic responses of the larynx. *Ann Otol Rhinol Laryngol*. 1995;104:13–18.
21. Madruga de Melo EC, Lemos M, Aragão Ximenes Filho J, Sennes LU, Nascimento Saldiva PH, Tsuji DH. Distribution of collagen in the lamina propria of the human vocal fold. *Laryngoscope*. 2003;113(12):2187–2191.
22. Prades JM, Dumollard JM, Duband S, et al. Lamina propria of the human vocal fold: histomorphometric study of collagen fibers. *Surg Radiol Anat*. 2010;32(4):377–382.
23. Hirano M, Kurita S, Nakashima T. Growth, development of aging of human vocal folds. In: Bless DM, Abbs JH, eds. *Vocal Fold Physiology*. San Diego, CA: College Hill Press; 1983:22–43.
24. Hirano M, Nakashima T. Vascular network of the vocal fold. In: Stevens KN, Hirano M, eds. *Vocal Fold Physiology*. Tokyo, Japan: University of Tokyo Press; 1981:45–59.
25. Sato K. Functional fine structures of human vocal fold mucosa. In: Rubin JS, Sataloff RT, Korovin G, eds. *Diagnosis and Treatment of Voice Disorders*. 2nd ed. Albany, NY: Singular Thomson Learning; 2003:41–48.

26. Kurita S, Nagata K, Hirano M. Comparative histology of mammalian vocal folds. In: Kirchner JA, ed. *Vocal Fold Histopathology: A Symposium*. San Diego, CA: College Hill Press; 1986:1–10.

27. Stiblar-Martincic D. Histology of laryngeal mucosa. *Acta Otolaryngol Suppl* (Stockh).1997;527:138–141.

28. Friedrich G, Kainz J, Freidl W. Zur funktionellen Struktur der menschlichen Stimmlippe. *Laryngorhinootologie*. 1993;72(5):215–224.

29. Tucker JA, Tucker ST. Posterior commissure of the human larynx revisited. *J Voice*. 2010;24(3):252–259.

30. Hirano M, Kurita S, Kiyokawa K, Kiminori S. Posterior glottis. Morphological study in excised human larynges. *Ann Otol Rhinol Laryngol*. 1986;95:576–581.

31. Hirano M. Surgical anatomy and physiology of the vocal folds. In: Gould WJ, Sataloff RT, Spiegel JR, eds. *Voice Surgery*. St. Louis, MO: Mosby; 1993:135–258.

32. Sato K, Hirano M, Nakashima T. Stellate cells in the human vocal fold. *Ann Otol Rhinol Laryngol*. 2001;110: 319–325.

33. Sato K, Hirano M, Nakashima T. Vitamin A—storing stellate cells in the human vocal fold. *Acta Otolaryngol*. 2003;123:106–110.

34. Sato K, Hirano M, Nakashima T. 3D structure of the macula flava in the human vocal fold. *Acta Otolaryngol*. 2003;123:269–273.

35. Sato K, Hirano M, Nakashima T. Age-related changes of collagenous fibers in the human vocal fold mucosa. *Ann Otol Rhinol Laryngol*. 2003;111:15–20.

36. Sato K, Hirano M. Age-related changes of elastic fibers in the superficial layer of the lamina propria of the vocal folds. *Ann Otol Rhinol Laryngol*. 1997;106: 44–48.

37. Hirano M, Kurita S, Sakaguchi S. Ageing of the vibratory tissue of the human vocal folds. *Acta Otolaryngol* (Stockh). 1989;107:428–433.

38. Sato K, Sakaguchi S, Kurita S, Hirano M. A morphological study of aged larynges. *Larynx Jpn*. 1992;4:84–94.

39. Sato K, Shirouzu H, Nakashima T. Irradiated macula flava in the human vocal fold mucosa. *Am J Otolaryngol*. 2008;29(5):312–318.

40. Fuja TJ, Probst-Fuja MN, Titze IR. Transdifferentiation of vocal-fold stellate cells and all-trans retinol-induced deactivation. *Cell Tissue Res*. 2005;322(3):417–424.

41. Hirano M, Yoshida T, Kurita S, et al. Anatomy and behavior of the vocal process. In: Baer T, Sasaki C, Harris K, eds. *Laryngeal Function in Phonation and Respiration*. Boston, MA: College-Hill Press; 1987:1–13.

42. Gray S. Basement membrane zone injury in vocal nodules. In: Gauffin J, Hammarberg B, eds. *Vocal Fold Physiology: Acoustic, Perceptual and Physiologic Aspects of Voice Mechanics*. San Diego, CA: Singular Publishing Group; 1991:21–27.

43. Sundberg J. The acoustics of the singing voice. *Sci Am*. 1977;236(3):82–91.

44. Franz P, Aharinejad S. The microvascular of the larynx: a scanning electron microscopy study. *Scanning Microsc*. 1994;5:257–263.

45. Nakai Y, Masutani H, Moriguchi M, Matsunaga K, Sugita M. Microvascular structure of the larynx. *Acta Otolaryngol Suppl* (Stockh). 1991;486:254–263.

46. Hochman I, Sataloff RT, Hillman RE, Zeitels SM. Ectasias and varices of the vocal fold: clearing the striking zone. *Ann Otol Rhinol Laryngol*. 1999;108:10–16.

47. De Biase NG, Pontes PA. Blood vessels of vocal folds: a videolaryngoscopic study. *Arch Otolaryngol Head Neck Surg*. 2008;134(7):720–724.

48. Frenzel H, Kleinsasser O. Ultrastructural study on the small blood vessels of human vocal cords. *Arch Otorhinolaryngol*. 1982;236:147–160.

49. Sanders I. Microanatomy of the vocal fold musculature. In: Rubin JS, Sataloff RT, Korovin GS, eds. *Diagnosis and Treatment of Voice Disorders*. 2nd ed. Albany, NY: Delmar Thomson Learning; 2003:49–68.

50. de Campos D, do Nascimento PS, Ellwanger JH, et al. Histological organization is similar in human vocal muscle and tongue—a study of muscles and nerves. *J Voice*. 2012;26(6):811,e19–26.

51. Brandon CA, Rosen C, Georgelis G, Horton MJ, Mooney MP, Sciote JJ. Staining of human thyroarytenoid muscle with myosin antibodies reveals some unique extrafusal fibers, but no muscle spindles. *J Voice*. 2003;17(2):245–254.

52. Asanau A, Timoshenko AP, Prades JM, Galusca B, Martin C, Féasson L. Posterior cricoarytenoid bellies: relationship between their function and histology. *J Voice*. 2011;25(2):e67–73.

53. Brooke MH, Engle WK. The histographic analysis of human muscle biopsies with regard to fibre types. 1. Adult male and female. *Neurology*. 1969;19:221–233.

54. Sadeh M, Kronenberg J, Gaton E. Histochemistry of human laryngeal muscles. *Cell Mol Biol*. 1981;27:643–648.

55. Lindestad P. *Electromyographic and Laryngoscopic Studies of Normal and Disturbed Vocal Function*, Stockholm, Sweden: Suddinge University;1994:1–12,

56. English DT, Blevins CE. Motor units of laryngeal muscles. *Arch Otolaryngol*. 1969;89:778–784.

57. Faaborg-Andersen K. Electromyographic investigation of intrinsic laryngeal muscles in humans. *Acta Physiol Scand Suppl*. 1957;41(suppl 140):1–149.

58. Rossi G, Cortesina G. Morphological study of the laryngeal muscles in man: insertions and courses of the muscle fibers, motor end-plates and proprioceptors. *Acta Otolaryngol* (Stockh). 1965;59:575–592.

59. Wu YZ, Crumley RL, Armstrong WB, Caiozzzo VJ. New perspectives about human laryngeal muscle: single fiber analyses and interspecies comparisons. *Arch Otolaryngol Head Neck Surg*. 2000;126:857–864.

60. Malmgren LT, Lovice DB, Kaufman MR. Age-related changes in muscle fiber regeneration in the human thyroarytenoid muscle. *Arch Otolaryngol Head Neck Surg*. 2000;126:851–856.

61. Sataloff RT. Vocal aging. *Curr Opin Otolaryngol Head Neck Surg*. 1998;6:421–428.

62. Davis PJ, Nail BS. On the location and size of laryngeal motoneurons in the cat and rabbit. *J Comp Neurol*. 1984;230:13–22.

63. Yoshida Y, Miyazaki O, Hirano M, et al. Arrangement of motoneurons innervating the intrinsic laryngeal muscles of cats as demonstrated by horseradish peroxidase. *Acta Otolaryngol.* 1982;94:329–334.

64. Yoshida Y, Miyazaki T, Hirano M, Kanaseki T. Localization of the laryngeal motoneurons in the brain stem and myotopical representation of the motoneurons in the nucleus ambiguus of cats—an HRP study. In: Titze I, Scherer R, eds. *Vocal Fold Physiology: Biomechanics, Acoustics and Phonatory Control.* Denver, CO: Denver Center for the Performing Arts; 1983:75–90.

65. Zhang SP, Bandler R, Davis P. Integration of vocalization: the medullary nucleus retroambigualis. *J Neurophysiol.* 1995;74:2500–2512.

66. Bandler R. Induction of "rage" following microinjections of glutamate into midbrain but not hypothalamus of cats. *Neurosci Lett.* 1982;30:183–188.

67. Kelly AH, Beaton LE, Magoun HW. A midbrain mechanism for facio-vocal activity. *J Neurophysiol.* 1946;9: 181–189.

68. Adametz J, O'Leary JL. Experimental mutism resulting from periaqueductal lesions in cats. *Neurology.* 1959; 9;636–642.

69. Skultety FM. Experimental mutism in dogs. *Arch Neurol.* 1962;6:235–241.

70. Esposito A, Demeurisse G, Alberti B, Fabbro F. Complete mutism after midbrain periaqueductal gray lesion. *Neuroreport.* 1999;10:681–685.

71. Bandler R, Shipley MT. Columnar organization in the midbrain periaqueductal gray: modules for emotional expression? *Trends Neurosci.* 1994;17:379–389.

72. Zhang SP, Davis PJ, Bandler R, Carrive P. Brain stem integration of vocalization: role of the midbrain periaqueductal gray. *J Neurophysiol.* 1994;72:1337–1356.

73. Bandler R, Carrive P. Integrated defence reaction elicited by excitatory amino acid microinjection in the midbrain periaqueductal grey region of the unrestrained cat. *Brain Res.* 1988;439:95–106.

74. Bandler R, Depaulis A. Midbrain periaqueductal gray control of defensive behavior in the cat and the rat. In: Depaulis A, Bandler R, eds. *The Midbrain Periaqueductal Gray Matter: Functional, Anatomical and Immunohistochemical Organization.* New York, NY: Plenum Press; 1991:175–198.

75. Bandler R, Keay K, Vaughan C, Shipley MT. Columnar organization of PAG neurons regulating emotional and vocal expression. In: Fletcher N, Davis P, eds. *Vocal Fold Physiology: Controlling Complexity and Chaos.* San Diego, CA: Singular Publishing Group; 1996:137–153.

76. Shipley MT, Ennis M, Rizvi TA, Behbehani MM. Topographical specificity of forebrain inputs to the midbrain periaqueductal gray: evidence for discrete longitudinally organized input columns. In: Depaulis A, Bandler R, eds. *The Midbrain Periaqueductal Gray Matter: Functional, Anatomical and Immunohistochemical Organization.* New York, NY: Plenum Press; 1991: 417–448.

77. Davis P, Zhang SP. What is the role of the midbrain periaqueductal gray in respiration and vocalization? In: Depaulis A, Bandler R, eds. *The Midbrain Periaqueductal Gray Matter: Functional, Anatomical and Immunohistochemical Organization.* New York, NY: Plenum Press; 1991:57–66.

78. Davis P, Zhang SP, Winkworth A, Bandler R. The neural control of vocalization: respiratory and emotional influences. *J Voice.* 1996;10:23–38.

79. Davis PJ, Zhang SP, Bandler R. Midbrain and medullary control of respiration and vocalization. *Prog Brain Res.* 1996;107:315–325.

80. Davis PJ, Zhang SP, Bandler R. Pulmonary and upper airway afferent influences on the motor pattern of vocalization evoked by excitation of the midbrain periaqueductal gray of the cat. *Brain Res.* 1993;607: 61–80.

81. Ambalavanar R, Tanaka Y, Damirjian M, Ludlow CL. Laryngeal afferent stimulation enhances Fos immunoreactivity in periaqueductal gray in the cat. *J Comp Neurol.* 1999;409(3):411–423.

82. Nonaka S, Takahashi R, Enomoto K, Katada A, Unno T. Lombard reflex during PAG-induced vocalization in decerebrate cats. *Neurosci Res.* 1997;29:283–289.

83. Penfield W, Roberts L. *Speech and Brain Mechanisms.* Princeton, NJ: Princeton University Press; 1959.

84. Perry DW, Zatorre RJ, Petrides M, Alivisatos B, Meyer E, Evans AC. Localization of cerebral activity during simple singing. *Neuroreport.* 1999;10:3979–3984.

85. Perrodin C, Kayser C, Logothetis NK, Petkov CI. Voice cells in the primate temporal lobe. *Current Biology: CB.* 2011;21(16):1408–1415.

86. Simonyan K, Horwitz B. Laryngeal motor cortex and control of speech in humans. *Neuroscientist.* 2011;17(2): 197–208.

87. Kleber B, Veit R, Birbaumer N, Gruzelier J, Lotze M. The brain of opera singers: experience-dependent changes in functional activation. *Cereb Cortex.* 2010; 20(5):1144–1152.

88. Chuang FJ, Chen JY, Shyu JF, et al. Surgical anatomy of the external branch of the superior laryngeal nerve in Chinese adults and its clinical applications. *Head Neck.* 2010;32(1):53–57.

89. Cernea CR, Ferraz AR, Nishio S, et al. Surgical anatomy of the external branch of the superior laryngeal nerve. *Head Neck.* 1992;14:380–383.

90. Aina EN, Hisham AN. External laryngeal nerve in thyroid surgery: recognition and surgical implications. *ANZ J Surg.* 2001;71:212–214.

91. Hurtado-Lopez LM, Zaldivar-Ramirez FR. Risk of injury to the external branch of the superior laryngeal nerve in thyroidectomy. *Laryngoscope.* 2002;112: 626–629.

92. Friedman M, Losalvio P, Ibrahim H, et al. Superior laryngeal nerve identification and preservation in thyroidectomy. *Arch Otolaryngol Head Neck Surg.* 2002; 128:296–303.

93. Kierner A, Ainger M, Burian M. The external branch of the superior laryngeal nerve: its topographical anatomy as related to surgery of the neck. *Arch Otolaryngol Head Neck Surg.* 1998;124:301–303.

94. Furlan JC, Cordeiro AC, Brandao LG. Study of some "intrinsic risk factors" that can enhance an iatrogenic injury of the external branch of the superior laryngeal nerve. *Otolaryngol Head Neck Surg*. 2003;128:396–400.

95. Bellantone R, Boscherini M, Lombardi CP, et al. Is the identification of the external branch of the superior laryngeal nerve mandatory in thyroid operation? Results of a prospective randomized study. *Surgery*. 2001;130:1055–1059.

96. Wu BL, Sanders I, Mu L, Biller HF. The human communicating nerve: an extension of the external superior laryngeal nerve that innervates the vocal cord. *Arch Otolaryngol*. 1994;120(12):1321–1328.

97. Sanders I, Mu L. Anatomy of human internal superior laryngeal nerve. *Anat Rec*. 1998;252:646–656.

98. Yoshida Y, Tanaka Y, Mitsumasu T, Hirano M, Kanaseki T. Peripheral course and intramucosal distribution of the laryngeal sensory nerve fibers of cats. *Brain Res Bull*. 1986;17(1):95–105.

99. Yoshida Y, Tanaka Y, Hirano M, Nakashima T. Sensory innervation of the pharynx and larynx. *Am J Med*. 2000; 108(suppl 4a):51S–61S.

100. Harrison D. Fibre size frequency in the recurrent laryngeal nerves of men and giraffe. *Acta Otolaryngol*. 1981;91:383–389.

101. Malmgren L, Gacek R. Peripheral motor innervation of the larynx. In: Blitzer A, Brin MF, Sasaki CT, Fahn S, Harris KS, eds. *Neurologic Disorders of the Larynx*. New York, NY: Thieme Medical Publishers; 1992:36–44.

102. Jotz GR, de Campos D, Rodrigues MF, Xavier LL. Histological asymmetry of the human recurrent laryngeal nerve. *J Voice*. 2011;25(1):8–14.

103. Scheid SC, Nadeau DP, Friedman O, Sataloff RT. Anatomy of the thyroarytenoid branch of the recurrent laryngeal nerve. *J Voice*. 2004;8(3):279–284.

104. Eller RL, Miller M, Weinstein J, Sataloff RT. The innervations of the posterior cricoarytenoid muscle: exploring clinical possibilities. *J Voice*. 2009;23(2):229–234.

105. Sato K, Hirano M. Fine three-dimensional structure of pericytes in the vocal fold mucosa. *Ann Otol Rhinol Laryngol*. 1997;106:490–494.

106. Heman-Ackah YD, Goding GS Jr. Laryngeal chemoreflex severity and end-apnea $PaO_2$, and $PaCO_2$. *Otolaryngol Head Neck Surg*. 2000;123(3):157–163.

107. Heman-Ackah YD, Goding GS Jr. The effects of intralaryngeal carbon dioxide and acetazolamide on the laryngeal chemoreflex. *Ann Otol Rhinol Laryngol*. 2000; 109(10):921–928.

108. Heman-Ackah YD, Rimell F. Current progress in understanding sudden infant death syndrome. *Curr Opin Otolaryngol Head Neck Surg*. 1999;7(6):320–327.

109. Abo-el-Enein M. Laryngeal myotactic reflexes. *Nature*. 1966;209:682–685.

110. Tomori Z, Widdicomb J. Muscular bronchomotor and cardiovascular reflexes elicited by mechanical stimulation of the respiratory tract. *J Physiol*. 1969;200:25–49.

111. Gould WJ, Okamura H. Static lung volumes in singers. *Ann Otol Rhinol Laryngol*. 1973;82:89–95.

112. Hixon TJ, Hoffman C. Chest wall shape during singing. In: Lawrence V, ed. *Transcripts of the Seventh Annual Symposium, Care of the Professional Voice*. New York, NY: The Voice Foundation; 1978;9–10.

113. Sundberg J, Leanderson R, von Euler C. Activity relationship between diaphragm and cricothyroid muscles. *J Voice*. 1989;3(3):225–232.

114. Hunter EJ, Titze IR. Individual subject laryngeal dimensions of multiple mammalian species for biomedical models. *Ann Otol Rhinol Laryngol*. 2005;114(10): 809–818.

115. Scott TM. How we teach anatomy efficiently and effectively. *Med Teach*. 1993;15:67–75.

116. McLachlan JC, Bligh J, Bradley P, et al. Teaching anatomy without cadavers. *Med Educ*. 2004;38:418–424.

117. Parker LM. What's wrong with the dead body? Use of the human cadaver in medical education. *Med J Aust*. 2002;176(2):74–76.

118. Prince KJAH, Mameren H van, Hylkema N, et al. Does problem-based learning lead to deficiencies in basic science knowledge? An empirical case on anatomy. *Med Educ*. 2003;37:15–21.

119. American Association of Medical Colleges Institute for Improving Medical Education. *Effective Use of Educational Technology in Medical Education*. Washington, DC: Association of American Medical Colleges; 2007:3.

120. Hu A, Wilson T, Ladak H, et al. Three-dimensional educational computer model of the larynx: voicing a new direction. *Arch Otolaryngol Head Neck Surg*. 2009; 135(7):677–682.

121. Hu A, Wilson T, Ladak H, Haase P, Doyle P, Fung K. Evaluation of a three-dimensional educational computer model of the larynx: voicing a new direction. *J Otolaryngol Head Neck Surg*. 2010;39(3):315–322.

122. Fritz D, Hu A, Wilson T, Ladak H, Haase P, Fung K. Long-term retention of a three dimensional educational computer model of the larynx. *Arch Otolaryngol Head Neck Surg*. 2011;137(6):598–603.

123. Tan S, Hu A, Wilson T, Ladak H, Haase P, Fung K. Role of computer generated 3D-visualization in laryngeal anatomy teaching for advanced learners. *J Laryngol Otol*. 2012;126(4):395–401.

# Genetics of the Voice

*Robert Thayer Sataloff and Mary J. Hawkshaw*

The genetics of voice is a fascinating subject for speculation. Unfortunately, it has been a challenging area of research, and exciting progress has been made only in the last several years. When this chapter was written for the second edition of this book, a computer search of 8 009 307 references in four databases (MEDLINE, Health, AIDS Line, and Cancer Lit) was carried out using the key words: hereditary, genetics, voice, voice disorders, and familial. The computer search produced only 5 references,[1–5] only 3 of which really discussed hereditary voice disorders.[2,3,5]

Other conditions discussed in earlier versions of this chapter were identified through the author's clinical experience, various articles, and a valuable text.[6] Fortunately, for the fourth edition, review of the content and references contained in numerous medical and speech-language pathology textbooks, reference texts on human genetics, and numerous publications that have appeared during the last 2 decades has shown substantial progress in our mastery of traditional medical genetics of voice disorders. In addition, remarkable achievements have begun in voice-related molecular genetics and genomics.

## Normal Voice

Genetic factors do influence vocal quality. This has been recognized anecdotally in families and even nationalities (Italians, Welsh, Russians, and others). If one assumes that function is related to structure, the association of voice quality and genetic factors is intuitively comfortable. It is generally accepted that physical characteristics are genetically determined. If these include the size of the laryngeal cartilages, vocal fold length and structure, size and shape of the supraglottic vocal tract, and phenotypic similarities elsewhere in the vocal mechanism, then one might expect similarities in voice quality. If we postulate additional similarities in brain development, musical perception, and neuromotor control, the notion becomes even more attractive. However, in order to be credible, these issues require further study, and careful separation of genetic factors from environmental influences on development.

Some of the most interesting studies to date have looked at voice function in twins. In general, monozygotic twins have similar voices. Dizygotic twins appear to show the same differences that would be expected among any children of the same age.[7] Coon and Carey[8] studied genetic and environmental determinants of musical ability in twins. Because there is more to vocal quality and ability than vocal fold structure alone, such studies are relevant when studying the genetics of voice. Coon and Carey examined monozygotic and dizygotic twins and found evidence of hereditable variation, although environment appeared to be a more important factor than heredity. Kalmus and Fry[9] studied dysmelodia (inability to sing on tune) and found it to be hereditable as an autosomal dominant trait with imperfect penetrance. They speculated that their findings seemed to indicate the existence of some deep structure of tonality perception, comparable with Chomsky's deep language structure.

Although Bernstein and Schlaper[10] began looking at the genetic influences on the voice as early as 1922, and Schilling,[11,12] Seeman,[13] Gedda, Bianchi, and Bianchi-Neroni,[14] and others carried out subsequent work, the complexities of genetic research in humans have left most of the relevant questions unanswered.

## Pathological Voice and Syndromes

In addition to the voice quality characteristics that appear to be genetically transmitted in healthy individuals, many pathological conditions are associated with specific genetic voice dysfunctions.[15] For example, raspy voice quality has been recognized in hyalinosis cutis et mucosae,[16–18] Opitz BBB/G compound syndrome,[19–22] pachyonychia congenita syndrome,[23–25] Werner's syndrome,[26,27] William's syndrome,[28–31] and other conditions. High-pitched voice occurs in Bloom syndrome,[32–35] chondrodystrophic myotonia,[36–39] deletion (5p) syndrome,[40] Dubowitz syndrome,[41,42] and Seckel syndrome.[43] Low-pitched voice has been observed in cutis laxa syndrome,[44–46] de Lange syndrome,[47–49] deletion (18q) syndrome,[50–53] mucopolysaccharidoses (types I-H, II, III, VI), and Weaver syndrome.[54,55] Other voice abnormalities have been observed in myotonic dystrophy syndrome,[15,56] and in hereditary dystonias that may be associated with spasmodic dysphonia. A dominant form of spinal muscular atrophy associated with distal muscle atrophy, vocal fold paralysis, and sensorineural hearing loss has been reported. Familial vocal fold dysfunction associated with digital anomalies also exists. Verma et al described familial male pseudohermaphroditism with female external genitalia, male habitus, and male voice.[2] Urbanova reported familial dysphonia,[3] and Friol-Vercelletto et al reported familial oculopharyngeal muscular dystrophia with associated abnormal voice.[5] A variety of other genetic conditions have been associated with voice abnormalities, including Cri du Chat syndrome,[57,58] Plott syndrome,[59] Ehlers-Danlos syndrome,[60] Huntington's chorea,[61,62] von Recklinghausen's neurofibromatosis[63] (hoarseness and dysphagia), Hunter's and Hurler's syndromes (hoarseness due to laryngeal deposition of mucopolysaccharide metabolites),[64] a variety of craniofacial anomalies (Down's syndrome, Crouzon disease, and others), and various short stature syndromes.[65] Hence, evidence for the existence of a genetic component to vocal quality is compelling, and fascinating new studies reflect exciting growth in this important field. Richmon et al[66] reported 2 cases of patients presenting to an otolaryngologic clinic for evaluation of dysphonia. Both patients were found to have tongue hypermobility; both patients were diagnosed subsequently with Ehlers-Danlos syndrome, a group of related hereditary connective tissue diseases.

Spring et al[67] evaluated 2 families known to have autosomal dominant hereditary sensory neuropathy (HSN-1), a genetically heterogeneous group of disorders associated with chronic cough and gastroesophageal reflux disease (GERD). Many patients with chronic cough develop dysphonia from vocal fold trauma. Thirty-eight individuals provided clinical information and blood for genetic analysis. Linkage to chromosome 3p22-p24 was found in both families. However, there was no linkage to loci for HSN-1 (known). The authors described this family as a novel variant of HSN-1 with distinctive coughs associated with involvement of the upper aerodigestive tract.

Sharma and Franco[68] reported that several genetic mutations have been identified as associated with different forms of dystonia and may result in spasmodic dysphonia. They pointed out that the pathogenesis of spasmodic dysphonia is not well understood. However, the research of dystonia genetics is ongoing.

Sidtis et al[69] examined the speech characteristics associated with 3 genotypes of spinocerebellar ataxia (SCA). They obtained voice samples from 26 individuals known to have SCA. The 3 genotypes included were SCA-1, SCA-5, and SCA-6. Speech tasks included diadochokinesis, word repetition, picture description, and sentence reading. The authors found the SCA-6 genotype to be the most prevalent with articulation being the most impaired. They suggested that voice characteristics might be significant in the differentiation of ataxic subtypes; however, a greater understanding of genetic disorders that affect speech and voice is still needed.

Solot et al[70] reported that communication disorders are some of the common features of the 22q11.2 microdeletion syndrome. They pointed out that children with the 22q11.2 microdeletion syndrome have multiple medical and developmental issues. The communication disorders include articulation, resonance and voice abnormalities, and language problems. In addition to communication, feeding disorders are often a presenting feature of this syndrome.

Chang and Yung[71] reported a case of a 40-year-old male with hereditary hemorrhagic telangiectasia (HHT) who presented with a 2-year history of hoarseness. They noted that this patient was on anticoagulation therapy. Laryngeal examination revealed vocal fold telangiectasia, vocal fold scar, evidence of previous vocal fold hemorrhage, and dysphonia plica ventricularis. Dysphonia and vocal fold telangiectasia are common in HHT, with this population being at high risk for vocal fold hemorrhage.

In a 2011 report,[72] Martins et al found evidence of autosomal dominant hereditary transmission of sulcus vocalis. They reported the finding of sulcus vocalis in 4 dysphonic patients from 3 generations of the same family with vertical transmission, affecting both males and females. The authors reported that the findings were consistent with an autosomal dominant inheritance pattern.

Moore et al[73] reported that untreated growth hormone deficiency (GHD) is due to genetic GHRH receptor deficiency in adult males, causing high pitch and raspy voice. Their sample size was small (4), and it included untreated adult males. However, they suggested that growth hormones' effect on vocal fold compliance and size results in a high-pitched voice. Additionally, they pointed out that the time of GHD onset (congenital or acquired) is a determining factor in the voice abnormalities seen.

In 2006, Shriberg et al[74] reported their evaluation of a mother and daughter known to have 7;13 translocation causing disruption of the transcription gene *FOXP2*, and both mother and daughter had acquired apraxia of speech and spastic dysarthria, although dysphonia was not a key feature.

Several other studies have reported a correlation between genetic and environment effects on symptoms of dysphonia.[75,76]

In 2011, Wilcox et al[77] described an Australian family with whispering dysphonia that had been assigned the designation of DYT4, a familiar form of dysphonia. They stated that a comprehensive analysis of the causes of the dysphonia was not carried out, nor was the finding of Wilson disease (WND) in 2 siblings in this family explored fully. They obtained DNA samples from 18 family members. Linkage analysis was performed with microsatellite markers, and 6 genes were sequenced: *THAP1* (DYT6), *PRKRA* (DYT16), and *ATP7B* (WND). Results identified 9 living affected members in this family. Neurological evaluation revealed isolated spasmodic dysphonia to severe, generalized dystonia. All loci tested were excluded from genetic analysis. Haplotype analysis of *ATP7B* (WND) region, revealed 2 parental alleles in 8 siblings of the 2 WND patients (deceased). Two mutated alleles were identified in the WND patients only. The authors identified a missense (c.2297C>G; p.T766R) on these 2 alleles. Five DYT4 family members had neither mutation. The authors concluded that *ATP7B* did not segregate the dystonia, but suggested 2 separate genetic diseases in this family.

In 2013, Lohmann et al[78] performed genome-wide linkage analysis in 14 members of the Australian family previously studied in 2011. Findings showed a mutation in *TUBB4* (tubulin beta-4; Arg2Gly) caused the DYT4 dysphonia, suggesting that other mutations in *TUBB4* might contribute to the development of spasmodic dysphonia, and that abnormal microtubule function has a role in the pathophysiology of dysphonia.

Tanner et al[79] reported a case of two 79-year-old monozygotic male twins with vocal fold bowing and severe dysphonia. DNA samplings by cheek swabs were obtained, confirming monozygosity for DNA polymorphisms with 10 of 10 concordance for *STR* DNA markers. Both patients underwent surgical intervention to improve glottic closure, as well as voice therapy. Vocal fold bowing was more pronounced in Twin 1, and Twin 2 obtained greater improvement following treatment. The authors suggested response to voice therapy might have affected outcomes.

An interesting study by Worthey et al[80] examined the use of whole-exome sequencing (WES) in the assessment of heterogeneous genetic origins in children with childhood apraxia of speech (CAS). Children with CAS, a rare, severe disorder, have deficits of motor speech, cognition, affect, language, and other functions. CAS has been studied widely and found to be a disorder segregating with a mutation in *FOXP2*. WES findings in a group of 10 unrelated subjects with CAS ranging in age from 13 to 19 years were reported. WES was performed using the Illumina Genome Analyzer IIx Sequencing System. They found reportable variants on 5 chromosomes (Chr3, Chr6, Chr7, Chr9, and Chr17), including 6 genes strongly associated with CAS (FOXP1 and CNTNAP2). Of this study population of 10, 80% were found to have variants in 1 or 2 of the 6 genes studied. The most prevalent variants were in ATP13A4, KIAA0319, and CNTNAP2. Their research shows support for heterogeneous genetic origins of the complex disorder of childhood apraxia of speech. They suggested that whole-exome sequencing for gene identification is useful in the diagnostic evaluation of children with disorders of motor speech. Although these children have speech problems primarily, the effort involved in speaking can lead to secondary dysphonia.

Pal et al[81] reported genome-wide linkage of centrotemporal sharp wave (CTS) on EEGs in families with Rolandic epilepsy (RE) to chromosome 11p13. They fine-mapped this locus to variants in the *ELP4* gene. Speech sound disorder (SSD) and verbal and oral motor apraxia are mutations commonly seen with Rolandic epilepsy; however, the etiology and neuromechanisms are unknown. The authors performed genome-wide linkage analysis for SSD in 38 families having a proband with RE, and acoustic analysis of recordings to assess dyspraxia as the potential mechanism for SSD. They found abnormalities in voice onset time, which they suggest proved evidence of spatial/temporal properties of articulation consistent with a dyspraxic mechanism. Furthermore, they suggested a pleiotropic role of the 11p13 locus in development of CTS and SSD, and a dyspraxic mechanism for SSD linked to 11p13.

Parkinson's disease is associated with voice and swallowing problems that often manifest in the early stages of the disease and can be challenging to treat medically.[82] The pathology of Parkinson's disease is the accumulation of presynaptic protein a-synuclein (aSyn) and the degeneration of substantia nigra dopaminergic neurons. Grant et al point out that it remains unclear how this process affects voice and swallowing functions. In a rat model, the authors examined the effect of loss of function of the phosphatase and tensin homolog-induced putative kinase 1 gene (PINK1[-/-]), considered as a model of autosomal receptive Parkinson's disease. Behavioral measurements were made at ages 2, 4, 6, and 8 months. Vocalization and oromotor deficits; reduced TH-ir in the locus that correlates with vocal loudness and tongue force; and aSYN neuropathology in brain areas critical for sensorimotor control were reported. They proposed that utilizing a PINK1[-/-] genetic model of Parkinson's disease will aid in defining biomarkers of behaviors and aid in therapeutic management of patients with Parkinson's disease.

Floating Harbor syndrome (FHS) includes expressive language delay and high-pitched voice in addition to short stature, triangular face, prominent nose, and deep-set eyes. High gliadin antibodies suggestive of celiac disease were found in 3 of 15 reported cases of Floating Harbor syndrome.[83]

Williams syndrome (WS) and supravalvular aortic stenosis (SVAS) patients have significant abnormalities of voice quality.[84] Research has shown that these individuals have a lack of 1 normal ELN (human elastin gene) allele, suggesting that heterozygous ELN abnormalities might have a negative effect on vocal fold biomechanics. Moreover, research suggests that ELN requires 2 functioning alleles for normal, structural development of the lamina propria.

An excellent review of the literature on genetic disorders affecting voice was prepared by Mette Pedersen for the *European Manual of Phoniatrics*.[85] She pointed out that the human genome sequence has been completed, and suggested that genetics offers great promise in the management of patients, and for developing a better understanding of the variability of individual's response to medical and surgical treatments. She also indicated that gene transcript profiling, modern sequencing platforms, microarrays, among others, will be instrumental in developing individualized treatment in the rehabilitation of voice. She acknowledged, however, that phenotypes can be difficult to differentiate based on polymorphism and heterogeneity. Her research focused on genetics and personalized medicine, which she defined as "a medical model emphasizing in general the customization of health, with all practices being tailored to individual patients." Applications of genetics and tissue engineering are new tools being used in voice

research in addition to microarray analysis and gene expression profiling (fundamental to biochip development), and are used commonly in some voice laboratories. Pedersen provided a comprehensive review of the relationship between genetics and neurological speech/voice disorders, and the related language and genetic speech deficits, including articulation disorders, verbal dyspraxia, aphasia, stuttering, and dyslexia, reporting that many disorders are seen in members of the same families. She cited that mutation in genes GNPTAB, NAGPA, and GNPTG associated with lysosomal targeting pathways have been reported to cause stuttering. Other studies have demonstrated that genetic variations of the transcription factor FOXP2 are instrumental in the development of speech. Candidate genes regulated by this transcription factor have been identified: CMIP and ATP2C2 with language disorders, and ROBO1, DCDC2, and KIAAO319 with dyslexia. Pedersen pointed out also that tissue engineering science has advanced our understanding of laryngeal fibroblasts. She discussed hyalinosis of skin and mucosa, which is a rare autosomal receptive disorder that causes deposition of hyalin material in the basement membranes of skin and mucous membranes. Hoarseness is a common and often incurable symptom of this disorder. The underlying defect is thought to be mutations within the extracellular matrix protein ECMI.

Much research in voice has focused on restoring normal voice, with attention on fibroblast function and elastin genetics, which are crucial to the vocal folds' microstructures critical to vibration. Pedersen stated that "vibration is a crucial positive factor in restoring ECM structure. It may provide basis for reducing vocal scarring and improvement of voice quality." The genetic influences on ability to heal or tendency to scar remain largely unknown.

Pedersen outlined several other genetic disorders that impact vocal fold function in voice, emphasizing what we know and what we do not know, yet. A few are discussed here, but interested readers are encouraged to review her article in totality, which also contains an extensive list of references on this very important topic.

Other research methods include analysis of lymphocytes and leukocytes in humans, DNA concordance analysis, stem cell research, genetic microarray analysis, and proteomic investigation. Basic genetics and proteomics are discussed in greater detail in another chapter.

Pedersen pointed out that advances have been made in genetic studies of vocal fold carcinoma. RNA segment studies have been utilized, and epidermal growth factor studies have shown efficacy of therapeutic treatments. Gene therapies for cancers include colon phytoreduction to induce death of cells, corrective therapy to repair genetic defects related to the malignancy, and immune modulation to aid in the body's immune response to the cancer.

She also cited the meta-analysis report of Van,[86] which identified voice and resonance disorders in 299 different genetic syndromes. Pederson highlighted the need for greater understanding of the role of genetics in voice and the need for documented, randomized, controlled studies.

## Molecular Genetic Considerations

Developments in genetic research in recent years are exciting and have largely moved from clinical to molecular studies, as discussed above. Unfortunately, although substantial progress is being made, close scrutiny still reveals discouraging complexities. Much of today's genetic research is involved with gene mapping. This methodology is elegant, but of limited clinical value for broad conditions associated with one major gene. They used to require an extremely specific phenotypic description. Indeed, without specification of not only a phenotype but also a candidate gene, linkage studies used to be extraordinarily difficult and time consuming. Recent technological advances such as the development of microassay technology have facilitated this process greatly.

Because the basement membrane matrix proteins are found on the long arm of chromosome 1, and other materials may be localized to specific chromosomes, locating genes responsible for voice phenomena was recognized as practical in selected cases even before the development of newer techniques. For example, Mace et al[87] described a family with hereditary, congenital, bilateral adductor vocal fold paralysis inherited as an autosomal dominant, with linkage with HLA, a syndrome localized to chromosome 6, position 21.3–23. However, for many questions regarding voice traits and problems, more gene mapping remains to be done. Important research in this and other areas of molecular genetics and genomics is ongoing; but acquiring all of the information needed will take many years. In the meantime, it appears worthwhile to continue the study of pathological conditions known to be hereditary and associated with voice abnormalities. This research should include genetic, structural, physiologic, and epidemiologic studies. Such investigations, together with advances in molecular genetic research, should eventually lead us to the kind of information we seek about normal and exceptional voices. Later research efforts are likely to be facilitated by

building a database of pedigree information now. A national registry to coordinate this information may even be appropriate, as suggested by the late Dr Stephen Gray (personal communication, June 1993). Clinicians should be encouraged to acquire much more meticulous family histories focusing on voice quality, skills, peculiarities, and other non-voice-distinguishing features and diseases. This type of clinical research is also likely to provide information that will help us clarify the genetic nature of voice traits, not just pathology. In addition, it may give us insight into disease susceptibility. This has been recommended in the past for cancer. However, questions about benign disease still remain to be answered. For example, in families with vocal nodules, we have always assumed that environmental factors were causal. Perhaps there are also genetic deficiencies in healing patterns in response to phonotrauma that can be identified. If so, preventive measures may be possible and may guide medical, genetic, and surgical therapy.

## Conclusion

Despite many exciting breakthroughs, much remains to be learned about how the voice functions, what causes phonatory dysfunction, and how voice characteristics (normal and abnormal) are transmitted within families and larger groups. Genetic research has barely begun to address these problems.

Considerable additional study should be encouraged to elucidate the genetics of voice. This research should investigate not only vocal tract structure and function, but also genetic aspects of cortical function, perception, and neurological control, which are so inextricably involved in voice production.

Although questions involving heredity are associated with somewhat discouraging difficulties in research design and implementation, they must be addressed along with the more limited anatomic and physiologic questions studied to date. Clinical and molecular genetic research should provide important new insights into healthy and pathological phonation, the relationship between vocal tract structure (such as basement membrane ultrastructure) and function, and valuable contributions to the physician's armamentarium for treating voice disorders.

## References

1. Rudiger RA, Schmidt W, Loose DA, Passarge E. Severe developmental failure with coarse facial features, distal limb hypoplasia, thickened palmar creases, bifid

uvula, and ureteral stenosis: a previously unidentified familial disorder with lethal outcome. *J Pediatr.* 1971;79(6):977–981.

2. Verma IC, Sansi PK, Kumar V, Ahuja MM. Familial male pseudohermaphroditism with female external genitalia, presence of labial testes, male habitus and voice, and complete absence of Muellerian structures and lack of breast development. *Birth Defects.* 1975;11(4):145–152.

3. Urbanova O. Familial occurrence of dysphonia [Czech]. *Cesk Otolaryngol.* 1973;22(3):180–183.

4. Shriberg LD. Four new speech and prosody-voice measures for genetics research and other studies in developmental phonological disorders. *J Speech Hear Res.* 1993;36(11):105–140.

5. Friol-Vercelletto M, Mussini JM, Dumas-Guillemot A, Denis G, Lavenant-Oger F, Feve JR. Familial cases of oculopharyngeal muscular dystrophy. A case. [Czech]. *Rev Otoneuroophtalmol.* 1983;55(4):329–336.

6. Ludlow CL, Cooper JA. *Genetic Aspects of Speech and Language Disorders.* New York, NY: Academic Press; 1983:3–218.

7. Luchsinger R, Arnold GE, eds. Genetics of the voice. In: Luchsinger R, ed. *Voice-Speech-Language.* Belmont, CA: Wadsworth Publishing; 1965:122–130.

8. Coon H, Carey G. Genetic and environmental determinants of musical ability in twins. *Behav Genet.* 1989; 19(2):183–193.

9. Kalmus H, Fry DB. On tone deafness (dysmelodia): frequency, development, genetics and musical background. *Ann Hum Genet.* 1980;43:369–382.

10. Bernstein F, Schlaper B. Über die Tonlage der menschlichen Singstimme. *Sitzungsberichte der Preuss. Akad Wiss, Math-physikal. Klasse*; 1922.

11. Schilling R. Über die Stimme erbgleicher Zwillinge. *Klin Scher.* 1936;15:756 [cited in Luchsinger and Arnold, see reference 7].

12. Schilling R. Über die Stimme erbgleicher Zwillinge. *Folia Phoniatr.* 1950;2:98–119.

13. Seeman M. Die Bedeutung der Zwillingspathologie für die Erforschung von Sprachleiden. *Arch Sprach-Stimmheilk.* 1937;1:88.

14. Gedda L, Bianchi A, Bianchi-Neroni L. La voce dei gemelli I: prova di identificazione intrageminale della voce in 104 coppie (58 Mz e 46 Dz). *Acta Gerontol* (Milano). 1955;4:121–130.

15. Gorlin R, Cohen MM, Levin LS. *Syndromes of the Head and Neck.* 3rd ed. New York, NY: Oxford University Press; 1990:48, 53, 99, 106, 108, 113, 143, 298, 300, 304, 314, 316, 339, 423, 446, 485, 507, 632, 792.

16. Finkelstein MW, Hammond HL, Jones RB. Hyalinosis cutis et mucosae. *Oral Surg Oral Med Oral Pathol.* 1982;54:49–58.

17. Hofer P-Å, Öhman J. Laryngeal lesions in UrbachWiethe disease. *Acta Pathol Microbiol Scand.* 1974;82A:547–558.

18. Ward WQ, Bianchine J, Hambrick GW. Lipoid proteinosis. *Birth Defects.* 1971;7(8):288–291.

19. Cordero JF, Holmes LB. Phenotypic overlap of the BBB and G syndromes. *Am J Med Genet.* 1978;2:145–152.

20. Funderburk SJ, Stewart R. The G and BBB syndromes: case presentations, genetics, and nosology. *Am J Med Genet.* 1978;2:131–144.

21. Opitz JM. G syndrome (hypertelorism with esophageal abnormality and hypospadias or hypospadias-dysphagia, or "Opitz-Frias" or "Opitz-G" syndrome)—perspective in 1987 and bibliography. *Am J Med Genet.* 1987;28:275–285, Editorial Comment.

22. Opitz JM, Summit RL, Smith DW. The BBB syndrome. Familial telecanthus with associated congenital anomalies. *Birth Defects.* 1969;5(2):86–94.

23. Cohn AM, McFarland JR. Pachyonychia congenita with involvement of the larynx. *Arch Otolaryngol.* 1976; 102:233–235.

24. Jackson ADM, Lawler SK. Pachyonychia congenita: a report of six cases in one family. *Ann Eugen.* 1951–1952;16:142–146.

25. Laing CR, Hayes JR, Scharf G. Pachyonychia congenita. *Am J Dis Child.* 1966;111:649–652.

26. Epstein CJ, Martin GM, Schultz AL, Motlusky AG. Werner's syndrome. *Medicine.* 1966;45:177–221.

27. Zucker-Franklin D, Rifkin H, Jacobson HG. Werner's syndrome. An analysis of ten cases. *Geriatrics.* 1968; 23(8):123–135.

28. Beuren AJ, Apitz J, Harmjanz D. Supravalvular aortic stenosis in association with mental retardation and a certain facial appearance. *Circulation.* 1962;26: 1235–1240.

29. Beuren AJ, Schultz C, Eheril P, Harmjanz DM, Apitz J. The syndrome of supravalvular aortic stenosis, peripheral pulmonary stenosis, mental retardation and similar facial appearance. *Am J Cardiol.* 1964;13:471–483.

30. Jones KL, Smith PW. The Williams' elfin facies syndrome: a new perspective. *J Pediatr.* 1975;86:718–723.

31. Kivalo E, Autio L, Palo A, Amnell G. Mental retardation, typical facies and aortic stenosis syndrome. *Ann Med Intern Fenn.* 1965;54:81–87.

32. Bloom F. The syndrome of congenital telangiectatic erythema and stunted growth. *J Pediatr.* 1966;68:103–113.

33. German J. Bloom's syndrome. VIII. Review of clinical and genetic aspects. In: Goodman RM, Motulsky AG, eds. *Genetic Diseases Among Ashkenazi Jews.* New York, NY: Raven Press; 1978:121–139.

34. Katzenellenbogen I, Laron Z. A contribution to Bloom's syndrome. *Arch Dermatol.* 1960;82:609–616.

35. Keutel J, Marghesco S, Teller W. Bloom-Syndrom. *Z Kinderheilkd.* 1967;101:165–180.

36. Aberfeld DC, Hinterbuchner LP, Schneider M. Myotonia, dwarfism, diffuse bone disease and unusual ocular and facial abnormalities (a new syndrome). *Brain.* 1965;88:313–322.

37. Aberfeld DC, Namba T, Vye MV, Grob D. Chondrodystrophic myotonia: report of two cases. Myotonia, dwarfism, diffuse bone disease and unusual ocular and facial abnormalities. *Arch Neurol.* 1972;22:455–462.

38. Mereu TR, Porter IH, Hug G. Myotonia, shortness of stature, and hip dysplasia. Schwartz-Jampel syndrome. *Am J Dis Child.* 1969;117:470–478.

39. Pavone L, LaRosa M, LiVolti S, Mallica F. Immunologic abnormalities in Schwartz-Jampel syndrome. *J Pediatr*. 1981;98:512.

40. Manning KP. The larynx in the cri-du-chat syndrome. *J Laryngol Otol*.1977;91:887–892.

41. Wilheim OL, Méhes K. Dubowitz syndrome. *Acta Paediatr Hung*. 1986;27:67–75.

42. Wilroy RS Jr. Tipton RE, Summitt RL. The Dubowitz syndrome. *Am J Med Genet*. 1978;2:275–284.

43. Muller W, Frisch H, Gassner I, Kofler J. Seckel-Syndrom. *Monatsschr Kinderheilkd*. 1978;126:454–456.

44. Beighton P. The dominant and recessive forms of cutis laxa. *J Med Genet*. 1972;9:216–221.

45. Goltz RW, Hult A, Goldfarb M, Gorlin RJ. Cutis laxa, a manifestation of generalized elastolysis. *Arch Dermatol*. 1965;92:373–387.

46. Wilsch L, Schnmid G, Haneke E. Spätmanifeste Dermatochalasis. *Dtsch Med Wochenschr*. 1977;102:1451–1454.

47. Berg JM, McCreary BD, Ridler MAC, Smith GF. *The de Lange Syndrome*. New York, NY: Pergamon; 1970.

48. Breslau EJ, Disteche C, Hall JG, Thuline H, Cooper P. Prometaphase chromosomes in five patients with the Brachmann-de Lange syndrome. *Am J Med Genet*. 1981; 10:179–186.

49. Fraser WI, Campbell BM. A study of six cases of de Lange Amsterdam dwarf syndrome, with special attention to voice, speech and language characteristics. *Dev Med Child Neurol*. 1978;20:189–198.

50. Gorlin RJ. 18q-syndrome. In: Yunis JJ, ed. *New Chromosomal Syndromes*. New York, NY: Academic Press; 1977: 72–74.

51. Rethoré MO. Deletions and ring chromosomes. In: Vinken JP, Bruyn GW, eds. *Handbook of Clinical Neurology*. Amsterdam: North-Holland Publishing; 1977: 26–27.

52. Schinzel A, Hayashi K, Schmid W. Structural aberrations of chromosome 18 II. The 18q syndrome. Report of three cases. *Humangenetik*. 1975;26:123–132.

53. Wilson MG, Towner JW, Forsman I, Siris E. Syndromes associated with deletion of the long arm of chromosome 18[del(18q)]. *Am J Med Genet*. 1979;3:155–174.

54. Bosch-Banyeras JM, Saleedo S, Lucaya J, Laverde R, Boronat M, Marti-Henneberg C. Acceleration du developpment postnatal, hypertome, elargissement des phalanges médianes et des metaphyses distales du femur, facies particuliar: s'agit-il d'un syndrome de Weaver? *Arch Fr Pédiatr*. 1978;35:177–183.

55. Weisswichert PH, Knapp G, Willich P. Accelerated bone maturation syndrome of the Weaver type. *Eur J Pediatr*. 1981;137:329–333.

56. Salomonson J, Kawamoto H, Wilson L. Velopharyngeal incompetence as the presenting symptoms of myotonic dystrophy. *Cleft Palate J*. 1988;25:296–300.

57. Joan K I. *Smith's Recognizable Patterns of Human Malformation*. 5th ed. Philadelphia, PA: WB Saunders; 1997: 44–46.

58. Aronson A. *Clinical Voice Disorders: An Interdisciplinary Approach*. New York, NY: Thieme-Stratton;1980:57–61.

59. Plott D. Congenital laryngeal abductor paralysis due to nucleus ambiguus dysgenesis in three brothers. *N Engl J Med*. 1964;271:593–596.

60. Scott-Brown WG. *Scott-Brown's Otolaryngology*. Vol 5. 5th ed. London: Butterworth's; 1987:119–144.

61. Darley F, Aronson A, Brown J. Differential diagnostic patterns of dysarthria. *J Speech Hear Res*. 1969;12: 246–269.

62. Darley F, Aronson A, Brown J. Clusters of deviant speech dimensions in the dysarthrias. *J Speech Hear Res*. 1969;12:462–496.

63. Ramig LA, Scherer RC, Titze IR, Ringel SP. Acoustic analysis of voices of patients with neurological disease: rational and preliminary data. *Ann Otol Rhinol Laryngol*. 1988;97:164–172.

64. Ramig LA. Acoustic analyses of phonation in patients with Huntington's disease: preliminary report. *Ann Otol Rhinol Laryngol*. 1986;95:288–293.

65. Heuer RJ, Sataloff RT, Spiegel JR, et al. Voice abnormalities in short stature syndromes. *Ear Nose Throat J*. 1995;74:622–628.

66. Richmon JD, Wang-Rodriguez J, Thekdi AA. Ehlers-Danlos syndrome presenting as dysphonia and manifesting as tongue hypermobility: report of 2 cases. *Ear Nose Throat J*. 2009 Feb;88(2):E8–E12.

67. Spring PJ, Kok C, Nicholson GA, et al. Autosomal dominant hereditary sensory neuropathy with chronic cough and gastro-oesophageal reflux: clinical features in two families linked to chromosome 3p22-p24. *Brain* 2005 Dec;128(pt 12):2797–2810.

68. Sharma N, Franco RA Jr. Consideration of genetic contributions to the risk for spasmodic dysphonia. *Otolaryngol Head Neck Surg*. 2011 Sep;145(3):369–370.

69. Sidtis JJ, Ahn JS, Gomez C, Sidtis D. Speech characteristics associated with three genotypes of ataxia. *J Commun Disord*. 2011 Jul-Aug;44(4):478–492.

70. Solot CB, Knightly C, Handler SD, et al. Communication disorders in the 22q11.2 microdeletion syndrome. *J Commun Disord*. 2000 May-Jun;33(3):187-203.

71. Chang J, Yung KC. Dysphonia and vocal fold telangiectasia in hereditary hemorrhagic telangiectasia. *Ann Otol Rhinol Laryngol*. 2014 Nov;123(11):769–770.

72. Martins RH, Goncalves TM, Neves DS, et al. Sulcus vocalis: evidence for autosomal dominant inheritance. *Genet Mol Res*. 2011 Dec 19;10(4):3163–3168.

73. Moore C, Shalet S, Manickam K. Voice abnormality in adults with congenital and adult-acquired growth hormone deficiency [published online May 3, 2005]. *J Clin Endocrinol Metab*. 2005 Jul;90(7):4128–4132.

74. Shriberg LD, Ballard KJ, Tomblin JB, et al. Speech, prosody, and voice characteristics of a mother and daughter with a 7;13 translocation affecting FOXP2. *J Speech Lang Hear Res*. 2006 June;49(3):500–525.

75. Simberg S, Santtila P, Soveri A, et al. Exploring genetic and environmental effects in dysphonia: a twin study. *J Speech Lang Hear Res*. 2009 Feb;52(1):153–163.

76. Nybacka I, Simberg S, Santtila P, et al. Genetic and environmental effects on vocal symptoms and their

intercorrelations. *J Speech Lang Hear Res.* 2012 Apr;55(2): 541–553.

77. Wilcox RA, Winkler S, Lohmann K, Klein C. Whispering dysphonia in an Australian family (DYT4): a clinical and genetic reappraisal. *Mov Disord.* 2011 Nov; 26(13):2404–2408.

78. Lohmann K, Wilcox RA, Winkler S. Whispering dysphonia (DYT4 dystonia) is caused by a mutation in the TUBB4 gene. *Ann Neurol.* 2013 Apr;73(4):537–545.

79. Tanner K, Sauder C, Thibeault SL, et al. Vocal fold bowing in elderly male monozygotic twins: a case study. *J Voice.* 2010 Jul;24(4):470–476.

80. Worthey EA, Raca G, Laffin JJ, et al. Whole-exome sequencing supports genetic heterogeneity in childhood apraxia of speech. *J Neurodev Disord.* 2013 Oct 2;5(1):29.

81. Pal DK, Li W, Clark T, et al. Pleiotropic effects of the 11p13 locus on developmental verbal dyspraxia and EEG centrotemporal sharp waves. *Genes Brain Behav.* 2010 Nov;9(8):1004–1012.

82. Grant LM, Kelm-Nelson CA, Hilby BL, et al. Evidence for early and progressive ultrasonic vocalization and oromotor deficits in a PINK1 gene knockout rat model of Parkinson's disease [published online July 31, 2015]. *J Neurosci Res.* 2015;93(11):1713–1727.

83. AlaMello S, Peippo M. Two more diagnostic signs in the Floating Harbor syndrome. *Clinical Dysmorphology.* 1996 Jan;5(1):855.

84. Morris CA. Introduction: Williams syndrome. *Am J Med Genet C Semin Med Genet.* 2010 May 15;154C(2): 203–208.

85. Pedersen M. (2017). Genetics. In: Zehnhoff-Dinnesen A, Wiskirska-Woznica B, Neumann K, Nawka T, eds. *Phoniatrics; Voice, Swallowing, Speech, Language, Pediatric Hearing Disorders, European Manual of Medicine, Springer.* In press.

86. Van Borsel J. Voice and resonance disorders in genetic syndromes: a meta-analysis. *Folia Phoniatrica et Logopaedica.* 2004;56(2):83–92.

87. Mace M, Williamson E, Worgan D. Autosomal dominantly inherited adductor laryngeal paralysis—a new syndrome with a suggestion of linkage to HLA. *Clin Genet.* 1978;14:265–270.

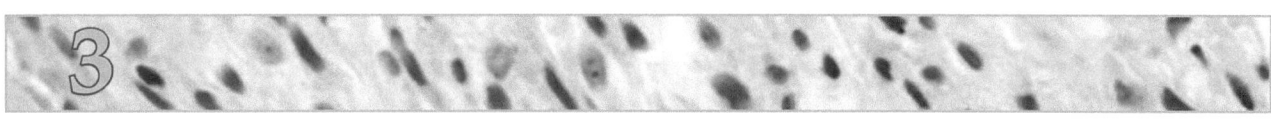

# Impact of Aging on the Voice

*Abdul-Latif Hamdan, Robert Thayer Sataloff, and Mary J. Hawkshaw*

Aging is inevitable. It is the end result of cumulative physiologic and pathologic events that lead to senility of structures within our body. It is a natural process that affects all systems leading to laxity, decrease in strength, instability, and weakness. Plato described the elderly Cepahlus in the opening of the *Republic* as physically withdrawn with reduction in his physical strength.[1] In his theory on gerotranscendence, the inner awakening for metaphysical contemplation in the elderly is triggered by the decline in physical function and its subsequent morphologic changes.

The function of the phonatory system, like any other system in the body, is affected by aging. The senile changes in the larynx result in an increase in its non-linear behavior, thus leading to changes in voice quality classified as presbysphonia.[2] This condition is on the rise nowadays with the increase in the aging population. It is estimated to reach up to 30% based on numerous epidemiologic reports, with a chronicity rate of 60%.[3–5] Social and behavioral factors may contribute to its high prevalence. In a large cross-sectional study looking at prevalence of dysphonia in elderly subjects, the odds ratio for urban residence and poor social status were reported to be 1.83 and 2.99, respectively.[6]

## Dysphonia in the Elderly

Dysphonia is common in the elderly. Based on an epidemiologic study by Roy et al, the life prevalence of dysphonia has been estimated to be 47%.[3] However, it is important to note that age-related change in voice quality is not the only cause of dysphonia in the elderly. The prevalence of presbyphonia is markedly surpassed by other causes of dysphonia.[3,7,8] In an investigation on dysphonia in 151 elderly individuals, Woo et al reported the presence of systemic diseases and the use of chronic medications in 53.6% and 40.3% of the cases, respectively.[4] Similarly, the study by Gregory et al, on voice disorders in elderly patients, revealed the presence of one or more pathologic factors that contributed to dysphonia in all the subjects investigated. In that study, 91% had laryngopharyngeal reflux disease, 73% had muscle tension dysphonia, and 72% had vocal fold paresis.[9] In another study by Çiyiltepe and Şenkal conducted on 91 patients, vocal nodules, laryngopharyngeal reflux disease and vocal fold paresis were present in 23.9%, 10.8%, and 9.78% of the cases, respectively.[10] This high prevalence of co-morbidities emphasizes the need for an adequate laryngeal examination and a thorough investigation in an elderly patient presenting with dysphonia. Systemic diseases must be sought diligently even after diagnosing or excluding infectious, benign, and malignant causes of dysphonia as local and systemic disorders co-exists.[4,11,12] To that end, presbyphonia should be diagnosed only after all other diagnoses have been established or excluded.

## Presbyphonia

### Self-Reported Symptoms, Perceptual Properties, and Acoustic Findings In the Elderly

Patients with presbyphonia typically complain of roughness, change in vocal pitch, vocal instability, and weakness, in addition to inability to project the voice and loss of range. Symptoms such as throat clearing and excessive mucus also are often described.[13] These self-reported complaints, which may impact the ability to communicate in a noisy environment, also are perceived by trained listeners.[14–18] Perceptual evaluation of the elderly voice often reveals asthenia, breathiness, and/or straining. In a report by Honjo and Isshiki in 1980, the voices of elderly women aged between 69 and 85 years were described perceptually as rough and hoarse in comparison to young women.[19] Acoustic analysis reveals often an increase in perturbation parameters, namely, cycle-to-cycle variation in frequency (jitter) and intensity (shimmer), and an increase in noise-to-harmonic ratio.[20–22] In a report by Linville in 1987 on acoustic changes in elderly women, she reported an increase in frequency variability (standard deviation) with aging.[20] Similarly, Ferrand, in his investigation on acoustic measures in vocal aging, highlighted the high sensitivity of noise-to-harmonic ratio as an acoustic cue in comparison to other acoustic measures such as cycle-to-cycle variation in frequency.[21] In another study, Harnsberger et al reported that vocal tremor, degree of noise, and rate of speech can shift the perception of age by 12 years. The authors reached that conclusion by manipulating the degree of noise and tremor in resynthesized voice samples obtained from 10 young male subjects.[22]

The aging voice also is characterized by a change in the mean fundamental frequency (F0) and habitual pitch, with a consensus that there is an increase in men by an average of 35 Hz and a decrease in women by an average of 10 to 15 Hz,[23–25] although these data remain controversial. In the study by Honjo and Isshiki on 40 elderly women and men, the authors reported elevated fundamental frequency in men and reduced fundamental frequency in women.[19] The increase in F0 in men was attributed to atrophic changes in the vocal fold musculature and stiffening of the vocal ligament, whereas the decreased F0 in women was attributed primarily to edematous changes of the vocal folds. Similarly, in another longitudinal study of women using archival data, Russell et al reported significant lowering in speaking fundamental frequency with age. The results were obtained by comparing the recordings of women across a 50-year time span.[26] Numerous other studies reported different changes in F0 with aging.[27–29] Endres, Bambach, and Flosser reported a decrease in the mean pitch frequency with aging in a sample of four male voices and two female voices. The authors reported that with age formants moves toward lower frequencies.[28] Krook in 1988 reported data on speaking fundamental frequency in a group of 467 females and 198 males of different age groups. The results indicated that the mean SFF in the female group, which averaged 188 Hz, decreased until the age of 70 years but then tended to increase after that age. In men, the mean SFF averaged 116 Hz at a young age and

tended to rise after middle age.[27] In another study by Benjamin on frequency variability conducted on 20 males and 20 females, the author reported a decrease rather than an increase in modal frequency in elderly men with aging (110.3 Hz vs 103.0 Hz).[29] A possible explanation for these conflicting reports is the high within-subject variability in elderly subjects and the possible contributing factor of hormonal changes in women after menopause, the impact of which may mask or heighten other effects of aging on voice.

Variation in speech intensity with aging also has been thoroughly investigated in the literature. Morris and Brown in 1994 investigated the effect of aging on speech intensity in women. The study was performed on two groups of women, young (20–35 years) and elderly (70–90 years), who were asked to read the "Rainbow Passage "and to sustain the vowel / α / at different intensities. The results indicated that elderly women had higher minimum intensity level and lower maximum intensity level during vowel production compared to young women.[30] In addition to the changes in speech intensity with age, there are also changes in speech intensity modulation and control of vocal loudness. Elderly patients are described as having either decreased loudness, or increased loudness often attributed to impaired hearing. In the study by Baker et al on control of vocal loudness in adults, the authors reported lower sound pressure levels at three levels of loudness in elderly subjects compared to young subjects.[31] The similarity in subglottal pressure values and the dissimilarity in laryngeal electromyographic activities between both groups alluded to a laryngeal cause for these differences.[31] Similarly, an investigation by Hodge et al on vocal intensity in elderly versus a control group showed a significant difference between the two groups.[32] Sound pressure level and peak airflow were lower in the elderly compared to controls. However, there were no significant differences in the maximum flow declination, phonatory threshold pressure, or fundamental frequency between the two groups.

In conclusion, it is important to note that high intensity phonation plays an important role in accentuating the presence of phonatory changes, which may not be apparent when habitual intensity level is used.[33]

## Resonance with Aging

In addition to the aforementioned changes in F0 and perturbation parameters, formants' position and dispersion also may be affected with aging.[28] Acoustic measures extrapolated from sustained vowels and connected speech often reveal a shift of formants towards lower frequencies. A study by Linville and Fisher in 1985 on formant frequencies in a group of 75 women stratified into three age groups, showed a decrease in resonance peaks F1 and F2 with aging.[34] The analysis was performed on both sustained spoken and whispered vowels. Similar findings were reported few years later, in another investigation by Scukanec et al.[35] The authors reported significant lowering of F1 on four vowels and significant lowering of F2 on vowel / α / and /u/ with aging in women. In another study by Linville and Rens in 2001 measuring the first three spectral peaks during connected speech (reading the first paragraph of the Rainbow Passage), the authors showed clearly significant lowering of the first peak with age in both genders, and significant lowering of the second and third peaks in women. The decline in frequency for peaks 1, 2, and 3 in women compared to men were 29% versus 11%, 10% versus 2%, and 9% versus 2%, respectively. This gender effect on formant lowering with age has been attributed to a higher degree of the vocal tract lengthening in women compared to men.[36] The accentuated drop in the suspended position of the larynx secondary to weakening of the strap muscles is further enhanced by the loss of vertebral support in women with osteoporosis.[37] A study by Xue and Hao in 2003 on vocal tract changes with aging, revealed lengthening and enlargement of the oral cavity with significant increase in the volume of the vocal tract. Acoustic analysis of formant frequencies in groups of young and elderly men and women showed lowering of formant frequencies F1 for five vowels in men and for 7 vowels in women. Commensurate with these acoustic changes were anatomical differences in oral cavity length and volume, and in vocal tract volume but not length. The authors alluded to the importance of vocal tract volume as a determinant of formant measures in addition to vocal tract length. Two other important findings were the similarity in senile changes in both genders and the differential effect of aging on various segments of the vocal tract. Noteworthy is the enlargement and lengthening of the oral cavity and not the pharyngeal cavity.[38] A more recent study by Eichhorn et al on the effects of aging on the first four formants in a group of 43 men and 53 women, revealed a mild change in the formants frequencies of the corner vowels secondary to compensatory behavior.[39]

### Laryngeal Airflow Measurements with Aging

Studies on laryngeal airway resistance and airflow measures in the elderly are conflicting. Hoit and Hixon in their investigation on laryngeal valving

economy in a group of 70 women of different age groups (10 at each age of 25, 35, 45, 55, 65, 75, and 85 years) reported no significant difference in laryngeal airway resistance with aging, although there were lower values in the 45-year-old age group subjects.[40] The lack of significant changes in airflow measurements across the different age groups was attributed to slow adaptation and compensatory behavior. Similarly, in another investigation looking at "amplitude-based glottal airflow characteristics " in 60 women stratified according to six age groups (10 in each group from 20–,30–,40–,50–,60–,70–) Sapienza and Dutka reported that none of the airflow measures used, namely, "minimum glottal airflow, alternating glottal airflow, peak glottal airflow and minimum glottal airflow,"[41] was predictive of age.[41] However, other investigators described significant differences in glottal resistance and airflow rates in elderly compared to young subjects. The study by Hodge et al on the mechanism for intensity difference between elderly and control subjects demonstrated lower values for sound pressure level and peak airflow, and higher open quotient in the elderly.[32] In an investigation by Melcon et al on laryngeal valving in 60 men of different age groups, the authors reported lower mean airway resistance during sustained vowel production in elderly men (75 years old) compared to younger men.[42] In another study by Holmes et al on subjects of different age groups, including 10 males and 10 females, the authors investigated laryngeal airway resistance (RLAW) at four sound pressure levels (SPL). The results indicated significant difference in RLAW values at all sound pressure levels in women compared to men and in women across different ages, in addition to a significant difference between the oldest male group and the youngest at the 75th SPL percentile. The authors also reported "more linear changes in transglottal airflow and transglottal pressure as relative SPL increased in men."[43] They concluded that women, unlike men, seem to have less speech intensity variations, probably secondary to the high laryngeal airway resistance attributed to relatively small laryngeal size.

### Stroboscopy, Electroglottography, and High-Speed Imaging in the Elderly

In parallel with all the aforementioned perceptual, acoustic, and airflow alterations in the elderly, vocal folds changes are often observed on laryngeal examination. The most common laryngeal stroboscopic findings are vocal process prominence, bowing of the vocal folds with incomplete closure, vocal fold edematous changes, stiffening, reduced pliability of the vocal fold cover, irregular vibratory behavior, and aperiodicity.[19, 44–48] In the study in 1980 by Honjo and Isshiki, the authors reported evidence of vocal fold atrophy and edema in men and vocal fold edema in women.[19] Similar results were reported by Linville et al in a group of 20 elderly women.[44] However, they found vocal fold edema and inadequate glottic closure but in different frequencies in comparison to the report by Honjo and Isshiki in 1980.[44] A few years later, Linville, in her investigation on glottal gap configuration in relation to loudness and pitch, reported significant differences between elderly and young women. The young group displayed a posterior chink more often on stroboscopic examination, whereas elderly displayed more anterior gap with a spindle-shaped opening.[45] In another study on elderly women by Biever and Bless in 1989, stroboscopic examination revealed incomplete closure, vocal fold edema, and aperiodicity with alterations in both mucosal wave and amplitude.[46] Pontes et al examined the correlation between presbylaryngeal glottic signs of aging and vocal characteristics in 88 men and 122 women. The authors reported the prevalence of membranous spindle-shaped chinks in 37.6%, vocal process prominence in 29.5%, and vocal fold bowing in 23.8% of the total group.[47] Similarly, Pontes et al in their analysis of the senile larynx have reported significant differences in the prevalence of vocal process prominence in females (56 vs 8, $p$-value 0.0006) and a significant difference in the prevalence of vocal fold bowing in males (68 vs 0, $p$-value less than 0.0001) compared with younger subjects. The analysis was conducted on 100 laryngeal images taken from 50 elderly subjects compared with younger subjects (65–85 years) with no vocal complaints.[48] Likewise, in a study on 361 elderly, Takano et al reported the presence of vocal fold atrophy in 20% of the cases in his review of 361 patients (47 men and 25 women) above the age of 65 years. The authors demonstrated also a negative correlation between maximum phonation time and age, and a positive correlation between mean airflow rate and age.[49] Interestingly, the degree of vocal fold bowing seen during abduction does not always correlate with the glottal opening seen during phonation.[50]

Other diagnostic modalities such as electroglottography and high-speed laryngeal imaging confirm the presence of glottic changes in the elderly. Electroglottographic analysis often reveals an increase in the open quotient for vowels that correlate with the perceived age of the speaker. For example, Winkler and Sendlmeier showed an increased open quotient on vowels in elderly men, which correlated with perceived age.[51] In a study by Yamauchi et al using high-speed imaging in 46 elderly patients with vocal fold atrophy, the authors reported "larger open quotient, larger lateral phase difference, larger glottal width and smaller speed index" in comparison with a group of vocally healthy controls.[52] In another cross-sectional study on 20 elderly females, Ahmad et al examined the vibratory behavior of the vocal folds using high-speed imaging. The results indicated that glottal area waveform was consistent with pressed phonation and the presence of anterior glottal gap. These findings were associated with increased glottal perturbation parameters.[53] In a study by Vaca et al on 104 elderly subjects with reduced maximum phonation time, a spindle-shaped glottal gap was present in 47 patients. The authors concluded that vocal fold bowing and s/z ratio were sensitive in predicting glottal gap in 93.6% and 91.4% of the cases, respectively.[54]

We can conclude that there are glottic changes with aging that are commensurate with the audio-perceptual alterations reported by listeners and patients. However, although aging often is considered a primary etiology, laryngeal findings must be interpreted within the context of phonotraumatic events that accumulate with aging, as well as with other conditions including paresis, deconditioning, polypharmacy, and many more that can contribute to laryngeal and voice changes.

## Why These Audio-Perceptual Changes?

### Respiration and Aging

With aging, there is a decrease in lung tissue elasticity and thoracic cage compliance. These changes are associated with an increase in residual lung volume, a decrease in vital capacity, and decrease in inspiratory and expiratory reserve volume. There is also a decrease in the contractile force of respiratory muscles leading to a decrease in forced expiration and airflow rate. These effects may be compounded by postural changes and spinal abnormalities, all of which can markedly impair breathing support and control.[55] In study by Vaca et al in 2015 on the effect of aging on voice and respiration, the authors reported the presence of respiratory deficit in 37% of the cases. Patients were affected the most when a glottal gap was present concomitantly. The study was conducted on a group of 105 elderly subjects who were investigated using strobolaryngoscopy and spirometry.[56] In parallel with these respiratory changes, the coordination between phonation and respiration also may be affected by age. This is, for example, evident when the onset of dysphonia in an elderly patient is preceded by an upper respiratory tract infection.[2]

## Vocal Fold Epithelial Lining

The epithelial lining of the vocal folds undergoes changes with aging. Hirano et al conducted a histologic examination on 64 larynges of subjects between the age of 70 years and 104 years.[57] The authors reported overall thickening of the vocal fold cover with thickening of the mucosa around the free edge of the vocal fold. The increase in vocal fold mucosal thickness was present primarily in women and not in men. Many years later, Goncalves et al described the presence of atrophic changes in the vocal fold epithelium, reduced thickness (2–3 cells compared to 5–7 in young controls) with evidence of desquamation.[58] The study was conducted using electron microscopy in two groups of subjects, eight below the age of 50 years and eight above that age. A year later, the same author, using transmission electronic microscopic examination of 16 human larynges, reported widening of the epithelial intercellular junctions.[59]

## Vocal Fold Lamina Propria

The lamina propria of an elderly person differs from that of a youngster. There are changes in its thickness, layered structure, and extracellular matrix landscape. With aging, there is thickening of the superficial layer of the lamina propria, thinning of the intermediate layer, and fibrosis of its deep layer.[60] The lamina propria loses its layered architecture with subsequent change in its viscoelastic and rheologic properties. The senile changes affect predominantly the distribution, density, and shape of collagen fibers and elastic fibers as well as the concentration and spreading of hyaluronic acid. In young adults, collagen fibers are predominantly of type III and less of type I. These fibers are located primarily in the deep layer of the lamina propria adjacent to the vocalis muscle and less in the intermediate layer.[13] These fibers are intertwined to provide tensile strength and durability, allowing tissues to deform while stretching yet remain anchored to the deep layers of the vocal fold.[61] They also act as a scaffold that may contribute to the stability and sustainability of the vocal fold architecture.[62] With aging, these collagen fibers become less organized, dispersed, and hence less efficient. They thicken and aggregate in thick bundles that bring stiffness to the vocal folds. In a study by Roberts et al on the vocal folds of eight human cadavers, the authors demonstrated that with aging there is predominance of collagen type I in the lamina propria, whereas type III fibers become more plentiful in the superficial layer.[63] These findings corroborate the histologic study by Hirano et al which showed increased density and fibrosis of the collagen fibers in the deep layer of the lamina propria in elderly males.[57] Similarly, the electron microscopic study by Sato on 10 elderly subjects demonstrated an increase in the concentration of collagen in the lamina propria, loss of the layered structure, and a change in the architecture of the collagen fibers that develop a twisted, irregular outline.[64]

Similarly, there are significant histologic changes in the elastic fibers within the lamina propria. In young subjects, the elastic fibers run parallel to the vocal fold edge and are located primarily in the intermediate layer of the lamina propria. In the study by Ishii et al, the authors reported the importance of both the longitudinal orientation of the elastic fibers in the intermediate layer and their coil shape in the deep layer. Their concentration and distribution contribute to the elastic properties of the vocal folds and the ability to stretch with changes in vocal pitch.[62] In the elderly, there is a decrease in the concentration of elastic fibers, which become erratically distributed, amorphous, and lose their orientation along the long axis of the vocal folds.[65] In the study by Hirano et al on 64 human larynges, the authors demonstrated a decrease in the density of the elastic fibers in the intermediate layer of the lamina propria with age.[57] In another study on the vocal fold microstructure in the elderly by Roberts et al, the authors also reported scarcity of elastic fibers in the intermediate layer of the lamina propria and their increased density in the deep layer.[63]

Most of the aforementioned changes in the extracellular matrix of the lamina propria are attributed to reduction in the productivity of fibroblasts.[66] Awd et al in their investigation on the changes in morphologic features of fibroblasts across three different age groups, reported less development of the rough endoplasmic reticulum and Golgi apparatus in the elderly compared to younger adults and newborns.[67] This supports the results of the investigation by Sato and Hirano on the macula flava of the vocal folds in the elderly. Other researchers demonstrated that fibroblasts produce less hyaluronic acid and denser collagen with aging.[68] A transmission electron microscopic examination of the vocal folds of 16 larynges concurred with the aforementioned reports, showing thickening and condensation of the collagen fibers underneath the basement membrane, with the presence of numerous elongated fibroblasts.[59] All these changes lead us to believe that there is an element of aging of the fibroblasts with subsequent alterations in their productivity. As a result, there are changes in vocal fold viscoelastic properties with subsequent stiffening and reduced malleability of the vocal folds. These histologic changes are translated clinically as the need to increase effortful speech, as reported by elderly subjects.[69,70]

## Vocal Fold Muscles

At the muscular level, there are atrophic changes with a marked reduction in the number and diameter of the myofibrils. The decrease in muscle mass is accompanied by an increase in collagen concentration and fat deposition. In a cadaver study by Martins et al on 30 vocal folds using morphometric measures, the authors reported a gradual decrease in the mean diameter of the muscle fibers from 16.389 micrometers in subjects below the age of 50 years to 14.162 in those above the age of 76 years. The authors alluded to the importance of these findings as signs of muscle atrophy in elderly.[71] In another immunohistochemical and stereologic study performed on the thyroarytenoid muscle in comparison to limb muscles, Malmgren et al reported an "age related loss in the length density of type I fibers and age related decrease in surface density of type 2 fibers."[72] These histologic changes in the thyroarytenoid muscles are attributed partially to metabolic changes, reduced blood flow, and partially to degenerative changes in laryngeal innervation that occur with aging. Sataloff et al reported that dysfunctional mitochondria within the thyroarytenoid muscles of the elderly have been described together with a reduction in laryngeal blood flow.[73] There are laryngeal neural and neuromuscular changes very similar to those observed in neural denervation throughout the body. The study by Nakai et al on the right recurrent laryngeal nerve obtained from 16 human cadavers revealed not only disappearance of large axons but also a decrease in the diameter or thinning of the myelinated axons.[74] Similarly, the study by Connor et al on the architecture of neuromuscular junctions in rat thyroarytenoid muscles, revealed severe alteration in the axon terminal area. There was also an increased number of unoccupied post-synaptic acetylcholine receptors.[75] In parallel with these alterations, there is a shift in the myosin heavy chain composition with replacement of type IIB myosin heavy chain by a slower contracting isoform, specifically type IIX.[76] This new landscape in innervation and neuromuscular architecture partially contributes to the loss of fine muscle control and phonatory instability often reported by elderly subjects.

*Other changes*: Together with the aforementioned changes in the lamina propria and muscles, histologic alterations in the cartilages and joints of the laryngeal structures occur also. With aging, there is ossification of the cartilages, and thinning of the articular surfaces of the joints with erosion often leading to limited range of motion.[55] These histologic changes may contribute not only to the change in voice quality observed in elderly people, but also have clinical implication. As an example, ossification of the thyroid cartilage with age may preclude the transthyroid approach in injection laryngoplasty, it also may mandate the use of a drilling device while performing thyroplasty type I for the treatment of vocal fold paralysis, and it may preclude the use of some surgical options for pitch modification in transgender patients.

## Vocal Tract Changes

The manifestations of vocal tract changes in the elderly involve primarily changes in vocal resonance and articulation.[77–81] Articulatory changes, such as vowel centralization, have been investigated. The pattern or inclination toward vowel centralization seem to be more prevalent in men compared to women and more so in subjects with advanced age.[78] The second important consideration is elongation of the vocal tract. Based on the source-filter theory by Titze in 1994,[82] there is a strong correlation between vocal tract dimensions and formant frequencies. Acoustic outputs, including the formant frequencies, reflect the anatomical configuration of the vocal tract. According to this model there is an inverse relationship between vocal tract length and formant frequencies. This elongation of the vocal tract results in lowering of all formants. With aging there is elongation of the vocal tract due to lengthening in some of its segments such as the oral and pharyngeal cavities as reported by Xue and Hao in 2013, and due to the descent of the larynx.[38] Ferreri was the first to report lengthening of the vocal tract in elderly subjects, described as "laryngeal ptosis."[83] This senile effect has been attributed to several factors: atrophy of the strap muscles, stretching of attached ligaments, lowering of the lower respiratory tract and lungs due to thinning of the intervertebral spaces, and enlargement of craniocervical structures. Kahane et al described lengthening of the vocal tract as a result of the decrease in the support of the lower respiratory tract and laryngo-tracheo-bronchial tree.[84] Lowering of the formants also can be attributed to enlargement of vocal tract space, particularly oral cavity, pharyngeal, and supraglottic tract. In the study by Xue and Hao, enlargement in the volume of the vocal tract, rather than elongation, correlated with lowering of formants with aging.[38]

## Treatment of Presbyphonia

Dysphonia in the elderly is associated strongly with decreased quality of life. There is a significant association between the perception of quality of voice and that of an individual's quality of life.[85] Good health has a positive impact on voice in healthy elderly individuals exhibiting less vocal changes than those in poor health. Moreover, numerous studies have indicated that changes in voice quality that require repetition while talking often result in anxiety which in turn can lead to withdrawal of social events and subsequent social isolation.[3,85,86] In a study by Golub et al on the prevalence of perceived dysphonia in the aging population, one out of two elderly with dysphonia reported that the change in voice quality significantly impacted their quality of life.[7] The behavioral and social effects of the aging voice is emphasized further by the presence of associated comorbidities such as neurogenic disorders, which also can foster isolation from the society.

A multidisciplinary approach is needed for optimal treatment of dysphonia in the elderly. Behavioral modification and change in life style are often a good and rewarding start. Physical exercise may mitigate the aging changes within the different components of phonation. De Macahado et al in 2016 reported that aerobics can deter or slow down the effect of aging on voice.[87] Their study was performed on 58 elderly women using both broadband and narrowband spectrographic analysis.[87] Hence, management of presbyphonia should include attention to the power source of phonation, namely, breathing, and chest, abdomen, and back muscle strength. Speech-language pathologists also play a major role in the rehabilitation of the aging voice. Using breathing exercises, in addition to resonance therapy and tension releasing exercises, speech-language pathologists can help patients project their voice more efficiently with the least amount of laryngeal tension. The prognostic value of vocal therapy using various outcome measures is well documented in the literature.[88–90] Gorman et al demonstrated a significant improvement in both subjective and objectives measures following a 12-week program of voice therapy. There was a reduction in the amount of breathiness that was commensurate with an increase in the maximum phonation time by 15 seconds.[88] Similarly, Kaneko et al, in a retrospective study on 16 patients with presbyphonia, reported the beneficial effect of vocal fold exercise. There was a significant improvement in the perceptual evaluation, self-reported questionnaire, frequency perturbation parameters, as well as stroboscopic parameters such as mucosal waves and glottic closure.[89] In another review by Oates on the role of voice therapy and impact of behavioral treatment on the elderly voice, the authors strongly advocated the potential role of various vocal techniques in mitigating the effects of aging on voice.[90] The group led by Dr. Robert Sataloff at the Drexel University College of Medicine has taken therapy of the elderly voice to a new frontier. Since the 1980s, the team that manages the aging voice expanded to include a singing teacher and an acting voice specialist added in the 1990s in addition to the speech-language pathologist. The rationale behind this expanded approach is building more agility and flexibility in the phonatory apparatus, which bears significant usefulness for both speaking and singing. Singing, which is an athletic vocal exercise, also has been shown to circumvent or delay the aging effect on voice. Elderly who sing tend to have fewer acoustic changes compared to non-singers.[55] A study by Prakup on 30 singers and 30 non-singers between the age of 65 and 80 years showed that singers had significantly more sound intensity and lesser values for jitter compared to non-singers. Moreover, in addition to the aforementioned objective differences, the voice of both male and female singers were subjectively perceived as younger than those of non singers.[91] In another study looking at the effect of singing using acoustic measures in a group of 72 healthy adult singers with different singing backgrounds, the authors demonstrated that the frequency of singing was positively associated with increased vocal stability and improved voice quality. To that end, the moderating effect of singing on the aging voice was emphasized and suggested as an important behavioral exercise that can be used to delay or deter vocal aging change.[92]

Surgery in the form of injection laryngoplasty or thyroplasty type I is another useful intervention for some patients with presbyphonia. In a study by Sachs et al comparing these two options in a group of 22 patients, the authors reported that thyroplasty type I was superior to injection laryngoplasty using endoscopic evaluation, acoustic and airflow measurements, as well as self-rating questionnaires. A retrospective review of the endoscopic images revealed less vocal fold bowing and supraglottic activity post-thyroplasty compared to pre-injection laryngoplasty. Similarly, from the patient's perspective, those who underwent laryngeal framework surgery rated themselves as markedly better with significant improvement after treatment.[93] However, results of such studies need to be interpreted with great caution because of the major effects associated with the injection technique and especially the choice of material injected.

At the molecular level, regenerative medicine is gaining ground as a future therapeutic modality. Both animal and human studies have demonstrated promising results in the management of the aging vocal folds. Andreatta et al explored the effect of Neutrophin 4 injected either systemically or directly into the vocal folds in an animal study conducted on rats. The impetus for the study was the well-reported decrease in the number and size of the neuromuscular junctions that occurs with aging, and the known differentiating effect of neutrophins at these junctions in addition to their enhancing effect in the release of neurotransmitters.[94] Ohno et al investigated the regenerative effect of basic fibroblast growth factor on vocal fold atrophy in six patients. Using several outcome measures, both subjective such as VHI-10 and objective findings such as glottic closure and extent of mucosal waves, the authors reported significant improvement six months after the injection. The effect is thought to be mediated by the enhanced activity of the fibroblast cells in the lamina propria leading to increased concentration of hyaluronic acid and other extracellular matrix constituent.[95] One limitation of this study is the small number of patients studied. Further research is needed.

## References

1. Plato. The Republic. In Rouse WHD (Trans.) and Warmington EH & Rouse PG, eds.), *Great Dialogues of Plato*. New York, NY: Mentor Books. 1956.
2. Baken RJ. The aged voice: a new hypothesis. *J Voice*. 2005;19(3):317–325.
3. Roy N, Stemple J, Merrill RM, Thomas L. Epidemiology of voice disorders in the elderly: preliminary findings. *Laryngoscope*. 2007;117(4):628–633.
4. Woo P, Casper J, Colton R, Brewer D. Dysphonia in the aging: physiology versus disease. *Laryngoscope*. 1992;102(2):139–144.
5. Kandoğan T, Olgun L, Gültekin G. Causes of dysphonia in patients above 60 years of age. *Kulak Burun Bogaz Ihtis Derg*. 2003;11(5):139–143.
6. Ryu CH, Han S, Lee MS, et al. Voice changes in elderly adults: prevalence and the effect of social, behavioral, and health status on voice quality. *J Am Geriatr Soc*. 2015;63(8):1608–1614.
7. Golub JS, Chen P, Otto K, et al. Prevalence of perceived dysphonia in a geriatric population. *J Am Geriatr Soc*. 2006;54:1736–1739.
8. Turley R, Cohen S. Impact of voice and swallowing problems in the elderly. *Otolaryngol Head Neck Surg*. 2009;140:33–36.
9. Gregory ND, Chandran S, Lurie D, Sataloff RT. Voice disorders in the elderly. *J Voice*. 2012;26(2):254–258.
10. Çiyiltepe M, Şenkal ÖA. The aging voice and voice therapy in geriatrics. *Aging Clin Exp Res*. 2017;29(3):403–410.
11. Martins RH, do Amaral HA, Tavares EL, Martins MG, Goncalves TM, Dias NH. Voice disorders: etiology and diagnosis. *J Voice*. 2016;30(6) 761.e1–761.e9.
12. Ramig LA, Ringel RL. Effects of physiological aging on selected acoustic characteristics of voice. *J Speech Hear Res*. 1983;26(1):22–30.
13. Kendall K. Presbyphonia: a review. *Curr Opin Otolaryngol Head Neck Surg*. 2007;15(3):137–140.
14. Ptacek P, Sander E. Age recognition from voice. *J Speech Hear Res*. 1966;9:353–360.
15. Shipp T, Hollien H. Perceptions of the aging male voice. *J Speech Hear Res*. 1969;12:703–710.
16. Ryan W, Burk K. Perceptual and acoustic correlates in the speech of males. *J Commun Disord*. 1974;7:181–192.
17. Ryan W, Capadano H. Age perceptions and evaluative reactions toward adult speakers. *J Gerontol*. 1978;33:98–102.
18. Hartman D. The perceptual identity and characteristics of aging in normal male adult speakers. *J Commun Disord*. 1979;12:53–61.
19. Honjo I, Isshiki N. Laryngoscopic and voice characteristics of aged persons. *Arch Otolaryngol*. 1980;106(3):149–150.
20. Linville SE. Acoustic-perceptual studies of aging voice in women. *J Voice*. 1987;1(1):44–48.
21. Ferrand CT. Harmonics-to-noise ratio: an index of vocal aging. *J Voice*. 2002;16(4):480–487.
22. Harnsberger JD, Brown WS, Shrivastav R, Rothman H. Noise and tremor in the perception of vocal aging in males. *J Voice*. 2010;24(5):523–530.
23. Kahane JC. Connective tissue changes in the larynx and their effects on voice. *J Voice*. 1987;1(1):27–30.
24. Segre R. Senescence of the voice. *Eye Ear Nose Throat Mon*. 1971;50:62–68.
25. de Pinto O, Hollien H. Speaking fundamental frequency characteristics of Australian women: then and now. *J Phonetics*. 1982;10(4): 367–375.
26. Russell A, Penny L, Pemberton C. Speaking fundamental frequency changes over time in women: a longitudinal study. *J Speech Lang Hear Res*. 1995;38(1):101–109.
27. Krook MI. Speaking fundamental frequency characteristics of normal Swedish subjects obtained by glottal frequency analysis. *Folia Phoniatr Logopaed*. 1988;40(2):82–90.
28. Endres W, Bambach W, Flösser G. Voice spectrograms as a function of age, voice disguise, and voice imitation. *J Acoust Soc Amer*. 1971;49(6B):1842–1848.
29. Benjamin BJ. Frequency variability in the aged voice. *J Gerontol*. 1981;36(6):722–726.
30. Morris RJ, Brown Jr WS. Age-related differences in speech intensity among adult females. *Folia Phoniatr Logopaed*. 1994;46(2):64–69.
31. Baker KK, Ramig LO, Sapir S, Luschei ES, Smith ME. Control of vocal loudness in young and old adults. *J Speech Lang Hear Res*. 2001;44(2):297–305.
32. Hodge FS, Colton RH, Kelley RT. Vocal intensity characteristics in normal and elderly speakers. *J Voice*. 2001;15(4):503–511.
33. de Menezes KS, Master S, Guzman M, Bortnem C, Ramos LR. Differences in acoustic and perceptual

parameters of the voice between elderly and young women at habitual and high intensity. *Acta Otorrinolaringologica* (English ed). 2014;65(2):76–84.

34. Linville SE, Fisher HB. Acoustic characteristics of perceived versus actual vocal age in controlled phonation by adult females. *J Acoust Soc Amer*. 1985;78(1):40–48.

35. Scukanec GP, Petrosino L, Squibb K. Formant frequency characteristics of children, young adult, and aged female speakers. *Percep Motor Skills*. 1991;73(1):203–208.

36. Linville SE, Rens J. Vocal tract resonance analysis of aging voice using long-term average spectra. *J Voice*. 2001;15(3):323–330.

37. National Osteoporosis Foundation Washington, DC; 1998.

38. Xue SA, Hao GJ. Changes in the human vocal tract due to aging and the acoustic correlates of speech production: a pilot study. *J Speech Lang Hear Res*. 2003;46(3): 689–701.

39. Eichhorn JT, Kent RD, Austin D, Vorperian HK. Effects of aging on vocal fundamental frequency and vowel formants in men and women. *J Voice*. In press.

40. Hoit JD, Hixon TJ. Age and laryngeal airway resistance during vowel production in women. *J Speech Lang Hear Res*. 1992;35(2):309–313.

41. Sapienza CM, Dutka J. Glottal airflow characteristics of women's voice production along an aging continuum. *J Speech Lang Hear Res*. 1996;39(2):322–328.

42. Melcon MC, Hoit JD, Hixon TJ. Age and laryngeal airway resistance during vowel production. *J Speech Hear Dis*. 1989;54(2):282–286.

43. Holmes LC, Leeper HA, Nicholson IR. Laryngeal airway resistance of older men and women as a function of vocal sound pressure level. *J Speech Lang Hear Res*. 1994;37(4):789–799.

44. Linville SE, Skarin BD, Fornatto E. The interrelationship of measures related to vocal function, speech rate, and laryngeal appearance in elderly women. *J Speech Hear Res*. 1989;32(2):323–330.

45. Linville SE. Glottal gap configurations in two age groups of women. *J Speech Lang Hear Res*. 1992;35(6):1209–1215.

46. Biever DM, Bless DM. Vibratory characteristics of the vocal folds in young adult and geriatric women. *J Voice*. 1989;3(2):120–131.

47. Pontes P, Brasolotto A, Behlau M. Glottic characteristics and voice complaint in the elderly. *J Voice*. 2005; 19(1):84–94.

48. Pontes P, Yamasaki R, Behlau M. Morphological and functional aspects of the senile larynx. *Folia Phoniatr Logopaed*. 2006;58(3):151–158.

49. Takano S, Kimura M, Nito T, Imagawa H, Sakakibara KI, Tayama N. Clinical analysis of presbylarynx—vocal fold atrophy in elderly individuals. *Auris Nasus Larynx*. 2010;37(4):461–464.

50. Bloch I, Behrman A. Quantitative analysis of videostroboscopic images in presbylarynges. *Laryngoscope*. 2001; 111 (11 pt 1):2022–2027.

51. Winkler R, Sendlmeier W. EGG open quotient in aging voices—changes with increasing chronological age and its perception. *Logoped Phoniatr Vocol*. 2006;31(2):51–56.

52. Yamauchi A, Yokonishi H, Imagawa H, et al. Vocal fold vibration in vocal fold atrophy: quantitative analysis with high-speed digital imaging. *J Voice*. 2015;29(6): 755–762.

53. Ahmad K, Yan Y, Bless D. Vocal fold vibratory characteristics of healthy geriatric females—analysis of high-speed digital images. *J Voice*. 2012;26(6):751–759.

54. Vaca M, Cobeta I, Mora E, Reyes P. Clinical assessment of glottal insufficiency in age-related dysphonia. *J Voice*. 2017;31(1):128–e1.

55. Sataloff RT. The effects of age on the voice. In: Sataloff RT. *Professional Voice: The Science and Art of Clinical Care*. 4th ed. San Diego, CA: Plural Publishing: 2017: 585–604.

56. Vaca M, Mora E, Cobeta I. The aging voice: influence of respiratory and laryngeal changes. *Otolaryngol Head Neck Surg*. 2015;153(3):409–413.

57. Hirano M, Kurita S, Sakaguchi S. Ageing of the vibratory tissue of human vocal folds. *Acta Oto-laryngol*. 1989;107(5-6):428–433.

58. Gonçalves TM, dos Santos DC, Pessin AB, Martins RH. Scanning electron microscopy of the presbylarynx. *Otolaryngol Head Neck Surg*. 2016;154(6):1073–1078.

59. Gonçalves TM, Martins RH, Adriana BB. Transmission electron microscopy of the presbylarynx in the process of voice aging. *J Voice*. In press.

60. Hirano M, Kurita S, Nakashima T. Growth, development and aging of human vocal folds. *Vocal Fold Physiology: Contemporary Research and Clinical Issues*. 1983: 22–43.

61. Sivasankar M, Ivanisevic A. Atomic force microscopy investigation of vocal fold collagen. *Laryngoscope*. 2007; 117(10):1876–1881.

62. Ishii K, Zhai WG, Akita M, Hirose H. Ultrastructure of the lamina propria of the human vocal fold. *Acta Oto-laryngol*. 1996;116(5):778–782.

63. Roberts T, Morton R, Al-Ali S. Microstructure of the vocal fold in elderly humans. *Clin Anat*. 2011;24(5):544–551.

64. Sato K, Hirano M, Nakashima T. Age-related changes of collagenous fibers in the human vocal fold mucosa. *Ann Otol Rhinol Laryngol*. 2002;111(1):15–20.

65. Hirano M, Kurita S, Sakaguchi S. Aging of the vibratory tissue of human vocal folds. *Acta Otolaryngol (Stockh)*. 1989;107:428–433.

66. Ohno T, Yoo MJ, Swanson ER, Hirano S, Ossoff RH, Rousseau B. Regenerative effects of basic fibroblast growth factor on extracellular matrix production in aged rat vocal folds. *Ann Otol Rhinol Laryngol*. 2009;118(8): 559–564.

67. Awd Allah RS, Dkhil MA, Farhoud E. Fibroblasts in the human vocal fold mucosa: an ultrastructural study of different age groups. *Singapore Med J*. 2009;50(2):201.

68. Sato K, Hirano M. Age-related changes of the macula flava of the human vocal fold. *Ann Otol Rhinol Laryngol*. 1995;104(11):839–844.

69. Filho JA, do Nascimento PH, Tsuji DH, Sennes LU. Histologic changes in human vocal folds correlated with aging: a histomorphometric study. *Ann Otol Rhinol Laryngol*. 2003;112(10):894–898.

70. Chan RW, Titze IR. Viscoelastic shear properties of human vocal fold mucosa: measurement methodology and empirical results. *J Acoust Soc Am*. 1999;106(4):2008–2021.

71. Martins RH, Pessin B, Bueno A, et al. Aging voice and the laryngeal muscle atrophy. *Laryngoscope*. 2015;125(11):2518–2521.

72. Malmgren LT, Fisher PJ, Bookman LM, Uno T. Age-related changes in muscle fiber types in the human thyroarytenoid muscle: an immunohistochemical and stereological study using confocal laser scanning microscopy. *Otolaryngol Head Neck Surg*. 1999;121(4):441–451.

73. Sataloff RT, Kost KM. Voice disorders in the elderly. In: Sataloff RT, Johns MM, Kost KM, eds. *Geriatric Otolaryngology*. New York, NY: Thieme; 2015: 154–164.

74. Nakai T, Goto N, Moriyama H, Shiraishi N, Nonaka N. The human recurrent laryngeal nerve during the aging process. *Okajimas Folia Anat Jpn*. 2000;76(6):363–367.

75. Connor NP, Suzuki T, Sewall GK, Lee K, Heisey DM. Neuromuscular junction changes in aged rat thyroarytenoid muscle. *Ann Otol Rhinol Laryngol*. 2002;111(7):579–586.

76. Suzuki T, Bless DM, Connor NP, Ford CN, Lee K, Inagi K. Age-related alterations in myosin heavy chain isoforms in rat intrinsic laryngeal muscles. *Ann Otol Rhinol Laryngol*. 2002;111(11):962–967.

77. Benjamin B. Phonological performance in gerontologic speech. *J Psycholinguist Res*. 1982; 11: 159–167.

78. Benjamin B. Speech production of normally aging adults. *Sem Speech Lang*. 1997; 18: 135–141.

79. Rastatter M, Jacques R. Formant frequency structure of the aging male and female vocal tract. *Folia Phoniatr*. 1990; 42: 312–319.

80. Rastatter M, McGuire R, Kalinowski J, Stuart A. Formant frequency characteristics of elderly speakers in contextual speech. *Folia Phoniatr Logop*. 1997; 49: 1–8.

81. Liss J, Weismer G, Rosenbek J. Selected acoustic characteristics of speech production in very old males. *J Gerontol Psychol Sci*. 1990; 45: 35–45.

82. Titze IE. *Principles of Voice Production*. Englewood Cliffs, NJ:Prentice-Hall; 1994.

83. Ferreri G. Senescence of the larynx. *Ital Gen Rev Oto-Rhino-Laryngol*. 1959; 1: 640–709.

84. Kahane J. Age-related histological changes in the human male and female laryngeal cartilages: biological and functional implications. In: Lawrence V, ed. *Transcripts of the Ninth Symposium: Care of the Professional Voice*. New York, NY: The Voice Foundation; 1980.

85. Costa HO, Matias C. Vocal impact on quality of life of elderly female subjects. *Braz J Otorhinolaryngol*. 2005;71(2):172–178.

86. Verdonck-de Leeuw I, Mahieu H. Vocal aging and the impact on daily life: a longitudinal study. *J Voice*. 2004;18(2):193–202.

87. de Machado FC, Lessa MM, Cielo CA, Barbosa LH. Spectrographic acoustic vocal characteristics of elderly women engaged in aerobics. *J Voice*. 2016;30(5):579–586.

88. Gorman S, Weinrich B, Lee L, Stemple JC. Aerodynamic changes as a result of vocal function exercises in elderly men. *Laryngoscope*. 2008;118(10):1900–1903.

89. Kaneko M, Hirano S, Tateya I, et al. Multidimensional analysis on the effect of vocal function exercises on aged vocal fold atrophy. *J Voice*. 2015;29(5):638–644.

90. Oates JM. Treatment of dysphonia in older people: the role of the speech therapist. *Curr Opin Otolaryngol Head Neck Surg*. 2014;22(6):477–486.

91. Prakup B. Acoustic measures of the voices of older singers and nonsingers. *J Voice*. 2012;26(3):341–350.

92. Lortie CL, Rivard J, Thibeault M, Tremblay P. The moderating effect of frequent singing on voice aging. *J Voice*. 2017;31(1):112–e1.

93. Sachs AM, Bielamowicz SA, Stager SV. Treatment effectiveness for aging changes in the larynx. *Laryngoscope*. 2017;127(11):2572–2577.

94. Andreatta RD, Stemple JC, Seward TS, McMullen CA. Subcutaneous Neurotrophin 4 infusion using osmotic pumps or direct muscular injection enhances aging rat laryngeal muscles. *J Visual Exp*. 2017 (124).

95. Ohno T, Hirano S. Treatment of aging vocal folds: novel approaches. *Curr Opin Otolaryngol Head Neck Surg*. 2014;22(6):472–476.

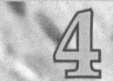

# Common Medical Diagnoses and Treatments in Patients With Voice Disorders: An Introduction and Overview

*Robert Thayer Sataloff, Mary J. Hawkshaw, and Johnathan B. Sataloff*

Laryngologists specializing in voice devote the majority of their practices to the medical management of benign voice disorders. Indeed, although most of us are active surgeons, the good voice specialist takes pride in avoiding the need for laryngeal surgery through expert medical management. Success depends not only on a good laryngologist but also on the availability of a voice team, including a speech-language pathologist, voice scientist, singing voice specialist, and medical consultants who have acquired special knowledge about voice disorders (neurologists, pulmonologists, endocrinologists, internists, allergists, and others). This chapter provides an overview of many of the benign voice problems encountered by otolaryngologists and current nonsurgical management concepts.

Numerous medical conditions adversely affect the voice. Many have their origins primarily outside the head and neck. This chapter is not intended to be all-inclusive but rather to highlight some of the more common and important conditions found in professional voice users seeking medical care.

In the 2286 cases of all forms of voice disorders reported by Brodnitz in 1971,[1] 80% were attributed to voice abuse or to psychogenic factors resulting in vocal dysfunction. Of these patients, 20% had organic voice disorders. Of women with organic problems, about 15% had identifiable endocrine causes. A much higher incidence of organic disorders, particularly reflux laryngitis, acute infectious laryngitis, and benign vocal fold masses, is found in one of the author's practice.

## Voice Abuse

When voice abuse is suspected or observed in a patient with vocal complaints, he or she should be referred to a laryngologist who specializes in voice, preferably a physician affiliated with a voice care team.

Common patterns of voice abuse and misuse will not be discussed in detail in this chapter. They are covered elsewhere in the literature[2] and elsewhere in this book. Voice abuse and/or misuse should be suspected particularly in patients who complain of voice fatigue associated with voice use, whose voices are worse at the end of a working day or week, and in any patient who is chronically hoarse. Technical errors in voice use may be the primary etiology of a voice complaint or may develop secondarily as a result of a patient's efforts to compensate for voice disturbance from another cause.

Speaking in noisy environments, such as cars and airplanes, is particularly abusive to the voice, as are backstage greetings, postperformance parties, choral conducting, voice teaching, and cheerleading, to name a few. With proper training, all these vocal activities can be done safely. However, most patients, surprisingly even singers, have little or no training for their speaking voice.

If voice abuse is caused by speaking, treatment should be provided by a licensed, certified speech-language pathologist in the United States or by a phoniatrist in many other countries. Training the speaking voice in many cases will benefit singers greatly not only by improving speech but also by indirectly helping singing technique. Physicians should not hesitate to recommend such training, but it should be performed by an expert speech-language pathologist who specializes in voice. Many speech-language pathologists who are well trained in swallowing rehabilitation, articulation therapy, and other techniques are not trained in voice therapy for the speaking voice, and virtually none are trained through their speech and language programs to work with singing.

Specialized singing training also may be helpful to some voice patients who are not singers, and it is invaluable for patients who are singers. Initial singing training teaches relaxation techniques, develops muscle strength, and is symbiotic with standard speech therapy. Abuse of the voice during singing is an even more complex problem, as discussed elsewhere in this book.

## Infection and Inflammation

### Upper Respiratory Tract Infection Without Laryngitis

Although mucosal irritation usually is diffuse, patients sometimes have marked nasal obstruction with little or no sore throat and a "normal" voice. If the laryngeal examination showed no abnormality, a singer or professional speaker with a "head cold" should be permitted to use his or her voice and be advised not to try to duplicate his or her usual sound but rather accept the insurmountable alterations in self-perception caused by the change in the supra-glottic vocal tract and auditory system. The decision as to whether performing under the circumstances is advisable professionally rests with the voice professional and his or her musical associates. The patient should be cautioned against throat clearing, as this traumatic and may produce laryngitis. If a cough is present, nonnarcotic medications should be used to suppress it. In addition, the patient should be taught how to "silent cough," which is less traumatic.

### Laryngitis With Serious Vocal Fold Injury

Hemorrhage in the vocal folds and mucosal disruption associated with acute laryngitis are contraindications to speaking and singing. When these are observed, treatment includes strict voice rest in addition to correction of any underlying disease. Vocal fold hemorrhage in voice professionals is most common in premenstrual women who are using aspirin products or nonsteroidal anti-inflammatory drugs (NSAIDS) for dysmenorrhea. Severe hemorrhage or mucosal scarring may result in permanent alternations in vocal fold vibratory function. In rare instances, surgical intervention may be necessary. The potential gravity of these conditions must be stressed, for singers are generally reluctant to cancel an appearance. As von Leden observed, it is a pleasure to work with "people who are determined that the show must go on when everyone else is determined to goof off."[3] However, patient compliance is essential when serious damage has occurred. At present, acute treatment of vocal fold hemorrhage is controversial. Most laryngologists allow the hematoma to resolve spontaneously. Because this sometimes results in an organized hematoma and scar formation requiring surgery, some physicians advocate incision along the superior edge of the vocal fold and drainage of the hematoma in selected cases. Further study is needed to determine optimal therapy guidelines (Figures 4–1 and 4–2).

### Laryngitis Without Serious Damage

Mild to moderate edema and erythema of the vocal folds may result from infection or from noninfectious causes. In the absence of mucosal disruption or hemorrhage, they are not absolute contraindications to voice use. Noninfectious laryngitis commonly is associated with excessive voice use in preperformance rehearsals. It may also be caused by other forms of voice abuse and by mucosal irritation produced by allergy, smoke inhalation, and other causes. Mucous stranding between the anterior and middle thirds of the vocal folds is seen commonly in inflammatory laryngitis. Laryngitis sicca is associated with dehydration, dry atmosphere, mouth breathing, and antihistamine therapy. Deficiency of mucosal lubrication causes irritation and coughing and results in mild inflammation. If no pressing professional need for performance exists, inflammatory conditions of the larynx are best treated with relative voice rest in addition to other modalities. However, in some instances, speaking and singing may be permitted. The patient should be instructed to avoid all forms of irritation and to rest the voice at all times except during warm-up and performance. Corticosteroids and other medications discussed later may be helpful. If mucosal secretions are copious, low-dose antihistamine therapy may be beneficial, but it must be prescribed with caution and should generally be avoided. Copious, thin secretions are better than scant, thick secretions or excessive dryness. The

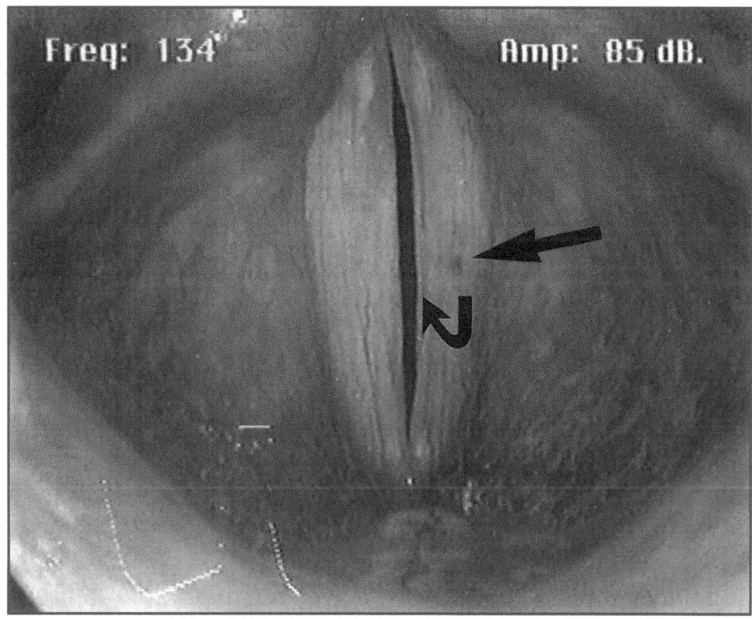

**Figure 4–1.** Video print obtained from a strobovideolaryngoscopic examination shows diffuse erythema from acute laryngitis. Additionally, there is a left sulcus vocalis. Also visible is an ecstatic vessel on the superior surface of the left vocal fold (*straight arrow*). (Figure 40–1 from Sataloff RT et al.[4])

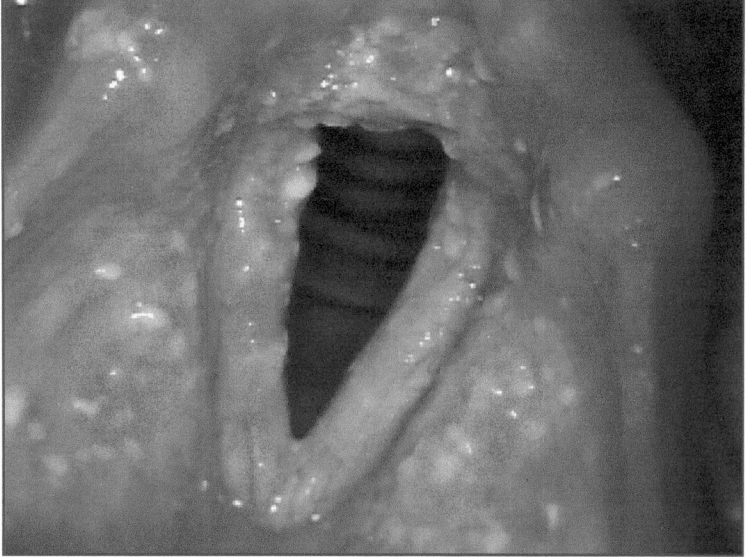

**Figure 4–2.** Strobovideolaryngoscopy in this 65-year-old female shows the white, lacy, diffuse plaques embedded in inflamed mucosal surfaces. This appearance is typical of fungal laryngitis, caused most commonly by *Candida albicans*. (Figure 45–1 from Sataloff RT et al.[4])

patient with laryngitis must be kept well hydrated to maintain the desired character of mucosal lubrication. The patient should be instructed to "pee pale," consuming enough water to keep urine diluted. Psychological support is crucial. For example, it is often helpful for the physician to intercede on a singer's behalf and to convey "doctor's orders" directly to agents or theater management. Such mitigation of exogenous stress can be highly therapeutic.

Infectious laryngitis may be caused by bacteria or viruses. Subglottic involvement frequently indicates a more severe infection, which may be difficult to control in a short period of time. Indiscriminate use of antibiotics must be avoided; however, when the physician is in doubt as to the cause and when a major voice commitment is imminent, vigorous antibiotic treatment is warranted. In this circumstance, the damage caused by allowing progression of a curable condition is greater than the damage that might result from a course of therapy for an unproven microorganism while culture results are pending. When a major concert or speech is not imminent, indications for therapy are the same as for the nonsinger or nonprofessional speaker.

Voice rest (absolute or relative) is an important therapeutic consideration in any case of laryngitis. When no professional commitments are pending, a short course of absolute voice rest may be considered, as it is the safest and most conservative therapeutic intervention. This means absolute silence and communication with a writing pad. The patient must be instructed not to whisper, as this may be an even more traumatic vocal activity than speaking softly. Whispering through the lips also involves vocal fold activity and should not be permitted. The playing of many musical wind instruments also should not be permitted. Absolute voice rest is *necessary* only for serious vocal fold injury such as hemorrhage or mucosal disruption (Figure 4–3). Even then, it is virtually never indicated for more than 7 to 10 days. Three days are often sufficient. Some excellent laryngologists do not believe voice rest should be used at all. However, absolute voice rest for a few days may be helpful in patients with laryngitis, especially those gregarious, verbal singers who find it difficult to moderate their voice use to comply with relative voice rest instructions. In many instances, considerations of finances and reputation mitigate against a recommendation of voice rest. In advising performers to minimize vocal use, Punt counseled, "Don't say a single word for which you are not being paid."[4] This admonition frequently guides the ailing singer or speaker away from preperformance conversations and backstage greetings and allows a successful series of performances. Patients should also be instructed to speak softly and as infrequently as possible, often at a slightly higher pitch than usual; to avoid excessive telephone use; and to speak with abdominal support as they would in singing. This is relative voice rest, and it is helpful in most cases. An urgent session with

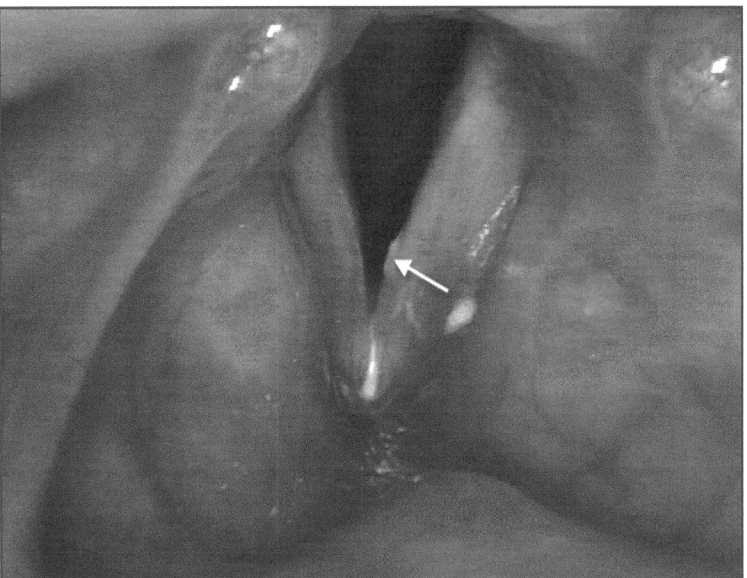

**Figure 4–3.** Mucosal tear (*arrow*) of the vibratory margin of the left vocal fold in a 27-year-old tenor with sudden voice change. This lesion resolved completely with voice rest. (Figure 58–1 from Sataloff RT et al.[4])

a speech-language pathologist is extremely helpful for discussing vocal hygiene and in providing guidelines to prevent voice abuse. Nevertheless, the patient must be aware that some risk is associated with performing with laryngitis even when performance is possible. Inflammation of the vocal folds is associated with increased capillary fragility and increased risk of vocal fold injury or hemorrhage. Many factors must be considered in determining whether a given speech or concert is important enough to justify the potential consequences.

Steam inhalations deliver moisture and heat to the vocal folds and tracheobronchial tree and may be useful. Some people use nasal irrigations, although these have little proven value. Gargling has no proven efficacy, but it is probably harmful only if it involves loud, abusive vocalization as part of the gargling process. Some physicians and patients believe it to be helpful in "moistening the throat," and it may have some relaxing or placebo effect. Ultrasonic treatments, local massage, psychotherapy, and biofeedback directed at relieving anxiety and decreasing muscle tension may be helpful adjuncts to a broader therapeutic program. However, psychotherapy and biofeedback, in particular, must be expertly supervised if used at all.

Voice lessons given by an expert teacher are invaluable. When technical dysfunction is suggested, the singer or actor should be referred to his or her teacher. Even when an obvious organic abnormality is present, referral to a voice teacher is appropriate, especially for younger actors and singers. Numerous "tricks of the trade" permit a voice professional to overcome some of the impairments of mild illness safely. If a singer plans to proceed with a performance during an illness, he or she should not cancel voice lessons as part of the relative voice rest regimen; rather, a short lesson to ensure optimal technique is extremely useful.

## Sinusitis

Chronic inflammation of the mucosa lining the sinus cavities commonly produces thick secretions known as postnasal drip. Postnasal drip can be particularly problematic because it causes excessive phlegm, which interferes with phonation, and because it leads to frequent throat clearing, which may inflame the vocal folds. Sometimes chronic sinusitis is caused by allergies and can be treated with medications. However, many medications used for this condition cause side effects that are unacceptable in professional voice users, particularly mucosal drying. When medication management is not satisfactory,

functional endoscopic sinus surgery may be appropriate.[5] Acute purulent sinusitis is a different matter. It requires aggressive treatment with antibiotics, sometimes surgical drainage, treatment of underlying conditions (such as dental abscess), and occasionally surgery.[5]

## Lower Respiratory Tract Infection

Lower respiratory tract infection may be almost as disruptive to a voice as upper respiratory tract infection. Bronchitis, pneumonitis, pneumonia, and especially reactive airway disease impair the power source of the voice and lead to vocal strain and sometimes injury. Lower respiratory tract infections should be treated aggressively, pulmonary function tests should be considered, and bronchodilators (preferably oral) should be used as necessary. Coughing is also a very traumatic vocal activity, and careful attention should be paid to cough suppression. If extensive voice use is anticipated, nonnarcotic antitussive agents are preferable because narcotics may dull the sensorium and lead to potentially damaging voice technique.

## Tonsillitis

Tonsillitis also impairs the voice through alterations of the resonator system and through technical changes secondary to pain. Although there is a tendency to avoid tonsillectomy, especially in professional voice users, the operation should not be withheld when clear indications for tonsillectomy are present. These include, for example, documented severe bacterial tonsillitis 6 times per year. However, patients must be warned that tonsillectomy may alter the sound of the voice, even though there is no change at the vocal fold (oscillator) level.

## Lyme Disease

Lyme disease, as it is known today, has been reported for over a hundred years, but the bacteria responsible for the disease was not identified until 1982. It was discovered in Lyme, Connecticut, when a group of children contracted arthritis inexplicably, and research was initiated to identify the cause.[6] Due to its ability to appear similar to many other diseases and its wide range of nonspecific symptoms, Lyme disease often goes undiagnosed. If not recognized and treated, this condition can have profound consequences including damage to the inner ear, the 8th cranial nerve, and the facial nerve as reviewed by Sataloff and Sataloff (from which a portion of this section has been modified, with permission)[7]. It can also affect laryngeal mewes.

Lyme disease is one of many common illnesses that can cause special problems for singers and other voice professionals. Lyme disease is an increasingly prevalent infection in many parts of the United States and elsewhere. It can affect the larynx directly by causing unilateral or bilateral vocal fold paresis/paralysis or interfere with other parts of the vocal tract by causing joint pains that impair posture and support, temporomandibular joint pain that leads to technical changes, and in other ways.[8] It is important for singing teachers and singers to be familiar with this common problem in order to improve the chances of prompt diagnosis and treatment.

### Epidemiology

In the United States, Lyme disease is known to be endemic particularly in northeastern, mid-Atlantic, and north-central states, with recent expansion into some parts of the southwest.[9] Approximately 60% of initial infections occur during the summer, when it's warm and people are outside.[10] Lyme disease has no sex or age predilection.

### Etiology

Lyme disease is an illness caused by a spirochete infection. Like syphilis, another spirochete infectious process, the clinical presentations may vary. Sir William Osler once termed syphilis "the great imitator," and likewise, Lyme disease has a broad clinical spectrum.

Lyme disease had many different names given to it until Steere, in 1977, recognized it as a multistage systemic disease.[11] In 1982, Burgdorfer et al isolated the infectious organism from the belly of a tick, while studying a group of children in Lyme, Connecticut, with unexplained arthritis.[12] He named this spirochete *Borrelia burgdorferi*. *Borrelia burgdorferi* is the primary cause of Lyme disease. However, *Borrelia garinii* and *Borrelia afzelii* also had been implicated and reported as common causes of Lyme neuroborreliosis in Europe.[13] Many different vectors have been listed as contributors to this disease. However, the tick seems to be the main culprit transmitting the spirochete. In the Northeast, the tick *Ixodes dammini* is the most common, and in the West, *Ixodes pacificus* has been named.[9] The ticks carry the disease in their stomachs and transmit it while feeding on the blood of their victims which can take up to 2 days. In many cases, the ticks are noticed and removed or washed away before the disease can be spread; but some-

times a tick is small enough to avoid notice. Even when definitive symptoms occur, the tick often is not found, and the classic target rash may have been absent or gone unnoticed, as well. Therefore, the opportunity for early diagnosis often is missed, and many people carry Lyme disease into later stages of the disorder, during which nerve and vascular problems can occur, before the condition is diagnosed.[7]

The tick life cycle has 3 stages: larva, nymph, and adult.[11] In each stage the tick acquires a blood meal and may obtain the spirochete from an infected host such as the white-tailed deer or white-footed mouse.

The exact nature of injury to the human is not known, but evidence exists for 3 possible mechanisms. These theories include direct invasion, immunological attack, and vasculitis.[14]

### Otolaryngologic Findings

The clinical spectrum of Lyme disease is broken down into 3 stages. In stage 1, a rash named erythema chronicum migrans follows the tick bite in 6% to 80% of cases.[15] The rash has an outer red circular or oval border with a clear central area. These lesions have led to the term "target rash." The outer red zone is felt to represent the best area for biopsy when trying to isolate the organism for culture. This rash may follow or precede cold or flu-like symptoms. The rash usually occurs within a few days of the tick bite but may show up as long as a month later.[16]

Other symptoms during this stage include fatigue, fever, chills, sore throat, headache, cough, chest pain, abdominal pain, muscle aches, loss of appetite, dizziness, lymphadenopathy, backache, conjunctivitis, enlarged liver and spleen, arthritis, and low-grade fever.

The patient usually calls on an otolaryngologist during stage 2 of Lyme disease. Although facial paralysis is the most common complaint in these patients, other symptoms may occur.[10,17] Patients may have symptoms such as hoarseness from involvement of the recurrent laryngeal nerve or inability to sustain a high note or project the voice due to injury to the superior laryngeal nerve. In 1988, Schroeter reported a case of a 45-year-old singer who developed a left vocal fold paralysis and had positive antibodies to *Borrelia burgdorferi*.[18] The patient was treated with antibiotics for 6 weeks, during which time there was resolution of the vocal fold paralysis and dramatic reduction of the Lyme titers.

Stage 2 also may include a skin lesion called lymphadenosis benigna cutis. This lesion has another name, Borrelia lymphocytoma, and is characterized by lymphocytic infiltration of the dermis or subcutaneous tissue.[19] The lesion has a blue-red color with gross swelling.

Patients may have involvement of the temporomandibular joint and complain of ear pain or pain when chewing. Other joints may be involved, such as the neck, knees, hips, shoulders, ankles, or elbows.

Patients also may have involvement of the cardiovascular system and may develop arrhythmias and/or lightheadedness. Failure to recognize any of these lesions may lead to increased morbidity and possible death.

Another skin lesion is seen in stage 3 of Lyme disease. It is termed *acrodermatitis chronic atrophicans*.[19] This lesion usually is seen in elderly patients and is often misdiagnosed as scleroderma or vascular insufficiency.

### Diagnosis and Treatment

The ELISA test is the most sensitive and is used widely for Lyme disease.[14] Western blot technique is used to confirm the diagnosis. Other assays such as immunofluorescence antibody and cultures have been utilized with varying success. Results of all of these studies vary from lab to lab, and blood samples should be sent to labs that do large volumes of testing and have experience. The IgM antibody is seen early and is less specific. However, it is useful when reinfection or reactivation is suspected. The IgG may take 6 weeks to appear and is good for assessing stages 2 and 3. False-positive tests occur in patients with mononucleosis, syphilis, or rheumatic fever.[9,14] False-negatives may be seen in patients on antibiotics or patients who are immunocompromised by diseases such as cancer or AIDS.

Antibiotics are the recommended treatment. For adults, doxycycline or tetracycline is effective. When intolerance to these medications is encountered, amoxicillin is used. Amoxicillin is preferred in children. Chloramphenicol may be used with allergy to cephalosporin or penicillin. When resistance to these medications is found, intravenous medication such as ceftriaxone is used. Lyme disease is complex; with proper recognition it is treatable and has an excellent prognosis.

### Autoimmune Deficiency Syndrome (AIDS)

AIDS is a lethal disease that is becoming more and more common. Its incidence in the artistic community is probably somewhat higher than in the general public. Physicians should consider this diagnosis along with other causes of chronic debilitation and recurrent infections in the proper clinical setting in professional voice users. Dry mouth and hoarseness are common complaints in patients with HIV infection. *Candida* infection of the oral cavity or tracheobronchial tree should make the clinician particularly suspicious. When fungal infections are encountered, particularly fungal laryngitis, it is important not only to treat the infection, but also to rule out serious predisposing causes such as HIV infection and other conditions that suppress the immune system. Recurrent respiratory tract infection and infection with unusual organisms also raise one's suspicions, but it should be remembered that infections with *Haemophilus influenza, Streptococcus pneumonia,* and common viruses are the most frequent pathogens in HIV-infected patients, just as they are in patients without HIV. Acute infectious laryngitis and epiglottis may occur in AIDS patients, but they are less common than mild chronic laryngitis, dry mouth, and frequent or persistent symptoms of a "cold."

## Other Diseases That May Affect the Voice

The larynx is subject to numerous acute and chronic infections. Some of them may be mistaken for malignancy and may be biopsied unnecessarily, exposing the patient (and sometimes the physician) to unnecessary risk. Tuberculosis, for example, is still seen in modern practice. Although laryngeal lesions used to be associated with extensive pulmonary infection, they are now usually associated with much less virulent disease, often only a mild cough. Laryngeal tuberculosis lesions usually are localized.[20,21] Sarcoidosis, another granulomatous disease, causes laryngeal symptoms in roughly 3% to 5% of cases.[22] Noncaseating granulomas are found in the larynx, and the false vocal folds are frequently involved, producing airway obstruction rather than dysphonia. Less common diseases including leprosy,[23,24] syphilis,[25] scleroderma,[26] typhoid,[27] typhus, anthrax, and other conditions, can produce laryngeal lesions that might lead the laryngologist to obtain an unnecessary biopsy. Confusing lesions also may be caused by a variety of mycotic infections including histoplasmosis,[28–30] coccidioidomycosis,[31] cryptococcosis,[32] blastomycosis,[30–34] actinomycosis,[35,36] candidiasis,[37] aspergillosis,[38–40] mucormycosis,[41] rhinosporidiosis,[42] and sporotrichosis.[43] Parasitic diseases may also produce laryngeal masses. The most prominent example is leishmaniasis.[44] More detailed information about most of the conditions discussed above is available in a text by Michaels[45] and elsewhere in this book.

Collagen vascular diseases and other unusual problems may produce laryngeal masses. Rheumatoid arthritis may produce not only disease of the cricoarytenoid and cricothyroid joints, but also consequent neuropathic muscle atrophy[46] and rheumatoid nodules of the larynx.[47] Rheumatoid arthritis with or without nodules may produce respiratory obstruction. Gout may cause laryngeal arthritis. In addition, gouty tophi may appear as white submucosal masses of the true vocal fold. They consist of sodium urate crystals in fibrous tissue and have been documented well.[48,49] Amyloidosis of the larynx is rare but well recognized,[50–53] as discussed in other chapters. Urbach-Wiethe disease (lipoid proteinosis)[54] often involves the mucous membrane of the larynx, usually the vocal folds, aryepiglottic fold, and epiglottis. Other conditions, such as granulomatosis with polyangiitis (Wegener granulomatosis) and relapsing polychondritis, also may involve the larynx. They are less likely to produce discrete nodules, but the diffuse edema associated with chondritis and necrotizing granulomas may produce substantial laryngeal and voice abnormalities. Unusual laryngeal masses also may be caused by trauma. Trauma is discussed in detail elsewhere in this book, but the physician must be careful to inquire about laryngeal trauma, the consequences of which may not be recognized until months or years after the injury.

A few rare skin lesions also may involve the larynx producing symptomatic lesions, and sometimes airway obstruction. These include pemphigus vulgaris, seen in adults between 40 and 60 years of age. Pemphigus lesions may involve the mucosa, including the epiglottis.[55] Epidermolysis bullosa describes a group of congenital vesicular disorders usually seen at birth or shortly thereafter. This condition may cause laryngeal stenosis, or large, bleb-like vocal fold masses. Some viral conditions may cause laryngeal structural pathology, most notably papillomata. However, herpes, variola, and other organisms also have been implicated in laryngeal infection.

There are numerous other conditions, many of which are not covered comprehensively in this book, that may affect voices adversely. Most of them are not common problems among professional voice users. However, the laryngologist should remember that laryngeal manifestations of many systemic diseases may cause voice changes that bring the patient to medical attention for the first time. We must remain alert for their presence and think of them particularly when more common, obvious etiologies are not identified, or when patients do not respond to treatment as expected. The voice may be affected by the following problems not discussed above (among others): acromegaly, Arnold-Chiari malformations, blood dyscrasias, neurologic disease (vocal fold paralysis), collagen vascular disease (including

rheumatoid arthritis, systemic lupus erythematosus, scleroderma, Sjögren's syndrome, and others), deafness, gout, Hodgkin's disease, leprosy, lymphoma, Madelung's disease, malignancies, myopathies, a myriad of infectious diseases (bacterial, viral, granulomatous, and fungal), mononucleosis, numerous syndromes (Basedow's, adrenogenital syndrome, Down's syndrome, hereditary angioedema, Kleinfelter's syndrome, Melkersson-Rosenthal syndrome, pachyonychia congenita, short stature syndromes, Shy-Drager syndrome, and many others), syphilis, sarcoidosis, tuberculosis, Crohn's disease, Wilson's disease, and other chronic diseases.

## Systemic Conditions

### Aging

This subject is so important that is has been covered extensively in other literature.[56] Many characteristics associated with vocal aging are actually deficits in conditioning, rather than irreversible aging changes. For example, in singers, such problems as a "wobble," pitch inaccuracies (singing flat), and inability to sing softly are rarely caused by irreversible aging changes, and these problems can usually be managed easily through voice therapy and training.

### Hearing Loss

Hearing loss is often overlooked as a source of vocal problems. Auditory feedback is fundamental to speaking and singing. Interference with this control mechanism may result in altered vocal production, particularly if the person is unaware of the hearing loss. Distortion, particularly pitch distortion (diplacusis), may also pose serious problems for the singer. This appears to cause not only aesthetic difficulties in matching pitch but also vocal strain, which accompanies pitch shifts.[57] Hearing impairment can cause vocal strain, particularly if a person has sensorineural hearing loss (involving the nerve or inner ear) and is unaware of it. This condition may lead people to speak or sing more loudly than they realize.

### Respiratory Dysfunction

The importance of "the breath" has been well recognized in the field of voice pedagogy. Respiratory disorders are discussed at length in other literature.[58] Even a mild degree of obstructive pulmonary disease can result in substantial voice problems. Unrecognized exercise-induced asthma is especially problematic in singers and actors, because bronchospasm may be precipitated by the exercise and airway drying that occurs during voice performance. In such cases, the bronchospastic obstruction on exhalation impairs support. This commonly results in compensatory hyperfunction.

Treatment requires skilled management and collaboration with a pulmonologist and a voice team.[59] Whenever possible, patients should be managed primarily with oral medications; the use of inhalers should be minimized. Steroid inhalers should be avoided altogether whenever possible. It is particularly important to recognize that asthma can be induced by the exercise of phonation itself,[60] and in many cases a high index of suspicion and methacholine challenge test are needed to avoid missing this important diagnosis.

## Allergy

Even mild allergies are more incapacitating to professional voice users than to others. This subject can be reviewed elsewhere.[61] Briefly, patients with mild intermittent allergies can usually be managed with antihistamines, although they should never be tried for the first time immediately prior to a voice performance. Because antihistamines commonly produce unacceptable side effects, trial and error may be needed in order to find a medication with an acceptable balance between effect and side effect for any individual patient, especially a voice professional. Patients with allergy-related voice disturbances may find hyposensitization a more effective approach than antihistamine use, if they are candidates for such treatment. For voice patients with unexpected allergic symptoms immediately prior to an important voice commitment, corticosteroids should be used rather than antihistamines, in order to minimize the risks of side effects (such as drying and thickening of secretions) that might make voice performance difficult or impossible. Allergies commonly cause voice problems by altering the mucosa and secretions and causing nasal obstruction. Management is not covered in depth in this brief chapter. However, it should be recognized that many of the medicines commonly used to treat allergies have side effects deleterious to voice function, particularly dryness and thickening of secretions. Consequently, when voice disturbance is causally related to these conditions, more definitive treatment through allergic immunotherapy should be considered. This is especially important to professional voice users.

## Gastroesophageal Reflux Laryngitis

Gastroesophageal reflux laryngitis is extremely common among voice patients, especially singers.[62] This is a condition in which the sphincter between the stomach and esophagus is inefficient, and acidic stomach secretions reflux (reach the laryngeal tissues), causing inflammation. The most typical symptoms are hoarseness in the morning, prolonged vocal warm-up time, halitosis and a bitter taste in the morning, a feeling of a "lump in the throat," frequent throat clearing, chronic irritative cough, and frequent tracheitis or tracheobronchitis. Any or all of these symptoms may be present. Heartburn is not common in these patients, so the diagnosis is often missed. Prolonged reflux also is associated with the development of Barrett esophagus, esophageal carcinoma, and laryngeal carcinoma.[62,63]

Physical examination usually reveals erythema (redness) of the arytenoids mucosa. A barium swallow radiographic study with water siphonage may provide additional information but is not needed routinely. However, if a patient complies strictly with treatment recommendations and does not show marked improvement within a month, or if there is a reason to suspect more serious pathology, complete evaluation by a gastroenterologist should be carried out. This is often advisable in patients who are older than 40 years or who have had reflux symptoms for more than 5 years. Twenty-four-hour pH monitoring of the esophagus is often effective in establishing a diagnosis. The results are correlated with a diary of the patient's activities and symptoms. Bulimia should also be considered in the differential diagnosis when symptoms are refractory to treatment and other physical and psychologic signs are suggestive.

The mainstays of treatment for reflux laryngitis are elevation of the head of the bed (not just sleeping on pillows), antacids, H2 blockers or proton pump inhibitors, and avoidance of eating for 3 to 4 hours before going to sleep. This is often difficult for singers and actors because of their performance schedule, but if they are counseled about minor changes in eating habits (such as eating larger meals at breakfast and lunch), they can usually comply. Avoidance of alcohol, caffeine, and specific foods is beneficial. Medications that decrease or block acid production may be necessary. It must be recognized that control of acidity is not the same as control of reflux. In many cases, reflux is provoked during singing because of the increased abdominal pressure associated with support. In these instances, it often causes excessive phlegm and throat clearing during the first 10 or

15 minutes of a performance or lesson, as well as other common reflux laryngitis symptoms, even when acidity has been neutralized effectively. Laparoscopic Nissen fundoplication has proven extremely effective and should be considered a reasonable alternative to lifelong medication in this relatively young patient population.[63]

**Endocrine Dysfunction**

Endocrine (hormonal) problems warrant special attention. The human voice is extremely sensitive to endocrinologic changes. Many of these are reflected in alterations of fluid content of the lamina propria just beneath the laryngeal mucosa. This causes alterations in the bulk and shape of the vocal folds and results in voice change. Hypothyroidism is a well-recognized cause of such voice disorders, although the mechanism is not fully understood.[64–67] Hoarseness, vocal fatigue, muffling of the voice, loss of range, and a sensation of a lump in the throat may be present even with mild hypothyroidism. Even when thyroid function tests results are within the low-normal range, this diagnosis should be entertained, especially if thyroid-stimulating hormone levels are in the high-normal range or are elevated. Thyrotoxicosis may result in similar voice disturbances.[68]

Voice changes associated with sex hormones are encountered commonly in clinical practice and have been investigated more thoroughly than have other hormonal changes. Although a correlation appears to exist between sex hormone levels and depth of male voices (higher testosterone and lower estradiol levels in basses than in tenors),[69] the most important hormonal considerations in males occur during the maturation process.

When castrato singers were in vogue, castration at about age 7 or 8 years resulted in failure of laryngeal growth during puberty, and voices that stayed in the soprano or alto range and boasted a unique quality of sound.[70] Failure of a male voice to change at puberty is uncommon today and is often psychogenic in etiology.[1] However, hormonal deficiencies such as those seen in cryptorchidism, delayed sexual development, Klinefelter syndrome, or Fröhlich syndrome may be responsible. In these cases, the persistently high voice may be the complaint that causes the patient to seek medical attention.

Voice problems related to sex hormones are most common in female singers.[71] Although vocal changes associated with the normal menstrual cycle may be difficult to quantify with current experimental techniques, unquestionably they occur.[2,71–75] Most of the ill effects seen in the immediate premenstrual period are

known as laryngopathia premenstrualis. This common condition is caused by physiologic, anatomic, and psychologic alterations secondary to endocrine changes. The vocal dysfunction is characterized by decreased vocal efficiency, loss of the highest notes in the voice, vocal fatigue, slight hoarseness, and some muffling of the voice. It is often more apparent to the singer than to the listener. Submucosal hemorrhages in the larynx are more common in the premenstrual period.[73] In many European opera houses, singers used to be excused from singing during the premenstrual and early menstrual days ("grace days"). This practice is not followed in the United States and is no longer in vogue in most European countries. Premenstrual changes cause significant vocal symptoms in approximately one-third of singers. Although ovulation inhibitors have been shown to mitigate some of these symptoms,[74] but in some women (about 5%),[76] birth control pills used to deleteriously alter voice range and character even after only a few months of therapy.[76–80] However, modern oral contraceptives usually do not produce such problems. Under crucial performance circumstances, oral contraceptives may be used to alter the time of menstruation, but this practice is justified only in unusual situations. Symptoms similar to laryngopathia premenstrualis occur in some women at the time of ovulation.

Pregnancy results frequently in voice alterations known as laryngopathia gravidarum. The changes may be similar to premenstrual symptoms or may be perceived as desirable changes. In some cases, alterations produced by pregnancy are permanent.[81–82] Although hormonally induced changes in the larynx and respiratory mucosa secondary to menstruation and pregnancy are discussed widely in the literature, the author has found no reference to the important alterations in abdominal support. Abdominal distention during pregnancy also interferes with abdominal muscle function. Any singer whose abdominal support is compromised substantially should be discouraged from singing until the abdominal impairment is resolved.

Estrogens are helpful in postmenopausal singers but generally should not be given alone. Sequential replacement therapy is the most physiologic regimen and should be used under the supervision of a gynecologist as potential systemic side effects have been described. Under no circumstances should androgens be given to female singers even in small amounts if any reasonable therapeutic alternative exists. Clinically, these drugs are most commonly used to treat endometriosis or postmenopausal loss of libido. Androgens cause unsteadiness of the voice, rapid changes of timbre, and lowering of the fundamental frequency (masculinization).[83–87] These changes are usually permanent.

Recently, we have seen increasing abuse of anabolic steroids among bodybuilders and other athletes. In addition to their many other hazards, these medications may alter the voice. They are (or are closely related to) male hormones; consequently, they are capable of producing masculinization of the voice. Lowering of the fundamental frequency and coarsening of the voice produced in this fashion are generally irreversible.

Other hormonal disturbances may also produce vocal dysfunction. In addition to the thyroid gland and the gonads, the parathyroid, adrenal, pineal, and pituitary glands are included in this system. Other endocrine disturbances may alter voice as well. For example, pancreatic dysfunction may cause xerophonia (dry voice), as in diabetes mellitus. Thymic abnormalities can lead to feminization of the voice.[88]

### Neurologic Disorders

Numerous neurologic conditions may adversely affect the voice. They are discussed in other literature[2] and elsewhere in this book. Some of them, such as myasthenia gravis, are amenable to medical therapy with drugs such as pyridostigmine (Mestinon). Such therapy frequently restores the voice to normal. An exhaustive neurolaryngologic discussion is beyond the scope of this chapter. Nevertheless, when evaluating voice dysfunction, laryngologists must consider numerous neurologic problems, including Parkinson disease, various other disorders that produce tremor, drug-induced tremor, multiple sclerosis, dystonias, and many other conditions. Spasmodic dysphonia (SD), a laryngeal dystonia, presents particularly challenging problems. This subject is covered in detail in another chapter. Stuttering also provides unique challenges. Although still poorly understood, this condition is noted for its tendency to affect speech while sparing singing.

### Vocal Fold Hypomobility

*Vocal fold hypomobility* may be caused by paralysis (no movement), paresis (partial movement), arytenoid dislocation, cricoarytenoid joint dysfunction, and laryngeal fracture. Differentiating among these conditions is often more complicated than it appears at first glance. A comprehensive discussion is beyond the scope of this chapter, and the reader is referred to other chapters in this book.[9] However, in addition to a comprehensive history and physical examination, evaluation commonly includes strobovideolaryngoscopy, objective voice assessment, laryngeal electromyography, and high-resolution computed tomography (CT) of the larynx. Most vocal fold motion disorders are amenable to treatment. Voice therapy should be used first in virtually all cases. Even in many patients with recurrent laryngeal nerve paralysis, voice therapy alone is often sufficient. When therapy fails to produce adequate voice improvement in the patient's opinion, surgical intervention is appropriate.

## General Health

As with any other athletic activity, optimal voice use requires reasonably good general health and physical conditioning. Abdominal and respiratory strength and endurance are particularly important. If a person becomes short of breath from climbing 2 flights of stairs, he or she certainly does not have the physical stamina necessary for proper respiratory support for a speech, let alone a strenuous musical production. This deficiency usually results in abusive vocal habits used in vain attempts to compensate for the deficiencies.

Systemic illnesses, such as anemia, Lyme disease, mononucleosis, AIDS, chronic fatigue syndrome, or other diseases associated with malaise and weakness, may impair the ability of vocal musculature to recover rapidly from heavy use and may also be associated with alterations of mucosal secretions. Other systemic illnesses may be responsible for voice complaints, particularly if they impair the abdominal muscles necessary for breath support. For example, diarrhea and constipation that prohibit sustained abdominal contraction may be reasons for the physician to prohibit a strenuous singing or acting engagement.

Any extremity injury, such as a sprained ankle, may alter posture and therefore interfere with customary abdominothoracic support. Voice patients are often unaware of this problem and develop abusive, hyperfunctional compensatory maneuvers in the neck and tongue musculature as a result. These technical flaws may produce voice complaints, such as vocal fatigue and neck pain, that bring the performer to the physician's office for assessment and care.

## Obesity

Singers, actors, and many other professional voice users are verbal, oral people. Most of us enjoy singing, talking, and a good bowl of pasta after the show. However, before indulging our passions for culinary excess, it is important to understand the impact of obesity not only on singing performance, but also on general health and longevity.

For medical reasons, when obesity becomes extreme, serious measures may be necessary to accomplish weight loss. The most severely overweight patients have an entity called "morbid obesity." This condition is diagnosed when a person is more than 100 pounds or 100% over ideal body weight (Table 4–1). Morbid obesity is a disease that is extremely common in our society. It is estimated that 34 million adult Americans (1 of every 5 people over the age of 19) have significant obesity. As little as 20% excess over desirable body weight may be enough to constitute a health hazard. Doctors have long been aware of the difficulty in controlling weight problems with medical treatment alone. Of all patients who lose weight,

90% regain it at some point in their lives, and many even exceed their original weight. This led doctors to consider surgery as an option in treating this problem in selected cases.

In February 1985, a panel of experts from the National Institutes of Health looked at health problems associated with obesity.[89] Opinions have not changed substantially since that time. They concluded that obesity has adverse effects on health and longevity.

1. Obesity creates enormous psychological stress, which is a problem not well understood by the general population. Large people are unpopular, discriminated against in the workplace, and considered lazy.
2. Obesity is associated with high blood pressure. Obese people have high blood pressure three times more often than nonobese people.
3. Obesity is associated with higher levels of cholesterol.
4. Obesity is associated with diabetes. As with high blood pressure, this is seen 3 times more commonly in obese individuals.
5. Obesity is a factor in the development of heart disease.
6. Obesity increases the risk of developing certain cancers, specifically those of the uterus, breast, cervix, and gall bladder in women and the colon, rectum, and prostate in men.
7. Obese individuals have a shorter life span.
8. Obesity is related to respiratory problems and arthritis.

With weight loss, all of these problems can be substantially improved, and prolongation of life is possible.

The best treatment for obesity is avoidance of the problem. Early in training, singers and other voice professionals should learn the importance of good physical and aerobic conditioning. This is important to the voice professional's general health, vocal health, and art. Even a moderate degree of obesity may affect the respiratory system adversely, undermining support. Weight reduction is recommended for people who are 20% or more above ideal weight. In the singer, weight should be lost slowly through modification of eating and lifestyle habits. Loss of 2 or 3 pounds per week is plenty. More rapid loss of weight causes fluid shifts and hormonal alterations that may result in changes in vocal quality and endurance. Although these changes appear to be temporary, the effects of weight loss on vocal function have not been studied adequately; therefore, we

**Table 4–1.** Weight Table

| Height | | Weight (in pounds) | |
|---|---|---|---|
| Feet/inches | Inches | Women | Men |
| 4'09" | 57 | 90 | 95 |
| 4'10" | 58 | 95 | 100 |
| 4'11" | 59 | 100 | 105 |
| 5'00" | 60 | 105 | 110 |
| 5'01" | 61 | 110 | 115 |
| 5'02" | 62 | 115 | 120 |
| 5'03" | 63 | 120 | 125 |
| 5'04" | 64 | 125 | 130 |
| 5'05" | 65 | 130 | 135 |
| 5'06" | 66 | 135 | 140 |
| 5'07" | 67 | 140 | 145 |
| 5'08" | 68 | 145 | 150 |
| 5'09" | 69 | 150 | 155 |
| 5'10" | 70 | 155 | 160 |
| 5'11" | 71 | 160 | 165 |
| 6'00" | 72 | 165 | 170 |
| 6'01" | 73 | 170 | 175 |
| 6'02" | 74 | 175 | 180 |
| 6'03" | 75 | 180 | 185 |
| 6'04" | 76 | 185 | 190 |
| 6'05" | 77 | 190 | 195 |

do not have answers to all the pertinent questions. It is certainly possible for a singer to lose weight too quickly, but we are not yet sure how much weight loss is too much. Studies should be encouraged to learn more about this problem. However, it appears that maintenance of ideal body weight is probably as healthy for the voice as it is for the rest of the body. For people 20% to 100% above ideal body weight, weight loss can be accomplished with a medically supervised diet. However, people who are morbidly obese frequently are unable to lose weight by dietary or medical means alone. Morbidly obese patients may be candidates for surgery to help control their weight problems.

Although several kinds of obesity operations exist, the older procedures have significant side effects. At present, the best methods are a form of gastric restrictive surgery, known as the gastric bypass and gastric banding. Postoperatively, weight loss occurs over 12 to 18 months and stops as ideal body weight is approached. In most cases, singing may be resumed at about 6 weeks following abdominal surgery. Although the effects on the voice are not yet documented fully, there does not appear to be any significant problem associated with weight loss in patients with morbid obesity. Although further study is necessary to confirm these impressions, in singers or actors with this degree of weight problem, considerations of longevity, heart condition, blood pressure, and other critical health matters may outweigh immediate vocal concerns.

For most singers, an extra 10, 20, or 30 pounds is not perceived as much of a problem. However, as 20 becomes 30, and 30 becomes 40, substantial adverse effects occur in the body in general and the vocal tract specifically. In training, singers and actors should be encouraged to treat their entire bodies with the same reverence with which they regard their vocal folds. Self-respect as a professional athlete is a sound basis for a longer vocal career—and a longer life.

### Anxiety

Voice professionals, especially singers and actors, are frequently sensitive and communicative people. When the principal cause of vocal dysfunction is anxiety, the physician can often accomplish much by assuring the patient that no organic problem is present and by stating the diagnosis of anxiety reaction. The patient should be counseled that anxiety is normal and that recognition of it as the principle problem frequently allows the performer to overcome it. Tranquilizers and sedatives are rarely necessary and are undesirable because they may interfere with fine

motor control. For example, beta-adrenergic blocking agents such as propranolol hydrochloride have become popular among performers for the treatment of preperformance anxiety. Beta-blockers are not recommended for regular use; they have significant effects on the cardiovascular system and many potential complications, including hypotension, thrombocytopenic purpura, mental depression, agranulocytosis, laryngospasm with respiratory distress, and bronchospasm. In addition, their efficacy is controversial. Although they may have a favorable effect in relieving performance anxiety, beta-blockers may produce a noticeable adverse effect on singing performance.[90]

Although these drugs have a place under occasional, extraordinary circumstances, their routine use for this purpose not only is potentially hazardous but also violates an important therapeutic principle. Performers have chosen a career that exposes them to the public. If such persons are so incapacitated by anxiety that they are unable to perform the routine functions of their chosen profession without chemical help, this should be considered symptomatic of an important underlying psychologic problem. (See Chapter 7 for further details.) For a performer to depend on drugs to perform is neither routine nor healthy, whether the drug is a benzodiazepine, a barbiturate, a beta-blocker, or alcohol. If such dependence exists, psychologic evaluation should be considered by an experienced arts-medicine psychologist or psychiatrist. Obscuring the symptoms by fostering the dependence is insufficient. However, if the patient is on tour and will only be under a particular otolaryngologist's care for a week or so, the physician should not try to make major changes in his or her customary regimen. Rather, the physician should communicate with the performer's primary otolaryngologist or family physician to coordinate appropriate long-term care.

As professional voice users constitute a subset of society as a whole, all the psychiatric disorders encountered among the general public are seen from time to time in voice professionals. In some cases, professional voice users require modification of the usual psychologic treatment, particularly with regard to psychotropic medications. Detailed discussion of this subject can be found elsewhere in the literature.[91]

When voice professionals, especially singers and actors, have a significant vocal impairment that results in voice loss (or the prospect of voice loss), they often go through a psychologic process similar to grieving.[92] In some cases, fear of discovering that the voice is lost forever may unconsciously prevent patients from trying to use their voices optimally following injury or treatment. This can dramatically impede or prevent recovery of function following a perfect surgical result, for example. It is essential that otolaryngologists, performers, and their teachers be familiar with this fairly common scenario, and it is ideal to include an arts-medicine psychologist and/or psychiatrist as part of the voice team.

### Other Psychologic Problems

Psychogenic voice disorders, incapacitating psychologic reactions to organic voice disorders, and other psychologic problems are encountered commonly in young voice patients. They are discussed in other literature and elsewhere in this book.[93]

### Substance Abuse

The list of substances ingested, smoked, or "snorted" by many people is disturbingly long. Whenever possible, patients who care about vocal quality and longevity should be educated about the deleterious effects of such habits upon their voice and upon the longevity of their careers by their physicians and teachers. A few specific substances have already been discussed.

## Structural Abnormalities

### Nodules

Nodules are callous-like masses of the vocal folds that are caused by vocally abusive behaviors and are a dreaded malady of singers or actors. Occasionally, laryngoscopy reveals asymptomatic vocal nodules that do not appear to interfere with voice production; in such cases, the nodules should not be treated. Some famous and successful singers have had untreated vocal nodules throughout their careers. However, in most cases, nodules result in hoarseness, breathiness, loss of range, and vocal fatigue. They may be caused by abusive speaking rather than improper singing technique. Voice therapy always should be tried as the initial therapeutic modality and will cure the vast majority of patients even if the nodules look firm and have been present for many months or years. Even apparently large, fibrotic nodules often shrink, disappear, or become asymptomatic with 6 to 12 weeks of voice therapy with good patient compliance. Even in those who eventually need surgical excision of the nodules, preoperative voice therapy is essential to prevent recurrence. Care must be taken in diagnosing nodules.

It is almost impossible to make the diagnosis accurately and consistently without strobovideolaryngoscopy and good optical magnification. Vocal fold cysts are commonly misdiagnosed as nodules, and treatment strategies are different for the 2 lesions. Vocal nodules are confined to the superficial layer of the lamina propria and are composed primarily of edematous tissue or collagenous fibers. Basement membrane reduplication is common. They are usually bilateral and fairly symmetric.

Caution must be exercised in diagnosing small nodules in patients who have been singing or speaking actively. In many singers, for example, bilateral, symmetric soft swellings at the junction of the anterior and middle thirds of the vocal folds develop after heavy voice use. No evidence suggests that patients with such "physiologic swelling" are predisposed to the development of vocal nodules. At present, the condition is generally considered to be within normal limits. The physiologic swelling usually disappears with 24 to 28 hours of rest from heavy voice use. The physician must be careful not to frighten the patient by misdiagnosing physiologic swellings as vocal nodules. Nodules carry a great stigma among voice professionals, and the psychologic impact of the diagnosis should not be underestimated. When nodules are present, these patients should be informed with the same gentle caution used in telling a patient that he or she has a life-threatening mass.

### Submucosal Cysts

Submucosal cysts of the vocal folds are probably also traumatic lesions that are the result of a blocked mucous gland duct in many cases. However, they may also be congenital or occur from other causes. They often cause contact swelling on the contralateral side and can be initially misdiagnosed as nodules. They can usually be differentiated from nodules by strobovideolaryngoscopy when the mass is observed to be obviously fluid filled. They may also be suspected when the nodule (contact swelling) on one vocal fold resolves with voice therapy while the mass on the other vocal fold does not resolve. Cysts may also be discovered on one side (occasionally both sides) when surgery is performed for apparent nodules that have not resolved with voice therapy. The surgery should be performed superficially and with minimal trauma, as discussed in a separate chapter. Cysts are ordinarily lined with thin squamous epithelium. Retention cysts contain mucus. Epidermoid cysts contain caseous material. Generally, cysts are located in the superficial layer of the lamina propria. In some cases, they may be attached to the vocal ligament.

## Polyps

Vocal *polyps,* another type of vocal fold mass, usu-ally occur on only one vocal fold. They often have a prominent feeding blood vessel coursing along the superior surface of the vocal fold and entering the base of the polyp. The pathogenesis of polyps cannot be proven in many cases, but the lesion is thought to be traumatic and sometimes starts as a hemorrhage. Polyps may be sessile or pedunculated. They are typ-ically located in the superficial layer of the lamina propria and do not involve the vocal ligament. In those arising from an area of hemorrhage, the vocal ligament may be involved with posthemorrhagic fibrosis that is contiguous with the polyp. Histologic evaluation most commonly reveals collagenous fibers, hyaline degeneration, edema, thrombosis, and often bleeding within the polypoid tissue. Cellular infiltration may also be present. In some cases, even sizable polyps resolve with relative voice rest and a few weeks of low-dose steroid therapy (e.g., methyl-prednisone 4 mg twice a day). However, most require surgical removal. If polyps are not treated, they may produce contact injury on the contralateral vocal fold. Voice therapy should be used to ensure good relative voice rest and prevention of abusive vocal behavior before and after surgery. When surgery is performed, care must be taken not to damage the leading edge of the vocal fold, especially if a laser is used, as discussed later. In all laryngeal surgery, delicate microscopic dis-section is now the standard of care. Vocal fold "strip-ping' is an out-of-date surgical approach formerly used for benign lesions that often resulted in scar and/or poor unserviceable voice function. It is no longer an acceptable surgical technique in most situations.

## Granulomas

*Granulomas* usually occur in the cartilaginous por-tion of the vocal fold near the vocal process or on the medial surface of the arytenoid. They are composed of collagenous fibers, fibroblasts, proliferated capil-laries, and leukocytes. They are usually covered with epithelium. Granulomas are associated with gastro-esophageal reflux laryngitis and trauma (including trauma from voice abuse and from intubation). Ther-apy should include reflux control, voice therapy, and surgery if the granuloma continues to enlarge or does not resolve after adequate time and treatment.

## Reinke's Edema

*Reinke's edema* is characterized by an "elephant ear," floppy vocal fold appearance. It is often observed during examination in many nonprofessional and professional voice users and is accompanied by a low, coarse, gruff voice. Reinke's edema is a condi-tion in which the superficial layer of lamina propria (Reinke's space) becomes edematous. The lesion does not usually include hypertrophy, inflammation, or degeneration, although other terms for the condition include *polypoid degeneration, chronic polypoid corditis,* and *chronic edematous hypertrophy.* Reinke's edema is often associated with smoking, voice abuse, reflux, and hypothyroidism. Underlying conditions should be treated. However, the condition may require sur-gery if voice improvement is desired. The surgery should be performed only if there is a justified high suspicion of serious pathology such as cancer, if there is airway obstruction, or if the patient is unhappy with his or her vocal quality. For some voice profes-sionals, abnormal Reinke's edema is an important component of the vocal signature. Although the con-dition is usually bilateral, surgery should generally be performed on one side at a time.

## Sulcus Vocalis

*Sulcus vocalis* is a groove along the edge of the mem-branous vocal fold. The majority are congenital, bilateral, and symmetric, although posttraumatic acquired lesions occur. When symptomatic (they often are not), sulcus vocalis can be treated surgi-cally if sufficient voice improvement is not obtained through voice therapy.

## Scar

*Vocal fold scar* is a sequela of trauma and results in fibrosis and obliteration of the layered structure of the vocal fold. It may markedly impede vibration and consequently cause profound dysphonia. Recent sur-gical advances have made this condition much more treatable than it used to be, but it is still rarely possi-ble to restore voices to normal in the presence of scar.

## Hemorrhage

*Vocal fold hemorrhage* is a potential disaster in sing-ers. Hemorrhages resolve spontaneously in most cases, with restoration of normal voice. However, in some instances, the hematoma organizes and fibro-ses, resulting in scar. This alters the vibratory pat-tern of the vocal fold and can result in permanent hoarseness. In specially selected cases, it may be best to avoid this problem through surgical incision and drainage of the hematoma. In all cases, vocal fold hemorrhage should be managed with absolute voice rest until the hemorrhage has resolved (usually about 1 week) and relative voice rest until normal vascular and mucosal integrity have been restored. This often takes 6 weeks and sometimes longer. Recurrent vocal fold hemorrhages are usually caused by weakness in a specific blood vessel, which may require surgical cauterization of the blood vessel using a laser or microscopic resection of the vessel.[94]

## Papilloma

*Laryngeal papillomas* are epithelial lesions caused by human papilloma virus. Histology reveals neoplastic epithelial cell proliferation in a papillary pattern and viral particles. At the present time, symptomatic papillomas are treated surgically, although alternatives have been recommended to the usual laser vaporization approach.[95–96] Cidofovir injected into the lesion has shown considerable promise.[97]

## Cancer

A detailed discussion of *cancer of the larynx* is beyond the scope of this chapter. The prognosis for small vocal fold cancers is good, whether they are treated by radiation or surgery. Although it may seem intuitively obvious that radiation therapy provides a better chance of voice conservation than even limited vocal fold surgery, later radiation changes in the vocal fold may produce substantial hoarseness, xerophonia (dry voice), and voice dysfunction. Consequently, from the standpoint of voice preservation, optimal treatments remain uncertain.[9] Prospective studies using objective voice measures and strobovideolaryngoscopy should answer the relevant questions in the near future. Strobovideolaryngoscopy is also valuable for follow-up of patients who have had laryngeal cancers. It permits detection of vibratory changes associated with infiltration by the cancer long before they can be seen with continuous light. Stroboscopy has been used in Europe and Japan for this purpose for many years. In the United States, the popularity of strobovideolaryngoscopy for follow-up of patients with cancer has increased greatly in recent years.

The psychologic consequences of vocal fold cancer can be devastating, especially in a professional voice user. They may be overwhelming for nonvoice professionals as well. These reactions are understandable and expected. In many patients, however, psychologic reactions may be as severe following medically "less significant" vocal fold problems such as hemorrhages, nodules, and other conditions that do not command the public respect and sympathy afforded to a cancer. In many ways, the management of related psychologic problems can be even more difficult in patients with these "lesser" vocal disturbances.

## Unusual Vocal Fold Masses

When vocal fold masses are mentioned, laryngologists usually think of nodules, cysts, polyps, and cancer. Although these are certainly the most common problems in clinical practice, many other conditions must be kept in mind. Collagen vascular diseases and other unusual problems may also produce laryngeal masses. Rheumatoid arthritis may produce not only disease of the cricoarytenoid and cricothyroid joints but also consequent neuropathic muscle atrophy[98] and rheumatoid nodules of the larynx.[99] Rheumatoid arthritis with or without nodules may produce respiratory obstruction. Gout may also cause laryngeal arthritis. In addition, gouty tophi may appear as white submucosal masses of the true vocal fold. They consist of sodium urate crystals in fibrous tissue and have been well documented.[100,101]

Amyloidosis of the larynx is rare but well recognized.[102–103] Amyloidosis is most common in the false vocal folds. Urbach-Wiethe disease (lipoid proteinosis)[104] often involves the mucous membrane of the larynx, usually the vocal folds, aryepiglottic fold, and epiglottis. Other conditions such as granulomatosis with polyangiitis (Wegener granulomatosis) and relapsing polychondritis may also involve the larynx. They are less likely to produce discrete nodules, but the diffuse edema associated with chondritis and necrotizing granulomas may produce significant laryngeal and voice abnormalities leading to surgical intervention. Granular cell tumors may involve the larynx and can be misdiagnosed easily as laryngeal granulomas. Unusual laryngeal masses may also be caused by trauma.

A few rare skin lesions may also involve the larynx, producing significant lesions and sometimes airway obstruction. These include pemphigus vulgaris, seen in adults between 40 and 60 years of age. Pemphigus lesions may involve the mucosa, including the epiglottis.[106] Epidermolysis bullosa describes a group of congenital vesicular disorders usually seen at birth or shortly thereafter. This condition may cause laryngeal stenosis.

## Other Conditions

Numerous other conditions could be included in this chapter. For a more comprehensive discussion of the subjects covered above, the reader is referred to other chapters in this book and to other literature.[2]

## Medical Management for Voice Dysfunction

Medical management of many problems affecting the voice involves not only care prescribed by the otolaryngologist but also voice therapy, which is provided by an interdisciplinary team. The roles and training of the principal members of the team are covered in detail elsewhere in this book. This chapter provides a brief introduction to their roles in the medical milieu.

### Speech-Language Pathologist

An excellent speech-language pathologist is an invaluable asset in caring for professional voice users and other voice patients. However, otolaryngologists and singing teachers should recognize that, like physicians, speech-language pathologists have varied backgrounds and experience in treatment of voice disorders. In fact, most speech-language pathology programs teach relatively little about caring for professional speakers and nothing about professional singers. Moreover, few speech-language pathologists have vast experience in this specialized area, and no fellowships in this specialty exist. Speech-language pathologists often subspecialize. A speech-language pathologist who expertly treats patients who have had strokes, stutter, have undergone laryngectomy, or have swallowing disorders will not necessarily know how to manage professional voice users optimally or even other less demanding voice patients. The otolaryngologist must learn the strengths and weaknesses of the speech-language pathologist with whom he or she works. After identifying a speech-language pathologist who is interested in treating professional voice users, the otolaryngologist should work closely with the speech-language pathologist in developing the necessary expertise. Assistance may be found through otolaryngologists who treat large numbers of singers or through educational programs such as the Voice Foundation's Symposium on Care of the Professional Voice. In general, therapy should be directed toward vocal hygiene, relaxation techniques, breath management, and abdominal support.

Speech (voice) therapy may be helpful even when a singer has no obvious problem in the speaking voice but significant technical problems singing. Once a person has been singing for several years, a singing teacher may have difficulty convincing him or her to correct certain technical errors. Singers are much less protective of their speaking voices, however. A speech-language pathologist may be able to teach proper support, relaxation, and voice placement in speaking. Once mastered, these techniques can be carried over fairly easily into singing through cooperation between the speech-language pathologist and singing teacher. This "back door" approach has been extremely useful. For the actor, coordinating speech-language pathology sessions with acting voice lessons, and especially with training of the speaking voice provided by the actor's voice teacher or coach, is often helpful. In fact, we have found this combination so helpful that we have added an acting voice trainer to our medical staff. Information from the speech-language pathologist, acting voice trainer, and singing teacher should be symbiotic and should not conflict. If major discrepancies exist, bad training from one of the team members should be suspected and changes should be made.

### Singing Voice Specialist

Singing voice specialists are singing teachers who have acquired extra training to prepare them for work with injured voices, in collaboration with a medical voice team. They are indispensable for singers.

In selected cases, singing lessons may also be extremely helpful to nonsingers with voice problems. The technique used to develop abdominal and thoracic muscle strength, breath control, laryngeal and neck muscle strength, and relaxation are similar to those used in speech therapy. Singing lessons often expedite therapy and appear to improve the outcome in some patients.

Otolaryngologists who frequently care for singers are often asked to recommend a voice teacher. This may put them in an uncomfortable position, particularly if the singer is already studying with someone in the community. Most physicians do not have sufficient expertise to criticize a voice teacher, and we must be extremely cautious about recommending that a singer change teachers. However, no certifying agency standardizes or ensures the quality of a singing teacher. Although one may be slightly more confident of a teacher associated with a major conservatory or music school or one who is a member of the National Association of Teachers of Singing (NATS), neither of these credentials ensures excellence, and many expert teachers have neither affiliation. However, with experience, an otolaryngologist can ordinarily develop valid impressions. The physician should record the name of the voice teacher of every patient and observe whether the same kinds of voice abuse occur with disproportionate frequency in the pupils of any given teacher. Technical problems can cause organic abnormalities such as nodules; therefore, any teacher who has a high incidence of nodules among his or her students should be viewed with cautious concern. The physician should be particularly wary of teachers who are reluctant to allow their students to consult a doctor. The best voice teachers usually are quick to refer their students to an otolaryngologist if they hear anything disturbing in a student's voice. Similarly, voice teachers and voice professionals should compare information on the nature and quality of medical care received and its success. No physician cures every voice problem in every patient, just as no singing teacher produces premiere stars from every student who walks through the studio. Nevertheless, voice professionals must be critical, informed consumers and accept nothing less than the best medical care.

After seeing a voice patient, the otolaryngologist should speak with and/or write a letter to the voice teacher (with the patient's permission) describing the findings and recommendations as he or she would to a physician, speech-language pathologist, or any other referring professional. An otolaryngologist seriously interested in caring for singers should take the trouble to talk with and meet local singing teachers. Taking a lesson or two with each teacher provides enormous insight as well. Taking voice lessons regularly is even more helpful. In practice, the otolaryngologist will usually identify a few teachers in whom he or she has particular confidence, especially for patients with voice disorders, and should not hesitate to refer singers to these colleagues, especially singers who are not already in training.

Pop singers may be particularly resistant to the suggestion of voice lessons, yet they are in great need of training. The physician should point out that a good voice teacher can teach a pop singer how to protect and expand the voice without changing its quality or making it sound "trained" or "operatic." It is helpful to point out that singing, like other athletic activities, requires exercise, warm-up, and coaching for anyone planning to enter the "big league" and stay there. Just as no major league baseball pitcher would play without a pitching coach and warm-up time in the bullpen, no singer should try to build a career without a singing teacher and appropriate strength and agility exercises. This approach has proved palatable and effective. Physicians should also be aware of the difference between a voice teacher and a voice coach.

A voice teacher trains a singer in singing technique and is essential. A voice coach is responsible for teaching songs, language, diction, style, operatic roles, and so on, but is not responsible for exercise and basic technical development of the voice.

## Acting-Voice Trainer

The use of acting-voice trainers (drama voice coaches) as members of the medical team is new. This addition to the team has been extremely valuable to patients and other team members. Like singing voice specialists, professionals with education in theatre arts use numerous vocal and body movement techniques that not only enhance physical function but also release tension and break down emotional barriers that may impede voice function. Tearful revelations to the acting-voice trainer are not uncommon, and, like the singing teacher, this individual may identify psychologic and emotional problems interfering with professional success that have been skillfully hidden from other professionals on the voice team and in the patient's life.

## Others

A psychologist, psychiatrist, neurologist, pulmonologist, and others with special interest and expertise in arts-medicine are also invaluable to the voice team. Every comprehensive center should seek out such people and collaborate with them, even if they are not full-time members of the voice team.

## Surgery

A detailed discussion of laryngeal surgery is beyond the scope of this chapter and may be found elsewhere in this book and other literature.[2] However, a few points are worthy of special emphasis. Surgery for vocal nodules should be avoided whenever possible and should almost never be performed without an adequate trial of expert voice therapy, including patient compliance with therapeutic suggestions. A minimum of 6 to 12 weeks of observation should be allowed while the patient is using therapeutically modified voice techniques under the supervision of a speech-language pathologist and ideally a singing voice specialist. Proper voice use rather than voice rest (silence) is correct therapy. The surgeon should not perform surgery prematurely for vocal nodules under pressure from the patient for a "quick cure" and early return to performance. Permanent destruction of voice quality is a very real complication.

Even after expert surgery, voice quality may be diminished by submucosal scarring, resulting in an adynamic segment along the vibratory margin of the vocal fold. This situation produces a hoarse voice with vocal folds that appear normal on indirect examination under routine light, although under stroboscopic light, the adynamic segment is obvious. No reliable cure exists for this complication. Even large, apparently fibrotic nodules of long standing should be given a chance to resolve without surgery. In some cases, the nodules remain but become asymptomatic and voice quality is normal. Stroboscopy in such patients usually reveals that the nodules are on the superior surface rather than the leading edge of the vocal folds during proper, relaxed phonation (although they may be on the contact surface and symptomatic when hyperfunctional voice technique is used and the larynx is forced down).

When surgery is indicated for vocal fold lesions, it should be limited as strictly as possible to the area of abnormality. Virtually no place exists for "vocal fold stripping" in patients with benign disease. Submucosal resection through a laryngeal microflap used to be advocated. In fact, the technique was introduced and first published by one of the authors (RTS). Microflap technique involved an incision on the superior surface of the vocal fold, submucosal resection, and preservation of the mucosa along the leading edge of the vocal fold. The concept that led to this innovation was based on the idea that the intermediate layer of the lamina propria should be protected to prevent fibroblast proliferation. Consequently, it seemed reasonable to preserve the mucosa as a biologic dressing. This technique certainly produced better results than vocal fold stripping. However, close scrutiny of outcomes revealed a small number of cases with poor results and stiffness beyond the limits of the original pathology. Consequently, the technique was abandoned in favor of a mini-microflap, or of local resection strictly limited to the region of pathology.[107] Lesions such as vocal nodules should be removed to a level even with the vibratory margin rather than deeply into the submucosa. This minimizes scarring and optimizes return to good vocal function. Naturally, if concern about a serious neoplasm exists, proper treatment takes precedence over voice preservation. Surgery should be performed under microscopic control. Preoperative and postoperative objective voice measures are essential to allow outcome assessment and self-critique. Only through such study can we improve surgical technique. Outcome studies are especially important in voice surgery as all our technical pronouncements

are anecdotal because there is no experimental model for vocal fold surgery. The human adult is the only species with a layered lamina propria.

Lasers are an invaluable adjunct in the laryngologists' armamentarium, but they must be used knowledgeably and with care. Considerable evidence suggests that healing time is prolonged and the incidence of adynamic segment formation is higher with the laser on the vibratory margin than with traditional instruments. Two early studies raised serious concerns about dysphonia after laser surgery.[108-109] Such complications may result from using too low a wattage, causing dissipation of heat deeply into the vocal fold; thus, high-power density for short duration has been recommended. Small spot size is also helpful. Nevertheless, many laryngologists caring for voice professionals avoid laser surgery in most cases pending further study. When biopsy specimens are needed, they should be taken before destroying the lesion with a laser. If a lesion is to be removed from the leading edge, the laser beam should be centered in the lesion, rather than on the vibratory margin, so that the beam does not create a divot in the vocal fold. The $CO_2$ laser may be particularly valuable for cauterizing isolated blood vessels responsible for recurrent hemorrhage. At the suggestion of Jean Abitbol, MD, the author has been placing a small piece of ice on the vocal fold immediately before laser use to help dissipate the heat and help prevent edema (personal communication, 1983). No studies on the efficacy of this maneuver exist, but the technique appears helpful.

Such vessels are often found at the base of a hemorrhagic polyp. Vascular lasers may be better than $CO_2$ lasers for management of these lesions and other vascular abnormalities. The 585-nm pulsed dye laser (PDL) has been used recently to treat vocal fold abnormalities. Pulsed dye lasers can be used through a flexible laryngoscope in an office or operating room. Typically, the laser is passed through a 1-mm fiber and delivers a spot size of 1 to 2 mm. In addition to treating abnormal vasculature, the PDL used to be used for papilloma,[109] dysplasia and papilloma. [110, 112]

The KTP/532 laser is an Nd-YAG laser. Its potential for use in surgery increased by 2 important improvements: doubling of the frequency of the wavelength and point of contact. Frequency doubling offers a technique to change the output wavelength from 1060 nm (infrared) to 532 nm (green) by means of a special crystal that combines 2 infrared photons to 1 green photon. A pulsed KTP laser has been used for treatment of vascular lesions of the vocal fold, in a manner similar to the pulsed dye laser (see below). The pulsed KTP laser has a wavelength of 532 nm. It has been advocated by some proponents as superior to the PDL because it may be less likely to cause hemorrhage of the vessels being treated because the 532-nm wavelength is more strongly absorbed by oxyhemoglobin than the 585-nm wavelength of the PDL. However, its tissue effects are different from the PDL, and it may be more likely to cause injury and stiffness of tissues adjacent to the blood vessels being treated. The KTP laser can be used either on an outpatient basis or in the operating room. It is delivered through a fiber. Although it is a "near-touch" laser, experience and skill are required to consistently achieve appropriate distance of the fiber from the vessel, in order to maximize vascular effect while minimizing adjacent tissue response. The pulsed KTP laser has been advocated for treatment of vascular lesions, as well as for treatment of papillomatosis and dysplasia.[113] A nonlaser technique (cold instrument) may be even better for managing some of these lesions.

Voice rest after vocal fold surgery is controversial. Although some laryngologists do not recognize its necessity at all, many physicians recommend voice rest for approximately 1 week or until the mucosal surface has healed. Even after surgery, silence for more than 7 to 10 days is nearly never necessary and represents a real hardship for many patients.

Too often, the laryngologist is controlled with a desperate patient whose voice has been "ruined" by vocal fold surgery, recurrent or superior laryngeal nerve paralysis, trauma, or some other tragedy. Occasionally, the cause is as straightforward as a dislocated arytenoid that can be reduced.[114–115] However, if the problem is an adynamic segment, decreased bulk of one vocal fold after "stripping," bowing caused by superior laryngeal nerve paralysis, or some other complication in a mobile vocal fold, great conservatism should be exercised. None of the available surgical procedures for these conditions is consistently effective. If surgery is considered at all, the procedure and prognosis should be explained to the patient realistically and pessimistically. The patient must understand that the chances of returning the voice to professional quality are very slim and that it may be made worse. Zyderm collagen (Xomed) injection has been studied and is helpful in some of these difficult cases.[116] Zyderm collagen, presently, is not approved by the Food and Drug Administration (FDA) for use in the vocal fold. If used at all, the material should be used under protocol with institutional review board approval. However, human collagen can be used and does not have the same shortcomings. Collagen may be particularly helpful for small adynamic segments. In one author's (RTS) opinion, the best technique

for extensive vocal fold scarring is autologous fat implantation into the vibratory margin.[117–118]

Occasionally, voice professionals inquire about surgery for pitch alteration. Such procedures have been successful in specially selected patients (such as those undergoing sex-change surgery), but they do not consistently provide good enough voice quality and range to be performed on a professional voice user.

## Discretion

The excitement and glamour associated with caring for voice patients, particularly a famous performer, naturally tempt the physician to talk about a distinguished patient. However, this tendency must be tempered. Having it known that he or she has consulted a laryngologist, particularly for treatment of a significant vocal problem, is not always in a voice professional's best interest. Famous singers, actors, politicians, and other professional voice users are ethically and legally entitled to the same confidentiality we ensure for our other patients.

## Voice Maintenance

Prevention of vocal dysfunction should be the goal of all professionals involved in the care of professional voice users. Good vocal health habits should be encouraged in childhood. Screaming, particularly outdoors at athletic events, should be discouraged. Promising young singers who join choirs should be educated to compensate for the Lombard effect. The youngster interested in singing, acting, debating, or other vocal activities should receive enough training to prevent voice abuse and should receive enthusiastic support for performing works and activities suitable for his or her age and voice. Training should be continued during or after puberty, and the voice should be allowed to develop naturally without pressure to perform operative roles prematurely.

Excellent regular training and practice are essential, and avoidance of irritants, particularly smoke, should be stressed early. Educating voice professionals about hormonal and anatomic alterations that may influence the voice allows him or her to recognize and analyze vocal dysfunction, compensating for it intelligently when it occurs. The body is dynamic, changing over a lifetime, and the voice is no exception. Continued vocal education, training, and monitoring are necessary throughout a lifetime, even in the most successful and well-established voice professionals. Vocal problems even in premiere singers are commonly caused by cessation of lessons, excessive schedule demands, and other correctable problems, rather than by irreversible alterations of aging. Anatomic, physiologic, and serious medical problems may affect the voices of patients of any age. Cooperation among the laryngologist, speech-language pathologist, acting teacher, and singing teacher provides an optimal environment for cultivation and protection of the vocal artist.

## References

1. Brodnitz F. Hormones and the human voice. *Bull NY Acad Med.* 1971;47:183–191.

2. Rubin JS, Sataloff RT, and Korovin GS. *Diagnosis and Treatment of Voice Disorders.* 4th ed. San Diego, CA: Plural Publishing; 2014.

3. von Leden H. Presentation at: Seventh Symposium on Care of the Professional Voice; June 16, 1978; The Juilliard School, New York, NY.

4. Punt NA. Applied laryngology—singers and actors. *Proc R Soc Med.* 1968;61:1152–1156.

5. Spiegel JR, Sataloff RT, Hawkshaw M, Hoover CA. Sinusitis. In: Sataloff RT. *Professional Voice: The Science and Art of Clinical Care.* 2nd ed. San Diego, CA: Singular Publishing; 1997:437–440.

6. Nachman SA, Pontrelli L. Central nervous system Lyme disease. *Semin Pediatr Infect Dis.* 2003;14(2):123–130.

7. Sataloff J, Sataloff RT. Otologic manifestations of Lyme disease. In: *Encyclopedia of Otolaryngology-Head and Neck Surgery.* New York, NY.

8. Goldfarb D, Sataloff RT. Lyme disease: a review for the otolaryngologist. *ENT.* 1994;73(11):824–829.

9. Kugeler KJ, Farley GM, Forrester JD, Mead P. Geographic distribution and expansion of human Lyme disease, United States. *Emerg Infect Dis.* 2015 Aug; 21(8):1455–1457.

10. Clark JR, Carlson RD, Sasaki CT, Pachner AR, Steere AC. Facial paralysis in Lyme disease. *NATS J.* 1995;95: 1341–1345.

11. Steere AC, Grodzick MS, Kornblatt AN, et al. The spirochetal etiology of Lyme disease. *New Engl J Med.* 1983;308:733–740.

12. Burgdorfer WA, Barbour AG, Hayes SF, Benach JL, Grunwaldt E, David JP. Lyme disease-tick-borne spirochetosis. *Science.* 1982;216:1317–1319.

13. Strle F, Ruzic-Sablijic E, Cimperman J, Lotric-Furlan S, Maraspin V. Comparison of findings for patients with *Borrelia garinii* and *Borrelia afzelii* isolated from cerebrospinal fluid. *Clin Infect Dis.* 43(6):704–710.

14. Magnarelli LA. Serologic diagnostics of Lyme disease. *Ann NY Acad Sci.* 1988;539:154–161.

15. Sehgal VN, Khurana A. Lyme disease/borreliosis as a systemic disease. *Clin Dermatol.* 2015;33:542–550.

16. Barbour AG. Diagnosis of Lyme disease: rewards and perils. *Ann Intern Med.* 1989;11(7):501–502.

17. Glassock ME, Pensak ML, Gulia AJ, Baker DC. Lyme disease: a cause of bilateral facial paralysis. *Arch Otolaryngol.* 1985;111:47–49.

18. Schroeter V. Paralysis of recurrent laryngeal nerve in Lyme disease. *Lancet.* 1988;2(8622):1245.

19. Steere AC, Malaawista SE, Hardin JA, Ruddy S, Askenase PW, Andiman WA. Erythema chronicum migrans and Lyme arthritis: the enlarging clinical spectrum. *Ann Intern Med.* 1988;86:685–698.

20. Bull TR. Tuberculosis of the larynx. *Br Med J.* 1966;2: 991–992.

21. Hunter AM, Millar JW, Wrightman AJ, Horne NW. The changing pattern of laryngeal tuberculosis. *J Laryngol Otol.* 1981;95:393–398.

22. Divine KD. Sarcoidosis and sarcoidosis of the larynx. *Laryngoscope.*1965;75:533–569.

23. Munor MacCormick CE. The larynx in leprosy. *Arch Otolaryngol.* 1957;66:138–149.

24. Binford CH, Meyers WM. Leprosy. In: Binford CH, Conor DH, eds. *Pathology of Tropical and Extraordinary Diseases,* Vol 1. Washington, DC: Armed Forces Institute of Pathology; 1976:205–225.

25. MacKenzie M. *A Manual of Diseases of the Throat and Nose, Vol. 1 Diseases of the Pharynx, Larynx, and Trachea.* London, England: J.& A. Churchill; 1884.

26. Astacio JN, Goday GA, Espinosa FJ. *Escleroma. Experiences en El Salvador.* Seconda Mongrafia de Dermatologia iberolatino-americana. Suplemento AO No. 1, Lisboa, Portugal, 1971.

27. Hajek M. *Pathologie unde Therapie der Erkrankungen des Kehlkopfes, der Luftrohre und der Bronchien.* Leipzig: Verlag von Curt Kabitzsch; 1932.

28. Withers BT, Pappas JJ, Erickson EE. Histoplasmosis primary in the larynx. Report of a case. *Arch Otolaryngol.* 1977;77:25–28.

29. Calcaterra TC. Otolaryngeal histoplasmosis. *Laryngoscope.* 1970;80:111–120.

30. Sataloff RT, Wilborn A, Prestipino A, Hawkshaw M, Heuer RJ, Cohn JR. Histoplasmosis of the larynx. *Amer J Otolaryngol.* 1993;14(3):199–205.

31. Friedmann I. Diseases of the larynx. Disorders of laryngeal function. In: Paparella MM, Shumrick DA, eds. *Otolaryngology.* 2nd ed. Philadelphia, PA: WB Saunders; 1980:2449–2469.

32. Reese MC, Conclasure JB. Cryptococcosis of the larynx. *Arch Otolaryngol.* 1975;101:698–701.

33. Bennett M. Laryngeal blastomycosis. *Laryngoscope.* 1964;74:498–512.

34. Hoffarth GA, Joseph DL, Shumrick DA. Deep mycoses. *Arch Otolaryngol.* 1973;97:475–479.

35. Brandenburg JH, Finch WW, Kirkham WR. Actinomycosis of the larynx and pharynx. *Otolaryngology.* 1978; 86:739–742.

36. Shaheen SO, Ellis FG. Actinomycosis of the larynx. *J R Soc Med.* 1983;76:226–228.

37. Tedeschi LG, Cheren RV. Laryngeal hyperkeratosis due to primary monilial infection. *Arch Otolaryngol.* 1968;82:82–84.

38. Rao PB. Aspergillosis of the larynx. *J Laryngol Otol.* 1969;83:377–379.

39. Ferlito A. Clinical records. Primary aspergillosis of the larynx. *J Laryngol Otol.* 1974;88:1257–1263.

40. Keir SM, Flint A, Moss JA. Primary aspergillosis of the larynx simulating carcinoma. *Hum Pathol.* 1983;14: 184–186.

41. Anand CS, Gupta MC, Kothari MG, Anand TS, Singh SK. Laryngeal mucormycosis. *Indian J Otolaryngol.* 1978;30:90–92.

42. Pillai OS. Rhinosporidiosis of the larynx. *J Laryngol Otol.* 1974;88:277–280.

43. Ferlito A. Clinical records. Primary aspergillosis of the larynx stimulating carcinoma. *Hum Pathol.* 1938; 14:184–186.

44. Zinneman HH, Hall WH, Wallace FG. Leishmaniasis of the larynx. Report of a case and its confusion with histoplasmosis. *Am J Med.* 1961;31:654–658.

45. Michaels L. *Pathology of the Larynx.* New York, NY: Springer-Verlag; 1984.

46. Wolman L, Darke CS, Young A. The larynx in rheumatoid arthritis. *J Laryngol.* 1965;79:403–434.

47. Bridger MWN, Jahn AF, van Nostrand AWP. Laryngeal rheumatoid arthritis. *Laryngoscope.* 1980;90:296–303.

48. Virchow R. Seltene Gichtablagerungen. *Virchows Arch Path Anat.* 1868;44:137–138.

49. Marion RB, Alperin JE, Maloney WH. Gouty tophus of the true vocal cord. *Arch Otolaryngol.* 1972;96: 161–162.

50. Epstein SS, Winston P, Friedmann I, Ormerod FC. The vocal cord polyp. *J Laryngol Otol Lond.* 1957;71:673–688.

51. Stark DB, New GB. Amyloid tumors of larynx, trachea or bronchi: report of 15 cases. *Ann Otol Rhinol Laryngol.* 1949;58:117–134.

52. Michaels L, Hyams VJ. Amyloid in localized deposits and plasmacytomas of the respiratory tract. *J Pathol.* 1979:128(1):29–38.

53. Pribtkin E, Friedman O, O'Hara B, et al. Amyloidosis of the upper aerodigestive tract. *Laryngoscope.* 2003; 113:2095–2101.

54. Urbach E, Wiethe C. Lipoidosis cutis et mucosae. *Virchows Arch Path Anat.* 1929;273:285–319.

55. Charow A, Pass F, Ruben R. Pemphigus of the upper respiratory tract. *Arch Otolaryngol.* 1971;93:209–210.

56. Sataloff RT, Johns MM, Kost KM. *Geriatic Otolaryngology.* New York, NY: Thieme; 2015.

57. Sundberg J, Prame E, Iwarsson J. Replicability and accuracy of pitch patterns in professional singers. In: David PJ, Fletcher NH, eds. *Vocal Fold Physiology: Controlling Chaos and Complexity.* Sydney, Australia: Singular Publishing; 1996:291–306.

58. Sataloff RT, Cohn JR, Hawkshaw M. Respiratory dysfunction. In: Sataloff RT. *Professional Voice: The Science and Art of Clinical Care.* 3rd ed. San Diego, CA: Plural Publishing; 2005:717–728.

59. Spiegel JR, Sataloff RT, Cohn JR, et al. Respiratory function in singers. Medical assessment, diagnoses and treatments. *J Voice.* 1988;2(1):40–50.

60. Cohn JR, Sataloff RT, Spiegel JR, et al. Airway reactivity-induced asthma in singers (ARIAS). *J Voice.* 1991;5(4): 332–337.

61. Cohn JR, Padams PA, Hawkshaw M, Sataloff RT. Allergy. In: Sataloff RT. *Professional Voice: The Science and Art of Clinical Care.* 3rd ed. San Diego, CA: Plural Publishing; 2005:711–716.

62. Sataloff RT, Katz PO, Sataloff DM, Hawkshaw MJ. *Reflux Laryngitis and Related Disorders.* 4th ed. San Diego, CA: Plural Publishing; 2013.

63. Sataloff RT, Katz PO, Sataloff DM, Hawkshaw MJ. *Reflux Laryngitis and Related Disorders.* 4th ed. San Diego, CA: Plural Publishing; 2013;60–64;89–91.

64. Ritter FN. The effect of hypothyroidism on the larynx of the rat. *Ann Otol Rhinol Laryngol.* 1964;67:404–416.

65. Ritter RN. Endocrinology. In: Paparella M, Shumrick D, eds. *Otolaryngology.* Vol 1. Philadelphia, PA: Saunders; 1973;727–734.

66. Michelsson K, Sirvio P. Cry analysis in congenital hypothyroidism. *Folia Phoniat.* 1976;28:40–47.

67. Gupta OP, Bhatia PL, Agarwal MK, Mehrotra ML, Mishr SK. Nasal pharyngeal and laryngeal manifestations of hypothyroidism. *Ear Nose Throat J.* 1977;56(9): 10–21.

68. Malinsky M, Chevrrie-Muller C, Cerceau N. Etude Clinique et electrophysiologique des alterations de la voix au cours des thyrotoxioses. *Ann Endocrinol.* 1977; 38:171–172.

69. Meuser W, Nieschlag E. Sexual hormone und Stimmlage des Mannes. *Deutsch Med Wochenschr.* 1977;102: 261–264.

70. Brodnitz F. The age of the castrato voice. *J Speech Hearing Disord.* 1975;40:291–295.

71. Anderson TD, Anderson DD, Sataloff RT. Endocrine dysfunction. In: Sataloff RT. *Professional Voice: The Science and Art of Clinical Care.* 3rd ed. San Diego, CA: Plural Publishing; 2005:537–550.

72. Schiff M. The influence of estrogens on connective tissue. In: Asboe-Hansen G, ed. *Hormones and Connective Tissue.* Copenhagen, Denmark: Munksgaard Press; 1967:282–341.

73. Lacina V. Der Einfluss der Menstruation auf die Stimme der Sangerinnen. *Folia Phoniatr.* 1968;20: 13–24.

74. Wendler J. Cyclicly dependent variations in efficiency of the voice and its influencing by ovulation inhibitors. Zyklusabhangige Leistungsschwankungen der Stimme und ihre Beeinflussung durch Ovulationshemmer. *Folia Phoniatr.* 1972;24(4):259–277.

75. von Gelder L. Psychosomatic aspects of endocrine disorders of the voice. *J Comm Disord.* 1974;7:257–262.

76. Carroll C. Arizona State University at Tempe. Personal communication with Dr. Hans von Leden. September 1992.

77. Dordain M. Etude Statistique de l'influence des contraceptifs hormonaux sur la voix. *Folia Phoniat.* 1972; 24:86–96.

78. Pahn V, Goretzlehner G. Stimmstorungen durch hormonale Kontrazeptiva. *Zentralb Gynakol.* 1978;100:341–346.

79. Schiff M. "The pill" in otolaryngology. *Trans Am Acad Opthalmol Otolaryngol.* 1968;72:76–84.

80. Brodnitz F. Medical care preventative therapy (panel). In: Lawrence V, ed. *Transcripts of the Seventh Annual Symposium, Care of the Professional Voice.* Vol 3. New York, NY: Voice Foundation; 1978:86.

81. Flach M, Schwickardi H, Simen R. Welchen Einfluss haben Menstruation und Schwangershaft auf die augsgebildete Gesangsstimme? *Folia Phoniatr.* 1968;21: 199–210.

82. Deuster CV. Irreversible Stimmstorung in der Schwangersheft. *HNO.* 1977;25:430–432.

83. Damste PH. Virilization of the voice due to anabolic steroids. *Folia Phoniatr.* 1964;16:10–18.

84. Damste PH. Voice changes in adult women caused by virilizing agents. *J Speech Hear Disord.* 1967;32:126–132.

85. Saez S, Francoise S. Recepteurs d'androgenes: mise en evidence dans la fraction cytosolique de muqueuse normale et d'epitheliomas pharyngolarynges humains. *C R Acad Sci (Paris).* 1975;280:935–938.

86. Vuorenkoski V, Lenko HL, Tjernlund P, Vuorenkoski L, Perheentupa J. Fundamental voice frequency during normal and abnormal growth, and after androgen treatment. *Arch Dis Child.* 1978;53:201–209.

87. Bourdial J. Les troubles de la voix provoques par la therapeutique hormonale androgene. *Ann Otolaryngol.* 1970;87:725–734.

88. Imre V. Hormonell bedingte Stimmstorungen. *Folia Phoniatr.* 1968;20:394–404.

89. National Institutes of Health. *Health Implications of Obesity.* Consensus Development Conference Statement. Bethesda, MD; 1986.

90. Gates GA, Saegert J, Wilson N, Johnson L, Sheperd A, Hearnd EM. Effects of beta-blockade on singing performance. *Ann Otol Rhinol Laryngol.* 1985;94:570–574.

91. Rosen DC, Sataloff RT. *Psychology of Voice Disorders.* San Diego, CA: Singular Publishing; 1997 .

92. Sataloff RT. Vocal fold scar. In: Sataloff RT. *Professional Voice: The Science and Art of Clinical Care.* 3rd ed. San Diego, CA: Plural Publishing; 2005:1309–1314.

93. Sataloff RT, Hawkshaw M. Vocal fold hemorrhage. In: Sataloff RT. *Professional Voice: The Science and Art of Clinical Care.* 3rd ed. San Diego, CA: Plural Publishing; 2005:1291–1308.

94. Hochman I, Sataloff RT, Hillman R, Zeitels S. Ectasias and varicies of the vocal fold: clearing the striking zone. *Ann Otol Rhinol Laryngol.* 1999;108(1):10–16.

95. Zeitels SM. Phonomicrosurgical techniques. In: Sataloff RT. *Professional Voice: The Science and Art of Clinical Care.* 3rd ed. San Diego, CA: Plural Publishing: 2005: 1215–1236.

96. Zeitels SM, Sataloff RT. Phonomicrosurgical resection of glottal papillomatosis. *J Voice.* 1999;13(1):123–127.

97. Wellens W, Snoeck R, Desloovere C, et al. Treatment of severe laryngeal papillomatosis with intralesional injections of cidofovir [(S)-1-(3-Hydroxy-Phosphonylmethoxypropyl) Cytosine, HPMPC, Vistide]. In: McCafferty G, Coman W, Carroll R, eds. *Proceedings of the XVI World Congress of Otorhinolaryngology Head and Neck Surgery.* Bologna, Italy: Monduzzi Editor; 1997:455–549.

98. Wolman L, Drake CS, Young A. The larynx in rheumatoid arthritis. *J Laryngol.* 1965;79:403–404.

99. Bridger MWM, Jahn AF, van Nostrand AWP. Laryngeal rheumatoid arthritis. *Laryngoscope.* 1980;90:296–303.

100. Virchow R. Seltene Gichtablagerungen. *Virchows Arch Pathol.* 1868;44:137–138.

101. Marion RB, Alperin JE, Maloney WH. Gouty tophus of the true vocal cord. *Arch Otolaryngol.* 1972;96:161–162.

102. Stark DB, New GB. Amyloid tumors of the larynx, trachea or bronchi; report of 15 cases. *Ann Otol Rhinol Laryngol.* 1949;58:117–134.

103. Michaels L, Hyams VJ. Amyloid in localized deposits and plasmacytomas of the respiratory tract. *J Pathol.* 1979;128:29–38.

104. Urbach E, Wiethe C. Lipoidosis cutis et mucosae. *Virchows Arch Pathol Anat.* 1929;273:285–319.

105. Sataloff RT, Hawkshaw M, Ressue J. Granular cell tumor of the larynx. *Ear Nose Throat J.* 1998;77(8):582–584.

106. Charow A, Pass F, Ruben R. Pemphigus of the upper respiratory tract. *Arch Otolaryngol.* 1971;93:209–210.

107. Sataloff RT, Spiegel JR, Heuer RJ, et al. Laryngeal mini-microflap: a new technique and reassessment of the microflap saga. *J Voice.* 1995;9(2):198–204.

108. Abitbol J. Limitations of the laser in microsurgery of the larynx. In: Lawrence VL, ed. *Transactions of the Twelfth Symposium: Care of the Professional Voice.* New York: NY: The Voice Foundation; 1984:297–302.

109. Strong MS, Jako GJ. Laser surgery in the larynx. Early clinical experience with continuous $CO_2$ laser. *Ann Otol Rhinol Laryngol.* 1972;81:791–798.

110. Cohen JT, Koufman JA, Postma GN. Pulsed-dye laser in the treatment of recurrent respiratory papillomatosis of the larynx. *ENT-J.* 2003;83(8):558.

111. Zeitels SM, Franco R, Dailey SH, Burns JA, Hillman RE, Anderson RR. Office-based treatment of glottal dysplasia and papillomatosis with the 585-nm pulsed dye laser and local anesthesia. *Ann Otol Rhinol Laryngol.* 2004;113(4):265–275.

112. Franco RA Jr, Zeitels SM, Farinelli WA, et al. 585-jm pulsed dye laser treatment of glottal dysplasia. *Ann Otol Rhinol Laryngol.* 2003;112(9):751–758.

113. Zeitels SM, Akst LM, Burns JA, et al. Office-based 532-nm pulsed-KTP laser treatment of glottal papillomatosis and dysplasia. *Ann Otol Rhinol Laryngol.* 2006;115(9):679–685.

114. Sataloff RT, Feldman M, Darby KS, Carroll LM, Spiegel JR. Arytenoid dislocation. *J Voice.* 1988;1(4):368–377.

115. Sataloff RT, Bough ID, Spiegel JR. Arytenoid dislocation: diagnosis and treatment. *Laryngoscope.* 1994; 104(10):1353–1361.

116. Ford CN, Bless DM. Collagen injected into the scarred vocal fold. *J Voice.* 1988;1(1):116–118.

117. Sataloff RT, Spiegel JR, Hawkshaw M, Rosen DC, Heuer RJ. Autologous fat implantation for vocal fold scar. *J Voice*. 1997;11(2):238–246.

118. Sataloff RT. Autologous fat implantation for vocal fold scar. *Curr Opin Otolaryngol Head Neck Surg*. 2010;18: 503–506.

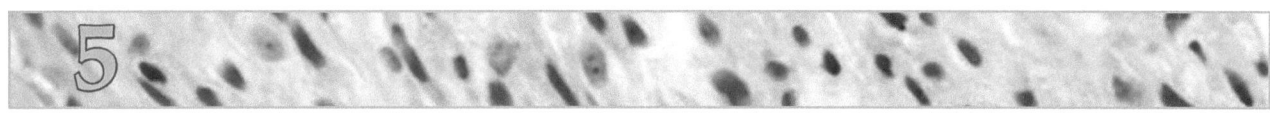

# Sleep, Body Fatigue, and Voice

*Abdul-Latif Hamdan, Robert Thayer Sataloff, and
Mary J. Hawkshaw*

Vocal fatigue is a broad term commonly used to describe voice impairment that develops with voice use. Kostyk and Rochet have considered vocal fatigue within a spectrum of symptoms that include specific complaints such as loss of voice, and non-specific ones such as running out of breath and throat tightness.[1] Professional voice users describe vocal fatigue differently. In a study by Kitch and Oates, actors reported vocal fatigue as "increased difficulty achieving adequate voice production," whereas singers reported it as "reduction in the pitch and dynamic range." These descriptions of vocal fatigue, which were retrieved in this study using a questionnaire, highlight the broad nature of this complaint and the multifaceted etiology behind it.[2] This chapter provides a brief review of vocal fatigue in the context of sleep deprivation and generalized body fatigue.

## Vocal Fatigue Pathophysiology

Vocal fatigue has been associated with various functional and organic voice disorders, with no clear consensus on which comes first. Vocal fatigue can be a symptom of a laryngeal pathology or a prelude to the development of such pathology. Further investigation is needed to understand this problem better. Its presence in patients with normal vocal folds and hyperfunctional supraglottic behavior may be associated with improper technique or repertoire, compensation for inefficiency in the vocal apparatus, or an underlying focal or systemic disease that may not be obvious at time of presentation. Welham and Maclagan reviewing current definitions and concepts of vocal fatigue, suggested five possible mechanisms for the development of vocal fatigue. In brief these include, neuromuscular fatigue, increased vocal fold

viscosity, reduced blood circulation, neuromuscular tissue strain and respiratory fatigue.[3] MacArdle et al, defined neuromuscular fatigue as "a reduction in the capacity of a muscle to sustain tension under repeated stimulation."[4] In phonation, hypothetically this translates into reduced ability of the adductors and longitudinal tensors to sustain the right amount of tension within the vocal folds during voice production. Neuromuscular fatigue can be either peripheral in origin secondary to inability to clear lactic acid or to replenish the glycogen storage, or centrally through an inhibitory pathway,[4] or a defective activator pathway (eg. paresis). Criticism of this hypothesis cite the high ratio of type I to type II fibers in the thyroarytenoid muscle which makes it highly resistant to vocal fatigue.[5] The increased vocal fold viscosity hypothesis is based on the relationship between lubrication and/or tissue viscosity and efficiency of vocal fold vibration. With an increase in vocal fold viscosity secondary to prolonged phonatory use or dehydration, there is an increase in the phonation threshold pressure (the pressure needed to initiate oscillation of the vocal folds). This theory has been substantiated by numerous animal and human studies.[6–10] Respiratory muscle fatigue is another plausible theory founded on the common knowledge that breathing energizes the oscillator. Reduced breathing capacity, as in patients with obstructive lung disease, may contribute to the development of vocal fatigue. This theory is particularly convincing in singers and other professional voice users in whom even a minor decrease in vital capacity may jeopardize vocal performance.[11] A thorough discussion of the association between breathing and phonation is presented in the chapter on respiratory diseases and voice in this book. Another suggested hypothesis for vocal fatigue is reduced blood circulation. A reduction in blood flow might hinder the removal of lactic acid, the dissipation of heat, and the transfer of adequate oxygenation. Last, neuromuscular strain also might contribute to vocal fatigability through repetitive mechanical stress to the non-muscular structures of the vocal folds. This phonation induced stress is particularly produced at high pitches and high intensities and may also affect other ligamentous structures of the larynx.

The self-reported complaint of vocal fatigue is often paralleled with acoustic and stroboscopic changes.[12–14] Mann et al showed an increase in perturbation parameters on the first day following the performance of vocally demanding tasks in 16 subjects out of 42. However the authors failed to demonstrate consistent acoustic changes over the course of 6 days, partially due to large intersubject variability and a large number of outliers. Laryngeal videostroboscopic examination proved more sensitivity in detecting effects of excessive vocalization. The most commonly reported findings were free edge irregularities, vocal fold edematous changes, and decrease in mucosal waves and amplitude.[13] In a study by Cho et al examining validated indicators of physical and mental fatigue, the authors reported that several acoustic parameters in addition to self-rated symptoms are indicative of the extent of fatigue using the Chalder Fatigue Scale score. VHI changed in association with physical fatigue in women and mental fatigue in men; and harmonic-to-noise ratio, shimmer, and F0 tremor correlated with mental fatigue in men only.[12] Thus, both acoustic analysis and stroboscopic examination are valuable tools in substantiating the self-reported symptom of vocal fatigue.

## Sleep Deprivation and Voice

Sleep duration has been related to quality of life and various health conditions. Sleep deprivation or excessive sleep may have adverse systemic effects leading to increased morbidity. Short sleep duration may exacerbate hypertension, diabetes, and cardiovascular diseases, in addition to oncologic diseases. Excessive sleep has been associated with autoimmune diseases, endocrine disorders, and many other medical conditions.[15–19] The importance of sleep on the functioning of various systems in the body has inspired numerous investigators to explore the possible effect of abnormal sleeping patterns on voice. In a cross-sectional study that involved 17,806 adults, Cho et al investigated the association between sleep duration and voice problems as reported by the patient using various questionnaires.[20] The results showed that the

lowest prevalence of dysphonia was associated with a 7 to 8 hours duration of sleep, whereas sleep duration of less than 5 hours and sleep duration of more than 9 hours were associated with higher prevalence of dysphonia. The impact of long sleep duration on voice was attributed to the possible inflammatory and immunologically mediated responses that can affect the respiratory system with subsequent vocal alterations. Similarly, short duration of sleep has been associated with dysphonia through its effect on overall body fatigability.[21,22] In a case-control study by O'Hara et al, the authors explored the level of fatigue in patients with functional dysphonia versus a control group matched by gender and within 5 years of age. The results showed that patients with functional dysphonia had higher mean fatigue scores compared to healthy subjects (17.0 vs 14.4, $p = 0.009$). Without inferring causality, the authors related fatigability to the worse overall health condition in patients with functional dysphonia.[21] Another intriguing study by Bagnall et al on the potential effect of sleep deprivation on voice substantiates the paramount effect of sleep on our ability to vocalize. By depriving 15 subjects of sleep for 24 hours, the authors demonstrated that sleep deprivation tires the voice and lowers its fundamental frequency. Sleep-deprived subjects sounded rough, "croaky," and not so "bright."[22] These results were in accordance with previous reports on the effect of sleep deprivation on voice and speech.[23–25] Harrison and Horne described the voices of sleep-deprived subjects as flat and monotonic. In addition to these vocal changes, there was decline or worsening of word generation.[24] The influence of sleep on voice also has been investigated by Rocha and Behlau in a descriptive and analytical study on 862 subjects.[26] Using various sleep and voice self-assessment questionnaires, the authors highlighted sleep as an important factor that influences vocal self-assessment. The results indicated that daytime sleepiness negatively influenced the perceived voice handicap (odds ratio less than 1). More severe forms of sleep disorders such as obstructive sleep apnea also have been shown to impact voice quality negatively. Atan et al, in their investigation on the effect of obstructive sleep apnea (OSA) on voice in a group of 27 patients, reported higher cycle-to-cycle variation in amplitude and higher values of Voice Handicap Index-10 in patients with OSA versus controls (13.11 in patients with OSA vs 1.18 in controls).[23]

In brief, sleep and voice are intimately related. As a sign of health, voice mirrors any threat to our well-being imposed by sleep deprivation. The importance of adequate sleep duration cannot be overemphasized in singers and professional voice users who are commonly challenged to perform under stressful conditions.[27]

## Body Fatigue and Voice

Body fatigue has many definitions and connotations associated with it. In research, it is defined as "reaction to a workload" that can be either psychological or physiological.[25] When fatigue persists for a long period of time, the term chronic fatigue syndrome (CFS) is used. This has been defined as "self-reported persistent or relapsing fatigue lasting 6 or more consecutive months."[28] Affected patients report fatigability that markedly impairs quality of life and productivity and that is not secondary to an ongoing exertion or relieved by rest.[28] Additional criteria for diagnosis include, among others, memory impairment, headache, muscular pain, and throat pain. Chronic fatigue syndrome has been associated with numerous medical conditions that include both psychologic and physiologic conditions. It has been associated with depression and somatic disorders, infectious diseases such as Epstein-Barr virus and infectious mononucleosis, cardiovascular diseases, and respiratory impairment. To that end, the definition of chronic fatigue syndrome has been linked in the literature with many terms such as neuroasthenia described by Abbey and Garfinkel[29] in relation to altered senses and cognitive impairment, or to neuromyasthenia in reference to muscular pain and fatigability.[30] Several authors also have reported reduced lung function, and abnormalities in gas exchange with decreased values for oxygen consumption in affected patients.[31-33]

Given the importance of physical fitness in phonation, patients and singers in particular who suffer from body fatigue may exhibit vocal dysfunction that can affect their performance. In addition to the compromise in physical endurance and muscular activity in patients with CFS, affected subjects may suffer from the associated morbidities of this syndrome. Decreased ability to concentrate and follow a conversation may affect the ability to communicate. Similarly, impaired breathing and decreased exercise tolerance associated with cardiopulmonary diseases may impact endurance and limit the duration of performance.

## References

1. Kostyk BE, Rochet AP. Laryngeal airway resistance in teachers with vocal fatigue: a preliminary study. *J Voice*. 1998;12:287–299.
2. Kitch JA, Oates J. The perceptual features of vocal fatigue as self-reported by a group of actors and singers. *J Voice*. 1994;8:207–214.
3. Welham NV, Maclagan MA. Vocal fatigue: current knowledge and future directions. *J Voice*. 2003;17(1): 21–30.
4. McArdle WD, Katch FI, Katch VL. *Exercise Physiology: Energy, Nutrition, and Human Performance*. 4th ed. Baltimore, MD: Williams & Wilkins; 1996.
5. Cooper DS, Rice DH. Fatigue resistance of canine vocal fold muscle. *Ann Otol Rhinol Laryngol*. 1990;99:228–233.
6. Finkelor BK, Titze IR, Durham PL. The effect of viscosity changes in the vocal folds on the range of oscillation. *J Voice*. 1988;1:320–325.
7. Jiang J, Ng J, Hanson D. The effects of rehydration on phonation in excised canine larynges. *J Voice*. 1999; 13:51–59.
8. Solomon NP, DiMattia MS. Effects of a vocally fatiguing task and systemic hydration on phonation threshold pressure. *J Voice*. 2000;14:341–362.
9. Verdolini K, Titze IR, Fennell A. Dependence of phonatory effort on hydration level. *J Speech Hear Res*. 1994; 37:1001–1007.
10. Verdolini-Marston K, Titze IR, Druker DG. Changes in phonation threshold pressure with induced conditions of hydration. *J Voice*. 1990;4:142–151.
11. Sataloff RT. Cohn JR, Hawshkaw M. Respiratory dysfunction. In: *Professinal Voice: The Science and Art of Clinical Care*. 4th ed. San Diego, CA; Plural Publishing: 2017; 751–764.
12. Cho SW, Yin CS, Park YB, Park YJ. Differences in self-rated, perceived, and acoustic voice qualities between high-and low-fatigue groups. *J Voice*. 2011; 25(5): 544–552.
13. Mann EA, McClean MD, Gurevich-Uvena J, et al. The effects of excessive vocalization on acoustic and videostroboscopic measures of vocal fold condition. *J Voice*. 1999;13(2):294–302.
14. Onofre F, de Almeida Prado Y, Rojas GV, Garcia DM, Aguiar-Ricz L. Measurements of the acoustic speaking voice after vocal warm-up and cool-down in choir singers. *J Voice*. 2017;31(1):129–e9.
15. Ikehara S, Iso H, Date C, et al. Association of sleep duration with mortality from cardiovascular disease and other causes for Japanese men and women: the JACC study. *Sleep*. 2009;32(3):295–301.
16. Gottlieb DJ, Redline S, Nieto FJ, et al. Association of usual sleep duration with hypertension: the Sleep Heart Health Study. *Sleep*. 2006;29(8):1009–1014.
17. Taheri S, Lin L, Austin D, Young T, Mignot E. Short sleep duration is associated with reduced leptin, elevated ghrelin, and increased body mass index. *PLoS Med*. 2004;1(3):e62.
18. Parish JM. Sleep-related problems in common medical conditions. *Chest*. 2009;135(2):563–572.
19. Nieto FJ, Peppard PE, Young T, Finn L, Hla KM, Farre R. Sleep-disordered breathing and cancer mortality: results from the Wisconsin Sleep Cohort Study. *Am J Respir Crit Care Med*. 2012;186(2):190–194.
20. Cho JH, Guilminault C, Joo YH, Jin SK, Han KD, Park CS. A possible association between dysphonia

and sleep duration: a cross-sectional study based on the Korean National Health and nutrition examination surveys from 2010 to 2012. *PloS One*. 2017;12(8): e0182286.

21. O'Hara J, Miller T, Carding P, Wilson J, Deary V. Relationship between fatigue, perfectionism, and functional dysphonia. *Otolaryngol Head Neck Surg*. 2011;144(6): 921–926.

22. Bagnall AD, Dorrian J, Fletcher A. Some vocal consequences of sleep deprivation and the possibility of "fatigue proofing" the voice with Voicecraft(R) voice training. *J Voice*. 2011;25(4):447–461.

23. Atan D, Özcan KM, İkincioğulları A, et al. The effect of obstructive sleep apnea syndrome and continuous positive airway pressure treatment on voice performance. *Sleep Breathing*. 2015;19(3):777–782.

24. Harrison Y, Horne JA. Sleep deprivation affects speech. *Sleep*. 1997;20(10):871–877.

25. Ruiz R, Legros C, Guell A. Voice analysis to predict the psychological or physical state of a speaker. *Aviation Space Environ Med*. 1990. 61: 266–271.

26. Rocha BR, Behlau M. The influence of sleep disorders on voice quality. *J Voice*. 2017.

27. Sataloff RT. Sleep and the vocal performer. In: Sataloff RT. *Professional Voice: The Science and Art of Clinical Care*. 4th ed. San Diego, CA: Plural Publishing: 2017: 863–876.

28. Fukuda K, Straus SE, Hickie I, Sharpe MC, Dobbins JG, Komaroff A. The chronic fatigue syndrome: a comprehensive approach to its definition and study. *Ann Int Med*. 1994;121(12):953–9.

29. Abbey SE, Garfinkel PE. Neurasthenia and chronic fatigue syndrome: the role of culture in the making of a diagnosis. *Am J Psychiatry*. 1991;148(12):1638.

30. Shorter E. Chronic fatigue in historical perspective. *Chron Fat Syn*. 1993; pp. 6–22.

31. Snell CR, Stevens SR, Davenport TE, Van Ness JM. Discriminative validity of metabolic and workload measurements for identifying people with chronic fatigue syndrome. *Phys Ther*. 2013;93(11):1484–1492.

32. Keller BA, Pryor JL, Giloteaux L. Inability of myalgic encephalomyelitis/chronic fatigue syndrome patients to reproduce VO 2 peak indicates functional impairment. *J Translat Med*. 2014;12(1):104.

33. Payne CB, Sloan HE. Pulmonary function and the chronic fatigue syndrome. *Ann Int Med*. 1989;111(10):860.

# 6

# Laryngeal Manifestations of Neurologic Disorders

*Abdul-Latif Hamdan, Robert Thayer Sataloff, and Mary J. Hawkshaw*

## Vocal Fold Paresis and Paralysis and Other Causes of Hypomobility

The larynx is a key player at three cross-cutting frontiers: breathing, phonation, and swallowing. In phonation, the airstream is chopped at the level of the vocal folds into glottal pulses with resulting harmonics, the position and dispersion of which are markedly affected by the configuration of the vocal tract. In breathing, the larynx acts as a resistor that controls the inspiratory and expiratory flow through its laryngeal inlet. In swallowing, the larynx becomes a sphincter that prohibits aspiration via the anterosuperior displacement of the hyoid bone, stretching of the hyoepiglottic ligament, and closure of the rima glottidis. In cases of vocal fold paralysis, the intertwining among these three complex aforementioned tasks is jeopardized. There is loss of the net abduction of the vocal folds with an alteration in the configuration of the vocal tract.

The etiology of vocal fold paralysis is broad and encompasses an array of conditions that includes infectious diseases such as viral neuritis, inflammatory diseases, lesions of the central nervous system, or peripheral masses compressing the recurrent laryngeal nerve along its course in the neck and chest. An equally important and common cause of vocal fold paralysis is iatrogenic injury to the recurrent laryngeal nerve during or in preparation for surgery.[1-5] The potential mechanisms of injury include right central venous catheterization, excessive traction on the esophagus, undue pressure of a large cuffed endotracheal tube, nasogastric tube syndrome, thermal injury, and last but not least is direct injury to the

nerve during dissection.[6-10] See Figures 6–1 and 6–2. Based on a study by Remacle in 1996, the most common causes of vocal fold paralysis include thyroidectomy in up to 58% of the cases, tumor compression, viral neuritis, thoracic surgery (tracheal surgery, esophagectomy), and peripheral neuropathy.[11] Other causes of vocal fold immobility such as cricoarytenoid joint ankylosis secondary to autoimmune diseases, radiotherapy and external trauma should be rule out.[12-14] See Figures 6–3 and 6–4.

The workup of patients with vocal fold paralysis starts by taking a good medical history inquiring about the presence of neurologic disorders, systemic diseases, history of malignancies, previous laryngeal manipulation, and last are surgeries to the neck or chest.[15] Equally important is the vocal history, learning about the patient's vocal habits and hygiene such as smoking and amount of water intake. Complaints related to phonation, breathing, and swallowing must be diligently solicited. In cases of unilateral vocal fold paralysis, patients may present with dysphonia, often described as breathiness, vocal fatigue, and inability to project the voice. Patients may also complain of dysphagia, aspiration with or without shortness of breath. In patients with bilateral vocal fold paralysis, the presentation is that of dyspnea, respiratory discomfort, and stridor. The voice is less commonly affected though many patients have vocal symptoms. The self-reported questionnaires, such as the Voice Handicap Index and Voice-Related quality of life VRQOL, in addition to perceptual evaluation are subjective tools that help markedly in deciding on the best treatment modality.[16] Patients with unilateral vocal fold paralysis presenting with a high-grade

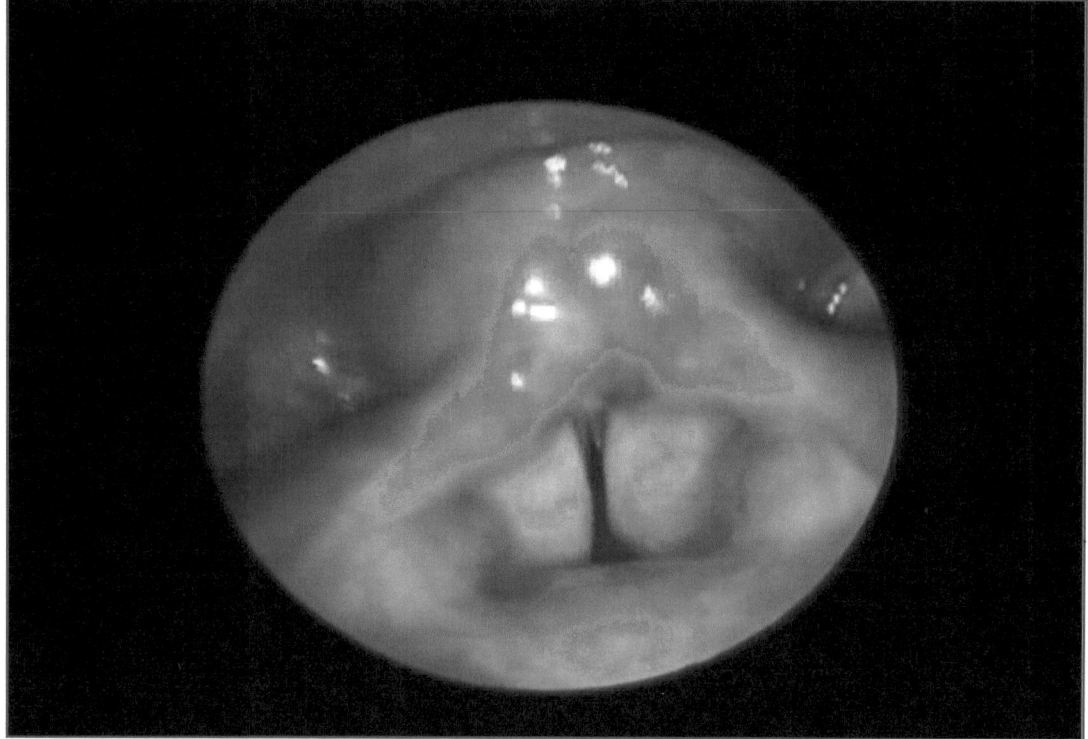

A

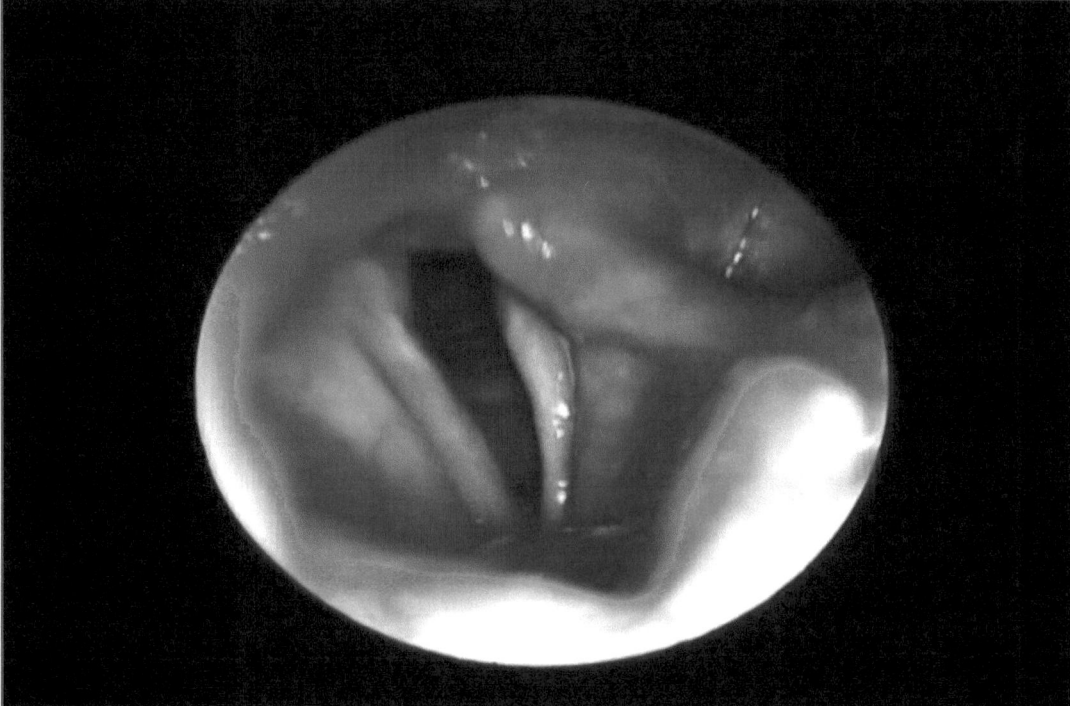

B

**Figure 6–1. A.** Compensatory supraglottic hyperfunctional behavior in a 76-year-old patient with unilateral vocal fold paralysis. Note the medialization of the false vocal fold and the anteroposterior shortening between the petiole and interarytenoid area. **B.** Bowing and shortening of the left vocal fold during inspiration.

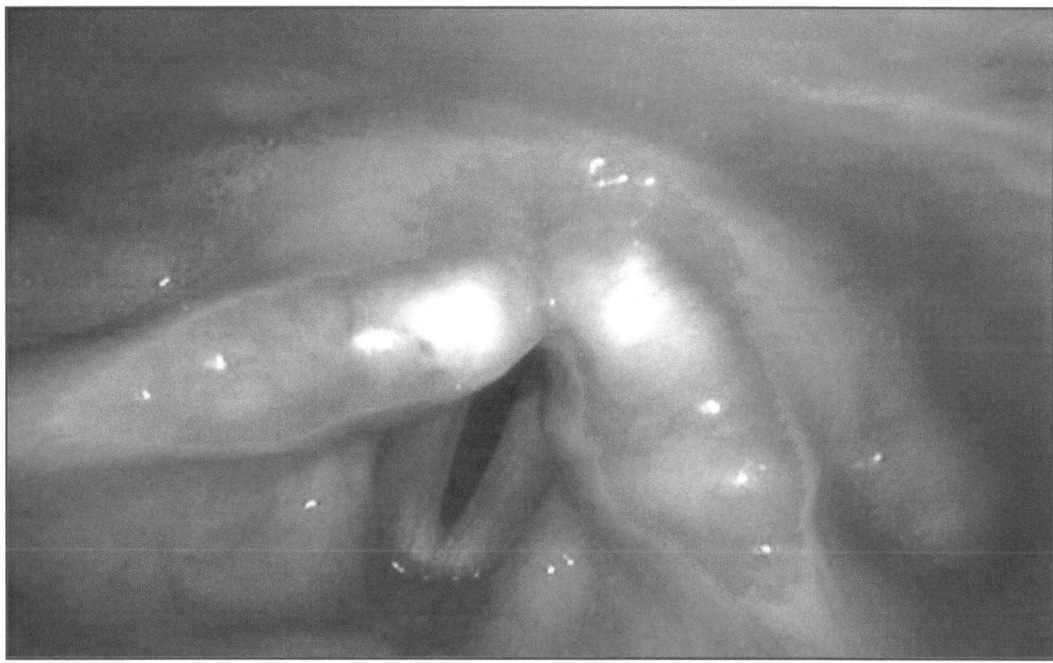

**Figure 6–2.** A 40-year-old woman presenting with bilateral vocal fold paralysis and a tracheotomy following thyroidectomy performed one year ago.

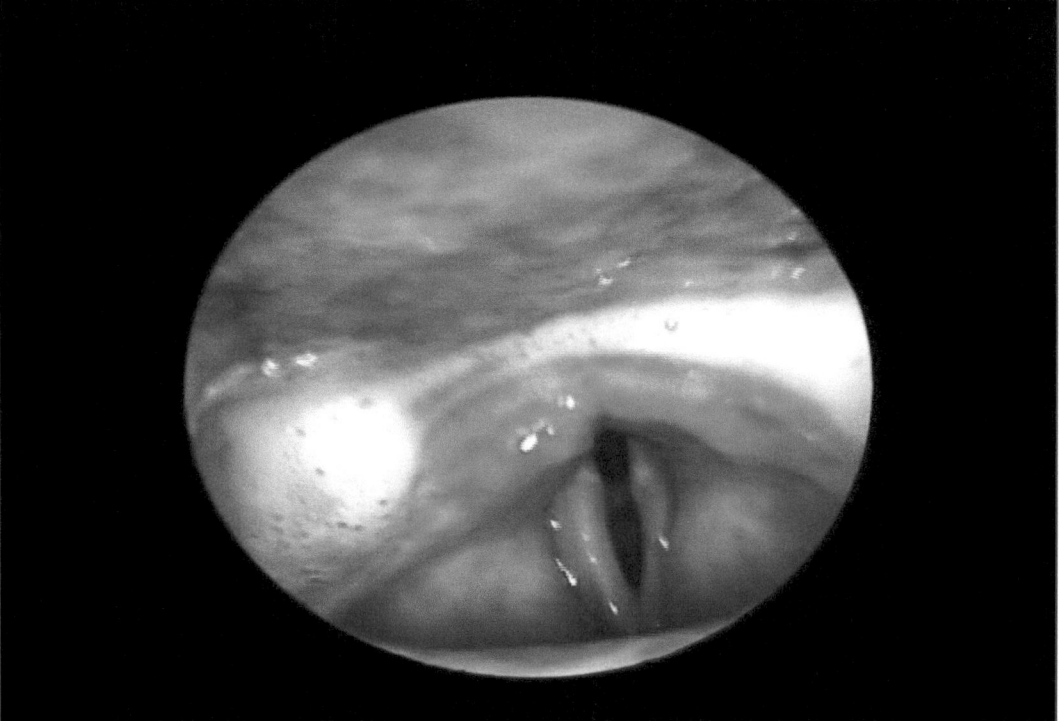

**Figure 6–3.** A 52-year-old man presenting with history of hoarseness of two years duration following chemoradiation treatment for nasopharyngeal carcinoma. On laryngeal examination there is impaired mobility and bowing of both vocal folds with pooling of mucus in both pyriform sinuses.

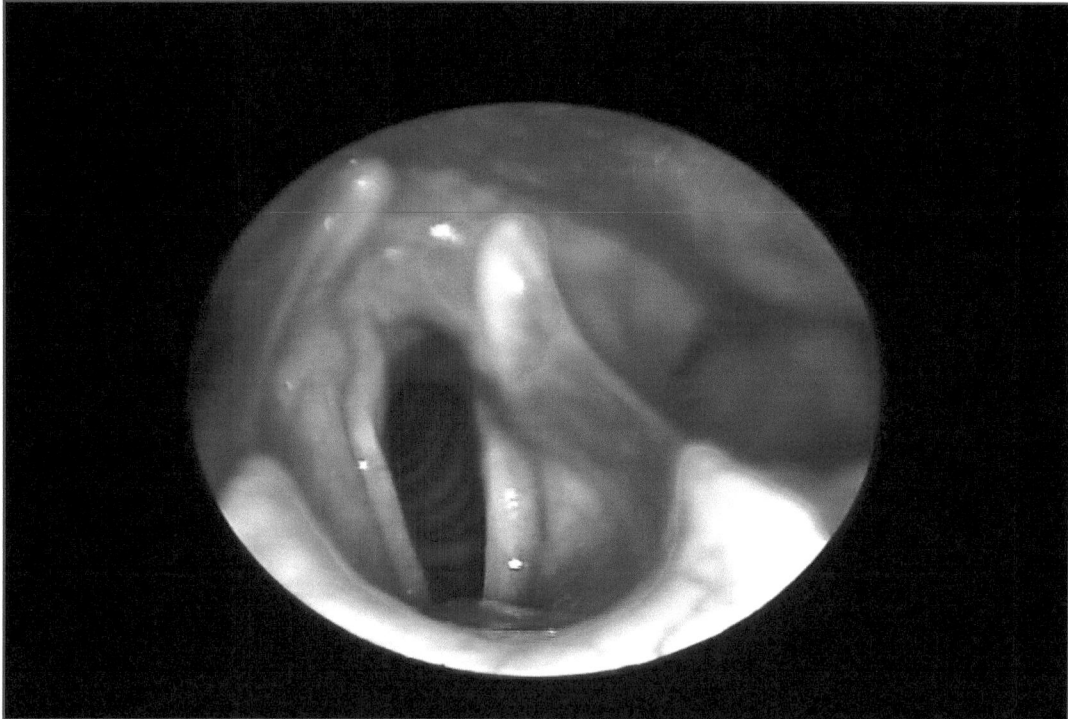

**Figure 6–4.** A 70-year-old man who presented with history of dysphonia and aspiration of sudden in onset following severe blunt trauma to his chest. On laryngeal examination there is complete paralysis of the left vocal fold.

dysphonia and a high VHI score will probably mandate early surgical intervention after few sessions of voice therapy, whereas patients with a low VHI score and mild change in voice quality may opt for voice therapy without surgical intervention. Similarly, in patients with bilateral vocal fold paralysis, the balance between having an adequate voice and comfortable breathing is a determining factor in designing the best management strategy. Having a chink wide enough to breathe through yet adequate for phonation cannot be overemphasized. To that end, the laryngeal examination is of paramount importance in making the right diagnosis and in assessing the position of the paralyzed vocal fold. Both fiberoptic laryngeal endoscopy for evaluation of the laryngeal biomechanics, and stroboscopic examination to rule out co-existing vocal fold pathology are mandatory. The position of the vocal folds, both in the vertical and horizontal dimensions, is often found to be disturbed leading to a large array of symptoms. The details of the laryngeal examination and the various phonatory tasks that the patient needs to perform during examination are discussed thoroughly in Chapter 22 of the fourth edition of *The Professional Voice: The Science and Art of Clinical Care*.[17]

The role of voice analysis is very limited with little added value when acoustic parameters are used in isolation. In a recent cross-sectional study by Lopes et al on 279 subjects with various laryngeal pathologies, only combined acoustic measures were useful in discriminating unilateral vocal fold paralysis form normal healthy larynges.[18] The incomplete closure of the vocal folds usually results in an increase in the perturbation parameters and in an increase in the first formant intensity.[19] In an acoustic and aerodynamic study by Hartl et al on eight men with unilateral vocal fold paralysis, the authors have demonstrated significantly higher jitter, shimmer, high-frequency–ratio, and significantly lower Cepstral peak prominence (CPP) in affected patients compared to controls.[20] Acoustic analysis may also be useful in assessing the follow-up of these patients after treatment. The study by Gillespie et al on 40 patients with various vocal fold pathologies among which was unilateral vocal fold paralysis, has shown "a disorder-specific response to frequency-based acoustic measures."[21] Similarly, Adams et al highlighted the usefulness of acoustic analysis, in combination with perceptual and aerodynamic measures, in the evaluation of patients with unilateral vocal fold paralysis following thyroplasty.

There was a significant improvement in vocal shimmer, s/z ratio, and signal-to-noise ratio.[22]

Airflow measurements are also markedly useful in assessing the extent of glottal insufficiency in patients with vocal fold paralysis. Patients will invariably have a reduced maximum phonation time and an increase in the mean airflow rate as reported by Makiyama et al and Kelchner et al.[23,24] These alterations in aerodynamic measures are attributed to inefficiency in the phonatory apparatus and decreased laryngeal control as a sequel to the paralysis. Kelchner et al has also demonstrated vocal fatiguing of patients with unilateral vocal fold paralysis following prolonged reading, a finding that correlated with changes in the aerodynamic measures. Post-prolonged loud reading, patients had further reduction in the maximum phonation time and an increase in the mean airflow rate at low, comfortable, and high pitches.[24]

Computerized tomography of the head and neck and chest is mandatory in order to rule out any central or peripheral lesions along the course of the recurrent laryngeal nerves. Based on a survey by the American Bronchoesophagological Association on the practice pattern among otolaryngologists in the workup of patients with undifferentiated unilateral vocal fold paralysis, computerized tomographic scan of neck and chest along the course of the recurrent laryngeal nerve was the most frequently requested test.[25] The main added value of this test has been further highlighted by two studies, one by Kang et al and another by Chin et al[26,27] where computerized tomography revealed previously unidentified causes for the paralysis in 23.5% and 15% of the cases, respectively. See Figure 6–5.

Laryngeal electromyography of the thyroarytenoid and lateral cricoarytenoid muscles is also of paramount importance in differentiating between neurogenic injury and ankylosis of the cricoaryetnoid joint.[15,28] A recent investigation by Chang et al on the quantitative electromyographic characteristics in patients with unilateral vocal fold paralysis has shown the added value of this diagnostic method

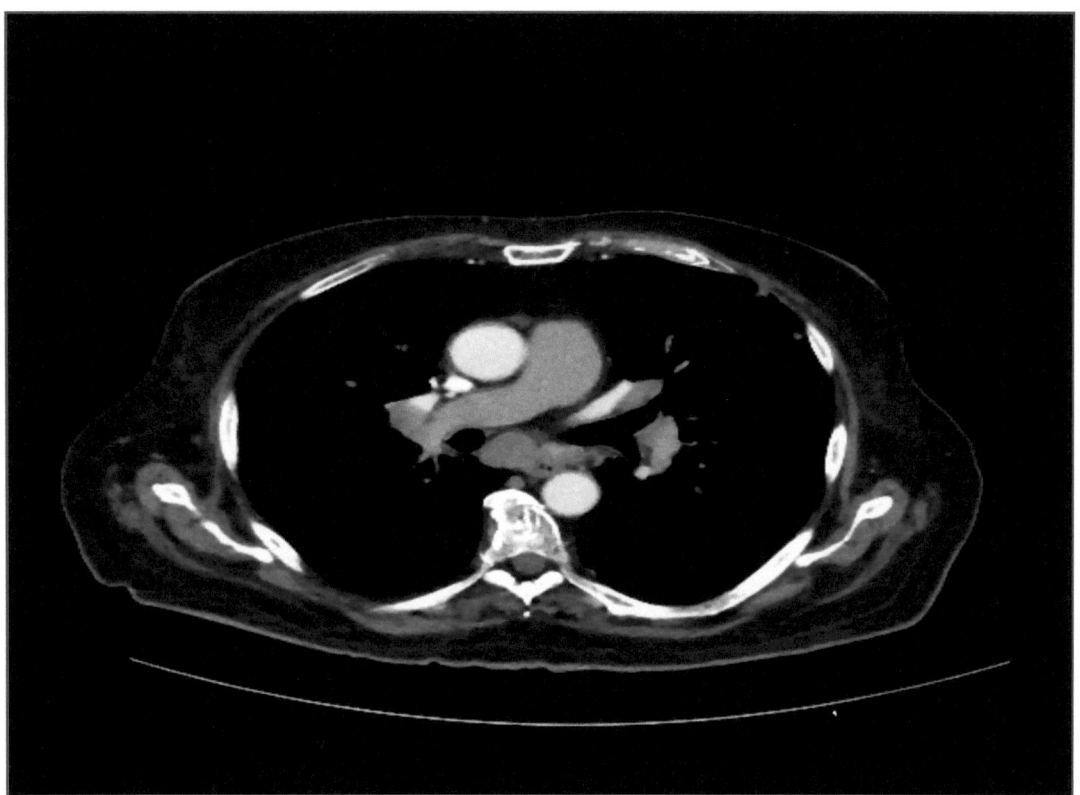

**Figure 6–5.** A 69-year-old man, diagnosed case of hepatocellular carcinoma, presented with dysphonia and aspiration of few month duration. Computerized tomography of the chest revealed enlarged mediastinal perivascular and paratracheal and paraesophageal lymph nodes the largest measuring 2.9 × 2.1 cm.

in differentiating iatrogenic causes from idiopathic ones. Those that were surgically induced had less recruitment of the thyroarytenoid-LCA complex compared to those who had idiopathic etiology.[29] Further information on laryngeal electromyography is available elsewhere.[30]

Before a management strategy is adopted whether for unilateral vocal fold paralysis or bilateral vocal fold paralysis, three important questions need to be answered in order to adopt the best therapeutic modality and optimize the surgical outcome;

*Question one*: "*Does the patient have a concomitant superior laryngeal nerve injury?*" Superior laryngeal nerve SLN paralysis is often unrecognized as many affected patients are being diagnosed with functional voice disorders.[31] The main reasons are the nonspecificity of the symptoms reported by the patient and the often nonconclusive laryngeal signs present on examination. Patients may complain of ill-defined vocal changes such as vocal fatigue and inability to project the voice. In professional voice users, symptoms such as loss of the high notes, lowered pitch, and contracted range are more noticeable and pronounced. These symptoms are partially attributed to the lost contraction of the cricothyroid muscle responsible for the increase in tension within the thyroarytenoid muscle, and partially to the hyperfunctional compensatory behavior and concomitant muscle tension dysphonia present in almost one out of four affected patients.[32] The laryngeal signs most commonly seen in patients with superior laryngeal nerve injury include bowing and flaccidity of the affected vocal fold, rotation of the posterior glottis toward the paralyzed side, and shortening of the ipsilateral aryepiglottic fold. See Figure 6–6. A more consistent finding as reported by Sataloff is sluggish movement and fatigability of the vocal fold after repeated adduction such as /i/-hi-/i/-hi-/i/-hi.[15] The presence of supraglottic constriction as a compensatory hyperfunctional behavior may also be observed and lead to delay in seeking therapy. Another reason why SLN palsy is underdiagnosed in the absence of history of neck surgery such as thyroidectomy, carotid endarterectomy, or anterior approach to cervical spine, is failure to correlate the presence of SLN palsy with other symptoms and signs of cranial polyneuropathies or recent viral infection.[32] Adour et al has reported the presence of laryngeal signs of SLN palsy, namely, laryngeal rotation and shortening of the vocal fold, in patients with vestibular neuritis, migraine headaches, and globus pharyngeus, thus alluding to the high prevalence of this entity in a wider and more diverse context than that of post-thyroidectomy patients.[33] In the

study by Dursun et al on 126 cases of SLN paresis, 93.6% had history of a recent viral infection prior to the development of phonatory complaints. To that end, the authors have emphasized the importance of a diligent and thorough history taking and the added value of both laryngeal videostroboscopy and laryngeal electromyography in the work-up of these patients.[32] Differences in the longitudinal tension of the vocal folds is often observed when the patient is asked to slide his or her voice from the low register to the high register in a glissando fashion. More so, voice range measurements may also be useful in analyzing the effect of SLN paresis on voice range profile and subsequently in monitoring the effect of voice therapy.[34]

Even in the presence of neck surgery, the diagnosis of SLN palsy is still being overlooked, more so in patients with unilateral or bilateral vocal fold paralysis where the main focus is on breathing and aspiration. For instance, in cases of thyroidectomy, superior laryngeal nerve paresis may be present either preoperatively or following the surgery itself. In a recent study on "Goiter and Laryngeal Sensory Neuropathy," the authors reported a significant difference in the prevalence of laryngeal sensory neuropathy in patients with goiter versus controls, 42% versus 12%, respectively. Patients with goiter had more frequently a constellation of symptoms such as throat clearing, cough, globus, and change in voice quality.[35] As goiter is one of the main indications for thyroidectomy, and thyroidectomy remains one of the most common causes of vocal fold paralysis, one ought to consider the rate of preoperative laryngeal sensory neuropathy and possible SLN palsy in patients who present with vocal fold paralysis status post-thyroidectomy. This is in agreement with the report of Jansson et al where three patients out of 20 undergoing thyroidectomy had SLN paresis preoperatively.[36] Indeed in that same report by Jansson et al, nine patients had postoperatively SLN paresis as evident by laryngeal electromyography. Injury occurs invariably during ligature of the superior vascular bundle flush with the thyrohyoid membrane as the superior laryngeal nerve courses deep to the superior thyroid artery and vein from superolateral to inferomedial and inserts at the cricothyroid muscle medial to the superior pole of the thyroid gland.[36] The presence or absence of SLN injury may mandate a change in the management strategy such as less widening of the rima glottidis in patients with bilateral vocal fold paralysis with fear of exacerbating aspiration, and the possible initiation of neuromodulators such as gabapentin or pregabalin.

*Question two*: "*Is the impaired mobility or fixed vocal fold the result of a systemic disease?*" The laryngeal

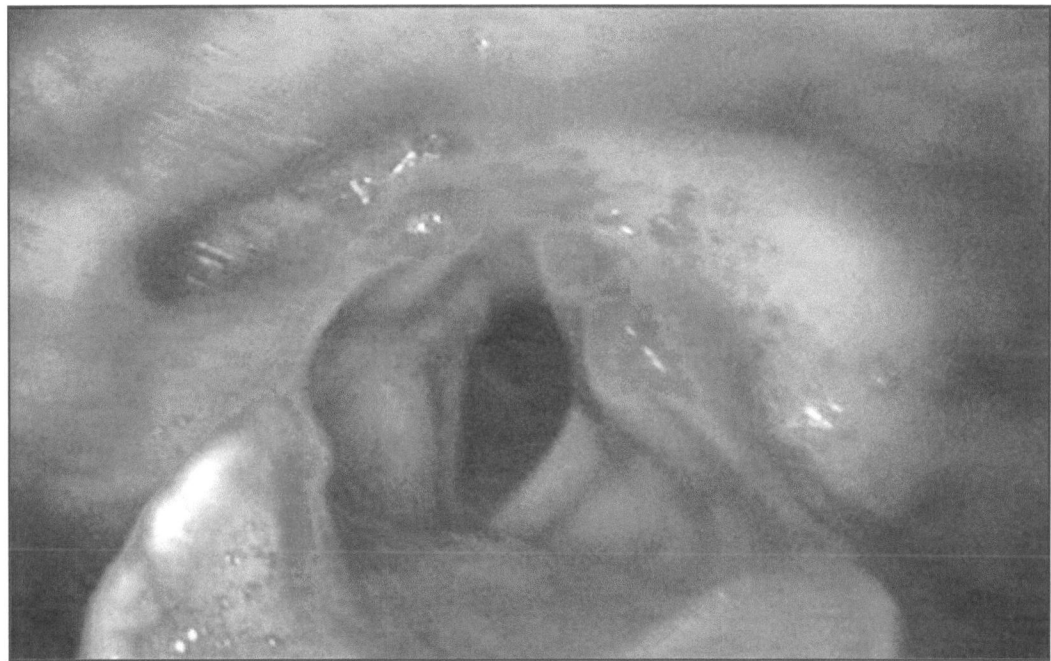

**A**

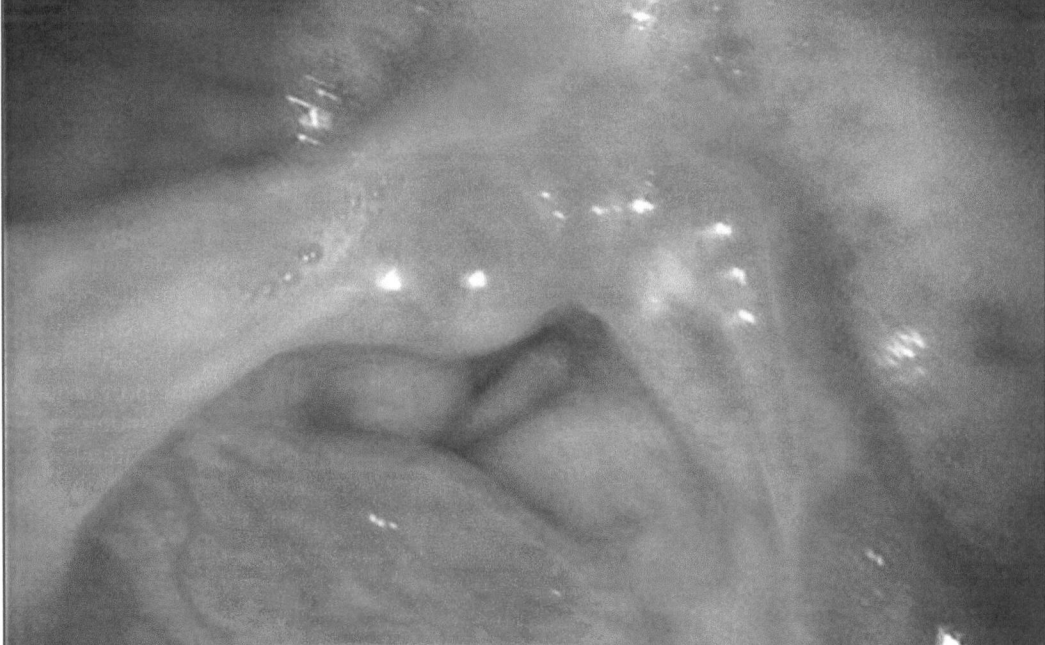

**B**

**Figure 6–6. A and B.** A 60-year-old man, presenting with roaring and pulsatile tinnitus of 3 months duration associated with dysphonia. Radiologic imaging revealed jugulotympanic paraganglioma eroding and widening the left jugular foramen. On laryngeal exam he had immobility of the left vocal fold with pooling of mucus in the left pyriform sinus and laryngeal lumen. Patient was diagnosed with recurrent laryngeal nerve and superior laryngeal nerve palsy. The upper picture is taken during inspiration and the bottom picture taken during sustained vowel /i/.

manifestations of systemic diseases are many and their prevalence is increasing in view of the advances in technology and increased physician's awareness. For instance, autoimmune diseases such as systemic lupus erythematosis and rheumatoid arthritis (RA) may affect the cricoarytenoid joint leading to impaired mobility and fixation of the vocal folds. Similarly, neurogenic disorders such as Parkinson's disease and amyotrophic lateral sclerosis may present with unilateral or bilateral vocal fold paralysis.[37–40] Diligent and early recognition of these manifestations may spare the patient unnecessary surgical intervention and morbidity. For example, the initiation of autoimmune therapy such as methotrexate in cases of advanced RA and or injecting periarticular steroids had shown promising results with regression of the pathology.[41]

*Question three*: "*When to intervene, when to operate?*" To answer this question there are five important factors to consider: One is the rate of spontaneous recovery which varies markedly with the etiology of the paralysis. For instance following thyroidectomy, Jatzko et al in 1994 has reported an 86% spontaneous recovery of vocal fold paralysis within a 6-month period, and as such has advocated laryngeal framework surgery at least 6 to 12 months post-surgery.[42] Whereas in cases of idiopathic vocal fold paralysis there is complete recovery of the voice in 25% to 87% of the cases in less than a year as reported by Sulica in 2008.[43] The second factor to consider is the degree of insult to the recurrent laryngeal nerve, which invariably is hard to estimate be it neuropraxia, axonotmesis, or neurotmesis.[44,45] The information whether the recurrent laryngeal nerve has been injured or not as well as the extent of its injury post-surgery is not always readily available. This can be attributed partially to the imperfect communication between the surgeon who has operated and the laryngologist who is taking care of the patient, and partially to the anatomical variations in the course of the recurrent laryngeal nerve which more often than not can be misleading. To that end, there are two important deviations to consider, one is the branching of the recurrent laryngeal nerve and second is its course and angulation before entering the larynx. The most vulnerable point of injury to the RLN is at its entrance into the larynx after splitting into anterior and posterior branches, although the number of branches can reach up to 8 with trifurcation being reported in one-third to two-thirds of the cases (left vs right).[46] Another equally important anatomical variation to consider, aside from the extralaryngeal splitting of the recurrent laryngeal nerve, is the angulation along its course which is more accentuated on the right compared to the left "45 degrees versus 30 degrees." The third important factor is the status of the cricoarytenoid joint. Although there have been debates in the literature as to whether there is fixation of the joint with time, which would mandate an adjunctive procedure to thyroplasty type I, recent reports indicate that the joint remains functional even up to 17 years after the injury to the recurrent laryngeal nerve.[47–49] The fourth important factor to consider in deciding when to operate is the position of the vocal fold at time of presentation keeping in mind that it might change. This latter is primarily determined by the synkinetic activity of the intrinsic laryngeal muscles, abductors and adductors. In an animal study by Shindo et al examining the histological and morphological changes of laryngeal muscles after sectioning the recurrent laryngeal nerve, the authors have demonstrated that denervation atrophy is only a phase following which there is reinnervation mainly from the sectioned recurrent laryngeal nerve.[50] These findings go in parallel with the shift in the topographic organization of the laryngeal motoneurons in the nucleus ambiguus following and after recurrent laryngeal nerve sectioning, as demonstrated by Flint et al.[51] An equally important factor to consider in that regard is the ubiquity in the anastomosis between the superior laryngeal nerve and the recurrent laryngeal nerve. To name a few, there is the Galen anastomosis between the dorsal branch of the internal branch of the superior laryngeal nerve and the dorsal branch of the recurrent laryngeal nerve, the anastomosis between the dorsal division of the internal branch of the superior laryngeal nerve and the ventral branch of the recurrent laryngeal nerve, and the anastomosis between the descending branch of the ventral branch of the internal branch of the superior laryngeal nerve and the ascending branch of the recurrent laryngeal nerve.[52]

Despite the difficulty in defining the exact time of intervention given the aforementioned factors, namely, the disparity in causes of denervation, the various degrees of injury and the hardship in predicting the final position of the affected vocal fold, early intervention, especially in cases of unilateral vocal fold paralysis have become common practice. The main reasons are the advances in technology that allow bedside intervention with little morbidity, and the marked improvement in quality of life following these interventions. In addition, there are few reports, namely, by Friedman et al and Prendes et al indicating that subjects who undergo early injection laryngoplasty have less need for permanent laryngeal framework surgery.[53,54] This has been attributed to the tactile stimulation of the paralyzed vocal folds which helps to improve its functional recovery. That being said, injection laryngoplasty has become the standard mode of therapy for patients with unilateral vocal fold paralysis and a viable alternative to laryngeal framework surgery. Nevertheless, there are many challenges to injection laryngoplasty, among which is the choice of material to use and the route of injection. The material used has to be biocompatible with reasonable longevity in order to serve its purpose. Teflon was commonly used in 1970s before it has been abandoned in view of the high complication rate such as extrusion and granuloma formation. Other materials used are calcium hydroxylapatite known as Radiesse, and hyaluronic acid (HA). Teflon lost its popularity in light of the increasing number of reports of inflammatory reactions and extrusion at the site of injections.[55] On the other hand, only few adverse reactions to hyaluronic acid have been reported in the literature and that is in view of its similar viscoelastic properties to the natural constituents of the lamina propria.[56] More so, experimental studies have shown that HA not only binds to water and loses less volume over time once injected, but also helps restore the vibratory malleability of the vocal fold cover. Fat has also been advocated as an alternative filling material given its long duration before it is absorbed and its high biocompatibility. With respect to the route of injection, there are many approaches performed as office-based procedures. These include the percutaneous approach, the perioral approach, the transnasal approach, and the transoral fiberoptic approach. The details of these approaches are not the subject of this chapter but it is important to note that the choice of approach is primarily determined by the surgeon's expertise, patient's tolerance and health, and last the patient's orofacial morphology of the patient. For instance, an obscure neck landmark would be unfavorable for the percutaneous approach whereas a septal deviation would prohibit the transnasal approach.

Laryngeal framework surgery, namely, thyroplasty type I is an alternative to injection laryngoplasty that offers a successful and more permanent solution to patients with unilateral vocal fold paralysis. Although the surgical details of this surgery is not the topic of this chapter, positioning of the implant through a thyroid cartilage window is the most crucial step of this procedure. Based on a recent presentation by Prof. Michael Benninger, individualized implants are being tailored in order to match the exact measures for medicalization.[57] Reinnervation procedures have also gained popularity as adjunctive procedures to laryngeal framework surgery. Several reinnervation procedures have been described, the most popular are the ansa-cervicalis by Crumley[47] and the nerve-muscle pedicle transfer by Tucker.[58,59] Crumley has reported improved tension and tonicity to the paralyzed intrinsic laryngeal muscles and Tucker has reported better voice quality especially if treated early.

For patients with bilateral vocal fold paralysis, various modalities of treatment have been advocated ranging from tracheotomy to laryngeal pacing and regenerative medicine. Today the primary treatment modality is a lateralization procedure that targets the posterior glottis and is based on tissue resection. Partial arytenoidectomy and or posterior cordotomy ultimately lead to a non-physiologic state where phonation and voice quality is being traded for a better breathing. There have been numerous modifications in the lateralization technique in attempt to improve the airway and yet preserve the premorbid voice quality. This refinement in surgery of the posterior glottis had led to improvement in voice quality with restoration of adequate loudness and clarity subjectively.[60] In the study by Remacle et al in 1996, 38% of his 41 patients had a near-normal voice based on high-resolution frequency analysis with a maximum phonation time of 8 + 4 seconds and a mean vocal intensity of 61 dB.[11]

## Future Alternatives

Given the limitations in the conventional therapeutic methods for the treatment of vocal fold paralysis, new strategies have evolved over the last two decades with emphasis on gene therapy, tissue engineering, and regenerative medicine. By delivering genes that encode growth factors responsible for the promotion and sprouting of neural structures, neuronal regeneration may be stimulated and degeneration may be halted. Rubin et al has reported the injection of these factors thru viral vectors to the central nervous system via the recurrent laryngeal nerve.[61] Similarly, Shiotani et al has reported reinnervation and decreased thyroarytenoid muscle atrophy after delivering IGF-I in a rat model.[62]

Alternatively, tissue engineering and regenerative medicine address the basic histopathologic changes that occur within the vocal fold in cases of paralysis. By using cells, scaffold, or regulatory factors, the architecture and distribution of the extracellular matrix constituents are restored and the function of its primary cells, namely, fibroblasts, is improved. Among these tissue engineering strategies, stem cell therapy has gained increasing attention in laryngology in view of its promising regenerative effect and ability to alter the biologic state of the paralyzed vocal fold. Since its introduction in 2003, many studies came forward in attempt to answer three main challenges: one is the viability of the implanted or injected stem cells in both animal and human models, second is their effect on the histology and architectural components of the injected site, and third is their capacity to enhance the current function of the paralyzed vocal fold in a favorable manner. This latter is translated by an improvement in the acoustic, aerodynamic, and rheologic properties of the vocal fold.

The first study on vocal fold tissue engineering was reported by Kanemaru et al on a canine model. The injection of 3-dimensional incubated mesenchymal stem cells resulted in regeneration of the injured vocal fold.[63] Two years later the same author investigated the viability of the autologous bone marrow-derived stromal cells in a rat vocal fold.[64] The results showed survival of the implanted cells with expression of markers of epithelium and muscle, alluding to the potential differentiation of the stem cells in vivo. In both studies there was evidence of survival of mesenchymal cells with further differentiation of these cells into epithelial and muscle. Hertegard et al investigated the viability and effect of injected human mesenchymal stem cells on the histologic properties of a scarred vocal fold in a rabbit model. There was persistence of human mesenchymal cells with reduced scarring and improved viscoelastic properties of the treated scarred vocal fold. These changes were attributed to the decrease in collagen content in comparison to the untreated vocal fold.[65] In 2008, Ohno et al group have looked at the therapeutic potential of bone marrow–derived stromal cells in restoring the injured vocal fold. Using reverse transcription polymerase chain reaction the authors reported alterations in the gene expression of HAS 2 and MMP 1.[66] In order to obtain optimum results of the bone marrow–derived mesenchymal cells implantation in the vocal folds, atelocollagen sponge was successfully used as a scaffold in an animal model.[63]

Among the regenerative therapeutic modes, growth factors have also been thoroughly investigated in laryngology with promising results both in the aged and paralyzed larynx.[67] The injection of βFGF has been successfully used as an alternative material to the conventional filling substances used and as an adjunctive procedure to thyroplasty as reported previously by Kanazawa et al.[68]

On a different front, functional electrical stimulation is equally gaining ground as a potential option for the treatment of vocal fold paralysis. Instead of changing the position of the paralyzed vocal fold using medialization or lateralization technique, the motor function of the paralyzed vocal fold is restored. This therapeutic alternative is based on the fact that synkinetic reinnervation of the laryngeal muscles following denervation has been proven to be amenable to selective electric stimulation and hence feasible for laryngeal pacing. This theory of laryngeal reanimation using electrical stimulation was initially described in the 1970s by Zealer and Dedo after having studied the keystones for its clinical application. Following numerous animal trials, abduction of the vocal folds in paralyzed larynges using rhythmic and regulated stimulation was successfully reported.[69] More so, histochemical studies have indicated that "greater appropriate reinnervation and less inappropriate reinnervation" is present in animals who had chronic electrical stimulation compared to controls.[70] Between 1995 and 1997, seven patients were implanted with the Itrel II device with limited success.[71] This has been attributed to some limitations and problems inherent to the translation of this technology to humans. These included the shift of the electrode position, electrochemical erosion, and last the lack of the sensor to align the respiratory rate with the pace of stimulation. A key element in the success of functional electrical stimulation is synchronization between an afferent input that signals inspiration and an efferent one connected to the denervated muscle through a nerve or a nerve-muscle–pedicle. To that end, human studies have been discontinued and newer animal studies using an implantable pulse generator initially designed for spinal cord stimulation have been started by numerous investigators[72–75] with emphasis on the positive impact of electrical stimulation on synkinetic reinnervation.

## Essential Tremor

Essential tremor is a movement disorder initially referred to as benign familial tremor due to its benign nature and lack of significant disability. Today this term is no longer being used given the increased morbidity associated with this disease. The estimated frequency ranges between 40 and 400 per 10,000 persons, reaching a figure of 20% in the elderly.[76,77] However it is important to note that the true prevalence is unknown as the majority of affected patients do not seek medical attention.[78,79] Despite the lack of a multiethnic population study, ethnicity seems to play a role given the fact that essential tremor is less common in African Americans compared to whites. Both men and women are equally affected with no predilection to gender. Based on a review of 350 patients with essential tremor, Lou and Jankovic have reported a bimodal age distribution, namely the second and sixth decades of life.[80] A family history is present in 17% to 100% of the cases based on numerous reports.[80–82] Genetic linkage has been identified at two sites, "chromosome 2p22-25 and 3q13" as reported by Higgins et al and Gulcher et al.[83,84] This genetic cause has been further supported by the higher prevalence of essential tremor in monozygotic twins compared to dizygotic twins (60% vs 27%).[85]

The pathophysiology of essential tremor remains a subject of investigation. Postmortem studies by Louis and Vonsattel indicated the presence of degenerative disease in the central nervous system.[86] As such essential tremor is considered as a central nervous system disorder that affects various sites such as the brainstem nuclei, cerebellum, and thalamus. There is growing evidence to support that the pathophysiology is heterogeneous, and many associated systemic disturbances are often overlooked by the physician whose main focus has been on tremor of the extremities.[87] Recent investigations have suggested that the Harmaline (beta-carboline) concentration was found to be high in cats with essential tremor. Montigny and Lamarre have demonstrated that Harmaline can induce rhythmic activity within the olivo-cerebello-bulbar system resulting in tremor.[88] This is in agreement with the study by Deuschl et al which suggests that the pathophysiology of essential tremor originates from the olivo-cerebellar circuit.[89] Another suggested pathophysiologic process is alteration in the somatosensory feedback and loop as reported by Elble et al.[90] Interestingly, Tomoda et al has also highlighted the possible impairment in the innervation of the voluntary expiratory muscles in the pathophysiology of voice tremor. In his report on two patients with voice tremor, the voice tremor was more pronounced during voluntary phonation or expiration and not during inspiration or involuntary phonation.[91]

The diagnosis of essential tremor is primarily made on clinical findings. Based on the diagnostic criteria set by the Movement Disorder Society on Tremor,[92] a patient is considered to have essential tremor if he or she has "Bilateral postural or kinetic tremor of the hands and forearms; or isolated head tremor without evidence of dysphonia." Evidently, other neurologic disorders associated with tremor such as Parkinson's disease, and or drug-induced tremor such as beta-adrenergic agonists, thyroxin, lithium, and tricyclic antidepressants must be ruled out. The body parts most commonly affected in essential tremor are the upper limbs in 95% followed

by the head in 34% and the lower extremities in 20%. The voice might be affected in almost 12% to 25% of the cases, although the true prevalence is unknown because only a minority seeks medical attention.[93,94] Thus, vocal tremor is often underdiagnosed for years and a high index of suspicion is needed to make the proper diagnosis. Many patients may be preoccupied and have overlooked their vocal tremor until it started affecting their communication. It is worth noting that a familial component may be present in almost half the patients, a fact that mandates a diligent family history taking.[95] When voice is affected, the entity is referred to as essential voice tremor or essential tremor of the voice. It is defined as "Periodic contraction of antagonistic adductor-abductor and/or superior-inferior laryngeal muscles in an alternating or synchronous fashion."[96] In consistency with essential tremor, vocal tremor has a gradual and slow onset leading to a delay of years before a diagnosis is made. It is often precipitated by stress, emotional disturbances, and vocal fatigue, leading the patient to seek medical attention.[97] Essential vocal tremor may be either isolated or accompanied by tremor in other parts of the body. Based on a cohort study by Sulica and Louis on 34 patients with essential vocal tremor, 32.3% were aware of having arm tremor.[95] Similarly the report by Brown and Simon on 31 patients with essential vocal tremor, concomitant tremor was present in the extremities in 90%, head in 52%, and face in 10%.[97] To that end, isolated vocal tremor in the absence of tremor in other parts of the body is rare. When present in isolation, vocal tremor is more often than not misdiagnosed. In the report by Sulica and Louis, essential vocal tremor was misdiagnosed as spasmodic dysphonia in 29.4% of the cases given the high prevalence of vocal tremor (25%) in patients with spasmodic dysphonia.[95] It is important to note that dysphonia in patients with SD is provoked by phrases that contain voiced onset such as counting from 80 to 90.

The diagnosis of essential voice tremor is based primarily on listening to the patient and visualization of the larynx while the patient is asked to perform various phonatory tasks. Invariably patients report a shaking voice that is weak, diminished, and unstable. Patient-reported outcome measures such as The Voice Handicap Index, the Voice-Related Quality of Life questionnaire, or the Quality of Life in Essential Tremor questionnaire, can also be used as a self-administered tool in order to evaluate the physical, functional, and emotional impact of the disease on speech intelligibility and quality of life as a whole.[98] By listening to a patient with essential vocal tremor, the periodicity of the tremor is the most important characteristic. There is a rhythmic variation in both intensity of voice as well as pitch which ranges in frequency between 5 to 7 Hz, and which makes it perceptually pathologic and noticeable unlike the physiologic frequency range of 8 to 12 Hz.[99] Acoustic analysis may also be useful in substantiating the perceptual evaluation in these patients. Periodic oscillation in amplitude and frequency with or without voice breaks are often seen in severe cases.[100] Laryngeal electromyography, in particular of the thyroarytenoid and lateral cricoarytenoid muscles can be used for further confirmation of the diagnosis of essential vocal tremor. Evidence of "periodic waxing and waning of muscular activation at a rate from 4 Hz to 10 Hz is usually diagnostic,"[95] Based on laryngeal EMG studies performed on eight patients with voice tremor, the intrinsic laryngeal muscles, and in particular the thyroarytenoid muscles revealed tremulous activity during respiration and speech.[101]

Laryngeal examination is essential for making the proper diagnosis though for decades the diagnosis of essential voice tremor has been based primarily on perceptual evaluation without laryngeal examination. This could have contributed to the reports of normal laryngeal findings in early series.[97] A kinetic laryngeal tremor that extends to involve the whole phonatory apparatus is invariably seen on fiberoptic laryngeal examination as reported by Sulica et al and Bove et al.[95,102] In their report on 34 cases of essential vocal tremor, 74% had some degree of vocal during respiration.[95] Similarly, in the report by Gurey et al three-fourths of patients with essential vocal tremor had both horizontal tremor and vertical tremor although the horizontal glottic tremor was more common than the vertical one (94% vs 81%).[103] It is important to note that essential vocal tremor, when present, must be differentiated from other forms of neurogenic tremors using specific phonatory tasks. In that regard, Moraes and Biase, have developed a phonatory task-specific protocol in order to distinguish essential vocal tremor from dystonic tremor syndromes. The most significant phonatory tasks used were production of /s/, production of a whistle, and falsetto.[104]

It is also worth noting that more than one intralaryngeal and extralaryngeal site are involved in patients with essential vocal tremor, with pharyngeal tremor being present in almost 31% of the cases.*[101,105–107] In a study by Koda and Ludlow evaluating laryngeal muscle activities in patients with vocal tremor, the thyrohyoid, thyroarytenoid, and sternothyroid muscles were most commonly involved.[101] Given that essential vocal tremor is not limited to the vocal folds and many anatomic areas within the vocal tract can be involved, a vocal tremor scoring system has been developed and

validated by Bove et al in order to better describe the anatomical site involved and the degree of involvement.[102] The "Vocal Tremor Scoring System" has also been helpful in selecting who are best candidates for injection by identifying the site of tremor. The system is being used to monitor the effect of treatment after Botulinum toxin injection as well.

The ultimate goal in the treatment of essential vocal tremor is control of symptoms. Alleviating the impact of the disease on the day-to-day activities and during a desired performance is the goal of therapy. To that end, treatment may be implemented either as needed or continuously. For intermittent usage, alcohol and or benzodiazepines can be prescribed in addition to beta-adrenergic blockers. By modulating the skeletal muscles beta-adrenergic receptors, there is improvement in 50% of the cases.[94,108,109] Justicz et al reported the use of propranolol in a group of 18 patients with essential vocal tremor. The average improvement in VRQOL score was 9.31 after taking propranolol for at least two weeks.[110]

Other medications include primidone, an anticonvulsant the efficacy of which has been reported by many despite the lack of clear understanding of its mechanism of action.[111,112] Based on a suggested algorithm by Pahwa and Lyons, if patients have insufficient improvement, other medications with potential benefits such as Gabapentin can be prescribed.[94] The study by Gironell et al has shown equal effect in controlling motor tasks using Gabapentin in comparison to propranolol.[113] Other suggested medications include Topiramate which is a sulfamate-substituted monosaccharide" the usage of which has been proven to be efficacious as well.[114]

For essential vocal tremor Botulinum toxin injection remains the gold standard therapy.[115–119] It is usually given in the thyroarytenoid and lateral cricoarytenoid muscles, unilaterally or bilaterally. Nevertheless, the treatment regimen should be individualized in order to optimize the outcome. Based on the report of Gurey et al, horizontal glottic tremor is best treated by injections in the thyroarytenoid muscles whereas vertical tremor mandates additional injections in the strap muscles.[103] The recommended dose and site of injection is mostly derived from the literature on spasmodic dysphonia.[115–119] It is advisable to adjust the dose based on the patient's response to therapy. It is important to note that Botulinum toxin injections only reduce the amplitude of the tremor but do not eliminate it. A major side effect to injection is dysphagia and breathiness which might be significant especially in elderly who have poor tolerance.

The inconsistency in the treatment of essential vocal tremor with Botulinum injection may be explained by the fact that the source of the vocal tremor is not confined to the vocal folds alone. Hence injecting the vocal folds, unilateral or bilateral, may not always be efficacious. In that regard, a crossover study of unilateral versus bilateral injection of Botulinum toxin, revealed substantial subjective improvement in most patients with essential vocal tremor at least perceptually despite the objective improvement in only a minority of patients, namely, 3 out of 10 for bilateral and 2 out of 9 for unilateral injection.[96] The disparity between the objective outcome measures and the subjective ones can be explained on the basis that the subjective reduction in vocal effort is linked to the reduction in laryngeal airway resistance.

Given the limited or focused effect of Botulinum toxin to the injected muscle and given the aforementioned side effects, alternative therapy, namely, surgical intervention in the form of thalamotomy or deep brain stimulation may be recommended.[120–122] Sataloff et al in 2002 reported the successful use of chronic stimulation of the thalamus in controlling vocal tremor in addition to upper limb tremor.[120] Recently Hagglund et al has published the effect of deep brain stimulation of Caudal Zona Incerta on voice tremor in a group of patients with essential tremor. The results indicated a reduction in vocal tremor as a group and the effect was more pronounced when the stimulation was bilateral. However, it is important to note that not all patients improved and that individual differences need to be accounted for.[122]

## Parkinson's Disease

Parkinson's disease is a neurodegenerative disease that affects more than a million persons in the United States. The prevalence is estimated to be 217 in 100,000 affecting men and women in their six and seventh decades of life.[123,124] The pathophysiology lies in the depletion or reduction in dopamine secretion in the substantia nigra leading to a large array of symptoms related mainly to the motor and autonomic systems. The course of the disease is very slow and many years may lapse before functional impairment becomes an issue. The symptoms most commonly reported are mainly tremor, rigidity in movement, hypokinesia, dyskinesia, and hyperkinesia, in addition to neuropsychiatric symptoms, dementia, and depression.

Affected patients more often than not complain of speech disturbances in up to 70% of cases. Speech is described as monopitch, monoloud, with loss of intonation. These speech alterations are partially due to reduced movement of the jaw and lips, which

may also affect the onset of speech, its prosodic features, and the duration of sentences. Patients may also suffer from motility disorders of both intrinsic and extrinsic laryngeal muscles as reported by Leopold and Kagel. In their study of 71 patients with Parkinson's disease (PD) who were stratified into stages based on their disability scale, the authors have reported a delay in vertical laryngeal excursion, and a delay in opening and closure of the vocal folds during deglutition in more than 90% of the patients, more so in those with advanced disease.[125] Given the aforementioned, affected patients may present with symptoms in relation to the laryngopharyngeal complex such as dysphagia, aspiration, and change in voice quality. These laryngopharyngeal symptoms are primarily due to dysfunction in the neural pathway from nucleus ambiguus to the intrinsic laryngeal muscles.[37,40,126,127] The depletion of dopamine in the substantia nigra pars compacta results in rigidity and alteration in laryngeal muscular control which ultimately leads to excessive tension in the phonatory system.[128] This impairment in the medullary ganglionic control results in impaired mobility, hypertonicity, and dysfunction of the laryngeal muscles.[38,129]

Phonatory and swallowing dysfunction may be the primary symptom of the disease. However, their presence is often masked by the hypokinetic and hyperkinetic dysarthria in affected patients. Therefore, the concomitant presence of articulatory, resonance, and/or respiratory dysfunction in these patients mandates a diligent history taking and laryngological examination in order to make the proper diagnosis. Careful perceptual evaluation of the phonatory complaints in patients with Parkinson's disease often reveals the presence of vocal tremor and pitch breaks in addition to impairment in voice onset and offset. Patients may also report volume disturbances with more effort to project their voice, symptoms that can be partially attributed to the higher subglottal pressure needed to produce the same vocal intensity given the inappropriate glottic closure during phonation.[130,131] Similarly, in the study by Ramig et al in 2001, the pre-treatment group of patients with PD had a weaker voice and a lower sound pressure level compared to controls.[132] This low volume or reduced ability to regulate the speech volume especially in a noisy environment has also been linked to inattention and lack of explicit instructions as to when speak loud or soft.[133] In a study by Midi et al on 20 patients with Parkinson's disease, roughness, breathiness, and asthenia were reported to be significantly higher in males compared to controls. Similarly, breathiness and asthenia were significantly higher in females compared to controls.[134] Acoustic analysis is often

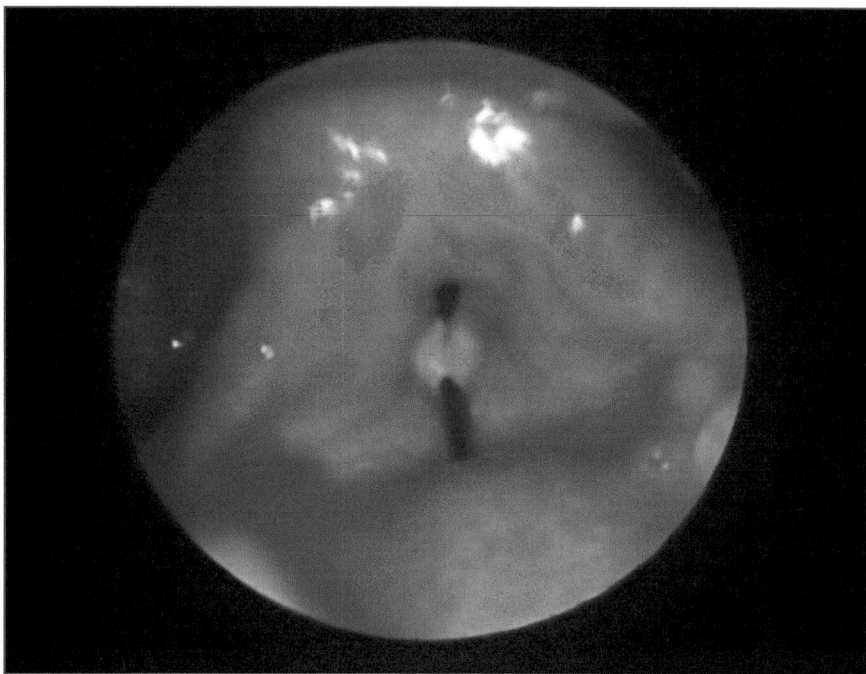

**Figure 6–7.** A 70-year-old male diagnosed case of Parkinson's disease presenting with vocal fatigue, loss of volume, and inability to control vocal pitch and loudness. On laryngeal endoscopy there is evidence of hypoadduction of the true vocal folds with compensatory hyperfunction of the false vocal folds.

useful in detecting acoustic perturbations that are commensurate with the perceptual evaluation of the phonatory changes in these patients. In 1997, Gamboa et al reported the acoustic measures in 41 patients with Parkinson's disease using the Computerized Speech Lab 4300 program and has shown higher perturbation parameters and lower harmonics to noise ratio as well as frequency and intensity variability compared to a control group.[135] In 2008, Midi et al reported the usage of the Multi-Dimensional Voice Program (MDVP) in his study on vocal abnormalities in patients with Parkinson's disease. His results failed to show any statistically significant difference in jitter, shimmer, and fundamental frequency compared to controls.[134] On the other hand a few years later Tanaka et al in his report on the vocal acoustic characteristics of 39 patients with idiopathic Parkinson's disease in comparison with 62 controls matched to age, indicated an increase in the perturbation parameters and noise-related measurements. The authors have also reported an increase in both fundamental frequency-tremor frequency and intensity index in males and fundamental frequency-tremor intensity index in females.[136] These gender-related vocal dysfunctions were also reported by Hertrich and Ackermann in their electrographic and acoustic analysis report in

patients with Parkinson's disease and vocal dysfunction. There were more abrupt F0 shifts and increased portions of subharmonic segments in females compared to males.[137] Many years later Bang et al analyzed the acoustic characteristics of four vowel sounds in seven female patients with Parkinson's disease using the Praat program. His investigation revealed a significant increase in cycle-to-cycle variation in frequency and in noise-to-harmonics ratio of patients with Parkinson's disease compared to controls. In addition there was asymmetric centralization of unrounded vowels /a/,/e/,/i/ with subsequent decrease in vowel space.[138]

All the aforementioned phonatory and acoustic disturbances can be attributed to abnormal laryngeal findings in affected patients. A study by Gallena et al in 2001 demonstrated an association between the endoscopic findings of vocal fold bowing and high muscular activity and the impairment in voice onset and offset seen in patients with idiopathic Parkinson's disease.[38] Indeed, laryngeal videoendoscopic and stroboscopic examination often reveals abnormalities in both abduction and adduction of the vocal folds during respiration and phonation.[129] See Figure 6–7. A study by Stelzig et al on 61 male patients and 39 female patients with Parkinson's disease revealed the prevalence of laryngeal movement abnormalities in 39% and 54% of the cases, respectively, with an obvious gender related vocal dysfunction. Other significant laryngeal findings included abnormal phase closure and asymmetry, vocal tremor, ventricular fold hypertrophy, vocal fold atrophy and bowing, and impaired mobility of the vocal folds.[129] Vocal tremor prevalence has been reported to vary between 14% to 55% based on the diagnostic method used and extent of disease.[135,139] As an example, the study by Perez et al revealed the presence of vertical laryngeal tremor in 55% of patients with idiopathic Parkinson's disease which was observed in the early course of the disease.[139] Similarly, vocal fold atrophy which is also a common finding in patients with Parkinson's disease, has been reported to be present in one-third of affected women and close to 50% of affected men.[129] On the other hand non-closure pattern, either in the form of spindle shape or posterior chink has been reported in 9 out of 12 male patients and eight of the eight female patients with Parkinson's disease according to Midi et al in 2008.[134]

There are also numerous reports on bilateral vocal fold paralysis in patients with Parkinson's disease who present with airway symptoms and respiratory distress often necessitating emergency tracheotomy. Vas et al in 1965 was the first to describe two cases who developed bilateral vocal fold palsy and laryngospasm. Both patients had stridor attacks that worsened over the years and ultimately led to intubation and tracheotomy.[140] In 1981, Plasse and Lieberman reported 2 more cases of Parkinson's disease who presented with stridor and on whom laryngeal examination revealed bilateral vocal fold paralysis and laryngeal spasm in one. Both patients underwent tracheotomy for alleviation of the respiratory symptoms.[141] Read and Young in 1983 reported the case of a 72-year-old female previously healthy who presented with a 6-month history of hoarseness, stridor, and salivation in addition to hoarseness. The patient was diagnosed with Parkinson's disease and started on medical therapy, the withdrawal of which caused severe exacerbation of stridor necessitating prophylactic tracheotomy.[142] Takayama et al in 1986 reported the case of a 66-year-old man with 20-year history of Parkinson's disease who presented with severe dyspnea and stridor and was found to have laryngeal carcinoma causing bilateral vocal fold paralysis.[143] Palesse et al in 1988 reported 2 cases of bilateral vocal fold abductor paralysis in patients with Parkinson's disease.[144] The cases were that of a 60-year-old and a 58-year-old man with 10-year and 2-year history of Parkinson's disease, respectively. Both patients were on L-Dopa and carbidopa

treatment when they presented to the hospital with attacks of asphyxia and severe nocturnal laryngeal stridor requiring emergent tracheotomy. Isozaki et al in 1995 reported the cases of 3 autopsy-proven Parkinson's disease patients who suffered from vocal fold abductor paralysis.[145] All three patients suffered from respiratory symptoms and stridor secondary to bilateral abductor paralysis which necessitated tracheotomy. Nakane et al in 1998 was the first to report the case of a 60-year-old female with juvenile Parkinson's disease diagnosed 30 years prior to presentation.[146] The patient was admitted for malignant syndrome that was induced by dehydration following which she developed progressive dyspnea and stridor. Endoscopic evaluation revealed bilateral vocal fold paralysis in the midline or paramedian position. Qayyum et al in 2005 reported the case of a 78-year-old woman with 4-year history of Parkinson's disease who was found to have bilateral vocal fold abductor paresis but normal adduction on phonation. The patient was admitted for acute shortness of breath and severe stridor leading to a tracheotomy followed by laser cordectomy and eventually decannulation.[147] Kim and Jeon in 2009 reported the case of a 49-year-old lady with a 19-year history of Parkinson's disease who after her admission for visual hallucinations developed severe inspiratory stridor, both awake and asleep, associated with oxygen desaturation and hypercapnia.[39] Fiberoptic laryngoscopy revealed immobile vocal folds and a subsequent tracheotomy relieved her respiratory difficulty. Similarly, Gan et al in 2010 reported a 73-year-old case who presented with difficulty in breathing and stridor secondary to immobile vocal folds fixed in the paramedian position causing airway obstruction.[40] The patient was intubated and had bedside percutaneous tracheotomy done later. Two years later, Lee et al in 2012 reported a case of bilateral vocal fold paralysis in a patient with Parkinson's disease that was treated with an urgent tracheotomy.[148] Recently the authors of this chapter have reported a case of unilateral vocal fold paralysis in an 83-year-old man with Parkinson's disease who presented with dysphonia and aspiration. See Figure 6–8.

Given the high morbidity of speech and voice dysfunction in patients with PD and their marked impact on quality of life often leading to isolation, the treatment should be initiated early and maintained throughout the progression of the disease. To that end, a multidisciplinary approach is a must in order to optimize the outcome of therapy. The tripod in the treatment of PD consists of medical therapy, speech therapy, and surgery.[149–152] In 1997, Angelis et al has reported the improvement in glottal efficiency

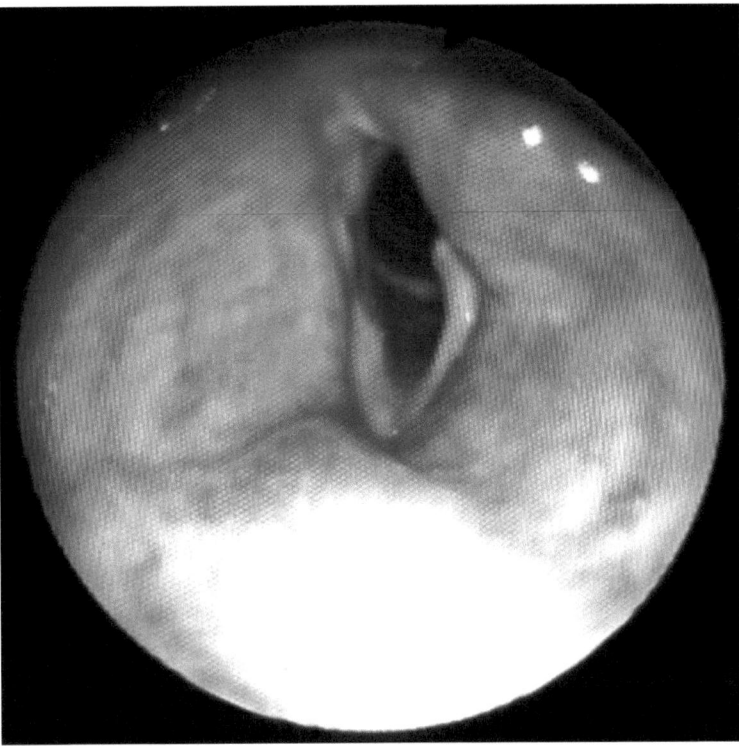

**Figure 6–8.** An 83-year-old man diagnosed with Parkinson's disease ten years ago presented with history of dysphonia, inability to project the voice, and aspiration of few month duration. On laryngeal exam there is evidence of left vocal fold paralysis.

in 20 patients treated with voice rehabilitation for one month. Patients had marked improvement in maximum phonation time and vocal intensity, and a marked reduction in vocal complaints such as strangulation and straining.[131] Ramig et al has also proven the successful treatment of patients with weak voice using the Lee Silverman Voice Treatment which consists primarily of putting high effort and speaking loud in order to enhance the function of all voice components. Treated subjects had an improvement in loudness by 8 dB which was perceptually audible.[132] An adjuvant to voice and speech therapy is the administration of levodopa, the impact of which on voice has been investigated by Jiang et al using both acoustic and glottographic measures.[153] Following therapy there was an improvement in sound pressure level and a decrease in the extent of tremor derived from acoustic intensity contours. It is worth noting that neither the perturbation in intensity, nor the extent of tremor extracted from airflow signal were affected after therapy. Another therapeutic option is injection laryngoplasty in an attempt to rectify the presence of any glottic insufficiency. In a study by Berke et al on 35 patients who underwent collagen

augmentation, 75% had reported satisfaction after the intervention.[154] More recent surgical procedures such as deep brain stimulation for the treatment of neurologic diseases with movement disorders have also been rewarding. By stimulating the subthalamic nucleus or globus pallidus, there is improvement in motor function, dyskinesia, and overall quality of life.[155,156]

## Multiple Sclerosis

Multiple sclerosis (MS) is a disease of the myelin sheath of the central nervous system characterized by the deposition of plaques at different sites of the brain white matter, spinal cord, and brainstem. It is believed to be autoimmune mediated but the exact etiology has not been elucidated yet. The prevalence ranges from 2.5 to 39 per 100,000 with a constant increase in view of the improved awareness and advances in radiologic imaging. Afflicted, patients may present with a large array of neurologic symptoms that can be either generalized such as numbness, spasticity, and weakness of the extremities or focal such as visual disturbances secondary to optic neuritis.[157] It is essential to note that the majority of patients fluctuate between remission and relapse and less than 10% have progressive disease.

The otolaryngologic manifestations of multiple sclerosis are many with various non-specific symptoms. Among those related to the laryngopharyngeal complex are dysarthria and dysphonia, the prevalence of which varies markedly and can reach up to 51% of the cases.[158–161] The discrepancy and variability in the prevalence of these symptoms are mainly attributed to differences in subject selection and to variations in study design. Higher figures have been reported in studies using acoustic analysis compared to those using self-reported questionnaires. In addition to the phonatory and swallowing dysfunction, patients with MS may describe speech alterations often referred to as "scanning speech" in view of the long pauses between words. In a review of the speech characteristics in 739 patients with MS, 9% had moderate to severe speech problems in constellation with other physical and psychological disabilities. These problems were more common and pronounced in patients who had progressive disease rather than the relapsing-remitting type.[162]

The pathophysiology of the phonatory symptoms in MS patients has been primarily attributed to neuronal alterations in the periaqueductal gray matter and nucleus ambiguus. Deposition of MS plaques in the corticobulbar pathway or in the brainstem region can result in weakness and loss of coordination of the intrinsic laryngeal muscles. In addition, patients may also suffer from a decrease in the laryngeal sensation due to dysfunction in the laryngeal afferent sensory input and feedback.[163,164] All the aforementioned motor and sensory disturbances lead to vocal dysfunction in affected patients.[165,166] What is interesting to note is that the occurrence of vocal symptoms does not correlate with the duration of the disease, meaning to say that MS patients may develop vocal symptoms anytime during the course of the disease. On the other hand, there is a correlation between the expanded disability status scale and vocal symptoms with a higher prevalence of these in patients with moderate to severe Expanded Disability Status Scale (EDSS) score.[167]

When present, vocal symptoms have a significant impact on quality of life.[168–172] In the study by Hamdan et al on 50 patients with MS, there was a positive correlation between VHI score, fatigue severity scale, and Hamilton rating scale of depression.[168] These results corroborate the findings of other studies on the strong correlation between quality of life and severity and progression of the disease. In the study by Rudick et al there was a correlation between the SF-36 scores and expanded disability status.[169] Similarly the study by Amato et al showed a moderate inverse relationship between the Multiple Sclerosis Quality of Life-54 composite score and disability level in affected patients.[170] Last is the study by Bauer et al which showed no correlation between the EDSS and the VHI score or any of its components nor between EDSS and the VRQL in a group of 36 patients with MS.[173]

The importance of noting the phonatory symptoms early in the course of the disease cannot be overemphasized as these can markedly impact the communication capability of the affected patient. These symptoms may also carry implications on the diagnosis and management strategy of MS patients. Nevertheless, phonatory disorders are still underdiagnosed in view of their subtle occurrence and intermittency, especially in the presence of speech alterations that can easily mask vocal changes when present. The most common vocal symptoms in MS patients are voice breaks, vocal fatigue, breathiness, and hypernasality, in addition to inappropriate control of pitch and loudness. In a large study of 40 patients by Yamout et al,[167] one out of four patients had at least one vocal symptom whereas none in the control group had voice breaks. Similarly, the study by Feijo et al revealed a significantly higher prevalence of dysphonia (70%) in MS patients compared to 33% in controls. More so, there was an association between MS and dysphonia (OR:2.2, CI 95%:.1.13–4.25) with the odds of having MS being almost twice in dysphonic patients.[174] The authors used both wideband and narrowband spectrographic analysis in their acoustic analysis. The discrepancy in the prevalence of phonatory symptoms among these studies can be attributed to the high variability in the duration of syllable and interstress intervals in addition to other factors such as patient selection and stage of disease.

Phonatory and speech disturbances in MS patients are easily perceived by both professional and non-professional listeners. In a study by Hartelius et al investigating the speech temporal characteristics of 14 MS patients with ataxic dysarthria, the results indicated instability and poor flexibility of temporal control of speech in MS patients.[175] More often than not, the voice is described as breathy and the speech as being hypernasal.[176] The prevalence of these phonatory and speech disturbances may reach up to 44% as reported by Hartelius et al.[161] Nevertheless, the degree of dysphonia may vary markedly among patients. In the study by Yamout et al the grade of dysphonia was rather low as 17 patients had grade one dysphonia and only one patient had grade two. The voice of affected patients was described as rough, asthenic, and breathy.[167] Similarly, in the study by Dogan et al on 27 MS patients, there was a statistically significantly higher asthenia and straining voice in the diseased group compared to controls.[177]

Acoustic analysis can obviously help substantiate the perceptual evaluation and at times detect early acoustic changes. In the acoustic analysis study conducted by Feijo et al, both the fundamental frequency and its deviation were higher in women with MS compared to controls. On the other hand, jitter (perturbation in intensity) was higher in men with MS compared to controls.[174] Similarly, the study by Dogan et al revealed higher jitter and shimmer percent and soft phonation index in MS patients compared to controls. However, there was no significant difference in the mean fundamental frequency and noise to harmonic ratio between the two groups.[177] On the other hand, the study by Yamout et al on 40 subjects with MS indicated a significantly lower fundamental frequency and a significantly higher shimmer in MS men compared to controls. There was no significant difference in any of the acoustic parameters in women compared to controls.[167] A year later, a study by Konstantopoulos et al using electroglottographic measures on 64 patients with MS and 64 pair-matched controls revealed a decrease in the fundamental frequency and its range and an increase in the standard deviation of fundamental frequency and in jitter. The increase in standard deviation of the fundamental frequency was more pronounced in the male group in MS patients compared to controls. More so, these findings were found to be associated with destructive MS lesions on magnetic resonance imaging.[178] The increase in the perturbation parameters in MS patients can be attributed to the high phonatory instability as reported by Hartelius et al.[179] Other possible mechanisms for the increased variation in perturbation parameters, specifically, variations in frequency, include fluctuations or irregular laryngeal muscle contraction[180,181] with fluctuation in subglottal pressure secondary to variation in glottal resistance.[182] With demyelination there is slowing of the electrical impulse with subsequent alteration in the speed and synchronization of electrical impulses leading to further instability in muscle contractions.[176] As a result, afflicted patients exhibit incoordination of the adductor muscles with spasticity during phonation that can be reflected as an abnormal frequency range, an increase in standard deviation of the fundamental frequency, and an increase in jitter.

It is also worth noting that MS patients, both men and women, exhibit significantly lower maximum phonation time compared to controls.[167,177] In the study by Dogan et al and the study by Yamout et al, the maximum phonation time values were significantly shorter in affected patients. This difference can be attributed either to glottic insufficiency or to the

known impact of MS on respiratory muscle.[167,177,183] A study by Natour et al on 39 MS patients revealed a significantly lower value for maximum expiratory pressure in the diseased subjects compared to control. As breathing is a major determinant of fundamental frequency, a decrease in expiratory flow may also explain the differences in F0 among subjects with MS compared to controls.[183]

Laryngeal videostroboscopic findings in patients with MS vary among different studies with no clear consensus. In the report by Dogan et al 23 out of 27 had incomplete glottis closure compared to only eight in the control group. The most common glottis configuration was posterior chink followed by spindle shaped.[177] In the study by Yamout et al, the stroboscopic findings in the MS and control group were comparable except for the presence of a posterior chink in only three female patients which may be a normal variant related to gender.[167]

The treatment of MS is multifaceted. It includes administration of steroids, Interferon beta-1a, Alemtuzumab, Daclizumab, or Natalizumab.[184,185] In the SELECT trial, Daclizumab high-yield process administered for 52 weeks had promising results.[184] Speech and voice therapy are also instrumental for the rehabilitation of swallowing difficulty and altered speech intelligibility. The treatment can improve the whole spectrum of laryngopharyngeal symptoms, such as tremor and dysphagia.[186] Other emerging modalities of treatment include deep brain stimulation which has been shown to have favorable effects on phonation. Lyons and Pahwa have reported on the beneficial role of deep brain stimulation to the thalamus and subthalamic area in the treatment of tremor specifically in those resistant to medical therapy.[187] Similarly, Putzer et al two years later has also demonstrated that high-frequency electrical stimulation of the thalamic region can lead to strained phonation and reduction in the extent of breathiness.[188] At a more peripheral level, Botulinum toxin injection into the abductor muscles has been advocated as a manipulative procedure for the treatment of unilateral vocal fold paralysis. The outcome of such an intervention after one year was very successful as reported by Rontal et al.[189]

## Myasthenia Gravis

Mysathenia gravis is a disorder that affects the neuromuscular junction of striated muscles leading to progressive weakness and functional disability. It is primarily due to the production of antibodies against acetylcholine receptors leading to ineffective transmission. Any skeletal muscle may be affected and to various degrees. However, the most commonly affected are the ocular muscles and specifically the levator palpebrae, resulting in ptosis and binocular diplopia in 90% of the cases. Based on the review by Grob et al, only 14% remain localized whereas the remaining 86% reach the generalized form during which the clinical presentation can be non-specific. The predominant symptoms are those of overall fatigability, and decrease in muscle strength and mass. The fatigability worsens after exercise or toward the end of the day and improves following rest. The disease has a predilection to women in their third and fourth decades of life and to men in their sixth decade of life. The course of the disease seems to be more aggressive in men with a higher mortality compared to women.[190]

The laryngeal manifestations of myasthenia gravis (MG) may present in up to 60% of patients during the course of the disease.[191] In the review by Xu et al on the laryngeal characteristics of 32 patients with myasthenia gravis, eight had laryngeal complaints throughout the course of their disease although none of them had presented with these complaints.[192] In fact, based on a review by Neal and Clarke, in only a minority of cases (6%) the laryngeal symptoms are the onset symptoms of MG.[191] There are only few reports in the literature of myasthenia gravis presenting initially with phonatory disturbances. Nieman et al in 1975 reported a case of myasthenia gravis focal to the larynx who presented with complete aphonia and flaccid vocal folds in addition to other bulbar signs such as regurgitation and dysphagia.[193] A few years later Carpenter et al reported the prevalence of primary oral and laryngopharyngeal involvement in 30% of 99 patients diagnosed with MG. The laryngeal symptoms included vocal weakness, hoarseness, breathy phonation, and decreased loudness.[194] Two decades later, Michalska et al reported a series of 11 cases of myasthenia gravis who presented primarily with vocal fatigability and altered nasality of speech. The dysphonia preceded the diagnosis of myasthenia by months to years.[195] Mao et al has also reported 40 cases of MG who had dysphonia as their presenting symptom.[196] In a 2007 review of 1,520 patients with MG, Liu et al also reported exclusive laryngeal involvement in 0.46% of the cases.[197]

When present, the vocal symptoms may be subtle and require a high index of suspicion in order to make the diagnosis. Patients will complain of inability to project the voice, vocal instability, and fatigue with difficulty in sustaining a note. Hypernasality may also be noticed as a symptom of velopharyngeal incompetence. In a nice retrospective review by Mao

et al on 40 cases of laryngeal myasthenia gravis, the most common symptoms in order of frequency were hoarseness (65%), vocal fatigue (52.5%), difficulty with pitch (30%), decreased volume or projection (27.5%), and breathy voice (20%). Symptoms related to swallowing such as globus sensation, dysphagia, and odynophagia were present but to a lesser extent (less than 7.5%). Only 15% of patients had extralaryngeal symptoms such as generalized fatigue and lower extremities weakness.[196] Acoustic analysis and upper airflow measurements are invariably abnormal in patients with MG. The review by Xu et al showed an increase in shimmer and normalized noise energy with a decrease in maximum phonation time and harmonic-to-noise ratio, commensurate with the stroboscopic findings of glottis incompetence.[192] In another report by Liu et al in 2007, there was a drop in the average noise energy from −7.45 to −17.70 dB following the neostigmine test.[197]

In addition to the phonatory symptoms, patients may also present with airway symptoms such as respiratory discomfort and stridor often leading to airway distress. In 1984 Schmidt-Nowara et al reported a case of respiratory failure secondary to vocal fold paresis that responded to anticholinesterase therapy.[198] Several years later there were three more reports of MG presenting as stridor due to bilateral vocal fold involvement.[199–201] Jos et al reported two patients with stridor secondary to weakness of the abductor muscles and Fairley and Hughes highlighted the importance of early administration of pyridostigmine in order to avoid unnecessary tracheotomy or airway complications.[199,200]

Several criteria can be used to make the proper diagnosis of MG among which is the presence of excessive muscle weakness and rapid fatigability that are relieved by rest and alleviated by anticholinesterase drugs. Response to therapy, namely, to any anticholinesterase drug, can markedly confirm the diagnosis. In the study by Mao et al, 23 out of the 30 patients who were maintained on pyridostigmine had reported improvement.[196] In the study by Liu et al, all 7 cases had a positive response to neostigmine test as shown on fiberoptic endoscopy, although additional immunotherapy has been advocated for full recovery.[197] Electromyography is an equally important and integral diagnostic tests in myasthenia gravis. Various types are commonly performed by neurologists and otolaryngologists, among which are the single-fiber EMG and the repeated nerve stimulation test. Although single-fiber EMG has the highest sensitivity, it is not widely used because it requires expertise and patient's collaboration. Instead, repeated nerve stimulation (RNS) is more commonly used for the evaluation of MG patients with suspected laryngeal involvement. It is interesting to note that laryngeal EMG findings are not always in parallel with the vocal complaints. The study by Xu et al revealed a positive RNS for the laryngeal nerves in 87.5% of the cases whereas only 25% had laryngeal symptoms.[192] The muscles most commonly involved were the cricothyroid muscles (CT) and thyroarytenoid muscles (TA) in 92.9% and 50%, respectively. This was in parallel with shorter motor unit durations of the TA and CT and an increase in the corresponding EPs.[192]

Another imperative diagnostic test commonly ordered in the workup of patients with MG is serum antibodies to acetylcholine receptors. Based on a study by Vincent and Newsom-Davis using 2,967 diagnostic assays in 153 cases of MG, anti-acetylcholine receptor has been proven to be a valuable diagnostic test that is positive in 88% in patients with clinical symptoms of MG.[202] Nevertheless, its yield in cases of isolated MG is lower than in cases of generalized myasthenia gravis.[196] Xu et al in their review of 32 patients with MG, 10 patients had a blood test of serum levels of anti-AchR antibodies. The authors did not specify how many of these had laryngeal involvement.[192] Along the same line, Liu et al in their review of 1,520 patients with MG have also reported a low seropositivity rate of anti-acetylcholine-receptor antibodies. Only one patient out of the seven who had initial complaint of dysphonia was seropositive.[197] Similar findings have been previously reported in patients with restricted ocular myasthenia gravis where anti-acetylcholine receptors antibodies as well as anti-striational and antinuclear antibodies were found to be rare compared to patients with generalized myasthenia gravis. In fact the yield in generalized MG is estimated to be 90% compared to 60% in ocular MG.[202] Sommer et al in their critical review of clinical and pathophysiological aspects of ocular myasthenia gravis concur that the detection of acetylcholine receptors autoantibodies does not exceed 65% when the disease is confined to the extraocular muscles, which happens in only 20% of the cases.[203] In a report by Garlepp et al on patients with the ocular variant of MG, the specificity rate of anti-Ach-R antibodies did not exceed 17%.[204] Nevertheless it is important to note that seronegative patients have a similar clinical picture as those who are seropositive.[205]

These findings suggest differences in the pathogenic mechanisms between the two categories of patients, those with localized MG and those with generalized MG.[205] The relatively low prevalence of positive serum levels of anti-AchR antibodies in patients with primary laryngeal manifestation of MG can be attributed to one or two of the following factors: One, the relatively small size of the laryngeal muscles and the corresponding low content of AChR. Meaning to say that when the disease is well localized, although the antibodies are present at the neuromuscular junction in the larynx yet the circulating level is low. Two, the fact that there is a difference in the target antigen in patients with localized MG compared to those with generalized MG. This hypothesis is further supported by the low incidence of thymic pathology in this subgroup of patients.[205–207] In a review of 221 patients with myasthenia gravis, Soliven et al has reported that none of the seronegative patients with ocular myasthenia gravis had thymoma.[205] Evoli et al has also examined the clinical heterogeneity of seronegative patients in 38 cases of myasthenia gravis in relation to thymic disease. The majority of the cases which were primarily confined to ocular and bulbar muscles (33 out of 38) had no thymic pathology.[206]

The alarming laryngeal signs that should alert the physician to the diagnosis of myasthenia gravis are the fluctuation in the impaired mobility of the vocal folds with the presence of incomplete closure during phonation, and the presence of compensatory supraglottic hyperfunctional behavior that is often observed in a large percentage of these patients (75%).[196] See Figure 6–9. Indeed the review by Mao et al in 2001 on 40 patients with myasthenia gravis did reveal impaired mobility, unilateral and bilateral, in up to 92.5% of the cases. Laryngeal stroboscopic evaluation showed also incomplete closure in 65% with evidence of phase asymmetry and amplitude asymmetry in 52.5% and 42.5% of the cases, respectively.[196] Similarly in a retrospective review of 7 cases of primary laryngeal manifestation of MG among a total of 1,520 patients, the authors reported dysfunction in vocal fold mobility, incomplete closure, and muscle tension dysphonia in these cases.[197] These findings were also concurred with the review of the laryngeal manifestation of 32 cases of MG by Xu et al in 2009. In his report 50% of those with laryngeal symptoms, (4 out of eight patients) had abnormal stroboscopic findings, specifically incompetent glottis and impaired mobility of the vocal folds.[192]

The treatment of MG is primarily medical although a multidisciplinary approach is highly advocated during the progress of the disease. The most commonly used medications aside from steroids are pyridostigmine bromide in addition to cytotoxic drugs to a lesser extent. The use of intravenous immunoglobulin (IVIg) has been a controversial issue given the conflicting results in the literature.[196] In a nice review by Gajdos et al, only one randomized control

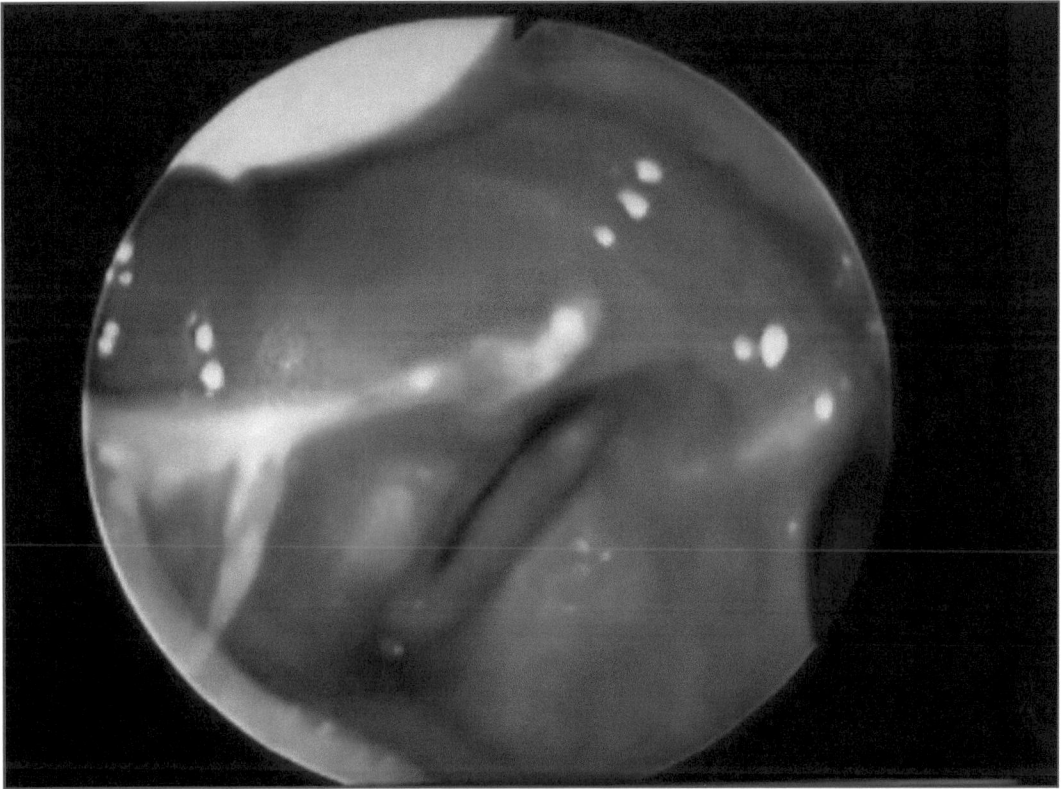

**Figure 6–9.** A 58-year-old man, diagnosed with myasthenia gravis four months ago after presenting to the neurology clinics with ptosis, double vision, and dysphagia. No dyspnea or choking sensation was noted at that time and the flexible laryngoscopy showed a right paretic vocal fold and a mobile left vocal fold. The diagnosis of myasthenia gravis was confirmed using nerve conduction studies and the patient was treated with intravenous immunoglobulin and steroids with a significant improvement of his symptoms.

study showed evidence of efficacy compared to placebo whereas another study showed no significant difference between IVIg and methylprednisolone.[208] Thymectomy is recommended in selective cases and not advocated in professional voice users given the inadvertent risk of recurrent laryngeal nerve injury.[186]

## Amyotrophic Lateral Sclerosis

Given its musculoskeletal structure, the larynx is highly susceptible to systemic diseases including those of the neurologic system. The high degree of coordination needed to perform a phonatory task mandates intricate neurologic control, the disruption of which can lead to vocal changes. Amyotrophic Lateral Sclerosis (ALS) is a degenerative disease that affects the neuromuscular system resulting in both spastic and atrophic muscular symptoms and signs. It is a disease of both upper and lower neurons that

manifests slowly with spasticity and hyperreflexia in addition to flaccidity and hyporeflexia. The etiology of ALS is multifactorial. Immunological, viral, neurotrophic, and oxidative stress factors have been incriminated in its development and progression.[209] One hundred thousand individuals are affected yearly between their fifth and seventh decades of life with a slight male preponderance (1.4:1 male to female ratio).[210] The overall survival rate is very low, with the 5-year survival being 25% to 30%, and less than 10% surviving more than 10 years.[211–213]

The diagnosis of ALS is clinical following the criteria of the World Federation of Neurology.[214] It is based on the presence of symptoms that result from degeneration of both upper and lower motor neurons in different anatomical regions, and on their progression along the course of the disease. Confirmation of the diagnosis may be made using electromyographic studies and neuroimaging. Imaging has added value in helping to exclude other diseases or neurologic disorders.[214-215] The presenting symptoms may either be bulbar or limbic or both, with the most common being limbic. Patients present with weakness of the lower extremities, spasticity, brisk reflexes, fasciculation, and muscular atrophy. Nevertheless, almost one out of four complains initially of bulbar symptoms such as dysphagia, dysarthria, or dysphonia.[216] The decrease in the strength and control of the oropharyngeal and laryngeal muscles manifests as a dysfunction in phonation, speech, and swallowing. This dysfunction has been attributed to involvement of the intrinsic laryngeal muscle with evidence of neurogenic atrophy as reported by Isozaki et al in his histological examination of the intrinsic laryngeal muscles.[37]

To that end the laryngologist plays a key role in the early diagnosis of ALS patients who present with bulbar symptoms at the onset of the disease. In a report by Tomik et al, in reference to the Krakow Motor Neuron Disease database, 19 out of 630 patients with ALS had presented initially with bulbar symptoms and were diagnosed primarily by an otolaryngologist.[217] In another review by Chen and Garrett, out of 220 ALS patients who presented to the neurology clinic, 44 had bulbar symptoms and 19 had presented initially to an otolaryngology clinic.[218] Despite the aforementioned, the diagnosis of ALS is not straightforward as many of the complaints related to the laryngopharyngeal complex may be subtle and ill defined. In a review by Watts and Vanryckeghem in 2001, the authors highlighted the salient feature of laryngeal dysfunction in patients with ALS. They emphasized the importance of critical examination of the bulbar nerves in patients presenting with swallowing or phonatory disorders in order to track early symptoms and signs of cranial neuropathies.[219]

That being said, otolaryngologists must be diligent in the evaluation of patients with dysphagia, dysarthria, and phonatory disturbances. The bulbar symptoms may include dysphagia, aspiration, dysarthria, and phonatory disturbances that can markedly impair communication and quality of life. Other complaints may include hypernasality secondary to velopharyngeal incompetence. The prevalence of dysarthria, dysphagia, and dysphonia varies in different reports. Carpenter et al in 1978 has reported the head and neck manifestations in 441 patients diagnosed with ALS. Primary head and neck symptoms were present in 28% of the cases, among which 14% had primary laryngeal involvement with hoarseness as the main symptom followed by dysphagia in 13% of the cases.[220] On the other hand, a recent review by Chen and Garret in 1,759 ALS patients indicated the presence of dysarthria in 93% of the cases followed

by dysphagia in 86% and dysphonia in 48%.[218] When present, phonatory symptoms are perceived as harsh vocal quality in up to 80% of the cases, breathy in two-thirds of cases, and hypernasal in three out of 4 patients.[221] Based on the review of Tomik et al in 2007, the voice quality may differ based on whether lower or upper motor neurons are affected. In the former case, the voice is husky, low, and diminished, whereas in the latter, the voice is more strained and strangled.[217] Another vocal feature in patients with ALS is rapid voice tremor described as "Flutter." Aronson et al investigated this vocal feature acoustically in eight patients with ALS, and the results indicated higher prevalence of frequency and amplitude modulations compared to controls. The origin of these modulations has been speculated to be of peripheral neural origin.[222]

Acoustic analysis may be helpful in substantiating the perceptual evaluation of the phonatory changes in ALS patients. A few reports also have alluded to the predictive value of acoustic analysis in the diagnosis of bulbar involvement in ALS patients with no bulbar symptoms.[180,181,223-226] The initial reports emphasized pitch and intensity abnormalities during connected speech in the presence of dysarthria which often masks vocal disturbances.[222, 227] These were followed by studies on acoustic changes in relation to dysarthria and type of ALS, whether limb or bulbar. Kent et al has demonstrated an increase in jitter, cycle-to-cycle variation in frequency, and shimmer, cycle-to-cycle variation in intensity, and signal-to-noise ratio in patients with ALS.[224] In a single longitudinal case study by Ramig et al, a 69-year-old ALS patient with no vocal symptoms exhibited abnormal acoustic findings, namely, an increase in the perturbation parameters and a decrease in the harmonics-to-noise ratio in his final vocal recording.[223] A year later, Kent et al investigated voice function in an ALS patient with bulbar signs and reported high variability in the acoustic measures across test sessions.[181] These acoustic findings were corroborated later by the results of Silbergleit et al in his analysis of ALS patients with perceptually normal voice. His findings indicated that acoustic changes such as reduced vocal range and phonatory instability may precede any perceptual change in habitual voice quality.[225] Later in 1999, Robert et al reported the acoustic and aerodynamic findings in two groups of ALS patients, 23 asymptomatic, that is, without bulbar symptoms and 40 symptomatic, that is, with at least one bulbar symptom such as dysphonia, dysphagia, or dysarthria. Five out of the eight acoustic parameters analyzed, namely, jitter, shimmer, coefficient for variation of frequency, harmonic number, and maximal phonatory frequency range (MPFR) were abnormal compared to controls. The authors concluded that acoustic analysis is predictive of bulbar involvement in 73% of the symptomatic group and in 52% of the asymptomatic group.[226] It is also worth noting that in this study the phonatory also airflow was reduced in the symptomatic group. Similarly, in 2001 Silbergleit et al reported the acoustic analysis of 20 patients with ALS and normal voice quality versus 26 control subjects, using jitter, shimmer, signal-to-noise ratio, and maximum phonation frequency range. The results indicated significantly elevated jitter in ALS patients and a significantly higher mean semitone range in controls.[225] The authors highlighted the importance of acoustic analysis in detecting early bulbar laryngeal involvement despite the presence of normal voice perceptually. Similar findings were reported by Xie et al using the multidimensional voice program on 21 patients with ALS. Affected patients had higher noise-to-harmonic ratio and abnormal cycle-to-cycle variation in frequency.[228] The authors emphasized the added value and usability of the MDVP in the analysis of both speech and sustained vowels in patients with ALS. The aforementioned studies offer many possible explanations for the abnormal acoustic findings. The increase in frequency perturbation parameter might be attributed to the irregularity in laryngeal muscle contraction during phonation and to the excessive accumulation of secretions and saliva at the glottis.[223,224] The decrease in the harmonic-to-noise ratio which correlates with dysphonia could be due to glottal insufficiency and unintentional escape of air during phonation.

The diagnosis of laryngopharyngeal disorders in patients with suspected ALS depends upon a high index of suspicion. It is based on proper examination of the oral cavity, tongue, pharynx, and larynx while the patient is asked to perform various non-vegetative and vegetative phonatory tasks such as coughing and swallowing. To that end, various instrumentation such as a flexible nasopharyngeal laryngoscope and or videofluoroscope may be used in order to detect laryngeal movement disorders, impaired mobility of the vocal folds, and/or decreased sensation of the laryngopharyngeal mucosa. Oropharyngeal findings may include tongue fasciculation and atrophy (45%), palatal weakness, and asymmetry (18–27%), and decreased pharyngeal reflexes (18%).[217] The laryngeal findings can include abnormal movement of the vocal folds, hypoadduction, hyperfunction, incomplete closure, impaired mobility during inspiration or phonation, and laryngeal spasm.[219,220,229,230] Aperiodicity and weakness of the vocal folds may also be documented by laryngeal videostroboscopy.

Based on a review by Chen and Garrett on 13 patients with ALS who had videostroboscopic evaluation, the most frequent finding was incomplete closure of the vocal folds during phonation in 50% of the cases, followed by bowing in one-third and hyperfunction of the supraglottic structures in one out of four patients. Other findings included signs of laryngopharyngeal reflux disease such as pooling of mucus and pachydermia.[218] See Figure 6–10. Tomik et al in 2005 examined laryngeal function in ALS patients with and without bulbar signs and demonstrated disturbed position of the vocal folds due to vagal neuropathy or dysfunction. These findings were more pronounced in patients with bulbar onset disease compared to those with limbic onset.[231] Similar findings were reported a year later by the same author on a larger number of patients (24 with bulbar onset and 11 with limbic onset), emphasizing the importance of impaired mobility and altered position of the vocal folds as early signs of vagal nerve dysfunction prior to obvious clinical onset of bulbar disease.[217] In this report, the laryngeal findings in the bulbar group were stratified further as upper motor and lower motor neuron subgroups based on their presentation. The lower motor neuron subgroup had incomplete closure or bowing of the vocal folds (hourglass) during phonation whereas the upper motor neuron subgroup had hypoadduction of the true vocal folds with a compensatory hyperadduction of the ventricular folds. The authors described the voice as being associated with hyperkinesis of the cervical muscles. It is interesting that the limbic group who perceptually had a normal voice had also some abnormal laryngeal findings on endoscopy.[217] Later in 2015, the same authors evaluated the phonatory function of 17 patients with ALS at three points in time during a 6-month interval using several measures including perceptual evaluation, acoustic analysis, airflow measures, and laryngeal videostroboscopy. The most frequent symptoms were hoarseness and breathiness which were associated with a decrease in vocal range and abnormal perturbation parameters, more so in females. On videoendostroboscopy, there was evidence of abnormal mucosal waves, glottal closure, and amplitude of vibration.[232]

Less frequently encountered laryngeal findings include paradoxical vocal fold movement and laryngospasm. This latter may occur during or following laryngeal manipulation such as intubation or extubation as reported by Kuhnlein et al.[233] In a report by Forshew and Bromberg, 19% of patients in later stages of ALS may experience laryngeal spasm.[234] Along the same line, van der Graaf et al also reported four cases of vocal fold dysfunction or vocal fold

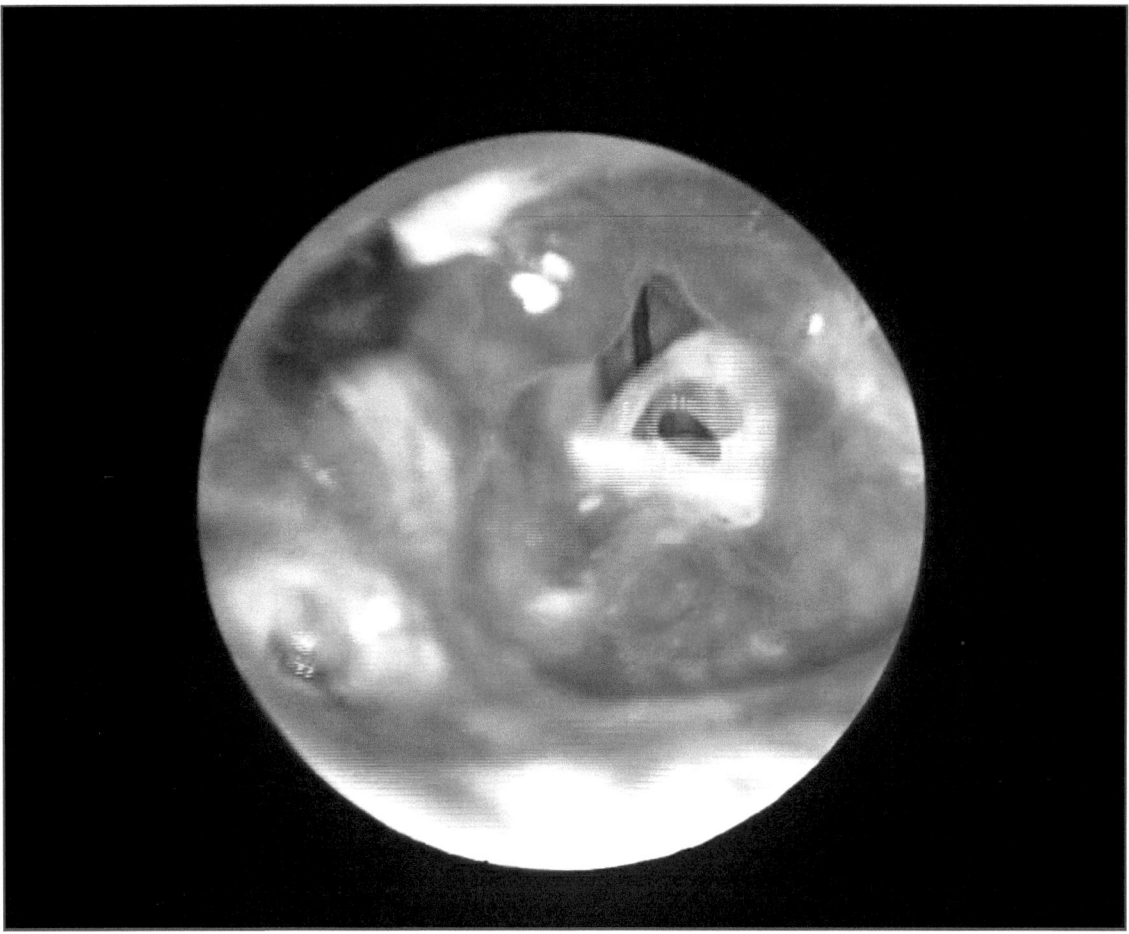

**Figure 6–10.** A 75-year-old male diagnosed case of amyotrophic lateral sclerosis presenting with history of dysphonia, aspiration, and dysphagia. On laryngeal examination there is hypoadduction of the vocal folds with signs of mucosal inflammation and pooling of mucus.

abductor paresis, three of whom developed these conditions over the course of the disease, and one of whom had them at the time of diagnosis. The mechanism of glottic narrowing in these patients is not clear given the lack of any autopsy studies on patients with ALS and vocal fold dysfunction. Nevertheless, the suggested nature of this glottic behavior can be of infranuclear or supranuclear origin, or both.[235] The weakness of the abductor muscles, together with the Venturi effect, may further accentuate the noisy breathing and stridor experienced by affected patients. The authors emphasized the need to secure the compromised airway which may occur irrespective of the stage of the disease.[235] Another rare laryngeal manifestation of ALS is spasmodic dysphonia. Roth et al reported a rare case who presented initially with typical symptoms of adductor SD and was found later to have ALS. The authors underscored the need for a diligent and comprehensive

neuromotor evaluation of patients with recent onset of movement disorders and symptoms of spasmodic dysphonia.[230]

An equally important and often underdiagnosed laryngeal manifestation of ALS is impaired laryngeal sensation. Amin et al investigated laryngeal sensation in 22 patients with ALS using a dysphagia questionnaire in addition to flexible endoscopic evaluation of swallowing using sensory testing (FEESST). The results indicated that although ALS is a motor neuron disease, close to 50% of patients had abnormal sensory threshold values with asymmetric findings in 75% of the cases. These sensory abnormalities did not correlate with disease duration or severity.[236]

The treatment of dysphonia in patients with ALS has many facets to it. Voice therapy is always a good start in order to address abnormalities in laryngeal functional behavior that can be either primary or secondary. Patterns of dysfunction are identified, and exercises for swallowing and breathing often are initiated. Vocal therapy to alleviate glottal incompetence and/or hyperkinetic laryngeal movement disorders also is beneficial. The importance of the otolaryngologist as a member of the multidisciplinary team in the management of these patients cannot be overemphasized. Rubin et al advocated early intervention of otolaryngologists rather than late in the approach to patients with bulbar symptoms.[237] Following a diligent head and neck examination, cranial nerve neuropathies when present can often be treated either surgically or using chemodenervation. For instance, Botulinum toxin A and B have been used successfully for the treatment of resting sialorrhea with ALS.[238,239] Alternative procedures may include resection of both submaxillary glands. Botulinum toxin injections also may be used for the treatment of spasmodic dysphonia that is secondary to hyperadduction of the vocal folds during phonation. On the other hand, augmentative alternative procedures can be offered for the treatment of glottic incompetence. Injection laryngoplasty using various filling materials such as hyaluronic acid, fat, or Gelfoam are used to help close any adductory gap during phonation. Caution must be exercised when considering medialization because of the risk of abductor weakness with ALS and the risk of airway compromise. Adjunctive procedures may include insertion of palatal prosthesis and pharyngeal flaps for the treatment of velopharyngeal incompetence. Other options include the performance of tracheotomy with or without a percutaneous gastrostomy. The main indication is recurrent aspiration despite patient having a percutaneous gastrostomy.[240,241] Alternatively, at times laryngeal diversion is needed in order to secure the airway and prevent aspiration to avoid life-threatening complications.[242]

## References

1. Crumley RL. Repair of the recurrent laryngeal nerve. *Otolaryngol Clin North Am.* 1990;23(3):553–563.
2. Jellish WS, Jensen RL, Anderson DE, Shea JF. Intraoperative electromyographic assessment of recurrent laryngeal nerve stress and pharyngeal injury during anterior cervical spine surgery with Caspar instrumentation. *J Neurosurg Spine.* 1999;91(2):170–174.
3. Slomka WS, Abedi E, Sismanis A, Barlascini Jr. Paralysis of the recurrent laryngeal nerve by an extracapsular thyroid adenoma. *Ear Nose Throat J.* 1989;68(11):855–856.
4. Jaffe R, Bogomolski-Yahalom V, Kramer MR. Vocal cord paralysis as the presenting symptom of sarcoidosis. *Respir Med.* 1994;88:633–636.
5. Tobias JK, Santiago SM, Williams AJ. Sarcoidosis as a cause of left recurrent laryngeal nerve palsy. *Arch Otolaryngol Head Neck Surg.* 1990;116: 971–972.
6. Ellis PD, Pallister WK. Recurrent laryngeal nerve palsy and endotracheal intubation. *J Laryngol Otol.* 1975;89:823–826.
7. Speicher CE, Ferrigan L, Wolfson SK, Erdsgon HV, Rawson AJ. Cold injury of myocardium and pericardium in cardiac hypothermia. *Surg Gynecol Obstet.* 1962;114:655–665.
8. Stern W, Saver W, Dauber W. Complications of central venous catheterization from an anatomical point of view. *Acta Anatomica.* 1990;138:137–143.
9. Baranyail L, Madarasz G. Recurrent laryngeal nerve paralysis following lung surgery. *J Thorac Cardiovasc Surg.* 1963;46:531.
10. Apostolakis LW, Funk GF, Urdaneta LF, McCulloch TM, Jeyapalan MM. The nasogastric tube syndrome: two case reports and review of the literature. *Head Neck.* 2001;23(1):59–63.
11. Remacle M, Mayné A, Lawson G, Jamart J. Subtotal carbon dioxide laser arytenoidectomy by endoscopic approach for treatment of bilateral cord immobility in adduction. *Ann Otol Rhinol Laryngol.* 1996;105(6): 438–445.
12. Shafei H, El Kholy A, Azmy S. Vocal cord dysfunction after cardiac surgery. An overlooked complication. *Eur J Cardiothorac Surg.* 1997;11(3):564–566.
13. Nishimaki T, Suzuki T, Suzuki S, Kuwabara S, Hatakeyama K. Outcomes of extended radical esophagectomy for thoracic esophageal cancer. *J Am Coll Surg.* 1998;186(3):306–312.
14. Johansson S, Lofroth PO, Denekamp J. Left-sided vocal cord paralysis: a newly recognized late complication of mediastinal irradiation. *Radiother Oncol.* 2001;58(3):287–294.
15. Sataloff RT. Vocal fold paresis and paralysis. In: Sataloff RT. *Professional Voice: The Science and Art of Clinical Care.* 4th ed. San Diego, CA: Plural Publishing; 2017.
16. Portone CR, Hapner ER, McGregor L, Otto K, Johns MM. Correlation of the Voice Handicap Index (VHI) and the Voice-Related Quality of Life measure (V-RQOL). *J Voice.* 2007;21(6):723–727.
17. Sataloff RT. The clinical voice laboratory. In: Sataloff RT. *Professional Voice: The Science and Art of Clinical Care.* 4th ed. San Diego, CA: Plural Publishing: 2017; 405–438.
18. Lopes LW, Simões LB, da Silva JD, et al. Accuracy of acoustic analysis measurements in the evaluation of patients with different laryngeal diagnoses. *J Voice.* 2017;31(3):382-e15.
19. Pinho CM, Jesus LM, Barney A. Aerodynamic measures of speech in unilateral vocal fold paralysis (UVFP) patients. *Logoped Phoniatr Vocol.* 2013; 38(1):19–34.
20. Hartl DM, Hans S, Vaissière J, Brasnu DF. Objective acoustic and aerodynamic measures of breathiness in paralytic dysphonia. *Eur Arch Oto-rhino-laryngol.* 2003;260(4):175–182.

21. Gillespie AI, Dastolfo C, Magid N, Gartner-Schmidt J. Acoustic analysis of four common voice diagnoses: moving toward disorder-specific assessment. *J Voice*. 2014;28(5):582–588.

22. Adams SG, Irish JC, Durkin LC, Wong DL, Brown DH. Evaluation of vocal function in unilateral vocal fold paralysis following thyroplastic surgery. *J Otolaryngol*. 1996;25(3):165–170.

23. Makiyama K, Kida A, Sawashima M. Evaluation of expiratory effort on dysphonic patients on increasing vocal intensity. *Otolaryngol Head Neck Surg*. 1998; 118(5):723–727.

24. Kelchner LN, Lee L, Stemple JC. Laryngeal function and vocal fatigue after prolonged reading in individuals with unilateral vocal fold paralysis. *J Voice*. 2003;17(4):513–528.

25. Merati AL, Halum SL, Smith TL. Diagnostic testing for vocal fold paralysis: survey of practice and evidence-based medicine review. *Laryngoscope*. 2006; 116(9):1539–1552.

26. Kang BC, Roh JL, Lee JH, et al. Usefulness of computed tomography in the etiologic evaluation of adult unilateral vocal fold paralysis. *World J Surg*. 2013;37(6):1236–1240.

27. Chin SC, Edelstein S, Chen CY, Som PM. Using CT to localize side and level of vocal cord paralysis. *Am J Roentgenol*. 2003;180(4):1165–1170.

28. Neel III HB, Harner SG, Benninger MS, et al. Evaluation and treatment of the unilateral paralyzed vocal fold. *Otolaryngol Head Neck Surg*. 1994;111(4):497–508.

29. Chang WH, Fang TJ, Li HY, Jaw FS, Wong AM, Pei YC. Quantitative electromyographic characteristics of idiopathic unilateral vocal fold paralysis. *Laryngoscope*. 2016;126(11).

30. Sataloff, RT, Mandel S, Heman-Ackah YD, Abaza MM. *Laryngeal Electromyography*. 3rd ed. San Diego, CA: Plural Publishing; 2017.

31. Ward PH, Berci G, Calcaterra TC. Superior laryngeal nerve paralysis an often overlooked entity. *Trans. Section Otolaryngol. American Academy Ophthalmol Otolaryngol*. 1977;84(1):78–89.

32. Dursun G, Sataloff RT, Spiegel JR, Mandel S, Heuer RJ, Rosen DC. Superior laryngeal nerve paresis and paralysis. *J Voice*. 1996;10(2):206–211.

33. Adour KK, Schneider GD, Hilsinger JR RL. Acute superior laryngeal nerve palsy: analysis of 78 cases. *Otolaryngol Head Neck Surg*. 1980;88(4):418–422.

34. Eckley CA, Sataloff RT, Hawkshaw M, Spiegel JR, Mandel S. Voice range in superior laryngealnerve paresis and paralysis. *J Voice*. 1998;12(3):340–348.

35. Hamdan AL, Jabour J, Azar ST. Goiter and laryngeal sensory neuropathy. *Int J Otolaryngol*. 2013.

36. Jansson S, Tisell LE, Hagne I, Sanner E, Stenborg R, Svensson P. Partial superior laryngeal nerve (SLN) lesions before and after thyroid surgery. *World J Surg*. 1988;12(4):522–526.

37. Isozaki E, Hayashi M, Hayashida T, Oda M, Hirai S. Myopathology of the intrinsic laryngeal muscles in neurodegenerative diseases, with reference to the mechanism of vocal cord paralysis. *Clin Neurol*. 1998;38 (8):711–718.

38. Gallena S, Smith PJ, Zeffiro T, et al. Effects of levodopa on laryngeal muscle activity for voice onset and offset in Parkinson disease. *J Speech Lang Hear Res*. 2001;44 (6):1284–1299.

39. Kim HJ, Jeon BS. Acute respiratory failure due to vocal cord paralysis in a patient with Parkinson's disease. *Mov Dis*. 2009; 24(12):1862–1863.

40. Gan EC, Lau DP, Cheah KL. Stridor in Parkinson's disease: a case of'dry drowning'?. *J Laryngol Otol*. 2010;124(6):668–673.

41. Habib MA. Intra-articular steroid injection in acute rheumatoid arthritis of the larynx. *J Laryngol Otol*. 1977;91(10):909–910.

42. Jatzko GR, Lisborg PH, Müller MG, Wette VM. Recurrent nerve palsy after thyroid operations—principal nerve identification and a literature review. *Surgery*. 1994;115(2):139–144.

43. Sulica L. The natural history of idiopathic unilateral vocal fold paralysis: evidence and problems. *Laryngoscope*. 2008;118(7):1303–1307.

44. Bridge PM, Ball DJ, Mackinnon SE, et al. Nerve crush injuries—a model for axonotmesis. *Exp Neurol*. 1994; 127(2):284–290.

45. Horn KL, Crumley RL. The physiology of nerve injury and repair. *Otolaryngol Clin North Am*. 1984; 17(2):321–333.

46. Shao T, Qiu W, Yang W. Anatomical variations of the recurrent laryngeal nerve in Chinese patients: a prospective study of 2,404 patients. *Sci Rep*. 2016;6.

47. Crumley RL. Update: ansa cervicalis to recurrent laryngeal nerve anastomosis for unilateral laryngeal paralysis. *Laryngoscope*. 1991;101(4):384–388.

48. Gacek M, Gacek RR. Cricoarytenoid joint mobility after chronic vocal cord paralysis. *Laryngoscope*. 1996; 106(12):1528–1530.

49. Colman MF, Schwartz I. The effect of vocal cord paralysis on the cricoarytenoid joint. *Otolaryngol Head Neck Surg*. 1981;89(3):419–422.

50. Shindo ML, Herzon GD, Hanson DG, Cain DJ, Sahgal V. Effects of denervation on laryngeal muscles: a canine model. *Laryngoscope*. 1992;102(6):663–669.

51. Flint PW, Downs DH, Coltrera MD. Laryngeal synkinesis following reinnervation in the rat: neuroanatomic and physiologic study using retrograde fluorescent tracers and electromyography. *Ann Otology Rhinol Laryngol*. 1991;100(10):797–806.

52. Naidu L, Ramsaroop L, Partab P, Satyapal KS. Galen's "Anastomosis" revisited. *Clin Anat*. 2012;25 (6):722–728.

53. Friedman AD, Burns JA, Heaton JT, Zeitels SM. Early versus late injection medialization for unilateral vocal cord paralysis. *Laryngoscope*. 2010;120(10):2042–2046.

54. Prendes BL, Yung KC, Likhterov I, Schneider SL, Al-Jurf SA, Courey MS. Long-term effects of injection laryngoplasty with a temporary agent on voice quality and vocal fold position. *Laryngoscope*. 2012; 122(10):2227–2233.

55. DeFatta RA, Chowdhury FR, Sataloff RT. Complications of injection laryngoplasty using calcium hydroxylapatite. *J Voice.* 2012;26(5):614–618.

56. Lisi C, Hawkshaw MJ, Sataloff RT. Viscosity of materials for laryngeal injection: a review of current knowledge and clinical implications. *J Voice.* 2013;27:119–123.

57. Abitbol J. Laser Voice Surgery and Voice Care 20th International Workshop. Paris. IFOS Congress. June, 2017, pp. 22–24.

58. Goding Jr GS. Nerve-muscle pedicle reinnervation of the paralyzed vocal cord. *Otolaryngol Clin North Am.* 1991;24(5):1239–1252.

59. Tucker HM. Long-term preservation of voice improvement following surgical medialization and reinnervation for unilateral vocal fold paralysis. *J Voice.* 1999;13(2):251–256.

60. Dennis DP, Kashima H. Carbon dioxide laser posterior cordectomy for treatment of bilateral vocal cord paralysis. *Ann Otol Rhinol Laryngol.* 1989;98(12):930–934.

61. Rubin AD, Hogikyan ND, Sullivan K, Boulis N, Feldman EL. Remote delivery of rAAV-GFP to the rat brainstem through the recurrent laryngeal nerve. *Laryngoscope.* 2001;111(11):2041–2045.

62 Shiotani A, O'malley BW, Coleman ME, Flint PW. Human insulinlike growth factor 1 gene transfer into paralyzed rat larynx: single vs multiple injection. *Arch Otolaryngol Head Neck Surg.* 1999;125(5):555–560.

63. Kanemaru S, Nakamura T, Omori K, et al. Regeneration of the vocal fold using autologous mesenchymal stem cells. *Ann Otol Rhinol Laryngol.* 2003;112:915–920.

64. Kanemaru S, Nakamura T, Yamashita M, et al. Destiny of autologous bone marrow-derived stromal cells implanted in the vocal fold. *Ann Otol Rhinol Laryngol.* 2005;114:907–912.

65. Hertegård S, Cedervall J, Svensson B, et al. Viscoelastic and histologic properties in scarred rabbit vocal folds after mesenchymal stem cell injection. *Laryngoscope.* 2006;116(7):1248–1254.

66. Ohno T, Hirano S, Kanemaru SI, et al. Expression of extracellular matrix proteins in the vocal folds and bone marrow–derived stromal cells of rats. *Eur Arch Oto-Rhino-Laryngol.* 2008;265(6):669–674.

67. Hirano S, Tateya T, Nagai H, Ford CN, Tateya I, Bless DM. Regeneration of aged vocal folds with basic fibroblast growth factor in a rat model: a preliminary report. *Ann Otol Rhinol Laryngol.* 2005;114(4):304–308.

68. Kanazawa T, Komazawa D, Indo K, et al. Single injection of basic fibroblast growth factor to treat severe vocal fold lesions and vocal fold paralysis. *Laryngoscope.* 2015;125(10).

69. Zealear DL, Dedo HH. Control of paralysed axial muscles by electrical stimulation. *Acta Otolaryngol.* 1977; 83:514–527.

70. Zealear DL, Billante CR. Neurophysiology of vocal fold paralysis. *Otolaryngol Clin North Am.* 2004; 37: 1–23.

71. Zealear DL, Rainey CL, Herzon GD, et al. Electrical pacing of the paralyzed human larynx. *Ann Otol Rhinol Laryngol.* 1996; 105:689–693.

72. Zealear DL, Kunibe I, Nomura K, et al. Rehabilitation of bilaterally paralyzed canine larynx with implantable stimulator. *Laryngoscope.* 2009; 119:1737–1744.

73. Katada A, Van Himbergen D, Kunibe I, et al. Evaluation of a deep brain stimulation electrode for laryngeal pacing. *Ann Otol Rhinol Laryngol.* 2008; 117:621–629.

74 Katada A, Ota R, Arakawa T, et al. Laryngeal pacing with an advanced generation implantable stimulator. In: *Proceedings of the 15th World Congress for Bronchology (Wcb) and 15th World Congress for Bronchoesophagology (Wcbe).* 2008: 133–137, 275.

75. Nomura K, Kunibe I, Katada A, et al. Bilateral motion restored to the paralyzed canine larynx with implantable stimulator. *Laryngoscope.* 2010; 120:2399–2409.

76. Louis ED, Ottman R, Hauser WA. How common is the most common adult movement disorder? Estimates of the prevalence of essential tremor throughout the world. *Mov Disord.* 1998;13:5–10.

77. Findley LJ. Epidemiology and genetics of essential tremor. *Neurology.* 2000;54(suppl):S8–S13.

78. Rautakorpi I, Takala J, Marttila RJ, Sievers K, Rinne UK. Essential tremor in a Finnish population. *Acta Neurol Scand.* 1982; 66(1): 58–67.

79. Benito-Leon J, Bermejo-Pareja F, Louis ED; Neurological Disorders in Central Spain (NEDICES) Study Group. Incidence of essential tremor in three elderly populations of central Spain. *Neurology.* 2005; 64(10): 1721–1725.

80. Lou JS, Jankovic J. Essential tremor: clinical correlates in 350 patients. *Neurology.* 1991; 41(2 (pt 1)): 234–238.

81. Louis ED, Ottman R. How familial is familial tremor? The genetic epidemiology of essential tremor. *Neurology.* 1996; 46(5): 1200–1205.

82. Louis ED, Ottman R, Ford B, et al. Washington Heights-Inwood. Genetic study of essential tremor: methodologic issues in essential-tremor research. *Neuroepidemiology.* 1997; 16(3): 124–133.

83. Higgins JJ, Loveless JM, Jankovic J, Patel P. Evidence that a gene for essential tremor maps to chromosome 2p in four families. *Mov Disord.* 1998;13:972–977.

84. Gulcher JR, Jonsson P, Kong A, et al. Mapping of a familial essential tremor gene, FET1, to chromosome 3q13. *Nat Genet.* 1997;17:84–87.

85. Tanner CM, Goldman SM, Lyons KE, et al. Essential tremor in twins: an assessment of genetic vs environmental determinants of etiology. *Neurology.* 2001;57: 1389–1391.

86. Louis ED, Vonsattel JP. The emerging neuropathology of essential tremor. *Mov Dis.* 2008;23(2):174–182.

87. Elble RJ. What is essential tremor? *Curr Neurol Neurosci Rep.* 2013;13(6):353.

88. Montigny C de, Lamarre Y. Rhythmic activity induced by harmaline in the olivocerebello-bulbar system of the cat. *Brain Res.* 1973; 53: 81–95.

89. Deuschl G, Raethjen J, Lindemann M, Krack P. The pathophysiology of tremor. *Muscle Nerve.* 2001;24(6): 716–735.

90. Elble RJ, Higgins C, Hughes L. Phase resetting and frequency entrainment of essential tremor. *Exp Neurol.* 1992; 116: 355–361.

91. Tomoda H, Shibasaki H, Kuroda Y, Shin T. Voice tremor dysregulation of voluntary expiratory muscles. *Neurology*. 1987;37(1):117–122.

92. Deuschl G, Bain P, Brin M. Consensus statement of the Movement Disorder Society on Tremor. Ad Hoc Scientific Committee. *Mov Disord*. 1998;13:2–23.

93. Elble RJ. Diagnostic criteria for essential tremor and differential diagnosis. *Neurology*. 2000;54(suppl):S2–S6

94. Pahwa R, Lyons KE. Essential tremor: differential diagnosis and current therapy. *Am J Med*. 2003;115(2): 134–142.

95. Sulica L, Louis ED. Clinical characteristics of essential voice tremor: a study of 34 cases. *Laryngoscope*. 2010;120(3):516–528.

96. Warrick P, Dromey C, Irish JC, Durkin L, Pakiam A, Lang A. Botulinum toxin for essential tremor of the voice with multiple anatomical sites of tremor: a crossover design study of unilateral versus bilateral injection. *Laryngoscope*. 2000;110(8):1366–1374.

97. Brown JR, Simonson J. Organic voice tremor. A tremor of phonation. *Neurology*. 1963;13:520–525.

98. Louis ED, Gerbin M. Voice handicap in essential tremor: a comparison with normal controls and Parkinson's disease. *Tremor Other Hyperkin Mov*. 2013;3.

99. Elble RJ, Higgins C, Leffler K, Hughes L. Factors influencing the amplitude and frequency of essential tremor. *Mov Dis*. 1994;9(6):589–596.

100. Winholtz WS, Ramig LO. Vocal tremor analysis with the vocal demodulator. *J Speech Lang Hear Res*. 1992; 35(3):562–573.

101. Koda J, Ludlow CL. An evaluation of laryngeal muscle activation in patients with voice tremor. *Otolaryngol Head Neck Surg*. 1992;107(5):684–696.

102. Bove MJ, Daamen N, Rosen C, Wang CC, Sulica L, Gaertner-Schmidt J. Development and validation of the vocal tremor scoring system. *Laryngoscope*. 2006:116: 1662–1667.

103. Gurey LE, Sinclair CF, Blitzer A. A new paradigm for the management of essential vocal tremor with botulinum toxin. *Laryngoscope*. 2013;123(10):2497–2501.

104. de Moraes BT, de Biase NG. Laryngoscopy evaluation protocol for the differentiation of essential and dystonic voice tremor. *Brazil J Otorhinolaryngol*. 2016; 82(1):88–96.

105. Findley LJ, Gresty MA. Head, facial and voice tremor. *Adv Neurol*. 1988;49:239–253.

106. Andran G, Kinsbourne M, Rushworth G. Dysphonia due to tremor. *J Neurol Neurosurg Psychiatry*. 1966;29: 219–223.

107. Hachinski VC, Thomsen IV, Buch NH. The nature of primary vocal tremor. *J Can Neurol Sci*. 1975;2:195–197.

108. Larsen TA, Teraväinen H, Calne DB. Atenolol vs propranolol in essential tremor. A controlled, quantitative study. *Acta Neurol Scand*. 1982;66:547–554.

109. Calzetti S, Findley LJ, Gresty MA, et al. Effect of a single dose of propranolol on essential tremor: a double-blind controlled study. *Ann Neurol*. 1983;13:165–171.

110. Justicz N, Hapner ER, Josephs JS, Boone BC, Jinnah HA, Johns MM. Comparative effectiveness of pro-

111. Gorman WP, Cooper R, Pocock P, Campbell MJ. A comparison of primidone, propranolol, and placebo in essential tremor using quantitative analysis. *J Neurol Neurosurg Psychiatr*. 1986;491:64–68.

112. Koller WC, Royse V. Efficacy of primidone in essential tremor. *Neurology*. 1986;36:121–124.

113. Gironell A, Kulisevsky J, Barbanoj M, et al. A randomized placebo controlled comparative trial of gabapentin and propranolol in essential tremor. *Arch Neurol*. 1999;56:475–480.

114. Connor GS. A randomized double-blind placebo controlled trial of topiramate treatment for essential tremor. *Neurology*. 2002;59:132–134.

115. Langeveld TP, Drost HA, Baatenburg de Jong RJ. Unilateral versus bilateral botulinum toxin injections in adductor spasmodic dysphonia. *Ann Otol Rhinol Laryngol*. 1998;107:280–284.

116. Adams SG, Hunt EJ, Irish JC, et al. Comparison of Botulinum toxin injection procedures in adductor spasmodic dysphonia. *J Otolaryngol*. 1995;24:345–351.

117. Zwirner P, Murry T, Woodson GE. A comparison of bilateral and unilateral botulinum toxin treatments for botulinum toxin treatments for spasmodic dysphonia. *Eur Arch Otorhinolaryngol*. 1993;250:271–276.

118. Adams SG, Hunt EJ, Charles DA, Lang AE. Unilateral versus bilateral botulinum toxin injections in spasmodic dysphonia: acoustic and perceptual results. *J Otolaryngol*. 1993;22:171–175.

119. Tsui JKC. Botulinum toxin as a therapeutic agent. *Pharmacol Ther*. 1996;72:13–24.

120. Sataloff RT, Heuer RJ, Munz M, Yoon MS, Spiegel JR. Vocal tremor reduction with deep brain stimulation: a preliminary report. *J Voice*. 2002;16(1):132–135.

121. Yoon MS, Munz M, Sataloff RT, Spiegel JR, Heuer RJ. Vocal tremor reduction with deep brain stimulation. *Stereotac Func Neurosurg*. 1999;72(2–4):241–244.

122. Hägglund P, Sandström L, Blomstedt P, Karlsson F. Voice tremor in patients with essential tremor: effects of deep brain stimulation of caudal zona incerta. *J Voice*. 2016;30(2):228–233.

123. Enders D, Balzer-Geldsetzer M, Riedel O, et al. Prevalence, duration and severity of Parkinson's disease in Germany: a combined meta-analysis from literature data and outpatient samples. *Eur Neurol*. 2017;78(3–4): 128–136.

124. Braunwald E, Fauci AS, Kasper DL, Hauser K, Longo DL, Jameson JL. *Harrison's Manual of Medicine*. McGraw-Hill Professional; 2001.

125. Leopold NA, Kagel MC. Laryngeal deglutition movement in Parkinson's disease. *Neurology*. 1997;48(2): 373–375.

126. Guindi GM, Bannister R, Gibson WP, Payne JK. Laryngeal electromyography in multiple system atrophy with autonomic failure. *J Neurol Neurosurg Psychiatry*. 1981; 44(1):49–53.

127. Isozaki E, Matsubara S, Hayashida T, Oda M, Hirai S. Morphometric study of nucleus ambiguus in multiple

system atrophy presenting with vocal cord abductor paralysis. *Clin Neuropathol.* 1999;19(5):213–220.

128. Duffy JR. Motor speech disorders: Substrates, *Differential Diagnosis and Management.* 2nd ed. St Louis, MO: Elsevier Mosby; 2005.

129. Stelzig Y, Hochhaus W, Gall V, et al. Laryngeal manifestations in patients with Parkinson disease. *Laryngorhinootologie.* 1999; 78:544–551.

130. Ho AK, Bradshaw JL, Iansek R. Volume perception in parkinsonian speech. *Mov Dis.* 2000;15(6):1125–1131.

131. Angelis ED, Mourao LF, Ferraz HB, Behlau MS, Pontes PA, Andrade LA. Effect of voice rehabilitation on oral communication of Parkinson's disease patients. *Acta Neurolog Scand.* 1997;96(4):199–205.

132. Ramig LO, Sapir S, Fox C, Countryman S. Changes in vocal loudness following intensive voice treatment (LSVT®) in individuals with Parkinson's disease: a comparison with untreated patients and normal age-matched controls. *Mov Dis.* 2001;16(1):79–83.

133. Ho AK, Bradshaw JL, Iansek R, Alfredson R. Speech volume regulation in Parkinson's disease: effects of implicit cues and explicit instructions. *Neuropsychologia.* 1999;37(13):1453–1460.

134. Midi I, Dogan M, Koseoglu M, Can G, Sehitoglu MA, Gunal DI. Voice abnormalities and their relation with motor dysfunction in Parkinson's disease. *Acta Neurolog Scand.* 2008; 117(1):26–34.

135. Gamboa J, Jiménez-Jiménez FJ, Nieto A, et al. Acoustic voice analysis in patients with Parkinson's disease treated with dopaminergic drugs. *J Voice.* 1997; 11(3): 314–320.

136. Tanaka Y, Nishio M, Niimi S. Vocal acoustic characteristics of patients with Parkinson's disease. *Folia Phonia Logopaed.* 2011; 63(5):223–230.

137. Hertrich I, Ackermann H. Gender-specific vocal dysfunctions in Parkinson's disease: electroglottographic and acoustic analyses. *Ann of Otol Rhinol Laryngol.* 1995;104(3):197–202.

138. Bang YI, Min K, Sohn YH, Cho SR. Acoustic characteristics of vowel sounds in patients with Parkinson disease. *NeuroRehabil.* 2013; 32(3):649–654.

139. Perez KS, Ramig LO, Smith ME, Dromey C. The Parkinson larynx: tremor and videostroboscopic findings. *J Voice.* 1996; 10(4):354–361.

140. Vas CJ, Parsonage MA, Lord OC. Parkinsonism associated with laryngeal spasm. *J Neurol Neurosurg Psychiatry.* 1965; 28(5):401–403.

141. Plasse HM, Lieberman AN, Bilateral vocal cord paralysis in Parkinson's disease. *Arch Otolaryngol,* 1981; 107(4): 252–253.

142. Read D, and Young A, Stridor and parkinsonism. *Postgrad Med J.* 1983; 59(694): 520–521.

143. Takayama H, Sato H, Ota Z, Nishizaki K, Ogawa N. Bilateral vocal cord paralysis due to laryngeal carcinoma in Parkinson's disease. *J Med.* 1986;18 (3–4):251–258.

144. Palesse N, Marelli A, Legge MP. Bilateral abductor paralysis of the vocal cords in the course of neurologi-cal diseases: report of 5 cases. *Ital J Neurolog Sci.* 1988; 9(1):59–62.

145. Isozaki E, Shimizu T, Takamoto K, et al. Vocal cord abductor paralysis (VCAP) in Parkinson's disease: difference from VCAP in multiple system atrophy. *J Neurolog Sci.* 1995;130(2):197–202.

146. Nakane S, Motomura M, Furuya T, Shirabe S, Nakamura T. A case of juvenile Parkinson disease with vocal cord abductor paralysis in the course of malignant syndrome. *Clin Neurol.* 1998; 39(2–3):370–372.

147. Qayyum A, Mierzwa K, See M, Sharma A, Montgommery PQ. Laser arytenoidectomy for bilateral vocal fold palsy in Parkinson's disease. *J Laryngol Otol.* 2005;119(10):831–833.

148. Lee DH, Lim SC, and Lee JK, Bilateral vocal cord paralysis in a patient with Parkinson's disease. *B-ENT.* 2012; 8(2): 141–142.

149. Hoberman S. Speech techniques in aphasia and Parkinsonism. *J Mich State Med Soc.* 1958;57:1720–1723.

150. LeDorze G, Doinne L, Ryalls J, Julien M, Oullet L. The effects of speech and language therapy for a case of dysarthria associated with Parkinson's disease. *Europ J Disord Communic.* 1992;27:213–224.

151. Sarno M. Speech impairment in Parkinson's disease. *Arch Phys Med Rehabil.* 1968;49:269–275.

152. Weiner W, Singer C. Parkinson's disease and non-pharmacological treatment programs. *J Am Geriatr Soc.* 1989;37:359–363.

153. Jiang J, Lin E, Wang J, Hanson DG. Glottographic measures before and after levodopa treatment in Parkinson's disease. *Laryngoscope.* 1999;109(8):1287–1294.

154. Berke GS, Gerratt B, Kreiman J, Jackson K. Treatment of Parkinson hypophonia with percutaneous collagen augmentation. *Laryngoscope.* 1999;109(8):1295–1299.

155. Surgical treatment of Parkinson's disease. Parkinson's Disease Clinic and Research Center. University of California at San Fancisco. Retrieved December 27, 2016, from Pdcenter.neurology.ucsf.edu/professionals -guide/surgical-treatment.

156. Weaver FM, Follett K, Stern M, et al. Bilateral deep brain stimulation vs. best medical therapy for patients with advanced Parkinson disease: a randomized controlled trial. *JAMA.* 2009;301(1):63–73.

157. Langer-Gould A, Popat RA, Huang SM, et al. Clinical and demographic predictors of long-term disability in patients with relapsing-remitting multiple sclerosis: a systematic review. *Arch Neurol.* 2006;63(12):1686–1691.

158. Beukelman DR, Kraft GH, Freal J. Expressive communication disorders in persons with multiple sclerosis: a survey. *Arch Phys Med Rehabil.* 1985;66(10):675–677.

159. Darley FL, Brown JR, Goldstein NP. Dysarthria in multiple sclerosis. *J Speech Lang Hear Res.* 1972;15(2): 229–245.

160. Hartelius L, Runmarker BO, Andersen O. Prevalence and characteristics of dysarthria in a multiple-sclerosis incidence cohort: relation to neurological data. *Folia Phoniatr Logopaed.* 2000;52(4):160–177.

161. Hartelius L, Svensson P. Speech and swallowing symptoms associated with Parkinson's disease and

multiple sclerosis: a survey. *Folia Phoniatr Logopaed.* 1994;46(1):9–17.

162. Yorkston KM, Klasner ER, Bowen J, et al. Characteristics of multiple sclerosis as a function of the severity of speech disorders. *J Med Speech-Lang Pathol.* 2003; 11(2):73–85.

163. Matthews WB, Compston A, Allen IV, et al. *McAlpine's Multiple Sclerosis.* 2nd ed. London, UK: Churchill; 1991:43–105.

164. Holstege G, Ehling T (1996) Two motor systems involved in the production of speech. In: Davis PJ, Fletcher NH, eds. *Vocal Fold Physiology—Controlling Complexity and Chaos.* San Diego, CA: Singular; 153–169.

165. Waxman SG. Editorial: Demyelinating diseases—new pathological insights, new therapeutic targets. *New Engl J Med.* 1998;338(5):323.

166. Poser CM, Paty DW, Scheinberg L, et al. New diagnostic criteria for multiple sclerosis: guidelines for research protocols. *Ann Neurol.* 1983;13(3):227–231.

167. Yamout B, Fuleihan N, Hajj T, Sibai A, Sabra O, Rifai H, Hamdan AL. Vocal symptoms and acoustic changes in relation to the expanded disability status scale, duration and stage of disease in patients with multiple sclerosis. *Eur Arch Oto-Rhino-Laryngol.* 2009;266(11):1759–1765.

168. Hamdan AL, Farhat S, Saadeh R, El-Dahouk I, Sibai A, Yamout B. Voice-related quality of life in patients with multiple sclerosis. *Autoimmune Diseases.* 2012.

169. Rudick RA, Miller D, Hass S, et al. Health-related quality of life in multiple sclerosis: effects of natalizumab. *Ann Neurol.* 2007;62(4):335–346.

170. Amato MP, Ponziani G, Rossi F, Liedl CL, Stefanile C, Rossi L. Quality of life in multiple sclerosis: the impact of depression, fatigue and disability. *Mult Scler J.* 2001;7(5):340–344.

171. Cutajar R, Ferriani E, Scandellari C, et al., Cognitive function and quality of life in multiple sclerosis patients, *J NeuroVirol.* 2000: 6(2): S186–S190.

172. Nortvedt MW, Riise T, Myhr KM, Landtblom AM, Bakke A, Nyland HI. Reduced quality of life among multiple sclerosis patients with sexual disturbance and bladder dysfunction. *Mult Scler J.* 2001;7(4): 231–235.

173. Bauer V, Aleric Z, Jancic E, Knezevic B, Prpic D, Kacavenda A. Subjective and perceptual analysis of voice quality and relationship with neurological dysfunction in multiple sclerosis patients. *Clin Neurol Neurosurg.* 2013;115:S17–20.

174. Feijó AV, Parente MA, Behlau M, Haussen S, De Veccino MC, de Faria Martignago BC. Acoustic analysis of voice in multiple sclerosis patients. *J Voice.* 2004; 18(3):341–347.

175. Hartelius L, Runmarker B, Andersen O, Nord L. Temporal speech characteristics of individuals with multiple sclerosis and ataxic dysarthria: 'Scanning speech' revisited. *Folia Phoniatr Logopaed.* 2000;52(5): 228–238.

176. Smith ME, Ramig LO. Neurological disorders and the voice. In: Rubin JS, Sataloff RT, Korovin GS, eds. *Diag-*

nosis and Treatment of Voice Disorders.* New York, NY: Singular; 1995:203–224.

177. Dogan M, Midi I, Yazıcı MA, Kocak I, Günal D, Sehitoglu MA. Objective and subjective evaluation of voice quality in multiple sclerosis. *J Voice.* 2007; 21(6):735–740.

178. Konstantopoulos K, Vikelis M, Seikel JA, Mitsikostas DD. The existence of phonatory instability in multiple sclerosis: an acoustic and electroglottographic study. *Neurolog Sci.* 2010;31(3):259–268.

179. Hartelius L, Buder EH, Strand EA. Long-term phonatory instability in individuals with multiple sclerosis. *J Speech Lang Hear Res.* 1997;40(5):1056–1072.

180. Ramig LA, Sherer RC, Titze IR, Ringel SP. Acoustic analysis of voices of patients with neurologic disease: a rationale and preliminary data. *Ann Otol Rhinol.* 1988; 97: 164–172.

181. Kent RD, Sufit RL, Rosenbek JC, et al. Speech deterioration in amyotrophic lateral sclerosis: a case study. *J Speech Hear Res.* 1991; 34: 1269–1275.

182. Baer T. Vocal jitter: a neuromuscular explanation. In: *Transcripts of the Eighth Symposium on the Care of the Professional Voice.* New York, NY: The Voice Foundation; 1980: 19–24.

183. Natour Y, Marie B, Aljunidy L. The respiratory muscle capabilities of Jordanian patients with multiple sclerosis. *J Voice.* 2012;26(6):811–e15.

184. Giovannoni G, Gold R, Selmaj K, et al. Daclizumab high-yield process in relapsing-remitting multiple sclerosis (SELECTION): a multicentre, randomised, double-blind extension trial. *Lancet Neurol.* 2014;13(5):472–481.

185. Comi G, De Stefano N, Freedman MS, et al. Comparison of two dosing frequencies of subcutaneous interferon beta-1a in patients with a first clinical demyelinating event suggestive of multiple sclerosis (REFLEX): a phase 3 randomised controlled trial. *Lancet Neurol.* 2012;11(1):33–41.

186. Sataloff RT. Respiratory dysfunction. In: *Professional Voice: The Science and Art of Clinical Care.* Vol 2. 4th ed. San Diego, CA: Plural Publishing: 2017.

187. Lyons KE, Pahwa R. Deep brain stimulation and tremor. *Neurotherapeut.* 2008;5(2):331–338.

188. Pützer M, Wokurek W, Moringlane JR. Evaluation of phonatory behavior and voice quality in patients with multiple sclerosis treated with deep brain stimulation. *J Voice.* 2016 Nov 30.

189. Rontal E, Rontal M, Wald J, Rontal D. Botulinum toxin injection in the treatment of vocal fold paralysis associated with multiple sclerosis: a case report. *J Voice.* 1999;13(2):274–279.

190. Grob D, Arsura EL, Brunner NG, Namba T. The course of myasthenia gravis and therapies affecting outcome. *Ann NY Acad Sci.* 1987;505(1):472–499.

191. Neal GD, Clarke LR. Neuromuscular disorders. *Otol Clin North Am.* 1987;20(1):195–201.

192. Xu W, Han D, Hou L, Hu R, Wang L. Clinical and electrophysiological characteristics of larynx in myasthenia gravis. *Ann Otol, Rhinol Laryngol.* 2009;118(9): 656–661.

193. Nieman RF, Mountjoy JR, Allen EL. Myasthenia gravis focal to the larynx: report of a case. *Arch Otolaryngol.* 1975; 101(9):569–570.

194. Carpenter RJ, Mcdonald TJ, Howard FM. The otolaryngologic presentation of myasthenia gravis. *Laryngoscope.* 1979;89(6):922–928.

195. Michalska T, Rowińska-Marcińska K, Strugalska H, Maniecka-Aleksandrowicz B, Emeryk-Szajewska B. Myasthenia preceded by dysphonia. Clinical and electrophysical study. *Neurolog Neurochir Polska.* 1995; 30(5):783–796.

196. Mao VH, Abaza M, Spiegel JR, Mandel S, Hawkshaw M, Heuer RJ, Sataloff RT. Laryngeal myasthenia gravis: report of 40 cases. *J Voice.* 2001;15(1):122–130.

197. Liu WB, Xia Q, Men LN, Wu ZK, Huang RX. Dysphonia as a primary manifestation in myasthenia gravis (MG): a retrospective review of 7 cases among 1520 MG patients. *J Neurolog Sci.* 2007;260(1):16–22.

198. Schmidt-Nowara WW, Marder EJ, Feil PA. Respiratory failure in myasthenia gravis due to vocal cord paresis. *Arch Neurol.* 1984;41:567–568.

199. Jos A, Raman R, Gnanamuthu C. Laryngeal stridor in myasthenia gravis. *J Laryngol Otol.* 1992;106:633–634.

200. Fairley JW, Hughes M. Acute stridor due to bilateral vocal fold paralysis as a presenting sign of myasthenia gravis. *J Laryngol Otol.* 1992;106:737–738.

201. Hanson JA, Lueck CJ, Thomas DJ. Myasthenia gravis presenting with stridor. *Thorax.* 1996;51:108–109.

202. Vincent A, Newsom-Davis J. Acetylcholine receptor antibody as a diagnostic test for myasthenia gravis: results in 153 validated cases and 2967 diagnostic assays. *J Neurol Neurosurg Psychiatry.* 1985;48(12): 1246–1252.

203. Sommer N, Melms A, Weller M, Dichgans J. Ocular myasthenia gravis. *Doc Ophthalmolog.* 1993;84(4): 309–333.

204. Garlepp MJ, Dawkins RL, Christiansen FT, et al. Autoimmunity in ocular and generalised myasthenia gravis. *J Neuroimmunol.* 1981;1(3):325–332.

205. Soliven BC, Lange DJ, Penn AS, et al. Seronegative myasthenia gravis. *Neurology.* 1988;38(4):514.

206. Evoli A, Batocchi AP, Lo Monaco M, et al. Clinical heterogeneity of seronegative myasthenia. *Neuromuscul Disord.* 1996;6:155–161.

207. Oh SJ. Electrophysiological characteristics in seronegative myasthenia gravis. *Ann NY Acad Sci.* 1993; 681:584–587.

208. Gajdos P, Chevret S, Toyka KV. Intravenous immunoglobulin for myasthenia gravis. *Cochr Lib.* 2012 Jan 1.

209. Strong MJ. The basic aspects of therapeutics in amyotrophic lateral sclerosis. *Pharmacol Therapeut.* 2003;98(3): 379–414.

210. Howard RS, Orrell RW. Management of motor neurone disease. *Postgrad Med J.* 2002;78(926):736–741.

211. McGuirt WF, Blalock D. The otolaryngologist's role in the diagnosis and treatment of amyotrophic lateral sclerosis. *Laryngoscope.* 1980;90(9):1496–1501.

212. Haverkamp LJ, Appel V, Appel SH. Natural history of amyotrophic lateral sclerosis in a database population: validation of a scoring system and a model for survival prediction. *Brain.* 1995;118(pt 3):707–719.

213. Chancellor AM, Slattery JM, Fraser H, Swingler RJ, Holloway SM, Warlow CP. The prognosis of adult-onset motor neuron disease: a prospective study based on the Scottish Motor Neuron Disease Register. *J Neurol.* 1993;240(6):339–346.

214. Brooks BR. El Escorial World Federation of Neurology criteria for the diagnosis of amyotrophic lateral sclerosis. *J Neurolog Sci.* 1994;124:96–107.

215. Kalra S, Arnold D. Neuroimaging in amyotrophic lateral sclerosis. *Amyotroph Lat Scler Other Motor Neur Dis.* 2003;4(4):243–248.

216. Faubel SM, Pardo ML, Perez CF, et al. Amyotrophic lateral sclerosis that begins with voice and deglution alterations. *Anal Otorrinolaringol Ibero-Amer.* 2005;33(3): 273–280.

217. Tomik J, Tomik B, Partyka D, Skladzien J, Szczudlik A. Profile of laryngological abnormalities in patients with amyotrophic lateral sclerosis. *J Laryngol Otol.* 2007;121(11):1064–1069.

218. Chen A, Garrett CG. Otolaryngologic presentations of amyotrophic lateral sclerosis. *Otolaryngol Head Neck Surg.* 2005;132(3):500–504.

219. Watts CR, Vanryckeghem M. Laryngeal dysfunction in amyotrophic lateral sclerosis: a review and case report. *BMC Ear Nose Throat Dis.* 2001;1(1):1.

220. Carpenter III RJ, McDonald TJ, Howard Jr FM. The otolaryngologic presentation of amyotrophic lateral sclerosis. *Otolaryngology.* 1978;86(3):479.

221. Carrow E, Rivera V, Mauldin M. Deviant speech characteristics in motor neuron disease. *Arch Otolaryngol.* 1974; 100: 212–218.

222. Aronson AE, Winholtz WS, Ramig LO, Silber SR. Rapid voice tremor, or "flutter," in amyotrophic lateral sclerosis. *Ann Otol, Rhinol Laryngol.* 1992;101(6): 511–518.

223. Ramig LA, Scherer RC, Klasner ER, Titze IR, Horii Y. Acoustic analysis of voice in amyotrophic lateral sclerosis: a longitudinal study. *J Speech Hear Dis.* 1990; 55: 2–14.

224. Kent JF, Kent RD, Rosenbek JC, et al. Quantitative description of the dysarthria in women with amyotrophic lateral sclerosis. *J Speech Hear Res.* 1992; 35: 723–733.

225. Silbergleit AK, Johnson AF, Jacobson BH. Acoustic analysis of voice in individuals with amyotrophic lateral sclerosis and perceptually normal voice quality. *J Voice.* 1997; 11: 222–231.

226. Robert D, Pouget J, Giovanni A, Azulay JP, Triglia JM. Quantitative voice analysis in the assessment of bulbar involvement in amyotrophic lateral sclerosis. *Acta Oto-laryngol.* 1999 ;119(6):724–731.

227. Darley FL, Aronson AE, Brown JR. Differential diagnosis patterns of dysarthria. *J Speech Hear Res.* 1969; 12: 246–269.

228. Xie HS, Ma FR, Fan DS, Wang LP, Yan Y, Lu PQ. Acoustic analysis for 21 patients with amyotrophic lateral sclerosis complaining of dysarthria. *J Peking Univ Health Sci.* 2014;46(5):751–755.

229. Hillel A, Dray T, Miller R, et al. Presentation of ALS to the otolaryngologist/head and neck surgeon: getting to the neurologist. *Neurology*. 1998;53(8 suppl 5): S22–S25.

230. Roth CR, Glaze LE, Goding GS, David WS. Spasmodic dysphonia symptoms as initial presentation of amyotrophic lateral sclerosis. *J Voice*. 1996;10(4):362–367.

231. Tomik J, Tomik B, Wiatr M, Składzień J. Laryngological presentation of patients with amyotrophic lateral sclerosis (ALS). *Przeglad Lekarski*. 2005;63(11):1198–1200.

232. Tomik J, Tomik B, Wiatr M, Składzień J, Stręk P, Szczudlik A. The evaluation of abnormal voice qualities in patients with amyotrophic lateral sclerosis. *Neurodegen Dis*. 2015;15(4):225–232.

233. Kühnlein P, Gdynia HJ, Sperfeld AD, et al. Diagnosis and treatment of bulbar symptoms in amyotrophic lateral sclerosis. *Nature Clin Prac Neurol*. 2008; 4(7):366–374.

234. A Forshew D, B Bromberg M. A survey of clinicians' practice in the symptomatic treatment of ALS. *Amyotroph Lat Scler Other Motor Neu Dis*. 2003;4(4):258–263.

235. van der Graaff MM, Grolman W, Westermann EJ, et al. Vocal cord dysfunction in amyotrophic lateral sclerosis: four cases and a review of the literature. *Arch Neurol*. 2009;66(11):1329–1333.

236. Amin MR, Harris D, Cassel SG, Grimes E, Heiman-Patterson T. Sensory testing in the assessment of laryngeal sensation in patients with amyotrophic lateral sclerosis. *Ann Otol Rhinol Laryngol*. 2006;115(7): 528–534.

237. Rubin AD, Griffin GR, Hogikyan ND, Feldman EL. A new member of the multidisciplinary ALS team: the otolaryngologist. *Amyotroph Lat Scler*. 2012;13(2): 229–232.

238. Elluru RG, Kumar M. Physiology of the salivary glands. In: Haughey BH, edit. *Cummings Otolaryngology Head and Neck Surgery*. 4th ed. Philadelphia, PA: Elsevier Mosby; 2005: 1293–1302.

239. Guidubaldi A. Botulinum toxin A versus B in sialorrhea: a prospective, randomized, double-blind, crossover pilot study in patients with amyotrophic lateral sclerosis or Parkinson's disease. *Mov Disord*. 2001;26: 313–319.

240. Vianello A, Arcarao G, Palmieri A, et al. Survival and quality of life after tracheostomy for acute respiratory failure in patients with amyotrophic lateral sclerosis. *J Crit Care*. 2011;26;7–14.

241. Sancho S, Servera E, Banuls P, Marin J. Prolonging survival in amyotrophic lateral sclerosis: efficacy of non-invasive ventilation and uncuffed tracheostomy tubes. *Am J Phys Med Rehab*. 2010;89:407–411.

242. Carter GT, Johnson ER, Bonekat HW, Lieberman JS. Laryngeal diversion in the treatment of intractable aspiration in motor neuron disease. *Arch Phys Med Rehab*. 1992;73(7):680–682.

# 7

# Psychological Aspects of Voice Disorders

*Deborah Caputo Rosen, Reinhardt J. Heuer, David A. Sasso, and Robert Thayer Sataloff*

Professional performers are not only demanding but also remarkably self-analytical. Like athletes, performers have forced health care providers to refine our definition of normalcy. Ordinarily, physicians, psychotherapists, and other professionals are granted great latitude in the definition of "normal." Arts-medicine practitioners have learned to recognize, often quantify, and sometimes restore very high levels of human performance, approaching perfection. The process has required advances in scientific knowledge, clinical management, technology for voice assessment, voice therapy, and surgical technique. The drive to expand our knowledge also has led to unprecedented teamwork and interdisciplinary collaboration.

As a result, voice care professionals have come to recognize important psychologic problems found commonly in patients with voice disorders. In 1971, Brodnitz[1] reported on 2286 cases of all forms of voice disorders and classified 80% of the disorders as attributable to voice abuse or psychogenic factors resulting in vocal dysfunction. Such psychologic problems were ignored routinely in past years. Now they are searched for diligently throughout evaluation and treatment. When identified, they often require intervention by a psychologic professional with special knowledge about voice disorders, as well as by a speech-language pathologist (SLP) and other voice team members.

Arts-medicine psychologists specializing in the management of performance anxiety are becoming more common, but there are still very few psychologic professionals with extensive experience in diagnosing and treating other psychologic concomitants of voice disorders. It is important for physicians and all other members of the voice care team to recognize the importance of psychologic factors in patients with voice disorders and to be familiar with mental health professionals in various disciplines in order to build a multidisciplinary team, generate appropriate referrals, and coordinate optimal patient care.

## The Voice Care Team

Otolaryngologists and other health care providers involved with patients with voice disorders should be able to recognize significant comorbid psychopathology and should be prepared to consult an appropriate mental health care professional. Psychologists and psychiatrists are responsible for psychologic diagnosis and treatment, but it is important to select a mental health professional with advanced understanding of the special problems associated with voice disorders (especially, but not exclusively, in professional voice users).

Psychiatrists are licensed physicians who have completed medical training, residency in psychiatry, and often additional training. They are qualified not only to establish medical and psychiatric diagnoses and provide psychotherapy but also to prescribe medications. Psychologists make mental health diagnoses, administer psychologic tests, and provide therapy. In most locations, they do not prescribe medications but often work closely with a physician (usually a psychiatrist) who may prescribe and help manage psychotropic medications during the course of psychotherapy. Clinical psychologists have a master's or doctoral degree in psychology and may have subspecialty training. Other clinical disciplines (ie, social work, nursing, counseling) license graduate-level practitioners to provide psychotherapy.

Laryngologists, phoniatrists, and SLPs are not mental health professionals, although all have at least limited training in psychologic diagnosis. Specialty definitions vary from country to country. In the United States, laryngologists are responsible for medical diagnosis and treatment and voice surgery. They also prescribe any medications needed to treat organic voice problems and occasionally take responsibility for prescribing psychoactive medications.

SLPs are responsible for behavioral therapy for speech, language, and swallowing disorders. In many other countries, phoniatrists perform behavioral therapy in addition to making diagnoses. Phoniatrists are physicians. Traditionally, in some countries, they have been members of an independent specialty that does not include laryngeal surgery. In other countries, they have been subspecialists of otolaryngology. The European Union recently determined that, in the future, phoniatry will be a subspecialty of otolaryngology in member countries.

Both speech-language pathologists and phoniatrists include at least some psychologic assessment and support in their therapeutic paradigms. However, they are not formally trained mental health professionals and must be constantly vigilant to recognize significant psychopathology and recommend appropriate referral for treatment by a mental health practitioner.

Finding a mental health professional familiar with the special needs and problems of voice patients, especially singers and actors, is not easy. Arts-medicine psychology is a relatively new field, as voice was in otolaryngology in the early 1980s. Nevertheless, it is usually possible to find a psychologic professional who is either knowledgeable about arts-medicine or the principles of mind-body medicine with whom to collaborate. Resources are available in the literature to assist the interested mental health professional,[2] and incorporating such a colleague into the voice care team is extremely beneficial.

## Psychology and Voice Disorders: An Overview

### Voice and Emotion

Patients seeking medical care for voice disorders come from the general population. Consequently, a normal distribution of comorbid psychopathology can be expected in a laryngology practice. Psychologic factors can be causally related to a voice dis-order and/or consequences of vocal dysfunction. In practice, they are usually interwoven.

The first task of the otolaryngologist treating any patient with a voice complaint is to establish an accurate diagnosis and etiology. Only as a result of a thorough, comprehensive history and physical examination (including state-of-the-art technology) can the organic and psychologic components of the voice complaint be elucidated. All treatment planning and subsequent intervention depend on this process.

However, even minor voice injuries or health problems can be disturbing for many patients and devastating to some professional voice users. In some cases, they even trigger responses that delay the return of normal voice. Stress and fear of the evaluation procedures often heighten the problem and may cloud diagnostic assessment. Some voice disorders are predominantly psychogenic, and psychologic assessment may be required to complete a thorough evaluation.

The essential role of the voice in communication of the "self" creates special potential for psychologic impact. Severe psychologic consequences of voice dysfunction are especially common in individuals in whom the voice is pathologically perceived to be the self, such as professional voice users. In all human beings, self-esteem comprises not only who we believe we are but also what we have chosen to do as our life's work. A psychologic double-exposure exists for performers who experience difficulty separating the two elements. The voice is in, is therefore of, and indeed is the self. Thus, performers in particular may experience a special intensification of psychologic distress in association with lapse in vocal health.

The interdependence between voice and emotion or psychologic health is explored in depth in several texts. Aronson's[3] extensive review of the literature has examined research supporting the maxim that the "voice is the mirror of personality," both normal and abnormal. Parameters such as voice quality, pitch, loudness, stress pattern, rate, pauses, articulation, vocabulary, syntax, and content are described as they reflect life stressors, psychopathology, and discrete emotions.[3] Sundberg[4] describes Fonagy's research on the effects of various states of emotion on phonation. These studies revealed specific alterations in articulatory and laryngeal structures and in respiratory muscular activity patterns related to 10 different emotional states. Vogel and Carter[5] include descriptive summaries of the features, symptoms, and signs of communication impairment in their text on neurologic and psychiatric disorders.

The mind and body are inextricably linked. Thoughts and feelings generate neurochemical transmissions that affect all organ systems. Therefore, disturbances of physical function can have profound emotional effects, and disturbances of emotion can also have profound bodily and artistic effects.

## Professional Voice Users: A Special Case

It is useful to understand in greater depth the problems experienced by professional voice users who have vocal injuries. Most of our observations in this population occur among singers and actors. However, although they are the most obvious and demanding professional voice users, many other professionals are classified as professional voice users. These include politicians, attorneys, clergy, teachers, salespeople, broadcasters, shop foremen (who speak over noise), football quarterbacks, secretaries, telephone operators, and others. Although we are likely to expect profound emotional reactions to voice problems among singers and actors, many other patients may also demonstrate similar reactions. If we do not recognize these reactions as such, they may be misinterpreted as anger, malingering, or other "difficult patient" behavior.

## Reactions to Emotional Stress

Some patients are unconsciously afraid that their voices are lost forever and are psychologically unable to make a full effort at vocal recovery after injury or surgery. This blocking of the frightening possibilities by rationalization (eg, "I haven't made a maximum attempt so I don't know yet if my voice will be satisfactory") can result in prolonged or incomplete recovery after technically flawless surgery. It is incumbent on the laryngologist and other members of the voice team to understand the psychologic consequences of voice disturbance and to recognize them not only in extreme cases but even in their subtler manifestations.[2]

Successful professional voice users (especially actors, singers, and politicians) may fall into a personality subtype that is ambitious, driven, perfectionistic, and tightly controlled. Externally, they present themselves as confident, competitive, and self-assured. Internally, self-esteem, the product of personality development, is often far more fragile.

All psychologic adjustment expresses itself through the personality of the patient, and it is essential to focus on the personality style of every performer who seeks psychologic help. This can best be done during psychologic assessment and evaluation by exploring daily activities, especially those pertaining to the performer's involvement with his or her art, the patient's growth and personality development as an artist, and relationships with people both within and outside his or her performing environment. Each developmental phase carries inherent coping tasks and responsibilities, which can play an important part in the patient's emotional response to vocal dysfunction.

## The Body's Role

Research into body image theory also provides a theoretical basis for understanding the special impact of stress or injuries to the voice in vocal performers.[6] The body is essential to perception, learning, and memory, and it serves as a sensory register and processor of sensory information. Body experience is deeply personal and constitutes a private world typically shared with others only under conditions of closest intimacy. Moreover, the body is an expressive instrument, the medium through which individuality is communicated verbally and nonverbally. It is therefore possible to anticipate direct correspondence between certain physical illnesses or injuries and body and self-image. Among these are psychosomatic conditions and/or body states with high levels of involvement of personality factors. In these cases, body illness or injury may reactivate psychopathologic processes that began in early childhood or induce an emotionally maladaptive reaction such as denial or prolonged depression.

Psychologic reactions to a physical injury are not uniformly disturbing or distressing and do not necessarily result in maladjustment. However, Shontz[6] notes that reactions to body injury are more a function of how much anxiety is generated by the experience than by the actual location, severity, or type of injury.

Patients are adaptive and capable of living with most types of difficulties, injuries, or disabilities if they feel there is a good reason for doing so. If one's life has broad meaning and purpose, any given disorder takes on less significance. When a physical disability or any given body part becomes the main focus of concern or has been the main source of self-esteem in a person's life, that life becomes narrowed and constricted. Patients adapt satisfactorily to a personal medical condition when the problems of living related to the injury cease to be the dominant element in their total psychologic life.

## Self-Image

A unique closeness exists between one's body and one's identity; this body-self is a central part of self-concept. The interdependence of body image and self-esteem means that distortion of one will affect the other.

The cognitive-behavioral model for understanding body image includes the perceptual and affective components, as well as attitudinal ones. From the cognitive perspective, any body image producing dysphoria results from irrational thoughts, unrealistic expectations, and faulty explanations.[7] Body-image constructs and their affective and cognitive outcomes relate to personality types and cognitive styles. For example, depressive personality types chronically interpret events in terms of deficiencies and are trapped by habitual self-defeating thoughts. Anxious personality types chronically overestimate risks and become hypervigilant. These types of cognitive errors generate automatic thoughts that intensify body image–related psychopathology.[2]

It is the task of personality theorists to explain the process of the genesis of the self. There are numerous coherent personality theories, all substantially interrelated. The framework of Karen Horney (1885–1952) is particularly useful in attempting to understand the creative personality and its vulnerabilities. In simplification, she formulated a "holistic notion of the personality as an individual unit functioning within a social framework and continually interacting with its environment."[8] In Horney's model, there are 3 selves:

- The *actual self* is the sum total of the individual's experience.
- The *real self* is responsible for harmonious integration.
- The *idealized self* sets up unrealistically high expectations, which, in the face of disappointment, result in self-hatred and self-alienation.[8]

We have chosen Horney's theory as a working model in evolving therapeutic approaches to the special patient population of professional voice users. They are the laryngologist's most demanding consumers of voice care and cling to their physician's explanations with dependency.[2,9]

## Psychologic Phases in Vocal Injury

For theoretical clarity, it is useful to divide the experience of vocal injury into several phases. In practice, however, these often overlap or recur, and the emotional responses are not entirely linear.

### Problem Recognition

The patient feels that something is wrong but may not be able to clearly define the problem, especially if the onset has been gradual or masked by a coexisting illness. Usually, personal first-aid measures will be tried, and when they fail, the performer will manifest some level of panic. This is often followed by the feelings of guilt when the distress is turned inward against the self, or rage or blame when externalized.

### Diagnosis

This may be a protracted period if an injured performer does not have immediate access to a laryngologist experienced in the assessment of vocal injury. He or she may have already consulted with voice teachers, family physicians, allergists, nutritionists, peers, or otolaryngologists and SLPs without specialized training in caring for professional voice users. There may have been several, possibly contradictory, diagnoses and treatment protocols. The voice dysfunction persists, and the patient grows more fearful and discouraged. If attempts to perform are continued, they may exacerbate the injury and/or produce embarrassing performances. The fear is of the unknown, but it is intuitively perceived as significant.

### Treatment: Acute/Rehabilitative

At this phase, fear of the unknown becomes fear of the known, and of its outcome. The performer, now in the sick role, initially feels overwhelmed and powerless. There is frequently a strong component of blame that may be turned inward. "Why me? Why now?" is the operant, recurrent thought. Vocal rehabilitation is an exquisitely slow, carefully monitored, often frustrating process, and many patients become fearful and impatient. Some will meet the criteria for major depression, which will be discussed in additional detail, as will the impact of vocal fold surgery.

### Acceptance

When the acute and rehabilitative treatment protocol is complete, the final prognosis is clearer. When there are significant lasting changes in the voice, the patient will experience mourning. Even when there is full return of vocal function, a sense of vulnerability lingers. These individuals are likely to adhere strictly, even ritualistically, to preventive vocal hygiene habits and may be anxious enough to become hypochondriacal.[2,9,10]

The psychology professional providing care to this special population must be well versed in developmental psychology, experience the world of the performer, and retain an unshakable empathy for the extraordinary psychologically disorganizing impact of potential vocal injury.

It is critical to harken back to one of the earliest lessons taught to all psychotherapists-in-training. That is, the therapist must, through accurate empathy, earn the right to make interpretations and interventions. When this type of insightful and accurate support is available to the professional voice user, the psychotherapist may well be the patient's rudder in the rough seas of diagnosis, treatment, and rehabilitation.

## Psychogenic Voice Disorders

Voice disorders are divided into organic and nonorganic etiologies. Various terms have been used interchangeably (but imprecisely) to label observable vocal dysfunction in the presence of emotional factors that cause or perpetuate the symptoms. Aronson[3] argues convincingly for the term *psychogenic*, which is:

> broadly synonymous with functional, but has the advantage of stating positively, based on an exploration of its causes, that the voice disorder is a manifestation of one or more types of psychological disequilibrium, such as anxiety, depression, conversion reaction, or personality disorder, that interfere with normal volitional control over phonation.

Psychogenic disorders include a variety of discrete presentations. There is disagreement over classification among SLPs, with some excluding musculoskeletal tension disorders from this heading. Aronson[3] and Butcher et al[11] conclude that the hypercontraction of extrinsic and intrinsic laryngeal muscles, in response to emotional stress, is the common denominator behind the dysphonia or aphonia in these disorders. In addition, the extent of pathology visible on laryngeal examination is inconsistent with the severity of the abnormal voice. They cite 4 categories:

- Musculoskeletal tension disorders, including vocal abuse, vocal nodules, contact ulcers, and ventricular phonation
- Conversion voice disorders, including conversion muteness and aphonia, conversion dysphonia, and psychogenic adductor "spasmodic dysphonia"
- Mutational falsetto (puberphonia)
- Childlike speech in adults.[3,11]

*Psychogenic dysphonia* often presents as total inability to speak, whispered speech, extremely strained or strangled speech, interrupted speech rhythm, or speech in an abnormal register (such as falsetto in

a male). Usually, involuntary vocalizations during laughing and coughing are normal. The vocal folds are often difficult to examine because of supraglottic hyperfunction. There may be apparent bowing of both vocal folds consistent with severe muscular tension dysphonia, creating anteroposterior squeeze during phonation. Long-standing attempts to produce voice in the presence of this pattern may even result in traumatic lesions associated with vocal abuse patterns, such as vocal fold nodules.

Normal abduction and adduction of the vocal folds may be visualized during flexible fiberoptic laryngoscopy by instructing the patient to perform maneuvers that decrease supraglottic load, such as whistling or sniffing. In addition, the singing voice is often more easily produced than the speaking voice in these patients. Tongue protrusion and stabilization during the rigid telescopic portion of the examination will often result in clear voice. The severe muscular tension dysphonia associated with psychogenic dysphonia can often be eliminated by behavioral interventions by the SLP, sometimes in one session. In many instances, moments of successful voice have been restored during stroboscopic examination.

Electromyography may be helpful in confirming the diagnosis by revealing simultaneous firing of abductors and adductors. Psychogenic dysphonia has been frequently misdiagnosed as spasmodic dysphonia, partially explaining the excellent "spasmodic dysphonia" cure rates in some series.

Psychogenic voice disorders are not merely the absence of observable neurolaryngeal abnormalities. This psychiatric diagnosis cannot be made with accuracy without the presence of a psychodynamic formulation based on "understanding of the personality, motivations, conflicts, and primary as well as; secondary gain" associated with the symptoms.[2,12]

*Conversion disorders* are a special classification of psychogenic symptomatology and reflect loss of voluntary control over striated muscle or the sensory systems as a reflection of stress or psychologic conflict. They may occur in any organ system, but the target organ is often symbolically related to the specifics of the unconsciously perceived threat. The term was first used by Freud to describe a defense mechanism that rendered an intolerable wish or drive innocuous by translating its energy into a physical symptom. The presence of an ego-syntonic physical illness offers *primary gain*: relief from the anxiety, depression, or rage by maintaining the emotional conflict in the unconscious. *Secondary gain* often occurs by virtue of the sick role.

Classic descriptions of findings in these patients include indifference to the symptoms, chronic stress, suppressed anger, immaturity and dependency, moderate depression, and poor sex role identification.[12,13] Conversion voice disorders also reflect a breakdown in communication with someone of emotional significance in the patient's life—wanting but blocking the verbal expression of anger, fear, or remorse, and significant feelings of shame.[2,3]

Confirmed neurologic disease and psychogenic voice disorders do coexist and are known as somatic compliance.[14,15] Of course, potential organic causes of psychiatric disorders must always be thoroughly ruled out. Insidious onset of depression, personality changes, anxiety, or presumed conversion symptoms may be the first presentation of central nervous system (CNS), endocrine, or other disease.[16]

## General Psychopathologic Presentations

Patterns of voice use may provide clues to the presence of psychopathology, although voice disturbance is certainly not the principal feature of a major psychiatric illness. Nevertheless, failure to recognize serious psychopathology in voice patients may result not only in errors in voice diagnosis and failures of therapy but, more important, in serious injury to the patient, sometimes even death.

### Depression

Although a full depressive syndrome can occur as a result of loss, it fulfills the criteria for a major depressive episode when the individual experiences 5 or more of the following symptoms (including depressed mood and/or loss of interest) present for at least 2 weeks:

1. Depressed mood
2. Markedly diminished interest or pleasure in activities
3. Significant weight loss or weight gain
4. Insomnia or hypersomnia
5. Marked psychomotor agitation or retardation
6. Fatigue or diminished energy
7. Preoccupation with feelings of worthlessness and guilt
8. Difficulty concentrating or indecisiveness
9. Recurrent thoughts of death or suicidal ideation

These symptoms should represent a change from previous functioning, result in significantly impaired social and/or occupational functioning, and not be due to the physiologic effects of a substance or other medical condition.[17]

Careful listening during the taking of a history will reveal a flat affect, including slowed rate of speech, decreased length of utterance, lengthy pauses, decreased pitch variability, mono-loudness, and frequent use of vocal fry.[1,2,5] William Styron[18] described his speech during his depressive illness as "slowed to the vocal equivalent of a shuffle."

Major depression may be part of the patient's past medical history, may be a comorbid illness, or may be a result of the presenting problem. The essential feature is a prominent, persistent dysphoric mood characterized by a loss of pleasure in nearly all activities. Appetite and sleep are disturbed, and there may be marked weight gain or loss, hypersomnia, or 1 of 3 insomnia patterns. Psychomotor agitation or retardation may be present. Patients may demonstrate distractibility, memory disturbances, and difficulty concentrating. Feelings of worthlessness, helplessness, and hopelessness are a classic triad. Suicidal ideation, with or without a plan, and/or concomitant psychotic features, may necessitate emergency intervention.

Major affective disorders are classified as unipolar or bipolar. Unipolar depression, as described above, is characterized by pervasive dark mood and accompanied by diminished self-worth as well as loss of pleasure and/or interest in previously and ordinarily enjoyable activities.[17] In bipolar disorder, the patient may or may not experience depressive episodes, but by definition experience periods of mania, a recurrent elated state. Manic episodes usually first occur in young adulthood (episodes presenting for the first time in patients older than 50 years may signal medical or CNS illness or the effects of drugs). The presentation of the illness includes the following major characteristics on a continuum of severity:

- Elevated mood
- Irritability/hostility
- Distractibility
- Inflated self-concept
- Grandiosity
- Physical and sexual overactivity
- Flight of ideas
- Decreased need for sleep
- Social intrusiveness
- Buying sprees
- Inappropriate collections of possessions

Manic patients demonstrate impaired social and familial behavior patterns. They are manipulative, alienate family members, and tend to have a very high divorce rate.[17,19] Vocal presentation will manifest flight of ideas (content), rapid-paced pressured speech, and often increased pitch and volume. There may be dysfluency related to the rate of speech, breathlessness, and difficulty interrupting the language stream.

Three major theories, based on neuroanatomy, neuroendocrinology, and neuropharmacology, are the most currently promulgated explanations for these disease states, but they are beyond the scope of this chapter.[19–21]

Treatment of affective disorders includes psychotherapy and/or psychopharmacology. The use of psychopharmacologic agents is a risk/benefit decision.

Major depression is a common medical condition, with a lifetime prevalence of 17%.[22] Recognition and treatment of depression are also known to improve adherence and patient outcomes in comorbid medical conditions.[23] It is important for health care professionals to have an index of suspicion for depression and to screen for it in patients who present signs or symptoms known to be associated with the disease. Among those relevant to performers who may present for voice care are unexplained somatic complaints, recent loss or bereavement, family history of depression, chronic medical illnesses, stressful life events, and, potentially, hormonally mediated mood states.[24]

It is also important to note that other psychiatric disorders may coexist with major depression. These are part of the differential diagnosis formulated by the clinician performing the evaluation and include social anxiety disorder, panic disorder, generalized anxiety disorder, obsessive-compulsive disorder, and posttraumatic stress disorder. The treatment plan must address any of these disorders that causes clinically significant distress or significantly impairs function in the performer.[25–28]

Because depression has such high prevalence, it is important to recognize it and to offer effective treatment as early in the course as possible. Persistent depressive symptoms lead to changes in personality, work habits, and effectiveness and restricted social interaction. This creates further social isolation. However, there is a debate within the behavioral health profession about approaches to treatment. DeRubeis and colleagues[29,30] have studied treatment outcomes with cognitive behavioral therapy and psychopharmacology since 1999. Their research has shown that, except in severe depression, cognitive therapy is as effective as antidepressants and continues to reduce the risk of relapse after therapy is discontinued.

The efficacy of antidepressant medications also is debated. The magnitude of benefit appears to vary with the severity of depressive symptoms. Compared with placebo in randomized, controlled clinical trials, the magnitude of benefit is significant in patients with severe depression. In those with mild or moderate symptoms, the benefits may be less certain.[31]

Patients must give informed consent to a course of treatment for depression. The risks and benefits of both antidepressant therapy and psychotherapy must be explained and discussed. Side effects of medication, and specifically their potential effects on voicing, must be explored. For some patients, a trial of medication, including its titration and appropriate monitoring, may be preferred. Others will eschew medication for skillful psychotherapy as a first intervention. Behavioral health professionals should monitor progress with symptom relief. It is the standard of care to add medication if psychotherapy alone does not provide sufficient improvement or to add psychotherapy if medication alone does not do so.

### Anxiety

Anxiety is an expected reaction to any medical diagnosis and the required treatment, but more pervasive anxiety disorders also may be seen in performers. Anxiety disorders may be classified into several forms, including generalized anxiety disorder, social phobia (which may include performance anxiety), other phobias, panic disorder, and obsessive-compulsive disorder.[17] Vocal presentations of anxiety vary with the continuum of psychiatric symptoms, ranging from depression to agitation and including impairment of concentration.

Treatment options include psychotherapeutic approaches, including desensitization, cognitive-behavioral techniques, stress management, hypnosis, and insight-oriented approaches. Patients must learn to tolerate their distress and identify factors that precipitate or intensify their symptoms (see Stress Management below). Medications may be used to treat underlying depression and decrease the frequency of episodes. However, it leaves the underlying conflict unresolved, and some side effects may negatively affect artistic quality.[2,9,32]

Psychopharmacology is often used in the treatment for anxiety disorders. The side effects of these medications and potential for abuse of certain classes of medications are further described in the section on medications. However, psychotherapeutic modalities, especially cognitive-behavioral therapy, have similar outcomes in many anxiety disorders. Neuroscience research is elucidating the brain structures and mechanisms of pharmacologic treatments.[33–35]

Some medical conditions are commonly associated with the presenting symptom of anxiety: CNS disease, Cushing syndrome, hyperthyroidism, hypoglycemia, minor head trauma, premenstrual syndrome, and cardiac disease (such as mitral valve prolapse and various arrhythmias). Medications prescribed for other conditions may have anxiety as a side effect. These include such drugs as amphetamines, corticosteroids, caffeine, decongestants, and antiasthma drugs, as well as drugs of abuse such as cocaine.[5]

## Performance Anxiety

This important topic has been reviewed in recent literature by the authors.[36] Much of that information is reviewed here, with permission. Of all the topics discussed in this chapter, performance anxiety has inspired the most writing, speculation, and even controversy in the field of performing arts medicine. Why does performance anxiety hold such fascination? How can one conceptualize its nature, and what obstacles exist to achieving a more complete understanding? Some practical wisdom, gleaned from a large and diffuse corpus of literature, may help the health practitioner attempting to confront this issue with a patient.

The ICSOM survey[37] revealed that "stage fright" was the single most prevalent medical problem among professional orchestral musicians, with 24% of respondents reporting it as a health problem and 16% as a severe problem. Other studies, albeit with smaller sample sizes, have indicated even higher prevalence rates. A study of professional and student performing artists in Britain found that 40% of 162 subjects suffered from performance anxiety.[38] A Dutch study of professional orchestra musicians found 59% of respondents reporting performance anxiety so serious that it affected their personal or professional lives.[39]

A survey of 302 musicians at the University of Iowa School of Music, most of them students, found 39.9% reporting moderate distress and 21.3% marked distress from performance anxiety.[40] In that study, 29.6% reported moderate impairment and 16.5% marked impairment in performance due to their anxiety, and more than one in three felt that performance anxiety had an effect on their career (19.1% moderate effect and 16.1% marked effect). Brodsky[41] cited a survey of the Organization of Canadian Symphony Musicians (OCSM) in which 96% of 204 respondents "reported experiencing stress related to performance." As a consequence of performance anxiety, Clark and Agras[42] reported that 77% of their sample had avoided performing, 19% had stopped performing, and 11% left the profession entirely. Statistics vary, but perfor-

mance anxiety sparks interest among researchers and clinicians in large part because it appears to be prevalent and can be severe.

More deeply, though, performance anxiety can be thought of as performing arts psychiatry's prototypical problem. It is an issue that affects and is affected by the very thing that performers do, namely, perform. Performance anxiety is right there, in the wings and on the stage.

Brandfonbrener[43] reflected on the level of excitement and controversy that the topic of performance anxiety seems to elicit and observed that it is to some degree universal, even to nonperformers (eg, in test-taking, public speaking, etc.), so it is something everyone is familiar with in some way.[44] Yet, Brandfonbrener wondered, could there be some element of personal stake or even voyeurism in the fascination with performance anxiety? Could it be in part a way to demystify or even dethrone performance genius? It is essential to recognize to what degree this may be the case and to attempt to adopt an objective approach to the problem.[43]

### Adaptive vs Maladaptive Anxiety

What is performance anxiety? And how does it differ from other senses of the word *anxiety*? To begin, some degree of what may be called performance anxiety is likely the norm among performing artists. The most common manifestations are well known and include various physical symptoms, as well as fears about making mistakes, having memory slips, or otherwise embarrassing oneself on stage. Among music students classified as "impaired" with performance anxiety, physical symptoms ranged from the common poor concentration (63.3%) and rapid heart rate (57.1%) to the less common nausea and dizziness (8.3% each) (Table 7–1).[40] But many performers are able to tolerate these symptoms, which may resolve as the performance proceeds.

Thus, some anxiety related to performing is perfectly natural and expected. Treating all performance anxiety as if it were a "mental illness" is clearly inappropriate. One would never conceive of transiently elevated blood pressure that occurs during exercise in the same way one regards a hypertensive urgency or chronic hypertension. The hypertension of exercise is adaptive, the result of intricate autoregulatory functions of the brain and cardiovascular systems, which, for the moment, appropriately provide increased blood flow to the muscles in use. In the same way, some performance anxiety may provide a certain level of arousal needed to facilitate performance.

**Table 7–1.** Common Physical Symptoms in Music Students Impaired With Performance Anxiety[a]

| Students Reporting Symptom | % |
| --- | --- |
| Poor concentration | 63.3 |
| Rapid heart rate | 57.1 |
| Trembling | 45.8 |
| Dry mouth | 42.6 |
| Sweating | 42.6 |
| Shortness of breath | 39.6 |
| Flushing | 16.3 |
| Quavering voice | 12.8 |
| Nausea | 8.3 |
| Dizziness | 8.3 |

[a]Adapted from Wesner et al.[40]

Powell,[45] using the terminology of Rafferty, Smith, and Ptacek,[46] distinguished *debilitating* performance anxiety from normal apprehension or anxiety that facilitates performance. Salmon contended that anxiety per se is never helpful for performance and advocates using the term *arousal* to describe what others have termed *adaptive anxiety*.[47] Wolfe explored in depth the distinctions between *facilitative* (adaptive) and *debilitating* (maladaptive) components of performance anxiety in amateur and professional musicians.[48] She delineated some of the characteristics of the two forms of anxiety and found that professional playing experience positively correlated with more adaptive as well as less maladaptive components of anxiety.

Other work supports this notion, which recalls the Yerkes-Dodson law with the classic inverted U-curve of motor skill performance vs arousal, as both low and high levels of arousal are a detriment to performance quality, while a moderate level of arousal predicts the best result.[49]

In a study of 29 professional violinists, while 83% believed that "every artist experiences some performance anxiety," 52% agreed that "some tension aided their performance."[50] Yet, clearly, some performance anxiety can be maladaptive. Failing to address the distinction between the facilitative and debilitating varieties confounds research on performance anxiety just as would including appropriate elevations in blood pressure during exercise as targets for antihypertensive treatment.

## Definitions

Several authors[41,49,51] have declared an urgent need to define performance anxiety, if not etiologically or mechanistically, then at least operationally. The wide variety of prevalence rates reported may be partly explained by such factors as differences in sample populations (eg, Steptoe and Fidler found that anxiety is higher in students than in professional musicians[52]), but it is also likely due in large part to the heterogeneity of terms used. The ICSOM study[37] asked about "performance anxiety," the British study[38] used the term "stage fright," and the OCSM survey[41] included the very broad "stress related to performance." Are these studies addressing the same thing? Beyond prevalence studies, how can intervention studies be compared if each one defines the problem differently?

Salmon[47] provided an often-quoted operational definition of musical performance anxiety: "the experience of persisting, distressful apprehension about, and/or actual impairment of, performance skills in a public context, to a degree unwarranted given the individual's aptitude, training, and level of preparation." Robson, Davidson, and Snell[53] make important distinctions between *"performance anxiety"* and *"audition anxiety."* Many performers who have little problem or may even revel on stage in front of a large, and mostly unknown, audience may have significant anxiety during auditions. Furthermore, auditions and juries may place different aspects of the performers' sense of self-worth, and even their very livelihood, on the line.

Brodsky[41] proposed the establishment of a *Diagnostic and Statistical Manual of Mental Disorders (DSM)*–like system of nomenclature for "music-performers' stress syndrome" (M-PSS), with specifiers for intensity and severity. He conceptualized a continuum of psychologically related problems of musicians, ranging from "career stress" to "tension in performance" to "performance anxiety" to "stage fright." However, it seems that this classification system conflates intensity with chronicity and at the same time ignores issues of etiology, which may be essential in understanding a particular performer's problem and selecting an appropriate treatment.

Yet the dilemma that Brodsky was attempting to solve is not simple and has not yet been adequately addressed in the literature. The question of how to come up with a meaningful and reproducible nomenclature while doing justice to the varieties of each individual's experience is the essence of the task at hand. An agreed-upon nomenclature to describe performance anxiety would go a long way toward improving communication within the field of performing arts psychiatry, enhance diagnostic reliability, and provide a framework for meaningful clinical research to proceed.

## Social Phobia and Performance Anxiety

The simple answer to the dilemma is to say that *DSM* has already solved it. Many would argue that performance anxiety as discussed here is simply a subtype of *social phobia* (also called *social anxiety disorder*). As described in the *DSM-IV-TR*, social phobia is a disorder characterized by marked fear of social or performance situations in which the individual is exposed to scrutiny by others and invariably becomes anxious that he or she will be humiliated or embarrassed (Table 7–2). The patient recognizes that the fear is

---

**Table 7–2.** Summary of DSM-IV-TR Diagnostic Criteria for Social Phobia[a]

- A marked and persistent fear of one or more social or performance situations in which the person is exposed to unfamiliar people or possible scrutiny by others. The individual fears that he or she will act in a way (or show anxiety symptoms) that will be humiliating or embarrassing.

- Exposure to the feared social situation almost invariably provokes anxiety, which may take the form of a situationally bound or situationally predisposed panic attack.

- The person recognizes that the fear is excessive or unreasonable. (Note: In children, this feature may be absent.)

- The feared social or performance situations are avoided or else are endured with intense anxiety or distress.

- The avoidance, anxious anticipation, or distress in the feared social or performance situation(s) interferes significantly with the person's normal routine, occupational (academic) functioning, or social activities or relationships, or there is marked distress about having the phobia.

- The fear or avoidance is not due to the direct physiological effects of a substance or general medical condition and it is not better accounted for by another mental disorder.

- Specify as "Generalized" if the fears include most social situations.

[a]Adapted from American Psychiatric Association.[17]

---

"excessive or unreasonable," and the symptoms lead to significant interference in daily functioning either by avoidance of the feared situation or by a degree of anxiety such that the feared situation is only endured with great distress. The anxiety may be "generalized" to multiple social domains, or it may be "specific" to one or two areas.

At face value, it appears that music performance anxiety fits the definition of a nongeneralized form of social phobia. However, some argue that performance anxiety as it manifests in the performing arts is in fact a distinct syndrome that the *DSM-IV* criteria for social phobia do not fully describe. Osborne and Franklin[54] noted that only 27% of those who self-report high music performance anxiety qualify for the *DSM-IV* diagnosis of social phobia, and Clark and Agras[42] found that only 4% of patients with music performance anxiety had generalized social phobia.

Powell[45] explored differences between debilitating performance anxiety, generalized social phobia, and specific anxiety seems to be secondary to the fear of not being able to perform up to one's own expectations, while in the *DSM*, the fear described is of scrutiny by others. Whereas in specific social phobia, patients are often ambivalent about or even actively avoidant of the feared situation, the opposite is the case in performance anxiety, where the individual is fiercely devoted to the challenge that provokes the anxiety.

Kenny[51] provided an extended discussion distinguishing music performance anxiety from trait anxiety. She also argued that the *DSM* criteria for social phobia may be too restrictive to capture those with music performance anxiety deserving of treatment and recalled that equating music performance anxiety with existing *DSM* diagnoses ignores the fact that some amount of anxiety or arousal is necessary for most performers to achieve their best performance.

In this light, it is not surprising that anecdotal evidence suggests that those with music performance anxiety may not endorse the *DSM* criterion that the fear be "excessive or unreasonable," which is necessary to make the diagnosis of social phobia.[49] For all these reasons, it remains unclear whether research evaluating treatments for social phobia may be rightly extended to the treatment of music performance anxiety.

## Etiology

Freud's original theories viewed anxiety as a buildup of psychic energy form either internal (instinctual) or external (traumatic) stimulation. In the 1920s, his shift from the topographical model of the mind to the structural model was accompanied by an adjustment of his understanding of anxiety. He began to describe the idea of "signal anxiety" (ie, anxiety as the reaction of the ego to a perceived danger situation and "a signal for help").[55] This view of anxiety, as a warning signal for a dangerous situation (reviewed by Wong[56]), can still be useful today in understanding performance anxiety in some patients.

Recent writings in efforts to describe the etiological and mechanistic underpinnings of performance anxiety have spanned the gamut from biological to psychological to social orientations. Sataloff, Rosen, and Levy[57] have provided a useful summary of the various approaches to understanding performance anxiety. A *physiological* explanation describes the sequence of events as follows: "Sympathetic activation produces physical symptoms, which the central nervous system interprets as anxiety and then reinforces with further sympathetic stimulation."[58] Performance anxiety may be viewed as a psychophysiological feedback loop in which activation of the autonomic nervous system leads to and maintains the subjective sense of anxiety.[59]

*Cognitive-behavioral* understandings[60] emphasize the distorted ways of thinking that lead to performance anxiety and the behaviors that reinforce them. Several authors, including Weisblatt[61] and Nagel,[62,63] have drawn on a long history of *psychoanalytic* thought and described an approach in which anxiety is understood as arising from unconscious desires that come into conflict in the context of a performance situation. Hamilton's book reviewed the role of *narcissism* in performance anxiety and the conflict a performer may feel in investing in a performance at the risk of potential loss of self-esteem.[64] Cox and Kenardy[65] focused on the impact of performance setting on anxiety, and Sternbach[66] described the *social conditions* of musicians as leading to a "total stress quotient" surpassing that seen in many other professions and contributing to situational anxiety on the stage.

It is critical not to forget basic differential diagnosis and to always rule out other possible causes for anxiety. A particular patient may complain chiefly of performance anxiety, while the real issue is a more pervasive underlying anxiety disorder (see below) or another psychiatric illness, such as a mood disorder. Substance abuse or withdrawal and many medical illnesses, such as metabolic or endocrine abnormalities, may also bring a patient to the clinic with anxiety as the only presenting symptom.

Many authors agree that the etiology of performance anxiety is most likely *multifactorial*[51] and unique for each individual. This view accounts for performance anxiety's distinctive manifestations in different performers as "loosely correlated constellation[s] of physiological, behavioral, and cognitive variables."[47] Salmon[47] argued that the effectiveness of any intervention is depending on tailoring the treatment to address the specific mix of variables in a particular patient's anxiety profile.

As with most other complex syndromes, the etiology of performance anxiety in a given performer is multiply determined by a combination of biological, developmental, cognitive, behavioral, and psychodynamic factors. These interact on a background of inherited predispositions, unique educational backgrounds, and individual skill levels and in the context of particular social, cultural, and situational performance environments.

## Treatment of Performance Anxiety

What is known about how to best treat performance anxiety is drawn from a diffuse body of literature with significant methodological limitations. Many studies are poorly controlled, and few randomized trials exist. Not surprisingly, these inquiries include vague and varied definitions of performance anxiety, impairing the ability to generalize the findings.

It is beyond the scope of this chapter to review the entire body of literature on the treatment of performance anxiety. This has been done meticulously in Kenny's recent paper,[51] the first broad "systematic review" of the literature on this topic. This review, as well as Brodsky's article,[39] also presents the major critiques of the field, some of which have been discussed here. McGinnis and Milling's recent review[49] focuses on psychological treatments of musical performance anxiety.

### Psychotherapy

Despite the deficiencies and controversies in the literature, some useful generalities may be drawn about the use of psychotherapy for performance anxiety (see descriptions of various psychotherapeutic approaches above).[49,51] Overall, *cognitive and behavioral treatments* appear to be effective, with various studies showing different combinations of effects on subjective anxiety, physiological parameters, and performance quality. While combined cognitive-behavioral therapies also seem to be effective, there is no evidence thus far that the combination is better than either component alone.[67]

As for psychodynamic treatments, which were not included in the above reviews, Nagel,[63] Plaut,[68] Ostwald,[69] and Weisblatt[61] all advocate *psychodynamic psychotherapy* as an effective treatment for performance anxiety.

Several other interventions, such as meditation, music therapy, hypnotherapy, and Alexander technique, have shown some promise, although in each case only one study has been undertaken thus far.[46]

### Beta-Blockers

Clinicians and research attempting to address performance anxiety with medications typically turn first to β-blockers. Nies[70] in 1986 provided a still-useful review of the clinical pharmacology of these medications for the performing arts medicine audience.

β-Blockers were first used in cardiac patients to block the effects of sympathetic activation of the heart, lowering blood pressure and reducing cardiac output. Because many of the physical symptoms of anxiety are mediated through the sympathetic nervous system, β-blockers have, over the years, become an extremely popular choice for the treatment of performance anxiety that includes somatic symptoms. Their popularity among performers is a strong testament to their effectiveness (and overall safety). However, a deeper reading of the literature reveals controversy among clinicians and researchers regarding the effects of this class of drugs on subjective anxiety and performance quality.

In his 1991 review, Nubé[71] concluded that β-blockers do improve somatic symptoms of anxiety, subjects' self-ratings of their performances, and overall jury assessment of musicality and technical quality. As such, these medications can be extremely helpful, even curative, for example, for the string player whose physical manifestations of, say, tremulousness, make him incapable of controlling his bow arm or vibrato.

However, there are some mixed data about β-blockers' effects on subjective anxiety and on specific components of performance, such as intonation, rhythmic control, dynamics, and emotional connection to the music. Nubé wondered whether the "gains relative to the peripheral somatic side effects are worth a potential decrease" in these areas related to performance.[71] Careful dose titration may be the key for some performers, based on the finding that low doses of a β-blocker improve performance whereas higher doses impair performance.[72]

Sataloff, Rosen, and Levy[57] advised that, for *singers* and wind instrumentalists who require "athletic stamina," β-blockers may not be appropriate (see also Gates et al[72]). Given that singing is an endeavor requiring physical effort leading to a kind of exercise-induced tachycardia, suppression of this physiologically normal response with β-blockers may hinder

optimal performance. Many singers in the study felt that higher doses of β-blockers were "energy-sapping." This argument has been extended to *dancers*, where the obvious need for athletic endurance may be frustrated by β-blocking medications. Harris explored this "dancer's dilemma" and cautioned that the literature on pharmacotherapy for orchestral musicians may not be generalized to dancers.[73]

So, β-blockers may be a "double-edged sword."[74] Nonetheless, they have undoubtedly been helpful to many performers struggling with debilitating performance anxiety. Lederman[75] clearly presents the pros and cons and advocates β-blockers as one alternative for treatment of performance anxiety if no contraindication exists. Brandfonbrener[43] offers a useful caution to use a test dose before the day of the big performance.

The most commonly used β-blocker for performance anxiety in clinical practice is *propranolol* at low doses of 10 to 20 mg 1 hour before a performance or audition. As with all other medical decisions, only when doctor and patient weigh the pros and cons of all possible treatments thoughtfully can an informed decision can be made.

In the real-world performing arts community, it is critical to recognize that many performers obtain β-blockers without a prescription. β-Blockers are not benign medications. They may exacerbate underlying conditions, such as asthma (symptoms of which may occasionally be mistaken for anxiety), or at higher doses may cause drops in blood pressure or heart rate. As with all medications, they should be used only under the care of a physician and should never be shared with colleagues. Furthermore, without a full medical evaluation, it is unknown whether the performer is suffering from run-of-the-mill performance anxiety or from another psychiatric or medical disorder that would not respond to β-blockers. Indeed, depression may be exacerbated by some β-blockers, although this association remains controversial.[76]

β-Blockers are widely used for performance anxiety. In the ICSOM survey,[37] 27% of respondents had taken β-blockers at some point in their lifetime. Of those, 70%, nearly 1 out of 5 in the entire sample (19%), took β-blockers without a prescription. Among nondaily users, 72% took β-blockers before auditions, 52% before solo recitals, 50% before difficult orchestral performances, and 42% before concerto performances. A small but not insignificant number, 4% of occasional users, took β-blockers before every orchestral performance; this translates to 0.9% of the entire cohort of orchestral musicians or nearly 1 in 100.

Of occasional β-blocker users in the ICSOM survey,[37] 96% reported some success in reducing performance anxiety. Interestingly, among those who reported stage fright as a severe problem, success was about half as common (46%) for those who used medications without a prescription as for those who used a prescribed medication (92%). Sixty percent of those performers who sought psychological counseling for severe stage fright found it effective. Several other interventions were reported, notably including aerobic exercise, which was felt to be effective in 70% of cases of severe stage fright. In another study, full-time professionals were more likely to use β-blockers (67%), than part-time professionals (37%), students (13%), and serious amateurs (13%).[42]

It is important to recognize that many performers obtain beta-blockers without a prescription from colleagues. Therefore, it is important to ask patients specifically whether they are taking medication without prescription. If used at all, β-blockers should be used only under the supervision of a physician who is able to rule out other causes of anxiety and monitor the dosage and side effects of these medications. Side effects may include bradycardia, hypotension, fatigue, and bronchospasm, particularly in those with asthma.[77]

In carefully selected patients, β-blockers may be extremely helpful. However, further exploration of the underlying etiology of performance anxiety is critical, as medications do not address any underlying psychologic conflict.

For singers and other performers, such as dancers, who require "athletic stamina" for their performance, β-blockers should be used with great care or avoided.[57,72] Singing is an endeavor requiring physical effort leading to a kind of exercise-induced tachycardia, which may be inappropriately suppressed by these medications.

## Nonrecommended Medications

*Benzodiazepines*, such as alprazolam, lorazepam, clonazepam, diazepam, and others, are commonly prescribed anxiolytics. However, these medications are generally *not indicated* for performance anxiety. First, they may cause side effects, such as sedation, dizziness, and weakness, possibly impairing performance parameters, such as intonation and rhythmic control.[78] Second, benzodiazepines often lead to tolerance and physiological addiction. Third, they may in fact impede the learning that takes place over repeated performances that could otherwise lead to extinction of performance anxiety over time.[79] The sensitive clinician must carefully distinguish performance anxiety from panic disorder (discussed below). Benzodiazepines, a common treatment for panic dis-

order, may be inappropriately used for situational performance anxiety that is mistaken for panic.

*Antidepressants* (discussed earlier) are often useful for patients who suffer from other anxiety disorders, such as generalized anxiety disorder, panic disorder, or posttraumatic stress disorder. There is also agreement that these medications are useful for those who clearly meet criteria for a diagnosis of social phobia.[80] However, there is no specific research on antidepressants for music performance anxiety.

Antidepressants also are discussed later in this chapter. Clark and Agras[42] found that 41% of musicians attempted to treat their performance anxiety with alcohol and 20% had tried benzodiazepines. However, in a study of mostly students, an encouraging 98.7% "never" or "infrequently" used drugs or alcohol for performance anxiety, and only 6.5% believed that drugs or alcohol were "justified" for that symptom.[40] Steptoe and Fidler[52] found that professional musicians with high performance anxiety were more likely to take sedatives (17%) than those with medium (4%) or low (0%) anxiety.

## Future Research

To help inform better treatment decisions in the future, more research on psychotherapeutic and psychopharmacologic treatment approaches is clearly needed. Notably, there is no study combining β-blockers with any psychological treatment.[49] As Kenny[51] noted, the current state of the literature on treatments for performance anxiety is "fragmented, inconsistent, and methodologically weak." But simply more research is not necessarily better. First steps include more sound research designs, larger sample sizes, more careful selection of sample populations (both in terms of level of anxiety and other factors, such as students vs professionals), and better agreement on a definition of performance anxiety.

Ideally, future studies will continue to look at mediating factors and predictors of response to particular treatments. This information will one day allow the clinician to select an individualized treatment that best addresses a particular patient's manifestation of performance anxiety. For example, one might select a behavioral approach for a patient who tends to catastrophize,[49] a pharmacological approach for a patient with prominent physiological symptoms and a psychodynamic approach for a patient whose unconscious conflicts seem to play a prominent role.

Clearly, some arousal or anxiety is necessary to a vital performance, just as some of Mahler's genius flowed from his unresolved conflicts. To move forward, we must acknowledge the utility of adaptive anxiety, come to a consensus about how to identify the maladaptive variety, and set to work on rigorous and coordinated studies in an evidence-based manner, never forgetting to treat each patient as an individual meriting an individualized approach.[81]

## Schizophrenia

Although psychotic behavior may be observed with major affective disorders, organic CNS disease, or drug toxicity, schizophrenia occurs in only 1% to 2% of the general population.[82] Its onset is most prominent in mid- to late adolescence through the late 20s. Its incidence is approximately equal for males and females, and schizophrenia has been described in all cultures and socioeconomic classes. This is a group of mental disorders in which massive disruptions in cognition or perception, such as delusions, hallucinations, or thought disorders, are present. The fundamental causes are not fully known, but the disease involves excessive amounts of neurotransmitters, chiefly dopamine. There is evidence of genetic predisposition.

The typical signs and symptoms include clear indications of deterioration in social or occupational function, changes in personal hygiene, changes in behavior and movement, an altered sense of self, and the presence of blunted or inappropriate affect. Somatic delusions may present as voice complaints. However, flattening or inappropriateness of affect, a diagnostic characteristic of schizophrenia, will produce voice changes similar to those described for depression and mania. When the hallucinatory material creates fear, characteristics of anxiety and agitation will be audible. Perseveration, repetition, and neologisms may be present.[52,82]

The disease is chronic and control requires consistent use of antipsychotic medications for symptom management. Social support and regulating activities of daily living are crucial in maintaining emotional control.

## Psychoactive Medications

There are a wide variety of medications in the psychiatric pharmacopeia that can effectively be used to treat various psychiatric symptoms. All members of the voice care team should become familiar with all types of medications that their patients with psychiatric diagnoses are taking. Treatment may be improved through frequent, open collaboration between the psychiatrist and other members of the voice care team. It is important, with the patient's consent, that the psychotherapist collaborate with the prescribing physician to help select the medications least likely to produce adverse effects on the voice while adequately controlling the psychiatric illness.[83]

All psychoactive agents have effects that can interfere with vocal tract physiology, some more severely than others. Patients must be informed of the likelihood of experiencing known side effects, and the patient and physicians need to weigh carefully the benefits and side effects of available medications. This is especially critical to the professional voice user who may be keenly aware of physical side effects of medications, especially those that affect vocal production.

### Antidepressants

Antidepressant medications include compounds from several different classes. The selective serotonin reuptake inhibitors (SSRIs), a group of antidepressant drugs that selectively inhibit the reuptake of neurotransmitter serotonin, include fluoxetine, paroxetine, sertraline, fluvoxamine, citalopram, escitalopram, and vilazodone. The SSRIs are effective in the treatment of major depressive disorder, especially in the moderate to severe range, and for many anxiety disorders.[83,84]

SSRIs have become popular first-line therapy for unipolar depression (nonbipolar) because of their relatively mild side effect profile compared with older antidepressant agents (described below). Patients often develop a small number of side effects, usually mild, which may abate over several weeks of continued therapy. The side effects will differ among patients. Those who do not respond to one agent or who experience intolerable side effects may try another agent with better results. It is important to remember that it may take 4 to 8 weeks to achieve the full benefit of an antidepressant medication when beginning therapy.

The most common initial side effects with SSRIs are restlessness, headache, gastrointestinal symptoms, and insomnia, but these symptoms generally subside in days. With all antidepressants, dry mouth may be a particularly bothersome symptom for voice professionals, and patients should be warned of this possibility. In the longer term, there exists the possibility of sexual dysfunction, which may be addressed by trying an alternate medication or by adding a medication to counteract the effect.

In 2004, a black box warning was added to antidepressants cautioning of the risk for increased suicidal thinking or behavior soon after initiating treatment in those younger than 24 years. While it is a rare occurrence, close and careful monitoring of younger patients starting these medications is critical.

Some controversy remains surrounding the risk of "switching" to mania if a patient with bipolar disorder is treated with a classic antidepressant, such as an SSRI.[85] These patients, especially at younger ages or with a history at all suggestive of bipolar disorder, should be monitored closely during the early weeks of treatment with an eye to this possibility.

Newer antidepressant medications include those with effects on multiple neurotransmitter systems: venlafaxine (Effexor), duloxetine (Cymbalta), and desvenlafaxine (Pristiq) on both the serotonin and noradrenergic systems, and bupropion (Wellbutrin) on the dopaminergic and noradrenergic systems. Venlafaxine carries a risk of increased blood pressure. Bupropion, which decreases the seizure threshold, should be used only with extreme caution in those with an increased baseline risk of seizures and is contraindicated in patients with bulimia. Mirtazapine (Remeron) is an antidepressant that has significant side effects of weight gain and sedation and therefore may be beneficial in patients whose depressive symptoms include poor appetite or insomnia.

Older antidepressant medications, such as the tricyclic antidepressants (TCAs; eg, amitriptyline [Elavil]) and monoamine oxidase inhibitors (MAOIs; eg, phenelzine [Nardil]), are as effective as the newer medications but are now typically reserved for treatment-refractory cases due to their less favorable side effect profile and potential drug-drug or drug-food interactions. Side effects of the TCA may include the following:

- Anticholinergic: dry mouth and nasal mucosa, constipation, urinary hesitancy, gastroesophageal reflux
- Autonomic: orthostatic hypotension, palpitations, increased cardiac conduction intervals, diaphoresis (sweating), hypertension, tremor
- Other: stimulation, sedation, nausea, weight gain, sexual side effects

The side effects of MAOIs also may be serious. In addition to the effects described above for other antidepressants, MAOIs interact with a long list of foods that have high levels of tyramine, such as certain cheeses and meats (among others); these foods must be carefully avoided while taking these medications to prevent dangerous hypertensive crises. Dangerous interactions can occur when MAOIs are taken with certain drugs, such as meperidine, over-the-counter cold preparations, SSRIs, and others.[83]

Many antidepressant medications produce bothersome and occasionally serious discontinuation effects if they are stopped suddenly. Medications should be discontinued only after a thorough discussion with the physician.

For severe depression that has not responded to multiple trials of psychotherapy and medication, as well as for other forms of severe, treatment-non-responsive psychiatric illness, electroconvulsive therapy (ECT) is a remarkably effective treatment, keeping in mind the risks of general anesthesia and the possibility of some cognitive side effects.[86]

## Mood-Stabilizing Drugs

The mood-stabilizing drugs are used to alleviate manic and hypomanic episodes and to prevent manic and depressive recurrences in patients with bipolar disorder. These medications include lithium salt formulations, various anticonvulsants, and antipsychotic medications.

Lithium, the classic mood stabilizer, is the only psychotropic medication that has been shown to decrease the risk of suicide.[78] Lithium has multiple side effects and a narrow therapeutic window, meaning that only a small range of blood levels is therapeutic, with higher levels placing the patient at risk for serious and potentially lethal toxicity. For these reasons, close clinical monitoring and routine blood level testing are important.

Side effects of lithium manifest in diverse organ systems. A common side effect is fine tremor, especially noticeable in the fingers. Some patients describe slowed thinking and memory deficit. Other patients gain weight progressively and may demonstrate increased thirst or appetite. Chronic nausea and diarrhea are usually related to gastrointestinal tract mucosal irritation but may be signs of toxicity. With toxic lithium levels, gross tremulousness, ataxia, dysarthria, and confusion or delirium may develop.

Lithium also may affect thyroid and renal function.[83] Polyuria and secondary polydipsia are complications and may progress to diabetes insipidus. In most cases, discontinuing the medication reverses the renal effects. There are important drug-drug interactions, including with certain diuretics, and lithium, like several other psychotropic medications, has clear teratogenic effects, should it be taken by pregnant women.

Anticonvulsant medications, such as valproic acid (Depakote), lamotrigine (Lamictal), and carbamazepine (Tegretol), among others, also may be used to treat bipolar disorder. Valproic acid, like lithium, requires regular blood level monitoring and may have effects on liver function and white blood cell counts. Sedation is common, and tremor, ataxia, weight gain, alopecia, and teratogenic fetal neural tube defects are all side effects that physicians and patients must discuss.

Lamotrigine, particularly useful for bipolar depression, carries a small but potentially lethal risk of severe rash. Carbamazepine carries a risk of agranulocytosis, and aplastic anemia and is monitored by complete blood counts.

Second-generation antipsychotics (see below) are now increasingly prescribed for their mood-stabilizing properties.

## Anxiolytics

Benzodiazepines, such as alprazolam, lorazepam, clonazepam, diazepam, and others, are commonly prescribed anxiolytics. These medications produce effective relief of acute anxiety but have a high addictive potential and can lead to physical symptoms of withdrawal and possibly seizures if stopped abruptly. These medications are unfortunately often available on the streets and from colleagues. The most common benzodiazepine side effects are dose-related sedation, followed by dizziness, weakness, ataxia, decreased motor performance, and mild hypotension.

Benzodiazepines generally are not indicated for the treatment of performance anxiety. In addition to the above side effects and risk for tolerance and dependence, they may impair performance parameters such as intonation and rhythmic control.[79] They also may impede the learning that takes place over repeated performances that could otherwise lead to extinction of anxiety over time.[80] The sensitive clinician must carefully distinguish performance anxiety from panic disorder (see below). Benzodiazepines, a common treatment for panic disorder, may be used inappropriately for situational performance anxiety that is mistaken for panic.

Antidepressants, such as SSRIs and others (see above), are often first-line choices for patients who have anxiety disorders, such as generalized anxiety disorder, obsessive-compulsive disorder, panic disorder, posttraumatic stress disorder, and social phobia. However, there is no little research on antidepressants used in the treatment of performance anxiety other than the studies reviewed above (see section on Performance Anxiety).

Clomipramine, a tricyclic antidepressant, was formerly a first-line choice for treating obsessive-compulsive disorder, although SSRIs have become more common, given the side effects of TCAs, described above.

Hydroxyzine, an antihistamine, is occasionally prescribed for mild anxiety. It does not produce physical dependence but does potentiate the effects of CNS sedatives.[84]

Buspirone is not sedating at its usual dosage levels and has little addictive potential. Its appears to be more useful for patients with generalized anxiety disorder who have not been on a benzodiazepine in the past.[83,81]

Beta-blockers are often used to treat physiologic symptoms of sympathetic arousal in performance anxiety. This may help alleviate the bothersome symptoms of upper respiratory tract dryness experienced by voice professionals with debilitating performance anxiety, along with somatic symptoms of anxiety that may impair optimal performance. However, they may also cause serious side effects and can impair performance. Moreover, requiring a drug to perform daily activities of one's chosen profession is problematic, and the underlying cause of anxiety should be identified. This important topic is reviewed in detail above in the section on performance anxiety.

## Antipsychotics

Antipsychotic drugs (also termed *neuroleptics*) are used in the treatment of schizophrenia and various forms of mania and bipolar disorders, as well as other disorders. Antipsychotic medications include the first-generation medications haloperidol, fluphenazine, perphenazine, and chlorpromazine, among others. To address some of the side effects of these drugs, over the past two decades, newer so-called second-generation or "atypical" antipsychotics have emerged. These include risperidone, olanzapine, quetiapine, ziprasidone, aripiprazole, paliperidone, iloperidone, asenapine, and lurasidone. The antipsychotic clozapine constitutes somewhat of a class of its own.

Antipsychotics are thought to act principally by blocking dopamine receptors in a particular part of the brain, but their action on dopamine receptors in others areas produces some of their most bothersome side effects. Also called extrapyramidal side effects (EPSs), these side effects include short-term effects, such as acute dystonia (involuntary and potentially dangerous muscle contractions), akathisia (a form a motor restlessness), and parkinsonian symptoms (which mimic those of Parkinson disease), and the long-term effect of tardive dyskinesia, an irreversible and potentially severe movement disorder. Important for vocal professionals, tardive dyskinesia and other EPSs often may involve the tongue, perioral, and even laryngeal musculature.

Second-generation antipsychotics appear to be as effective as their predecessors but were touted as having a lower risk of EPS. However, they come with a price of their own, including weight gain, hypercholesterolemia, and the potential of developing diabetes. Large studies in the past decade have questioned some of the assumptions made about the superiority of the second-generation antipsychotic.[87,88] Nevertheless, they often remain first-line treatment in clinical practice because of their presumed milder extrapyramidal side effect profile.

Clozapine (Clozaril) is the only medication that is consistently shown to be superior in efficacy to all other antipsychotics. It also has low likelihood of EPS. However, clozapine is generally reserved for refractory cases due to its low but significant 1% risk of agranulocytosis, a potentially fatal drop in white blood cells. Patients on clozapine need frequent monitoring of their blood counts for this complication.

Because antipsychotics are often effective adjunctive treatments for other psychiatric disorders (eg, obsessive-compulsive disorders, depression with psychotic features, bipolar disorders), it may be useful to discuss other side effects that would affect a voice professional using these medications. The pharmacology of antipsychotic medications is complex and unique to each medication and cannot fully be reviewed here. Suffice it to say that, in addition to blocking dopamine receptors, which can lead to EPS, each drug may cause side effects owing to actions on various other neurotransmitter systems:

- Hypotension from effects on the α-adrenergic system
- Weight gain and sedation due to effects on the histaminergic system
- Anticholinergic side effects such as dry mouth, blurred vision, and constipation
- A minor risk of cardiac arrhythmias, presumably mediated through effects on calcium channels in nerve and heart muscle cells
- Metabolic consequences, such as increased cholesterol or diabetes risk

All antipsychotics carry a small risk of the potentially lethal neuroleptic malignant syndrome, which presents with confusion, muscle rigidity, fever, and autonomic instability. Clozapine carries its particular risk for agranulocytosis and also may cause a troublesome increase in salivation.

Ongoing psychiatric treatment of patients with voice disorders mandates a careful evaluation of current and prior psychoactive drug therapy. In addition, numerous psychoactive substances are used in the medical management of such neurologic conditions as Tourette syndrome (antipsychotics), chronic pain syndromes (carbamazepine), and vertigo (diazepam, clonazepam). The vocal team thus must identify and avoid drug interactions. It is appropriate (with the patient's consent) to consult with the prescribing physician directly to advocate the use of the psychoactive drug least likely to produce adverse effects on the voice while adequately controlling the psychiatric illness.[83]

## Additional Psychologic Etiologies and Treatments

Rapport with voice team members may allow patients to reveal other psychiatric disorders. Among the most common in arts medicine are eating disorders and substance abuse. Comprehensive discussion of these subjects is beyond the scope of this chapter, but it is important for the health professional to recognize such conditions, not only because of their effects on the voice but also because of their potentially serious general medical and psychiatric implications.

### Eating Disorders

Bulimia nervosa and anorexia nervosa both involve disordered eating. Anorexia is a mental disorder that involves aversion to food and great fear of becoming obese, associated with disturbed body image. It afflicts young women most commonly and can be life threatening.[89] Bulimia involves episodes of rapid consumption of large quantities of food in short periods of time (binge eating) followed by purging using laxatives, diuretics, or self-induced vomiting. It also may be accompanied by vigorous exercise and fasting. Associated feelings of guilt are common, as is depression. It may occur sporadically or be a chronic problem.

Bulimia and binge eating may be more prevalent than is commonly realized. It is estimated to occur in as many as 1.5% to 3.5% of females, particularly adolescents and young adults (including female dancers). Males are also affected, although at lesser rates (0.5%–2%).[90] Bulimia also may be associated with anorexia nervosa.

Vomiting in bulimia produces signs and symptoms similar to severe chronic reflux as well as thinning of tooth enamel. In addition to posterior laryngitis and pharyngitis, laryngeal findings associated with bulimia include subepithelial vocal fold hemorrhages, superficial telangiectasia of the vocal fold mucosa, and vocal fold scarring. Clinicians must be attentive to the potential for anorexia or bulimia in the maintenance of a desirable body appearance in performers.

There is enormous popular interest in the use of appetite suppressants in weight management. Many myths persist about proper weight management approaches in singers and the value and/or risk of weight loss.

The availability and popularity of appetite suppressant drugs, and mass marketing approaches that made them available in franchised weight loss centers, led many Americans to explore the use of Fen-Phen (phentermine and fenfluramine) and dexfenfluramine HCI in the 1990s. These medications had limited efficacy in changing metabolism and craving, and many patients took these drugs in combinations that were never approved for concomitant use. These drugs were voluntarily withdrawn from the market by their manufacturers in 1997 due to a significant risk of cardiac valve damage and pulmonary hypertension.

Health professionals caring for singers and other performers should be certain to investigate the potential use of these medications, as well as other appetite suppressant or weight control drugs.

## Substance Abuse

Alcohol, benzodiazepines, stimulants, cocaine, narcotics, and other drugs are notoriously readily available in the performing arts community and on the streets.[91,92] In patients who demonstrate signs and symptoms of substance abuse, or who admit that these areas of their lives are out of control, these problems should be acknowledged while efficiently arranging treatment for them. The window of opportunity is often remarkably narrow. The physician should establish close ties to excellent treatment facilities, where specialized clinicians can offer confidential outpatient management, with inpatient care available when required for safety.[37]

## Neurogenic Dysphonia

Patients with neurologic disease are likely to experience psychiatric symptoms, especially depression and anxiety. These disorders cause physiologic changes that may exacerbate or mask the underlying neurologic presentation. Metcalfe and colleagues[93] cited the incidence of severe depression and/or anxiety in neurologic patients at one-third.

The site of neurologic lesion affects the incidence of depression and anxiety, with lesions of the left cerebral hemisphere, basal ganglia, limbic system, thalamus, and anterior frontal lobe more likely to produce these effects.[94] The same structures are important in voice, speech, and language production, and so depression and anxiety logically coexist with voice and language disorders resulting from CNS pathology.[94,95]

Dystonias and stuttering also are associated with both neurologic and psychogenic etiologies and must be carefully distinguished by the laryngologist before instituting interdisciplinary treatment.[96]

## Stress Management

Psychologic stress pervades virtually all professions in today's fast-moving society. A singer preparing for a series of concerts, a teacher preparing for presentation of lectures, a lawyer anticipating a major trail, a businessperson negotiating an important contract, or a member of any other goal-oriented profession, each must deal with myriad of demands on his or her time and talents. Stress is recognized as a factor in many types of illness and disease. It is estimated that 50% to 70% of all physician visits involve complaints of stress-related illness.[97]

Stress is a psychologic experience that has physiologic consequences. Stress-related problems are important and common among professional voice users. The stress may be physical or psychologic, and it often involves a combination of both. Either may interfere with performance. Stress represents a special problem for singers, because its physiologic manifestations may interfere with the delicate mechanisms of voice production.[37]

A brief review of some terminology may be useful:

- The term *stress* is used broadly. Our working definition is emotional, cognitive, and physiologic reactions to psychologic demands and challenges.
- Stress level reflects the degree of stress experienced. Stress is not an all-or-none phenomenon. The psychologic effects of stress range from mild to severely incapacitating.
- Stress response refers to the physiologic reaction of an organism to stress.
- A stressor is an external stimulus or internal thought, perception, image, or emotion that creates stress.[98]

Two other concepts are important in a contemporary discussion of stress: *coping* and *adaptation*. Lazarus and Folkman[99] have defined coping as "the process of managing demands (external or internal) that are appraised as taxing or exceeding the resources of the person." In the early 1930s, Hans Selye, an endocrinologist, discovered a generalized response to stressors in research animals. He described their responses using the term *general adaptation syndrome*. Selye (cited in Green and Snellenberger[98]) postulated that the physiology of the test animals was trying to adapt to the challenges of noxious stimuli. The process of adaptation to chronic and severe stressors was harmful over time. There were 3 phases to the observed response: *alarm, adaptation*, and *exhaustion*. These phases were named for physiologic responses during a sequence of events. The alarm phase is the characteristic fight-or-flight response. If the stressor continued, the animal appeared to adapt, where the physiologic responses were less extreme, but the animal eventually became more exhausted. In the exhaustion phase, the animal's adaptation energy was spent, physical symptoms occurred, and some animals died.[55]

### Physical Effects of Stress

Stress responses occur in part through the autonomic nervous system.[98] A stressor triggers particular brain centers, which in turn affect target organs through nerve connections. The brain has 2 primary pathways for the stress response, neuronal and hormonal, and these pathways overlap. The body initiates a stress response through 1 of 3 pathways:

- Sympathetic nervous system efferents that terminate on target organs such as the heart and blood vessels
- Release of epinephrine and norepinephrine from the adrenal medulla
- Release of various other catecholamines[98]

A full description of the various processes involved is beyond the scope of this chapter. However, stress has numerous physical consequences. Through the autonomic nervous system, it may alter oral and vocal fold secretions, heart rate, and gastric acid production. Under acute, anxiety-producing circumstances, such changes are to be expected. When frightened, a normal person's palms become cold and sweaty, the mouth becomes dry, heart rate increases, his or her pupils change size, and stomach acid secretions may increase. These phenomena are objective signs that may be observed by a physician, and their symptoms may be recognized by the performer as dry mouth and voice fatigue, heart palpitations, and heartburn.

More severe, prolonged stress is also commonly associated with increased muscle tension throughout the body (but particularly in the head and neck), headaches, decreased ability to concentrate, and insomnia. Chronic fatigue is also a common symptom. These physiologic alterations may lead not only to altered vocal quality but also to physical pathology. Increased gastric acid secretion is associated with ulcers, as well as reflux laryngitis and arytenoid irritation. Other gastrointestinal manifestations, such as colitis, irritable bowel syndrome, and dysphagia, are also described.

Chronic stress and tension may cause numerous pain syndromes, although headaches, particularly migraines in vulnerable individuals, are most common. Stress is also associated with more serious physical problems such as myocardial infarction, asthma, and depression of the immune system.[66,98,100]

Thus, the constant pressure under which many performers live may be more than an inconvenience. Stress factors should be recognized, and appropriate modifications should be made to ameliorate them.

### Stressors in Vocalists

Stressors may be physical or psychologic and often involve a combination of both. Either may interfere with performance.

There are several situations in which physical stress is common and important. Generalized fatigue is seen frequently in hard-working singers, especially in the frantic few weeks preceding major performances. To maintain normal mucosal secretions, a strong immune system to fight infection, and the ability of muscles to recover from heavy use, rest, proper nutrition, and hydration are required. When the body is stressed through deprivation of these essentials, illness (such as upper respiratory infection), voice fatigue, hoarseness, and other vocal dysfunctions may supervene.

Lack of physical conditioning undermines the power source of the voice. A person who becomes short of breath while climbing a flight of stairs hardly has the abdominal and respiratory endurance needed to sustain him or her optimally through the rigors of performance. The stress of attempting to perform under such circumstances often results in voice dysfunction.

Oversinging is another common physical stress. As with running, swimming, or any other athletic activity that depends on sustained, coordinated muscle activity, singing requires conditioning to build up strength and endurance. Rest periods are also essential for muscle recovery. Singers who are accustomed to singing for 1 or 2 hours a day stress their physical voice-producing mechanism severely when they suddenly begin rehearsing for 14 hours daily immediately prior to performance.

### Treatment Approaches for Stress

Medical treatment of stress depends on the specific circumstances. When the diagnosis is appropriate but poorly controlled anxiety rather than a physical problem, the physician's evaluation itself may reassure the patient. Under ordinary circumstances, once the singer's mind is put to rest regarding the questions of nodules, vocal fold injury, or other serious problems, his or her training usually allows compensation for vocal manifestations of anxiety, especially when the vocal complaint is minor.

Slight alterations in quality or increased vocal fatigue are seen most frequently. These are often associated with lack of sleep, oversinging, and dehydration associated with the stress-producing commitment. The singer or actor should be advised to modify these and to consult his or her voice teacher. The voice teacher should ensure that good vocal technique is being used under performance and rehearsal circumstances.

Frequently, young singers are not trained sufficiently in how and when to "mark." For example, many singers whistle to rest their voices, not realizing that active vocalization and potentially fatiguing vocal fold contact occur when whistling. Technical proficiency and a plan for voice conservation during rehearsal and performances are essential under these circumstances. A manageable stressful situation may become unmanageable if real physical vocal problems develop.

Several additional modalities may be helpful in selected circumstances. Relative voice rest (using the voice only when necessary) may be important not only to voice conservation but also to psychologic relaxation. Under stressful circumstances, a singer needs as much peace and quiet as possible, not hectic socializing, parties with heavy voice use in noisy environments, and press appearances. The importance of adequate sleep and fluid intake cannot be overemphasized. Local therapy, such as steam inhalation and neck muscle massage, may be helpful in some people and certainly does no harm.

The doctor may be very helpful in alleviating the singer's exogenous stress by conveying "doctor's orders" directly to theater management. This will save the singer the discomfort of having to personally confront an authority and violate his or her "show must go on" ethic. A short phone call by the physician can be highly therapeutic.

## Management of Chronic Stress

When stress is chronic and incapacitating, more comprehensive measures are required. If psychologic stress manifestations become so severe that they impair performance or necessitate the use of drugs to allow performance, psychotherapy is indicated. The goal of psychotherapeutic approaches to stress management includes changing external and internal stressors, affective and cognitive reactions to stressors, physiologic reactions to stress, and stress behaviors.

A psychoeducational model is customarily used. Initially, the psychotherapist will assist the patient in identifying and evaluating stressor characteristics. A variety of assessment tools are available for this purpose. Interventions designed to increase a sense of efficacy and personal control are designed. Perceived control over the stressor directly affects stress level, and it changes one's experience of the stressor. Laboratory and human research has determined that a sense of control is one of the most potent elements in the modulation of stress responses.[101–103] Concrete exercises that impose time management are taught and practiced. Patients are urged to identify and expand their network of support as well.

Psychologic intervention requires evaluation of the patient's cognitive model. Cognitive restructuring exercises are used, as well as classical conditioning tools that patients easily learn and utilize effectively with practice. Cognitive skills include the use of monitored perception, thought, and internal dialogue to regulate emotional and physiologic responses.

A variety of relaxation techniques are available and are ordinarily taught in the course of stress-management treatment. These include progressive relaxation, hypnosis, autogenic training and imagery, and biofeedback training. Underlying all of these approaches is the premise that making conscious normally unconscious processes leads to control and self-efficacy.[37]

As with all medical conditions, the best treatment for stress in singers is prevention. Awareness of the conditions that lead to stress and its potential adverse effect on voice production often allows the singer to anticipate and avoid these problems. Stress is inevitable in performance and in life. Performers must learn to recognize it, compensate for it when necessary, and incorporate it into their singing as emotion and excitement. Stress should be controlled, not pharmacologically eliminated. Used well, stress should be just one more tool of the singer's trade.

## Reactive Responses

Reaction to illness is the major source of psychiatric disturbance in patients with significant voice dysfunction. Loss of communicative function is an experience of alienation that threatens human self-definition and independence. Catastrophic fears of loss of productivity, economic and social status, and, in professional voice users, creative artistry contribute to rising anxiety. Anxiety is known to worsen existing communication disorders, and the disturbances in memory, concentration, and synaptic transmission secondary to depression may intensify other voice symptoms and interfere with rehabilitation.

The self-concept is an essential construct of Carl Rodger's theories of counseling.[45] Rodgers described self-concept as composed of perceptions of the characteristics of the self and the relationships of the self to various aspects of life, as well as the values attached to the perceptions. Rodgers suggested that equilibrium requires that patients' self-concepts be congruent with their life experiences. It follows, then, that it is not the disability per se that psychologically influences the person but rather the subjective meaning and feelings attached to the disability.

According to Rodgers, the 2 major psychologic defenses that operate to maintain consistent self-concept are denial and distortion.[45] Families of patients are affected as well. They are often confused about the diagnosis and poorly prepared to support the patient's coping responses. The resulting stress may negatively influence family dynamics and intensify the patient's depressive illness.[104]

As the voice-injured patient experiences the process of grieving, the psychologist may assume a more prominent role in his or her care. Essentially, the voice-injured patient goes through a grieving process similar to patients who mourn other losses, such as the death of a loved one. In some cases, especially among voice professionals, the patients actually mourn the loss of their self as they perceive it. The psychologist is responsible for facilitating the tasks of mourning and monitoring the individual's formal mental status for clinically significant changes.[37,44,105]

There are a number of models for tracking this process. The most easily understood is that of Worden,[106] as adapted by the author (DCR):

- Initially, the task is to accept the reality of the loss. The need for and distress of this is vestigial during the phase of diagnosis, is held consciously in abeyance during the acute and rehabilitative phases of treatment, but is reinforced with accumulating data measuring vocal function. As the reality becomes undeniable, the mourner must be helped to express the full range of the grieving effect. The rate of accomplishing this is variable and individual. Generally, it will occur in the style with which the person usually copes with crisis and may be florid or tightly constricted. All responses must be invited and normalized. The psychologist facilitates the process and stays particularly attuned to unacceptable, split-off responses or the failure to move through any particular response.
- As attempts to deny the loss take place and fail, the mourner gradually encounters the next task: beginning to live and cope in a world in which the lost object is absent. This is the psychoanalytic process of *decathexis*, which requires the withdrawal of

life energies from the other and the reinvesting of them in the self. For some professional voice users, this may be a temporary state as they make adjustments required by their rehabilitation demands. In other cases, the need for change will be lasting: change in fach (voice classification), change in repertoire, need for amplification, altered performance schedule, or, occasionally, change in career.[37,44,105]
- As the patient so injured seeks to heal his or her life, another task looms. Known as *recathexis*, it involves reinvesting life energies in other relationships, interests, talents, and life goals. The individual is assisted in redefining and revaluing the self as apart from the voice. The voice is then seen as the *product* of the self, rather than an equivalent to the self. For many performers, this is painfully difficult.[37,44,105,106]

Rosen and Sataloff[9] have described in detail research applying the various theoretical models of grief resolution to the perception of vocal injury in professional voice users.

## Psychologic Responses to Surgery

When vocal fold surgery is indicated, many individuals will demonstrate hospital-related phobias or self-destructive responses to pain. Adamson et al[107] describe the importance of understanding how the patient's occupational identity will be affected by surgical intervention. Vocal fold surgery affects the major mode of communication that all human beings utilize, and the impact is extraordinarily anxiety producing in professional voice users. Even temporary periods of absolute voice restriction may induce feelings of insecurity, helplessness, and dissociation from the verbal world. Carpenter[108] details the value of an early therapy session to focus on the fears, fantasies, misconceptions, and regression that frequently accompany a decision to undergo surgery.

A proper surgical discussion highlights vocal fold surgery as *elective*. The patient chooses surgery as the only remaining means to regaining the previously normal voice or to attain a different but desirable voice. Responsible care includes a thorough preoperative and written discussion of the limits and complications of surgery, with recognition by the surgeon that anxiety affects both understanding and retention of information about undesirable outcomes. Personality psychopathology or unrealistic expectations of the impact of surgery on their lives are elements for which surgical candidates can be screened.[48,109,110] Recognizing such problems preoperatively allows preoperative counseling and obviates many postoperative difficulties.

Although a thorough discussion is outside the scope of this chapter, surgically treated voice patients include those undergoing laryngectomy, with or without a voice prosthesis. The laryngectomized individual must make major psychologic and social adjustments. These include not only those adjustments related to a diagnosis of cancer but also to those of a sudden disability: loss of voice.

With the improvement in prognosis, research has begun to focus on the individual's quality of life after the laryngectomy. There is wide variability in the quality of preoperative and postoperative psychologic support reported by patients during each phase of care. Special psychologic issues in professional voice users diagnosed with laryngeal cancer are discussed in detail in other works.[37] Providing this support is a crucial role for the voice team's psychologist.[111–113]

## Voice Team's Roles in Treating Psychogenic Problems

### The Psychologic Professional

Both psychology and psychiatry specialize in attending to emotional needs and problems. Psychiatrists, as physicians, focus on the neurological and biological causes and treatment of psychopathology. Psychiatrists also may be trained to provide psychotherapy. Psychologists have advanced graduate training in psychologic function and therapy. They both concern themselves with cognitive processes, such as thinking, behavior, and memory; the experiencing and expression of emotions; significant inner conflict; characteristic modes of defense in coping with stress; and personality style and perception of self and others, including their expression in interpersonal behavior.

Other mental health professionals, such as social workers, also provide psychotherapy to performers. In the authors' practice, clinical psychologists serve as members of the voice team. They work directly with some patients and offer consultation to the physician and other professionals.[37]

In our center, patient assessment is done throughout the physician's history taking and physical examinations, as well as in a formal psychiatric interview when appropriate. Personality assessment, screening for or evaluating known psychopathology, and assessment of potential surgical candidates are performed. Occasionally, psychometric instruments are added to the diagnostic interview. Confidentiality of content is extended to the treatment team to maximize interdisciplinary care. Because of their special interest in voicing parameters, the voice team psychologists are especially attuned to the therapeutic use of their own voices for intensifying rapport and pacing/leading the patient's emotional state during interventions.[114–118]

Psychotherapeutic treatment is offered on a short-term, diagnosis-related basis. Treatment is designed to identify and alleviate emotional distress and to increase the individual's resources for adaptive functioning. Individual psychotherapeutic approaches include brief insight-oriented therapies, cognitive-behavioral techniques, Gestalt interventions, stress-management skill building, and clinical hypnosis.

After any indicated acute intervention is provided, and in patients whose coping repertoire is clearly adequate to the stressors, a psychoeducational model is used. The therapy session focuses on a prospective discussion of personal, inherent life stressors and predictable illnesses. Stress management skills are taught, and audiotapes are provided that offer portable skill building. Supplemental sessions may be scheduled by mutual decision during appointments at the center for medical examinations and speech or singing voice therapy.

A group therapy model, facilitated by the psychologist, has also been used to provide a forum for discussion of patient responses during the various phases of treatment. Participants benefit from the perspective and progress of other patients, the opportunity to decrease their experience of isolation, and the sharing of resources.

Long-term psychodynamic psychotherapy, chronic psychiatric care, and psychopharmacologic management are provided through referral to consultant mental health professionals with special interest and insight in voice-related psychologic problems. The voice team's psychologists also serve in a liaison role when patients already in treatment come to our center for voice care.

### The Speech-Language Pathologist

Speech-language pathology has its roots in psychology, as the original members of the field came primarily from psychology backgrounds. Early interest in the psychologic aspects of voicing are evidenced in texts such as *The Voice of Neurosis*.[119] Luchsinger and Arnold[120] present an excellent review of the early literature in their text, *Voice, Speech, Language*.

At the present time, speech-language pathologists (SLPs) need to be familiar with models of treatment from the psychologic tradition, the medical tradition, and the educational tradition. In defining the SLP's role in managing functional voice problems, it must be made clear that the SLP does not work in isolation but as a part of a team, which includes at a minimum a laryngologist and the SLP. Singing or acting instructors, stress specialists, psychologists, neurologists, and psychiatrists must be readily available and cognizant of the special needs to voice patients.

The SLP's role in treating voice-disordered patients is to normalize the patient's speaking and communication behavior. In this sense, many of the activities of SLPs with voice-disordered patients are "psychologic." This section does not intend to present a full description of the SLP's total function but instead focuses on areas in which the SLP must deal with issues not directly related to the physical vocal mechanism. Activities engaged in by the SLP with the patient can help to set the groundwork for discussion of psychologic issues. A more detailed description has been published elsewhere.[121]

### Preparation for Treatment

The SLP must be aware of, and be able to interpret, the findings of the laryngologist, including strobovideolaryngoscopy. Particular attention should be paid to findings demonstrating muscle tension or lack of glottic closure not associated with organic or physical changes. The perceptions of the laryngologist regarding organic and functional aspects of the patient need to be known.

A case history is taken, reviewing and amplifying the case history reported by the laryngologist (Table 7–3). Subjective and objective measures of the patient's vocal mechanism and communication skills need to be obtained, as outlined in Table 7–4. From these, the SLP should be able to develop a plan of behavioral changes.

During the patient interview, taking the case history provides the SLP with an ample sample of the patient's voice use, including his or her communication style and verbosity. It is important to note how the patient's voice changes when talking about certain topics and to note evidence of improvement or fatigue as the interview proceeds. It provides data on what speaking activities are most important to the patient and which may need to be addressed initially in therapy. It provides information on the patient's willingness to talk about stressful issues or needs beyond direct focus on voicing and speech skills, which may be important regarding referral to other specialists for stress and emotional or physical health.

The physical assessment (see Table 7–4) provides the SLP with objective support for what the clinician has heard and information about how the patient is producing the voice. Because any behavioral change instituted during therapy is based on eradicating symptoms of maladaptive voice or communication, the SLP should list and evaluate confirmed symptoms at this stage in order to develop an overall therapeutic plan. The focus should be on identifying the underlying behavior or behaviors responsible for maintaining the current voice in order to address these underlying behaviors first, which reduces the length of therapy and should predict improvement of voicing.

### Therapeutic Stage

Information giving is essential at the beginning of therapy and throughout the course of therapy. Patients need to know the reason for the activities in which they are engaging and why these activities are important in changing their current voice problem. Without a thorough understanding of the reasons for changing behavior, the probabilities of behavioral change are poor. The patient needs to know that a voice disorder is usually multifactorial and is maintained by a combination of physical changes (if present), communication demands on the voice, the patient's skills in producing speech, and the patient's attempts to compensate for vocal changes.

Initially, the goal in therapy is to manage communicative demands and improve the patient's ability to produce more normal voice. Reassessment of the need for medical and/or surgical interventions for physical changes is planned with the patient. The patient is reassured that the goal of therapy is not to change personality or limit communication opportunities but to return him or her at least to the level of communication enjoyed prior to the onset of the voice problem.

### Breathing Patterns

Information should be conveyed regarding the patient's current breathing pattern. It may be insufficient for the demands placed on the patient's voice or contribute to increased tension in the vocal mechanism.

Abdominal breathing is the natural and preferred method of breathing by the body. People are engaged in abdominal breathing when they are relaxed and when they are sleeping. Patients can be asked to observe or recall the breathing patterns of their pets, of babies engaging in comfort sounds vs painful or paroxysmal crying, or of significant others in repose.

**Table 7–3.** The History

1. **Circumstances surrounding the onset, development, and progress of the voice disorder, include the following:**
   - Illnesses of the patient
   - Recent changes in employment
   - Speaking responsibilities associated with the patient's employment
   - Effects of the voice disorder on employment
   - Employment environment
   - Speaking activities outside of employment
   - Environment in which social speaking activities occur
   - Effects of the voice disorder on social exchange and social activities
   - Activities the patient has had to give up because of voice disorder
   - Illness or difficulty among family members or friends
   - Stress factors at work and at home
   - Methods of dealing with stress

2. **The social structure of the patient and environment need to be explored:**
   - Family and living arrangements
   - Friends and social gathering places
   - Relationships with coworkers and superiors

3. **The patient's response to the voice disorder needs to be explored:**
   - What bothers the patient most about the voice disorder?
   - What has the patient done to change voicing and how effective have these attempts been?
   - Estimate the speaking times at work and socially, now and before the voice disorder.
   - How does the patient feel about speaking at the present time—stressed, indifferent, depressed, challenged?

4. **General health issues should be addressed:**
   - Chronic illness, including asthma, allergies, diabetes, thyroid dysfunction, chronic fatigue
   - Head and neck trauma, including whiplash, concussion, spinal degeneration, temporomandibular joint disease, facial injury
   - Surgery
   - High fevers
   - Nonvocal symptoms, including swallowing difficulty, pain on speaking or swallowing, numbness, neck stiffness or reduced range of motion, voice quality, speaking rate, movement limitations of the articulators, nasal regurgitation, tremor or shakiness

5. **Medications**
   - Prescription medications
   - Over-the-counter drugs, including nonsteroidal anti-inflammatory drugs (NSAIDs), cough drops, decongestants, antihistamines, mouthwash, vitamins, alcohol, tobacco and caffeine products, and water intake

Their observations can be discussed and used as confirmation of the primacy of abdominal breathing. Predominantly clavicular or thoracic breathing is usually the product of stress, societal preference toward tight clothing, and/or demands by parents, teachers, and society in maintaining a tight tucked-

**Table 7–4.** Vocal Function Assessment

1. **Average fundamental frequency and loudness of the patient's conversational voice**

2. **Average fundamental frequency, loudness, and speaking rate during a selected reading passage, both in normal reading and in the professional voice (if a professional speaker)**

3. **Acoustic and aerodynamic measures of sustained vowels, including**
   - Measures of perturbation
   - Measures of breathiness and noise
   - Measures of vocal breaks and quality change
   - Measures of airflow
   - Measures of glottic pressure

4. **Preferred breathing patterns for speech**
   - Shallow, deep, appropriate for phrase length
   - Clavicular, thoracic, abdominal, or mixed
   - Coordination with voicing—exhalation initiated before voicing, glottic closure prior to initiation of exhalation
   - Coordinated breath/voicing

5. **Neck and laryngeal use**
   - Positioning of the larynx during speech—high, low, inflexible
   - Tension in the extralaryngeal muscles, particularly the omohyoid
   - Laryngeal/hyoid space—present, reduced
   - Position of the hyoid—tipped, tense, discomfort on palpation of the cornu

6. **Use of the articulators**
   - Oral examination, including lip movements and symmetry, tongue movements and symmetry, palatal sufficiency in nonspeech contexts, diadochokinetic rates
   - Ability to separate jaw and anterior tongue activity during the production of /l/, /t/, /d/, /n/
   - Tongue tension during speech
   - Jaw tension and jaw jutting during speech
   - Looseness of temporomandibular joint during speech movements

in stomach. All of these factors lead to a reduction of abdominal release during inhalation that leads to restriction in diaphragmatic downward motion and maximal inflation of the lungs.

Patients are taught that taking a deep, high-chest breath increases air pressures in the lungs greatly, triggering a Valsalva response with closure of the glottis and laryngeal and chest muscle tension. The kind of breath the patient takes may influence tension in other parts of the vocal mechanism. High-chest breathing can contribute to a feeling of breathlessness and tightness in the chest. Abdominal breathing produces lesser increases in lung air pressure and removes the tension from the neck and larynx.

When speaking, the patient needs to know what he or she is about to say before he or she inhales the breath to say it, and this concept is discussed and practiced. This simple construct eliminates respiratory/laryngeal incoordination, reduces revisions and struggle during speaking, and allows the patient to focus on how he or she is saying something rather than on the content of what is being said. Speech should be a continuous breath event, beginning with inhalation of the appropriate amount of air and continuing through easy transition to exhalation and voicing to the end of the utterance.

Instruction and discussion of these matters before starting a program of breath support exercises increases the patient's willingness to change and turns the reluctant patient into an active participant. Specific breathing exercises to incorporate abdominal breathing are available in many other publications.

### Jaw and Tongue Positioning

Similarly, the patient needs to know that modification of articulation postures and open, relaxed jaw positioning improve loudness and acuity in noisy environments and can be invaluable in improving communication without effort and fatigue in most speaking circumstances. Tongue tension or pulling the tongue back in the mouth leads to tension in the hyoid and larynx region. These effects can be demonstrated and discussed by having the patient tense the tongue or retract the tongue while digitally monitoring tension under the chin and at the sides of the larynx. The same effects can be demonstrated during talking activities. Patients need to learn to explore the feelings associated with tension and extra-effort speaking.

### Phonation

Instruction in phonatory behavior helps the patient understand that the vocal folds are opened by the flow of air from the lungs and closed due to their own elasticity and the Bernoulli principle. The vocal folds are vibrating much too rapidly to be manipulated by laryngeal effort, and patients need to comprehend that the emotional system and the conscious speech system share control of voicing, which varies with emotional context. Laryngeal control is primarily automatic, and efforts to produce voice are counterproductive.

The quality of the patient's voice during physiologic sound making, such as laughter or a gentle cough, can predict the quality of sound when extra effort is removed. Humming and sighing can also effectively demonstrate the effect of reduced effort. Modeling by the SLP of easy, well-supported, well-resonated voice during these conversations can be a highly effective means of modifying the patient's vocal production in the therapy setting.

Closed, tense jaw articulation and substitution of jaw movement for tongue and lip movements increase tension and fatigue in the face and increase the amount of pulling on the temporomandibular joint (TMJ) capsule. The same methods of speaking reduce loudness in noisy speaking situations and impede the ability of listeners to read the speaker's lips. Patients learn that in American English, only 6 sounds (/s/ as in *see*, /z/ as in *zoo*, /ʃ/ as in *shoe*,

/ʒ/ as in *leisure*, /tʃ/ as in *chop*, /dʒ/ as in *judge*) require closure of the jaw. All other consonants and all vowels can be produced by modifying the position of the lips and tongue with no, or minor, jaw adjustment.

Most of speech can be produced with the jaw in a relaxed, partially open, neutral position. This can be demonstrated by monitoring tension in the masseter muscle—the patient places the fingers of both hands in front of the ears and alternately clenches and opens the jaw. The bulking of the masseter muscle fibers can be felt when the jaw is wide open. The neutral speaking position is identifiable by the absence of muscle bulk or stretched fibers. The patient needs to experience the feeling of relaxation associated with this speaking position.

The patient can then be instructed in producing the syllable /la/ by simply lifting the tongue and touching the roof of the mouth behind the upper front teeth and then dropping the tongue to a relaxed position behind, but touching, the lower front teeth. This is extended to other consonants (/ta/, /da/, /na/, and /ga/).

When the patient is proficient in eliminating jaw tension in these contexts, the effect of lip movement in addition to relaxed jaw and tongue is practiced by producing words such as *too*, *due*, *coo*, *load*, *coat*, and so on. Lip consonants without tensing the jaw are then added. The sounds /f/, /v/, /th/, and voiced /th/ need to be monitored for jaw jutting. An open relaxed jaw with improved oral resonance and a relaxed tongue can then be practiced in words, phrases, and finally in sentences.

### Practice Exercises

Initially, practice should be done while the patient monitors jaw position and movement with the fingers between the posterior molars and with a mirror. As the patient begins to feel comfortable with a relaxed jaw, the tactile monitoring and then the visual monitoring can be eliminated. At this point, the patient should identify phrases and sentences that he or she uses frequently, such as "Hello," "Put them away," or "I don't like that behavior," which can be used as frequent daily reminders in his or her normal speech of more normal oral resonance and speech production. This assists in carryover.

Practice continues with sentences including jaw closure sounds and open vowels, such as "He is going," "Let me have a piece of pie," "I chose two friends to go with me," and so on. The open relaxed jaw can then be extended into question-and-answer activities, monologue, and dialogue.

A pattern of frequent tension checks needs to be established with the cooperation of the patient. These need not be elaborate warm-up exercises or cool-down practices. The patient may decide to practice abdominal breathing in the shower, blowing the water away from his or her face or humming with a relaxed jaw while inhaling the warm steamy air. The patient may be able to stroke the face, jaw, or neck at each stoplight while driving to or from work or take an easy belly breath followed by a relaxed sigh. Jaw tension can be checked before picking up the telephone to say "hello."

Abdominal breathing can be practiced leaning over the desk while reading memos or correcting examination papers. A sip of water between tasks can help the patient focus on relaxation of the jaw and throat and can be preceded by a deep abdominal inhalation. Patients can be very creative and helpful in identifying times to practice correct vocal behavior. Multiple practices during the busy day can be more effective and are more likely to be done than a half-hour practice in the patient's home.

All of these exercises are helpful in aiding the patient to become aware of the subtle nature of tension in the speaking mechanism, but patients may be overwhelmed by overriding tension not associated directly with speaking behavior in the face and neck. The SLP should decide if he or she has the skill to develop a more stringent relaxation regimen or if the patient needs, and is amenable to, a referral to an expert in stress management.

### Behavior Modification

If the patient talks excessively, a discussion of relevant and irrelevant talking is necessary. The patient needs to know that total vocal rest, if extended past a week, can lead to muscle atrophy and an additional voice problem. The concept of vocal "naps" during the day and the possibility of reducing talking (or, more positively, becoming a better listener) in noisy environments should be introduced. The patient is more knowledgeable than the therapist in when and how long these quiet times can be inserted into his or her daily schedule.

Patients under stress will bring their "job-voice" home with them. Family members may complain about his or her use of too loud a voice, being too demanding, or giving too many directions. A vocal nap during the ride home with an added cool-down protocol can be helpful in providing a positive transition. The patient should be reminded that singing in the car over the traffic noise, radio, and engine noises can be abusive.

The patient needs to know that everyone lip-reads in noisy environments. If the patient has been successful in developing open oral resonance and articulation patterns, the ability of the patient's listeners to understand in noisy situations is enhanced. A slower rate of talking is also helpful in improving comprehension, and light can be used effectively to highlight his or her face during such conversations.

### Psychologic Referral

Voice patients under stress often violate the rules of conversation, including rules of relevance, brevity, and turn taking. A discussion of these rules may lead to an awareness of inappropriate communication patterns or the revelation of an underlying personality difficulty that may lead to a referral to a psychologic professional. Often, persons with difficulty in personal relationships or coping with their circumstances can admit to a voice disorder but not the underlying personal difficulties. The experience of voice therapy, especially supportive rather than prescriptive voice therapy, may lead to the acceptance of a referral to a professional trained in dealing with these underlying difficulties that might have been rejected at initial interview.

The combination of an inability to relax following focal voice exercises, an inability to modify communication behaviors, and a tendency for the patient to revert to discussions of personal problems rather than focus on the process of communication all assist the therapist in reinforcing the idea that the patient's problem lies outside the realm of traditional voice therapy. A statement by the therapist such as, "You have very real problems, but I am not trained to deal with them. I know someone who can help you" can be the beginning of a successful referral.

Finally, the patient needs to know that voice therapy is short term and finite. The goal of therapy is to identify underlying behavioral, emotional, and physical factors; modify current vocal behaviors; and develop better communication skills. The therapist must be aware that the stressed patient can develop inappropriate dependence on the therapist. If therapy sessions begin to focus more on the patient's day-to-day personal problems than on voice, the time for referral is long past. Patients need to know that voice therapy usually is successful in only a few sessions unless there are other problems that maintain the maladaptive vocal behavior. This is a difficult concept for some patients, particularly singers, who are used to taking ongoing singing lessons most of their lives. The therapeutic goal in these cases is to identify the underlying problems and make the appropriate referrals.

## Conclusions

Psychophysiological research informs our treatment and maximizes the benefits of medical interactions in every specialty.

- The rightful role of the arts-medicine psychologic professional is to possess mastery of the knowledge bases of psychology and medicine and also an experiential understanding of the performing arts, so that he or she may stand in alliance with the injured performer on the journey to explore, understand, and modify the psychologic impact of performance-related injuries.
- The speech-language pathologist must understand the psychologic factors that may cause, or be caused by, voice disorders. The SLP must be able to modify disordered voices into functional voices with sufficient stamina to endure the demands of their lifestyle and environment. The SLP provides a caring and supportive environment that allows patients to explore possible underlying causes. Also, he or she must recognize his or her limits as a psychotherapist and know when to refer to and collaborate with a mental health professional while maintaining responsibility for voice modification and some degree of psychologic support.
- The laryngologist must recognize the need for therapy in individual patients, accurately diagnose the presence of organic and functional disorders, select and coordinate the therapy team, and retain overall responsibility for the therapeutic process and the patient's outcome.

Those who are privileged to care for that uniquely human capability—the voice—quickly come to understand the essential role of psychologic awareness in our treatment failures and successes.

## References

1. Brodnitz FS. Hormones and the human voice. *Bull NY Acad Med*. 1971;47:183–191.
2. Rosen DC, Sataloff RT. *Psychology of Voice Disorders*. San Diego, CA: Singular Publishing; 1997.
3. Aronson AE. *Clinical Voice Disorders*. 3rd ed. New York, NY: Thieme; 1990:117–145, 314–315.
4. Sundberg J. *The Science of the Singing Voice*. DeKalb, IL: Northern Illinois University Press; 1985:146–156.
5. Vogel D, Carter J. *The Effects of Drugs on Communication Disorders*. San Diego, CA: Singular Publishing; 1995:31–143.
6. Shontz F. Body image and physical disability. In: Cash T, Pruzinsky T, eds. *Body Images: Development, Deviance and Change*. New York, NY: Guilford; 1990:149–169.
7. Freedman R. Cognitive behavioral perspectives on body image change. In: Cash TF, Pruzinsky T, eds. *Body Images: Development Deviance and Change*. New York, NY: Guilford; 1990:273–295
8. Horney K. Cited by: Meissner W. Theories of personality. In: Nicholi A, ed. *The New Harvard Guide to Psychiatry*. Cambridge, MA: Harvard University Press; 1988:177–199.
9. Rosen DC, Sataloff RT. Psychological aspects of voice disorders. In: Gould WJ, Rubin J, Korovin G, Sataloff RT, eds. *Diagnosis and Treatment of Voice Disorders*. New York, NY: Igaku-Shoin Medical; 1993:491–501.
10. Rodgers CA. A theory of personality and interpersonal relationships as developed in a client centered framework. In: Koch S, ed. *Psychology: A Study of a Science*. New York, NY: McGraw-Hill; 1959:184–256.
11. Butcher P, Elias A, Raven R. *Psychogenic Voice Disorders and Cognitive-Behavior Therapy*. San Diego, CA: Singular Publishing; 1993:3–22.
12. Nemiah J. Psychoneurotic disorders. In: Nicholi A, ed. *The New Harvard Guide to Psychiatry*. Cambridge, MA: Harvard University Press; 1988:234–258.
13. Ziegler FJ, Imboden JB. Contemporary conversion reactions: II. Conceptual model. *Arch Gen Psychiatry*. 1962;6:279–287.
14. Hartman DE, Daily WW, Morin KN. A case of superior laryngeal nerve paresis and psychogenic dysphonia. *J Speech Hear Disord*. 1989;54:526–529.
15. Sapir S, Aronson AE. Coexisting psychogenic and neurogenic dysphonia: a source of diagnostic confusion. *Br J Disord Commun*. 1987;22:73–80.
16. Cummings JL, Benson DF, Houlihan JP, Gosenfield LF. Mutism: loss of neocortical and limbic vocalization. *J Nerv Ment Dis*. 1983;171:255–259.
17. American Psychiatric Association. *Diagnostic and Statistical Manual of Mental Disorders–IV-TR*. Washington, DC: American Psychiatric Association; 2000.
18. Styron W. *Darkness Visible: A Memoir of Madness*. New York, NY: Random House; 1990.
19. Klerman G. Depression and related disorders of mood. In: Nicholi A, ed. *The New Harvard Guide to Psychiatry*. Cambridge, MA: Harvard University Press; 1988:309–336.
20. Ross E, Rush A. Diagnosis and neuroanatomical correlates of depression in brain-damaged patients: implications for a neurology of depression. *Arch Gen Psychiatry*. 1981;38:1344–1354.
21. Weissman MM. The psychological treatment of depression: evidence for the efficacy of psychotherapy alone, in comparison with, and in combination with pharmacotherapy. *Arch Gen Psychiatry*. 1979;38:1261–1269.
22. Depression Guideline Panel. *Depression in Primary Care: Vol. 1. Detection and Diagnosis—Clinical Practice Guideline No. 5*. Rockville, MD: Agency for Healthcare Policy and Research; 1993. No. 93–0550.

23. DiMatteo MR, Lepper HS, Croghan TW. Depression is a risk factor for noncompliance with medical treatment: meta-analysis of the effects of anxiety and depression on patient adherence. *Arch Intern Med.* 2000;160:2101–2107.

24. Culpepper L, Johnson P. In: Ciraulo D, ed. *Pharmacotherapy of Depression.* Totowa, NJ: Humana Press; 2010.

25. Kessler RC, Sonnega A, Bromet E, et al. Post-traumatic stress disorder in the National Comorbidity Survey. *Arch Gen Psychiatry.* 1995;52:1048–1060.

26. Van Ameringen M, Mancini C, Styan G, Donison D. Relationship of social phobia with other psychiatric illness. *J Affect Disord.* 1991;21:93–99.

27. Brawman-Mintzer O, Lydiard RB. Generalized anxiety disorder: issues in epidemiology. *J Clin Psychiatry.* 1996;57(suppl 7):3–8.

28. Stein MB, Kean YM. Disability and quality of life in social phobia: epidemiologic findings [published correction appears in *Am J Psychiatry.* 2000;157(12):2075]. *Am J Psychiatry.* 2000;157(10):1606–1613.

29. DeRubeis RJ, Gelfand LA, Tang TZ, Simons AD. Medications versus cognitive behavior therapy for severely depressed outpatients: mega-analysis of four randomized comparisons. *Am J Psychiatry.* 1999;156(7):1007–1013.

30. DeRubeis RJ, Siegle GJ, Hollon SD. Cognitive therapy versus medication for depression: treatment outcomes and neural mechanisms. *Nat Rev Neurosci.* 2008;9(10):788–796.

31. Fournier JC, De Rubeis RJ, Hollon SD, et al. Antidepressant drug effects and depression severity: a patient-level meta-analysis. *JAMA.* 2010;303(1):47–53.

32. Sataloff RT. Stress, anxiety and psychogenic dysphonia. In: Sataloff RT. *Professional Voice: The Science and Art of Clinical Care.* New York, NY: Raven Press; 1991:195–200.

33. LeDoux J. The emotional brain, fear, and the amygdala. *Cell Mol Neurobiol.* 2003;23(4–5):727–738.

34. Blair K, Shaywitz B, Smith RR, et al. Response to emotional expressions in generalized social phobia and generalized anxiety disorder: evidence for separate disorders. *Am J Psychiatry.* 2008;165:1193–1202.

35. Blair K, Geraci M, Devido J, et al. Neural response to self- and other referential praise and criticism in generalized social phobia. *Arch Gen Psychiatry.* 2008;65:1176–1184.

36. Sasso, DA. Psychiatric issues and performing artists. In: Sataloff RT, Branfanner AG, Letterman RJ. *Performing Arts Medicine.* 3rd ed. San Diego, CA: Science & Medicine, 2010.

37. Fishbein M, Middlestadt SE, Ottari V, et al. Medical problems among ICSOM musicians: overview of a national survey. *Med Probl Perform Art.* 1988;3(1):1–8.

38. Marchant-Haycox SE, Wilson GD. Personality and stress in performing artists. *Pers Individ Dif.* 1992; 13(10):1061–1068.

39. van Kemenade JFLM, van Son MJM, van Heesch NCA. Performance anxiety among professional musi-

cians in symphonic orchestras: a self-report study. *Psychol Rep.* 1995;77(2):555–562.

40. Wesner RB, Noyes R, David TL. The occurrence of performance anxiety among musicians. *J Affect Disord.* 1990;18(3):177–185.

41. Brodsky W. Music performance anxiety reconceptualized: a critique of current research practices and findings. *Med Probl Perform Art.* 1996;11(3):88–98.

42. Clark DB, Agras WS. The assessment and treatment of performance anxiety in musicians. *Am J Psychiatry.* 1991;148(5):598–605.

43. Brandfonbrener AG. Psychological issues in performing arts medicine [editorial]. *Med Probl Perform Art.* 1990;5(1):1.

44. Brandfonbrener A. Performance anxiety: different strokes for different folks. *Med Probl Perform Art.* 1999; 14(3):101.

45. Powell DH. Treating individuals with debilitating performance anxiety: an introduction. *J Clin Psychol.* 2004;60(8):801.

46. Rafferty BD, Smith RE, Ptacek JT. Facilitating and debilitating trait anxiety, situational anxiety, and coping with an anticipated stressor: a process analysis. *J Pers Soc Psychol.* 1997;72:892–906.

47. Salmon PG. A psychological perspective on musical performance anxiety: a review of the literature. *Med Probl Perform Art.* 1990;5(1):2–11.

48. Wolfe ML. Correlates of adaptive and maladaptive musical performance anxiety. *Med Probl Perform Art.* 1989;4(1):49–56.

49. McGinnis AM, Milling LS. Psychological treatment of musical performance anxiety: current status and future directions. *Psychother Theory Res Pract Train.* 2005;42(3):357–373.

50. Hiner SL, Brandt KD, Katz BP, et al. Performance-related medical problems among premier violinists. *Med Probl Perform Art.* 1987;2(2):67–71.

51. Kenny DT. A systematic review of treatments for music performance anxiety. *Anxiety Stress Coping.* 2005;18(3):183–208.

52. Steptoe A, Fidler H. Stage fright in orchestral musicians: a study of cognitive and behavioral strategies in performance anxiety. *Br J Psychol.* 1987;78(pt 2):241–249.

53. Robson B, Davidson J, Snell E. "But I'm not ready, yet": overcoming audition anxiety in the young musician. *Med Probl Perform Art.* 1995;10(1):32–37.

54. Osborne MS, Franklin J. Cognitive processes in musical performance anxiety. *Aust J Psychiatry.* 2002;54(2):86–93.

55. Freud S. Inhibitions, symptoms and anxiety. *Standard Edition.* 1926;20:87–174.

56. Wong PS. Anxiety, signal anxiety, and unconscious anticipation: neuroscientific evidence for an unconscious signal function in humans. *J Am Psychoanal Assoc.* 1999;47(3):817.

57. Sataloff RT, Rosen DC, Levy S. Medical treatment of performance anxiety: a comprehensive approach. *Med Probl Perform Art.* 1999;14(3):122–126.

58. Brantigan CO, Brantigan TA, Joseph N. Effect of β-blockade and β-stimulation on stage fright. *Am J Med*. 1982;72(1):88–94.

59. Zinn M, McCain C, Zinn M. Musical performance anxiety and high-risk model of threat perception. *Med Probl Perform Art*. 2000;15(2):65–72.

60. Kendrick MJ, Craig KD, Lawson DM, Davidson PO. Cognitive and behavioral therapy for musical-performance anxiety. *J Consult Clin Psychol*. 1982; 50(3):353–362.

61. Weisblatt S. A psychoanalytic view of performance anxiety. *Med Probl Perform Art*. 1986;1(2):64–67.

62. Nagel JJ. Stage fright in musicians: a psychodynamic perspective. *Bull Menninger Clin*. 1993;57(4):492–503.

63. Nagel JJ. Performance anxiety theory and treatment: one size does not fit all. *Med Probl Perform Art*. 2004; 19(1):39.

64. Hamilton LH. *The Person Behind the Mask: A Guide to Performing Arts Psychology*. Greenwich, CT: Ablex Publishing; 1997.

65. Cox WJ, Kenardy J. Performance anxiety, social phobia, and setting effects in instrumental music students. *J Anxiety Disord*. 1993;7(1):49–60.

66. Sternbach DJ. Musicians: a neglected working population in crisis. In: Sauter SL, Murphy LR, eds. *Organizational Risk Factors for Job Stress*. Washington, DC: American Psychological Association; 1995:283–302.

67. Sweeney GA, Horan JJ. Separate and combined effects of cue-controlled relaxation and cognitive restructuring in the treatment of musical performance anxiety. *J Counsel Psychol*. 1982;29:486–497.

68. Plaut EA. Psychotherapy of performance anxiety. *Med Probl Perform Art*. 1988;3(3):113–118.

69. Ostwald PF. Psychotherapeutic strategies in the treatment of performing artists. *Med Probl Perform Art*. 1987;2(4):131–136.

70. Nies AS. Clinical pharmacology of β-adrenergic blockers. *Med Probl Perform Art*. 1986;1(1):25–29.

71. Nubé J. β-blockers: effects on performing musicians. *Med Probl Perform Art*. 1991;6(2):61–68.

72. Gates GA, Saegert J, Wilson N, et al. Effect of β-blockade on singing performance. *Ann Otol Rhinol Laryngol*. 1985;94(6, pt 1):570.

73. Harris DA. Using β-blockers to control stage fright: a dancer's dilemma. *Med Probl Perform Art*. 2001; 16(1):72–76.

74. Packer CD, Packer DM. β-blockers, stage fright, and vibrato: a case report. *Med Probl Perform Art*. 2005; 20(3):126–130.

75. Lederman RJ. Medical treatment of performance anxiety: a statement in favor. *Med Probl Perform Art*. 1999; 14(3):117–121.

76. Steffensmeier JJ, Ernst ME, Kelly M, Hartz AJ. Do randomized controlled trials always trump case reports?: a second look at propranolol and depression. *Pharmacotherapy*. 2006;26(2):162–167.

77. Sataloff RT, Lawrence VL, Hawkshaw M, Rosen DC. Medications and their effects on the voice. In: Ben-

ninger MS, Jacobson BH, Johnson AF, eds. *Vocal Arts Medicine: The Care and Prevention of Professional Voice Disorders*. New York, NY: Thieme; 1994:216–225.

78. Baldessarini RJ, Tondo L, Davis P, et al. Decreased risk of suicides and attempts during long-term lithium treatment: a meta-analytic review. *Bipolar Disord*. 2006;8(5, pt 2):625–639.

79. James I, Savage I. Beneficial effect of nadolol on anxiety-induced disturbances of performance in musicians: a comparison with diazepam and placebo. *Am Heart J*. 1984;108(4, pt 2):1150–1155.

80. Birk L. Pharmacotherapy for performance anxiety disorders: occasionally useful but typically contraindicated. *J Clin Psychol*. 2004;60(8):867.

81. Chessick CA, Allen MH, Thase ME, et al. Azapirone for generalized anxiety disorder. *Cochrane Database Syst Rev*. 2006;3:CD006115.

82. Tsuang M, Faraone S, Day M. Schizophrenic disorders. In: Nicholi A, ed. *The New Harvard Guide to Psychiatry*. Cambridge, MA: Harvard University Press; 1988:259–295.

83. Schatzberg AF, Cole JO, DeBattista C. *Manual of Clinical Psychopharmacology*. 3rd ed. Washington, DC: American Psychiatric Association Press; 1997.

84. Arana GW, Rosenbaum JR. *Handbook of Psychiatric Drug Therapy*. 4th ed. Philadelphia, PA: Lippincott Williams & Wilkins; 2000:85–90.

85. Gijsman HJ, Geddes JR, Rendell JM, et al. Antidepressants for bipolar depression: a systematic review of randomized, controlled trials. *Am J Psychiatry*. 2004; 161(9):1537–1547.

86. UK ECT Review Group. Efficacy and safety of electroconvulsive therapy in depressive disorders: a systematic review and meta-analysis. *Lancet*. 2003;361(9360): 799–808.

87. Lieberman JA, Stroup TS, McEvoy JP, et al. Effectiveness of antipsychotic drugs in patients with chronic schizophrenia. *N Engl J Med*. 2005;353(12):1209–1223.

88. Jones PB, Barnes TR, Davies L, et al. Randomized controlled trial of the effect on quality of life of second- vs first-generation antipsychotic drugs in schizophrenia: cost utility of the latest antipsychotic drugs in schizophrenia study (CUtLASS 1). *Arch Gen Psychiatry*. 2006; 63(10):1079–1087.

89. Sullivan PF. Mortality in anorexia nervosa. *Am J Psychiatry*. 1995;152(7):1073–1074.

90. Hudson JI, Hiripi E, Pope HG, Kessler RC. The prevalence and correlates of eating disorders in the National Comorbidity Survey Replication. *Biol Psychiatry*. 2007;61:348–358.

91. Raeburn SD, Hipple J, Delaney W, Chesky K. Surveying popular musicians' health status using convenience samples. *Med Probl Perform Art*. 2003;18(3):113–119.

92. Chesky KS, Hipple J. Musicians' perceptions of widespread drug use among musicians. *Med Probl Perform Art*. 1999;14(4):187–195.

93. Metcalfe R, Firth D, Pollock S, Creed F. Psychiatric morbidity and illness behaviour in female neurologi-

cal inpatients. *J Neurol Neurosurg Psychiatry*. 1988;51: 1387–1390.

94. Gainotti G. Emotional behavior and hemispheric side of lesion. *Cortex*. 1972;8:41–55.

95. Alexander MP, LoVerne SR Jr. Aphasia after left hemispheric intracerebral hemorrhage. *Neurology*. 1980;30: 1193–1202.

96. Mahr G, Leith W. Psychogenic stuttering of adult onset. *J Speech Hear Res*. 1992;35:283–286.

97. Everly GS Jr. *A Clinical Guide to the Treatment of the Human Stress Response*. New York, NY: Plenum; 1989: 40–43.

98. Green J, Snellenberger R. *The Dynamics of Health and Wellness: A Biopsychosocial Approach*. Fort Worth, TX: Holt Reinhardt and Winston; 1991:61–64, 92, 98, 101–136.

99. Lazarus RS, Folkman S. *Stress Appraisal and Coping*. New York, NY: Springer-Verlag; 1984:283.

100. Stroudemire AG. *Psychological Factors Affecting Medical Conditions*. Washington, DC: American Psychiatric Press; 1995:187–192.

101. Averill JR. Personal control over aversive stimuli and its relationship to stress. *Psychol Bull*. 1973;80(4): 286–303.

102. Folkman S. Personal control and stress and coping processes: a theoretical analysis. *J Pers Soc Psychol*. 1984;46(4):839–852.

103. Judge T, Bono JE. Relationship of core self-evaluations traits—self-esteem, generalized self-efficacy, locus of control, and emotional stability—with job satisfaction and job performance: a meta-analysis. *J Appl Psychol*. 2001;86(1):80–92.

104. Zraick RI, Boone DR. Spouse attitudes toward the person with aphasia. *J Speech Hear Res*. 1991;34:123–128.

105. Rosen DC, Sataloff RT, Evans H, Hawkshaw M. Self-esteem and singing: singing healthy, singing hurt. *NATS J*. 1993;49:32–35.

106. Worden JW. *Grief Counseling and Grief Therapy*. New York, NY: Springer-Verlag; 1982:7–18.

107. Adamson JD, Hersuberg D, Shane F. The psychic significance of parts of the body in surgery. In: Howells JG, ed. *Modern Perspectives in the Psychiatric Aspects of Surgery*. New York, NY: Brunner/Mazel; 1976:20–45.

108. Carpenter B. Psychological aspects of vocal fold surgery. In: Gould WJ. Sataloff RT, Spiegel JR, eds. *Voice Surgery*. St Louis, MO: Mosby; 1993:339–343.

109. Macgregor FC. Patient dissatisfaction with results of technically satisfactory surgery. *Aesthetic Plast Surg*. 1981;5:27–32.

110. Ray CJ, Fitzgibbon G. The socially mediated reduction of stress in surgical patients. In: Oborne DJ, Grunberg M, Eisner JR, eds. *Research and Psychology in Medicine*. Vol 2. Oxford, UK: Pergamon; 1979:521–527.

111. Berkowitz JF, Lucente FE. Counseling before laryngectomy. *Laryngoscope*. 1985;95:1332–1336.

112. Gardner WH. Adjustment problems of laryngectomized women. *Arch Otolaryngol*. 1966;83:31–42.

113. Starm H, Koopmans J, Mathieson C. The psychological impact of a laryngectomy: a comprehensive assessment. *J Psychosoc Oncol*. 1991;9:37–58.

114. King M, Novick L, Citrenbaum C. *Irresistible Communication: Creative Skills for the Health Professional*. Philadelphia, PA: Saunders; 1983:21, 22, 115–127.

115. Bady SL. The voice as curative factor in psychotherapy. *Psychoanal Rev*. 1985;72:479–490.

116. Crasilneck HB, Hall J. *Clinical Hypnosis: Principles and Applications*. 2nd ed. Orlando, FL: Grune and Stratton; 1985:60–61.

117. Lankton S. *Practical Magic: A Translation of Basic Neurolinguistic Programming Into Clinical Psychotherapy*. Cupertino, CA: Meta Publications; 1980:174.

118. Watkins JG. *Hypnotherapeutic Techniques*. New York, NY: Irvington; 1987:114.

119. Moses PJ. *The Voice of Neurosis*. New York, NY: Grune and Stratton; 1954.

120. Luchsinger R, Arnold GE. *Voice, Speech, Language; Clinical Communicology: Its Physiology and Pathology*. Belmont, CA: Wadsworth; 1965.

121. Rulnick RK, Heuer RJ, Perez KS, et al. Voice therapy. In: Sataloff RT. *Professional Voice: the Science and Art of Clinical Care*. 2nd ed. San Diego, CA: Singular Publishing; 1997:699–720.

# Impact of the Auditory System on Voice*

*Morgan A. Selleck and Robert Thayer Sataloff*

## Introduction

The auditory system is believed to be a key component in the development and maintenance of excellent voice quality and accuracy. Individuals with profound hearing impairment or total deafness may have impaired voice quality, in addition to common abnormalities in resonance and speech. The possibility of the reverse scenario, a superb auditory system providing better-than-average voice quality, has not been studied well, and the effects of various levels of auditory performance on voice remain largely unknown. This review examines the literature on the effects of different auditory system characteristics on voice quality and accuracy. We believe that it is important to be familiar with what is known currently on this topic and to consider directions for future research.

## Methods

The following databases were searched from their inception to November 2013: PubMed, EBSCO, and CINAHL. The following keywords were used: "hearing impaired," "auditory system," "voice," "professional voice user," "hearing," "singing," and "hearing loss." The references of articles were studied to identify further relevant citations. Additionally, Internet searches of Google and Google Scholar were performed. Relevant articles in English were included for review. Studies were excluded on the basis of the search strategy followed, search keywords, search databases, and articles listed in the search that did not address the topic of interest.

## Background

The production of speech is still not understood fully, but it begins in the brain with a premotor process involving the integration of several kinds of information: auditory, somatosensory, and motor. This information is found in the temporal, parietal, and frontal lobes, including the areas of the brain specialized for speech such as Broca's and Wernicke's areas and elsewhere.[1] The premotor process consists of 3 general tasks: production of an idea, word finding, and then syllabification or production of sounds needed to make each of the words. After this process is complete, articulation is created through 3 key neural pathways: the cerebellar motor path, pyramidal, and extrapyramidal tracts. These tracts synapse in the medulla, which controls the muscles involved in speech such as those of the tongue, lips, and larynx.[2] The complex activities involving the larynx and vocal tract that result in phonation are well known.[3]

The auditory system provides 2 types of control over speech production: feedback control and feed-forward control. Feedback control allows for corrections in phonation using the sensory information acquired while the task is in progress. Feedback allows for a speaker or singer to increase volume in a noisy environment or modulate pitch to match a target.[4] Feed-forward control allows for speech or song to be produced based on previously learned commands without needing constant auditory feedback. Feedback is vital in developing and maintaining normal vocal production.[5] The auditory feedback system is thought to have 3 roles: (1) providing information regarding vocal targets, (2) providing feedback about environmental conditions that may affect the quality

---

*Republished from the *Journal of Voice* with permission from Elsevier.

of vocal production, and (3) contributing to the generation of internal models for the motor plans for voice production.[5] The first role of feedback is important for corrections in pitch, volume, and other attributes that may affect intelligibility of speech. The second role is important in noisy situations, for example, so that the speaker knows to enunciate more clearly, increase amplitude, and reduce speaking rate to increase intelligibility.[5] The third role is essential to the maintenance of a rapid speech rate through development of internal models, allowing for the vocal tract and related structures to be prepared before vocalization and for speech to continue without constant auditory feedback.[6,7]

Feed-forward control uses internal models to control speech speed and voice without dependence on real-time auditory feedback. Given the rapid rate of normal speech, it would be impossible for feedback to be processed and corrections set in place before each new segment of speech if the same rapid rate were to be maintained. Feed-forward control solves this problem.[6] Feed-forward control also allows for speech fluency in postlingually deafened individuals and for phonation in loud noise.[4] It is used by singers performing with orchestras or choirs that mask auditory feedback, for example.

## Discussion

### Hearing Impaired

Hearing impairment provides an obvious, if extreme, example of the importance of audition to phonation and speech. The changes found in the voices of severely hearing impaired people involve alterations in respiration, phonation, and articulation.[8,9]

### Respiration

The lungs provide airflow to allow for vocal fold oscillation. The chest, back, and abdominal musculature contribute to the production of this airflow. The respiratory system also plays a role in controlling pitch through modulating expiratory pressures, which can increase or decrease pitch.

Das et al[10] demonstrated that despite the presence of normal and healthy lung function, children with profound bilateral sensorineural hearing loss (SNHL) have a significantly lower vital capacity and maximum sustained phonation in comparison with normal hearing children. The reduction in vital capacity translates to these children having lower lung volumes to use for vocal production. Lower lung volumes force

these children to take more pauses during speech; hence, they are unable to produce the normal amount of syllables per breath or to sustain a song line for as long as normal. The reduction in maximum sustained phonation is a measure of the individual's ability to manage air supply effectively during voice production. These combined respiration issues lead to changes in pausing patterns during speech with the overall effect leading to a decrease in speech intelligibility.[10] It may be speculated that this relatively suboptimal performance in the power source of the voice also predisposes to phonatory inefficiency and possibly vocal injury, but studies of this possibility are needed.

### Phonation

Much of the literature on the hearing impaired and voice production focuses on phonation. Das et al[10] found uncoordinated contraction and relaxation of the intrinsic and extrinsic laryngeal muscles in the hearing impaired. They discovered a significant reduction in the fast adduction/abduction rate in children with profound bilateral SNHL compared with normal hearing children. From these results, the authors concluded that individuals with SNHL have difficulty in controlling subglottal pressure and tension of the vocal folds, and these difficulties affect phonation.

Ubrig et al[8] studied fundamental frequency and its variability in 40 postlingually deaf adults before and after cochlear implantation (CI). Despite the fact that these individuals have internal motor models and patterns based on their prior hearing experience, there was still a significant difference in phonation without feedback control of the auditory system. The authors noted a significant reduction in fundamental frequency (in males) and a significant reduction in variation in frequency during sustained vowel production (in both genders) after CI compared with their performance before CI. However, once these findings were compared with the control group without CI in both time periods, only the variability in males remained statistically significant. The reductions in variation with sustained vowel production after CI demonstrate that, with auditory feedback, individuals can control their voices better with fewer variations in frequency.

Xu et al studied 21 children, 7 perlingually deafened children with cochlear implants, and 14 children with normal hearing, and their ability to sing accurately. Each child sang one song, and the fundamental frequencies of each note were analyzed. Although there was no difference between the 2 groups in terms of rhythm, the children with CI had a significantly poorer performance in terms of pitch accuracy. Children with CI had a mean deviation of the pitch intervals of 2.86 semitones in comparison with those with normal hearing with a mean deviation of only 1.51 semitones. Despite this deficit in pitch, the authors comment on the achievement of singing in the CI children, given the obstacles of imperfect pitch information supplied by the CI. The authors speculated that deficits in singing skills are a result of poor pitch discrimination skills in the children with CI.[11]

## Articulation

The unique shape of each individual's vocal tract creates vocal individuality and affects audibility. Changes can be made to the voice by altering the position of the tongue and soft palate and the shape of the pharynx.[3] It is accepted generally that such adjustments are made based on auditory feedback and that excellent auditory and vocal abilities are present in elite professional voice users. However, there are no convincing data to confirm or refute this belief, although some findings in hearing impaired patients suggest that the link between audition and phonation can be confirmed at least in that population.

For example, Das et al[10] discovered that children with profound bilateral SNHL have more nasal speech than those with normal hearing. The hypernasality is caused by incomplete closure of the velopharyngeal sphincter during speech production. The additional air escape causes air supply to diminish rapidly, leading to the anomalous pausing for additional inspiratory breaths during speech. It is not known how or why hearing impairment is associated with this behavior.

Ubrig et al found that in men and women after cochlear implantation, there was a reduction in the number of hypernasal voices. These authors speculated that the hypernasality was likely a result of poor velopharyngeal control and suggest that this lack of control was from a lack of auditory feedback during vocal production.[8] However, there is no evidence to support this assumption.

## Hearing Enhanced

The literature on the hearing impaired demonstrates quite clearly the need for an adequately functioning auditory system to produce intelligible speech and "normal" voice. It is clear that faulty audition may be associated with impaired voice. So, it seems reasonable to ask whether an excellent auditory system might lead to a superior voice and whether there are subtle interrelationships along the spectrum of auditory and vocal performances.

## Auditory Discrimination Skills

Several studies have examined the question of a better "ear" leading to a better voice by examining auditory discrimination skills and vocal accuracy. The thought behind these studies is that potentially superior auditory skills would give an advantage in detecting smaller errors, missed by others, in voice production and then lead to a more accurate vocal output as a result of enhanced use of sensory feedback.[12] There is conflicting evidence on the existence of this relationship.

Amir et al[13] and Watts et al[14] found that subjects with superior auditory pitch discrimination had superior vocal pitch accuracy. However, neither study established a causal relationship. Amir et al[13] did find that all subjects with superior auditory skills had more accurate vocal production, but the reverse relationship was not found.

Estis et al[15] also studied pitch matching and discrimination in 40 individuals: 20 trained singers and 20 untrained singers. Trained singers' pitch matching and discrimination accuracy were significantly better than untrained singers' pitch. Interestingly, of the 20 untrained singers, 10 were considered accurate pitch matchers (a mean semitone difference score of <1 semitone from the target tone). The authors suggest that these findings indicate that inherent factors, and musical training, may play roles in pitch-matching skills. Results also suggested a relationship between pitch discrimination and pitch matching, but no significant correlation was found. Contrary to most of this study's data, 2 of the 10 untrained inaccurate singers (a mean semitone difference score >1 semitone from the target tone), despite the poor pitch-matching skills, had accurate pitch discrimination skills.[15]

Bradshaw et al,[16] Dalla Bella et al,[17] Pfordresher et al,[18] and Moore et al[19] studied this relationship but found no association between auditory discrimination and accurate vocal production. A study by Zarate et al[12] took this investigation a step further by looking for a direct cause-effect relationship between training-enhanced auditory discrimination and vocal accuracy. In nonmusicians, the training led to significantly enhanced auditory discrimination skills, but this training did not translate to an improvement in vocal accuracy. Interestingly, this study also examined the patients' singing tasks while the subjects underwent functional magnetic resonance imaging (fMRI). The fMRI demonstrated an increased functional connectivity among auditory cortical regions, but there was no increased connectivity among other regions thought to be involved in audio-vocal integration. It is possible that the training provided was not sufficient to improve vocal accuracy. The authors suggest that combined auditory and vocal motor training might be required to lead to improved vocal accuracy. Nevertheless, review of all these studies highlights continued uncertainty about the presence and nature of any relationship between auditory excellence and superior phonatory performance.

## Internal Model

The internal model is a neural pathway for motor patterns of voice production that allows for the interface of the output of pitch and the neural motor patterns that control the muscles of the voice creating the pitch. The production of these internal models relies on auditory feedback. Fundamental frequency control depends on both the internal model and the auditory feedback.[5] Studies have demonstrated that trained singers have superior pitch-matching abilities in comparison with untrained singers and demonstrate superior performance even in the presence of masking that interferes with auditory feedback.[7] This resistance to the effects of masking may be a result of the trained singers' greater-than-normal reliance on internal models.[5]

In a study by Jones and Keough,[5] 40 women, 20 of whom were trained singers, were asked to sing certain notes. Initially, they heard their F0 unaltered as a baseline; in the second phase, they were given frequency-altered feedback; and then in a third phase, they were able to hear their F0 unaltered again. In the presence of the altered feedback, both groups produced a higher mean F0 than F0 values produced at baseline, but trained singers had a mean F0 lower than that of the nonsingers. Interestingly, once exposed to their unaltered F0 in the third phase, the trained singers had after-effects that nonsingers did not experience. Their F0 values were significantly higher than those produced at baseline. These results demonstrate that the internal model can be altered easily, after even a brief exposure of 30 trials, as in this study, creating a false relationship between motor commands and the expected F0 output. These results also suggest that the internal model is relied on more in trained singers than in others, most likely as a result of singers' education and vocal training.

Zarate and Zatorre[20] studied the interface of the auditory system and the vocal motor system in the brain by examining the fMRI of nonmusicians and experienced singers. The authors hypothesized that to gain better control of pitch, experienced singers would need to recruit different regions within the brain compared with nonmusicians while singing. The study had subjects sing a single tone with either unaltered auditory feedback or pitch-shifted auditory feedback. When pitch-shifted feedback was presented, the subjects were told to either ignore or compensate for the changed auditory feedback, helping to identify the neural areas involved in the interaction of auditory information and vocal motor output. The results demonstrated that nonmusicians were less accurate than singers in the unaltered singing task, but both groups recruited similar neural areas: bilateral auditory areas, primary motor and premotor areas, right mid-dorsal insula, somatosensory areas, thalamus, and cerebellum. In the altered singing task when participants were asked to ignore the shifted auditory feedback, the singers were more accurate than the nonmusicians. Nonmusicians, during the ignore singing task, had statistically greater neural activity within the supramarginal gyrus and the mouth region of the primary motor cortex. Singers had significantly greater neural activity within the auditory cortices bilaterally and the left putamen compared with the nonmusicians during the ignore task. There was no significant difference between the two groups in the altered singing task when participants were asked to compensate for the difference. Nonmusicians in the compensate task had significantly greater activity in the left dorsal premotor cortex compared with singers. Singers had greater activity in the anterior cingulate cortex, superior temporal sulcus, and putamen. The authors suggest that these results indicate that vocal training allows for improved pitch control and a difference in approach and thus in the neural areas recruited to complete the vocal tasks. During both pitch-altered tasks, the singers had increased auditory activity. The putamen involvement for singers indicates that they are using a developed and ingrained vocal motor program to complete both the singing tasks. The authors propose that it is the dorsal premotor cortex that acts as the basic interface of the 2 systems, but with training the auditory cortices, putamen and anterior cingulated cortex are recruited as individuals monitor their auditory feedback more closely.

## Professional Singing

Professional singing relies on accuracy of intonation and excellent control of fundamental frequency. During normal speech, pitch targets are relative to the speaker's own voice, but in singing, pitch targets are absolute with fundamental frequencies expected to match nearly exactly the musical notes being played.[5]

Murbe et al[21] studied pitch control in 28 students, at the beginning of their professional singing education. Interested in how feedback of the auditory and kinesthetic systems plays a role in pitch control, they had participants sing a triad pattern with and without masking noise in legato and staccato, and at a slow and fast rates. The deviations of their tones from the standard were used as the measure of their accuracy of intonation. The results demonstrated that masking impaired mean pitch accuracy by 14% in all subjects. The authors suggest that this result indicates that the kinesthetic feedback system plays a significant role in pitch control. Additionally, the study found that, in the absence of auditory feedback, singers had increased mean deviations with both the staccato and the fast conditions in comparison with the legato and slow singing conditions. These results suggest that auditory feedback becomes more critical with increasing technical difficulty of the performance.

Murbe et al[22] again examined pitch control in the same group of 22 professional singers after 3 years of professional training. They had participants again sing the triad pattern with and without masking noise in legato and staccato and at slow and fast rates. They found that in the presence of masking, there was no significant difference in the mean deterioration of pitch accuracy when comparing the subjects before and after training. The authors suggest that this lack of a difference indicates that auditory feedback's contribution to pitch control is the same, with no change with training. However, this conclusion should be interpreted with caution in our opinion. Students accepted for professional singing training usually already have substantial singing experience. It is possible that there is a training effect, just that it had occurred already before their entering the study.

Nikjeh et al[23] examined difference limens for frequency (DLF) and pitch production accuracy (PPA) in 20 vocalists, 21 instrumentalists, and 21 nonmusicians. They found that musicians, both the vocalists and instrumentalists, had a PPA 6 times that of the nonmusicians, but there was no difference in PPA between the vocalists and instrumentalists. The authors suggest that these results indicate that any musical training, for either voice or instrument, develops in the musician an enhanced sensitivity for pitch. The lack of difference between the 2 groups, the authors feel, is a result of the simplicity of test used to determine PPA. The timing of the development of the pitch accuracy is unknown, and the study found no significant correlation between years of training or age when training began and pitch discrimination. Although the PPA was not significantly different between the vocalists and the instrumentalists, the

vocalists had minimal response variability in their group (0%–3%) in comparison with instrumentalists (0%–18%). According to the authors, these results imply that vocal training has an effect on laryngeal neuromuscular control, so that pitch is produced both accurately and consistently. The DLF for musical tones was 50% smaller in musicians compared with nonmusicians. The DLF did not differ significantly between the vocalists and the instrumentalists, with both groups additionally having minimal response variability. Nonmusicians scored worse in PPA in comparison with DLF, perhaps indicating that hearing pitch differences is easier than producing those differences. Considering all 3 groups, a significant positive correlation was found between PPA and DLF. However, after breaking down the results into their individual groups, only instrumental musicians and vocal musicians with instrumental training had significant correlations between PPA and DLF. The authors suggest that this result indicates that instrumental music training allows for an enhanced auditory perception-laryngeal musculature relationship.[23]

## Conclusions

### Hearing Impaired

Current literature on the hearing impaired suggests that the impaired auditory system leads to changes in respiration, phonation, and articulation affecting voice production. In terms of the respiratory changes, studies suggest that the hearing impaired have decreased speech intelligibility because low vital capacities force individuals to take more frequent pauses during speech. Current literature, however, does not address whether this phonatory inefficiency leads to vocal injury in these individuals. Studies also suggest that the hearing impaired have problems controlling their subglottal pressure and tension of the vocal folds leading to a reduction in the fast adduction/abduction rate of their vocal folds.

Studies focusing on articulation have found hypernasality in the voices of the hearing impaired and suggest a cause as lack of auditory feedback leading to poor closure of the velopharyngeal sphincter during speech production. Future research is indicated to further understand if these adjustments to the vocal tract are made based on auditory feedback. If a relationship does exist between the vocal tract musculature adjustments and the auditory feedback, is the professional voice user able to make these adjustments in a more effective manner than the average voice user? These issues should be studied further in the hearing impaired, untrained, and trained voice users with direct observation of the vocal tract musculature.

### Hearing Enhanced

The literature regarding those with a superior auditory system is much more limited in comparison with that on the hearing impaired. The exact relationship between auditory pitch discrimination and pitch accuracy in those with superior capabilities is uncertain with a great deal of conflicting evidence. Most of the studies are observational and thus unable to determine conclusively whether a cause-effect relationship exists between pitch discrimination and accuracy. Future studies must focus efforts on defining this relationship with prospective interventional studies that would allow for a determination of a cause-effect relationship. Outside factors, especially previous musical training, both instrumental and voice, must be controlled carefully to elucidate this relationship. Additionally, future research should address the underlying reasons, inherent factors, musical training, or both, for this potential relationship.

The internal model is an important part of voice production, the neural pathway that allows for the interface of auditory feedback and neural voice motor patterns. Current evidence suggests that trained singers may activate different neural components in comparison with the untrained while performing singing tasks. This superior neural combination may be responsible for singers' superior pitch accuracy in situations with a loss of auditory feedback. The understanding of the internal model and the key neural areas involved should be a focus of future research, to better understand how it interacts with auditory feedback and affects phonation. Studies should attempt to discern how the neural areas shift during training, examining students at the beginning and end of their instruction, to better understand how the shift in neural activity occurs and how it affects voice production.

The professional singer has additional demands placed on his or her vocal accuracy that require additional study and assist in further developing the relationship between the auditory system and the voice. Current evidence suggests that professional voice users use both auditory and kinesthetic feedbacks in producing accurate pitch, but with increasing difficulty of the performance, auditory feedback plays a more critical role. There is conflicting evidence on the role that training plays in developing auditory feedback. It also has been suggested

that training does not enhance auditory feedback skills, although future studies are warranted to better control for previous training experiences—for both instrumental and vocal education—as these may be potential confounding factors. The relationship between the auditory system and the voice production still remains largely unknown, despite its potentially great importance—especially to those at the extremes, the hearing impaired and professional voice users. Future research is critical to clarify this relationship and allow for better clinical intervention to improve the voices of those with hearing loss and cochlear implants and of professionals seeking vocal excellence.

## References

1. Guenther FH, Vladusich T. A neural theory of speech acquisition and production. *J Neurolinguistics*. 2012;25:408–422.
2. William S, Wang Y. Speech. AccessScience; 2012. http://www.accessscience.com.ezproxy2.library.drexel.edu. Accessed January 6, 2014.
3. Sataloff R. *Professional Voice: The Science and Art of Clinical Care*. 3rd ed. San Diego, CA: Plural Publishing; 2005:143–177, 237–291.
4. Tourville JA, Reilly KJ, Guenther FH. Neural mechanisms underlying auditory feedback control of speech. *Neuroimage*. 2008;39:1429–1443.
5. Jones JA, Keough D. Auditory-motor mapping for pitch control in singers and nonsingers. *Exp Brain Res*. 2008;190:279–287.
6. Borden GJ. An interpretation of research of feedback interruption in speech. *Brain Lang*. 1979;7:307–319.
7. Watts C, Murphy J, Barnes-Burroughs K. Pitch matching accuracy of trained singers, untrained subjects with talented singing voices, and untrained subjects with nontalented singing voices in conditions of varying feedback. *J Voice*. 2003;17:185–194.
8. Ubrig MT, Goffi-Gomez MV, Weber R, et al. Voice analysis of postlingually deaf adults pre- and postcochlear implantation. *J Voice*. 2011;25:692–699.
9. Yuba T, Itoh T, Kaga K. Unique technological voice method (The YUBA Method) shows clear improvement in patients with cochlear implants in singing. *J Voice*. 2009;23:119–124.
10. Das B, Chatterjee I, Kumar S. Laryngeal aerodynamics in children with hearing impairment versus age and height matched normal hearing peers. *ISRN Otolaryngol*. 2013;2013:394604.
11. Xu L, Zhou N, Chen X, Li Y, Schultz HM, Zhao X, Han D. Vocal singing by perlingually deafened children with cochlear implants. *Hear Res*. 2009;255:129–134.
12. Zarate JM, Delhommeau K, Wood S, Zatorre RJ. Vocal accuracy and neural plasticity following micromelody-discrimination training. *PLoS One*. 2010;5:1–15.

13. Amir O, Amir N, Kishon-Rabin L. The effect of superior auditory skills on vocal accuracy. *J Acoust Soc Am*. 2003;113:1102–1108.

14. Watts C, Moore R, McCaghren K. The relationship between vocal pitch-matching skills and pitch discrimination skills in untrained accurate and inaccurate singers. *J Voice*. 2005;19:534–543.

15. Estis JM, Dean-Claytor A, Moore RE, Rowell TL. Pitch-matching accuracy in trained singers and untrained individuals: the impact of musical interference and noise. *J Voice*. 2009;25:173–180.

16. Bradshaw E, McHenry MA. Pitch discrimination and pitch matching abilities of adults who sing inaccurately. *J Voice*. 2005;19:431–439.

17. Dalla Bella S, Giguere JF, Peretz I. Singing proficiency in the general population. *J Acoust Soc Am*. 2007;121:1182–1189.

18. Pfordresher P, Brown S. Poor-pitch singing in the absence of "tone deafness." *Music Perception*. 2007;25:95–115.

19. Moore RE, Estis J, Gordon-Hickey S, Watts C. Pitch discrimination and pitch matching abilities with vocal and nonvocal stimuli. *J Voice*. 2008; 22:399–407.

20. Zarate JM, Zatorre RJ. Experience-dependent neural substrates involved in vocal pitch regulation during singing. *Neuroimage*. 2008;40:1871–1887.

21. Murbe D, Pabst F, Hofmann G, Sundberg J. Significance of auditory and kinesthetic feedback to singers' pitch control. *J Voice*. 2002;16:44–51.

22. Murbe D, Pabst F, Hofmann G, Sundberg J. Effects of a professional solo singer education on auditory and kinesthetic feedback—a longitudinal study of singers' pitch control. *J Voice*. 2004;18:236–241.

23. Nikjeh DA, Lister JJ, Frisch SA. The relationship between pitch discrimination and vocal production: comparison of vocal and instrumental musicians. *J Acoust Soc Am*. 2009;125:328–338.

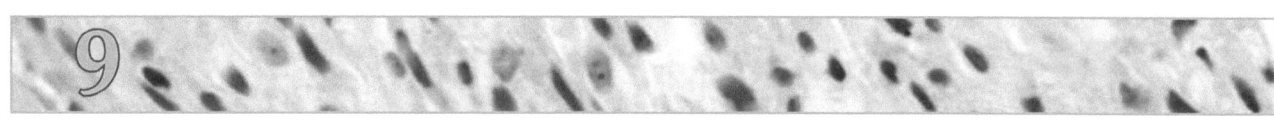

# Laryngeal Manifestations of Respiratory Disorders

*Abdul-Latif Hamdan, Robert Thayer Sataloff, and Mary J. Hawkshaw*

## Nose, Paranasal Sinuses, and Voice

Diseases and masses of the nose and paranasal sinuses may impact voice quality and phonation. Based on a review of the literature, the authors propose four possible mechanisms by which nasal and paranasal sinus disorders may cause phonatory changes.

### One: Alteration in Humidity

The nose acts as a humidifier that regulates the temperature and humidity of air during inspiration. Nasal obstruction secondary to a deviated septum, hypertrophic turbinates, nasal valve collapse, or lesion arising from the adjacent cavities, leads to mouth breathing which becomes the path of least resistance. The loss of nasal humidification results in drying of the pharyngeal and laryngeal mucosa. Given the crucial role of humidity in phonation, affected patients may complain of vocal changes. Sivasankar and Fisher have shown that breathing by mouth for 15 minutes can result in a change in phonation threshold pressure and self-perceived effort to talk.[1] The authors compared two groups of female subjects, oral breathers and nasal breathers, finding that nasal breathing reduced vocal effort in 70% of the cases. The increase in vocal effort witnessed in the oral breathing group was attributed to thinning of the mucous layer. This layer plays a key role in regulating the influx of water in and out of the vocal fold cover and, as such, is vulnerable to dehydration induced by mouth breathing. See Figure 9–1. Verdolini et al have demonstrated clearly that hydration and exposure to humidity at a concentration of 85% to 100% can decrease the phonation threshold pressure, the pressure needed to set the vocal folds into vibration.[2,3] Similarly, Solomon et al in more than one study have demonstrated that systemic hydration can attenuate the increase in phonation threshold pressure witnessed after prolonged phonatory tasks. One study was conducted on 4 women, 3 of whom exhibited an increase in self-perceived vocal effort following loud talking for 2 hours. The increase in vocal effort was attributed to glottic insufficiency seen on laryngeal videostroboscopy. In another study conducted on 4 men, the effect of vocal loading on the phonation threshold pressure was observed in all subjects, and the beneficial effect of systemic hydration was evident in two.[4,5]

Analogous to the aforementioned effects of dehydration and mouth breathing on voice, snoring caused by nasal obstruction also may predispose to vocal changes. The effect of snoring on voice has been investigated on 30 snorers compared with 30 controls. The results showed a significant difference in the prevalence of hoarseness between snorers and non-snorers.[6] Similarly, the usage of continuous positive airway pressure (CPAP) without a humidifier has been proven to impact voice quality negatively. A study on the impact of nasal continuous positive airway pressure revealed significantly higher prevalence of hoarseness, an increase in the cycle-to-cycle variations in intensity and frequency, and a decrease in the fundamental frequency and habitual pitch compared with controls. The acoustic changes were attributed to the drying effect of inhaling air without humidification.[7] These results corroborate the findings by Hemler et al that showed an increase in the perturbation parameters following inhalation of dry

159

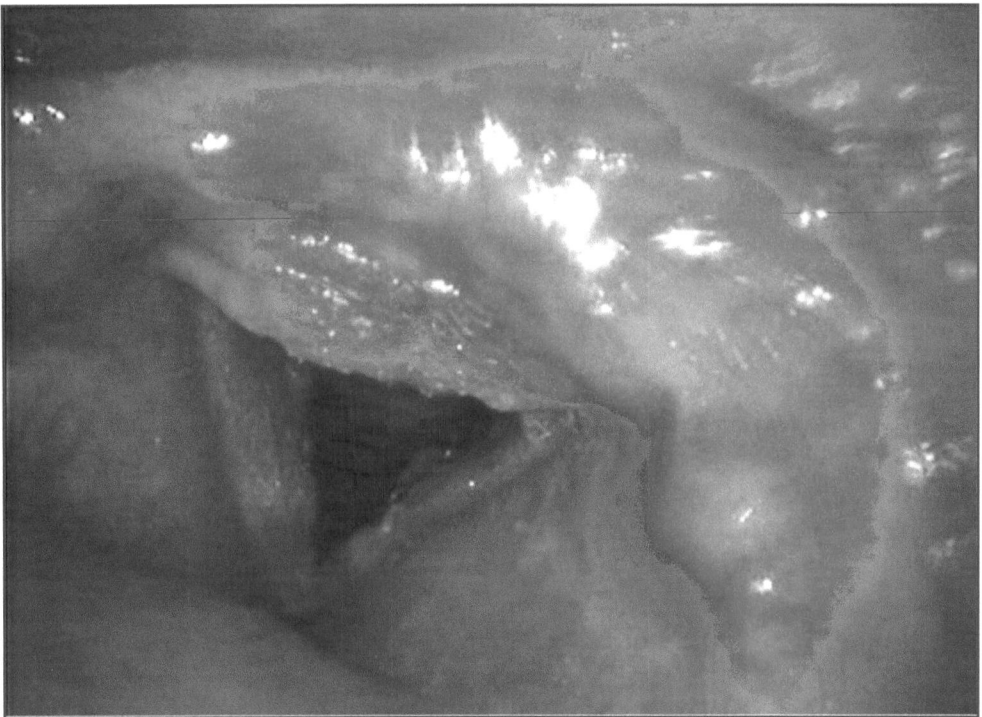

**Figure 9–1.** A 40-year-old women with symptoms of throat clearing, dryness, and change in voice quality. Laryngeal examination showing evidence of laryngitis sicca.

air for 10 minutes. The authors alluded to the crucial role of air humidity in phonation.[8]

## Two: Direct Irritation of the Vocal Folds By Inhaled Particles and Pathogens

The nose carries a thin mucociliary blanket (McB) that is secreted by the nasal and paranasal mucosal lining. The McB acts as a filter to inhaled pollutants and traps undesired pathogens and particles. Loss of this blanket secondary to bacterial infection, inherited diseases such as cystic fibrosis, diseases of the immune system, allergy, or following extensive sinus surgery, can lead to direct inhalation and deposition of these particles or pathogens in the upper and lower respiratory tract. As a result, patients may suffer from change in voice quality, vocal fatigue, and throat symptoms. As review, phonatory changes following inhalation of air pollutants may be the result of three mechanisms: One is the direct deposition of these particles on the vocal folds with subsequent edema and inflammation that may result in alterations in voice quality and phonatory disturbances. The second possible mechanism for the phonatory changes secondary to inhalation of air pollutants is cough. Although this is elicited as a defensive behav-

ior upon direct contact of the inhaled particles with the vocal folds, inadvertently it can lead to vocal fold surface damage, hemorrhage, and mucosal tears. See Figures 9–2 and 9–3. The third mechanism is through the effect of inhaled particles on the lower airway.[9] The impact of lower airway diseases is discussed more thoroughly later in this chapter.

## Three: Alteration in Resonance

The nose and, to a lesser extent, paranasal sinuses, in addition to the oral cavity, pharynx, and pyriform sinus, play a role as resonators. Resonance, defined as amplification of sound by reflection on various structures, is a component of voice production. In professional voice users, resonance is crucial in differentiating one's vocal timbre. It is also of crucial audibility and a focus of attention in vocal pedagogy and therapy. By using resonance properly, singers embrace the audibility and quality of their voices and learn how to project with minimal glottal effort.[10] The nasality of sound is often referred to as nasalance, an acoustic term that reflects "the ratio of nasal acoustic energy to nasal plus oral acoustic energy" in speech.[11] Patients may be stratified as being hyponasal as in cases of nasal polyposis and adenoid hypertrophy, or hypernasal as in cases of velopharyngeal incompetence. It is important to recognize that nasalance may vary with different languages, dialects, and with the ratio of vowels to consonants in a sentence.[12-14] Not surprisingly, nasal and paranasal sinus surgery can impact speech and vocal characteristics. In a study by Hosemann et al on the impact of endoscopic sinus surgery on voice, 6 out of the 21 patients with sinusitis who had surgery had noticeable change in voice quality. More so, there was a decrease in the bandwidth of the formants of vowel /a/ postoperatively. This effect was more pronounced in those who had total ethmoidectomy and bilateral surgery compared with those who had minor disease and had surgery on one side only.[15] Similarly, the study by Chen et al on the effect of sinus surgery on speech using voice recording before and one month after surgery, reported significant effect on nasality and on the acoustic signal in operated patients. There was a decrease in the nasality for the high vowel /i/ and an increase for the non-high vowel /ae/, which were commensurate with the spectral changes observed.[16]

## Four: By Affecting the Lower Airway

The coexistence of paranasal sinus disease and lower airway disease, often referred to as the "unified airway disease," as in patients with allergy and or asthma, has been an issue of investigation for many decades. The pathogenic relationship has been based on many mechanisms, perhaps the most important of which is postnasal drip with subsequent seeding of inflammatory and infectious secretions into the lower airway. The continuous postnasal discharge, swept posteriorly by the ciliary action of the nasal mucosa, may itself act as an irritant and as a source of infection to the larynx and lower airway. Other suggested mechanisms include presence of paranasal cell mediators, the nasal-bronchial reflex, decreased responsiveness of ß-agonist receptors due to infection in the sinuses, and stimulation of extrathoracic airway receptors thus provoking lower airway irritability.[17-19]

The pathogenic relationship between sinusitis and asthma has been underscored by the improvement in breathing following endoscopic sinus surgery. The long-term effect of functional endoscopic

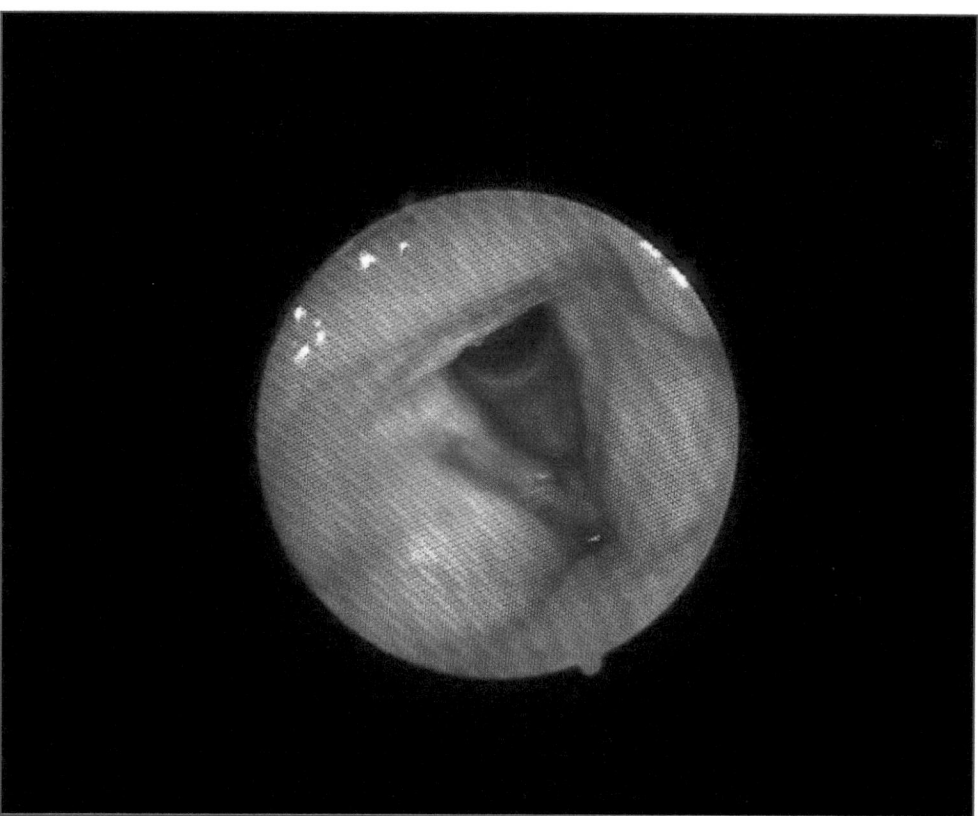

**Figure 9–2.** Right vocal fold hemorrhage and polyp in a professional voice user following a prolonged phonotraumatic behavior.

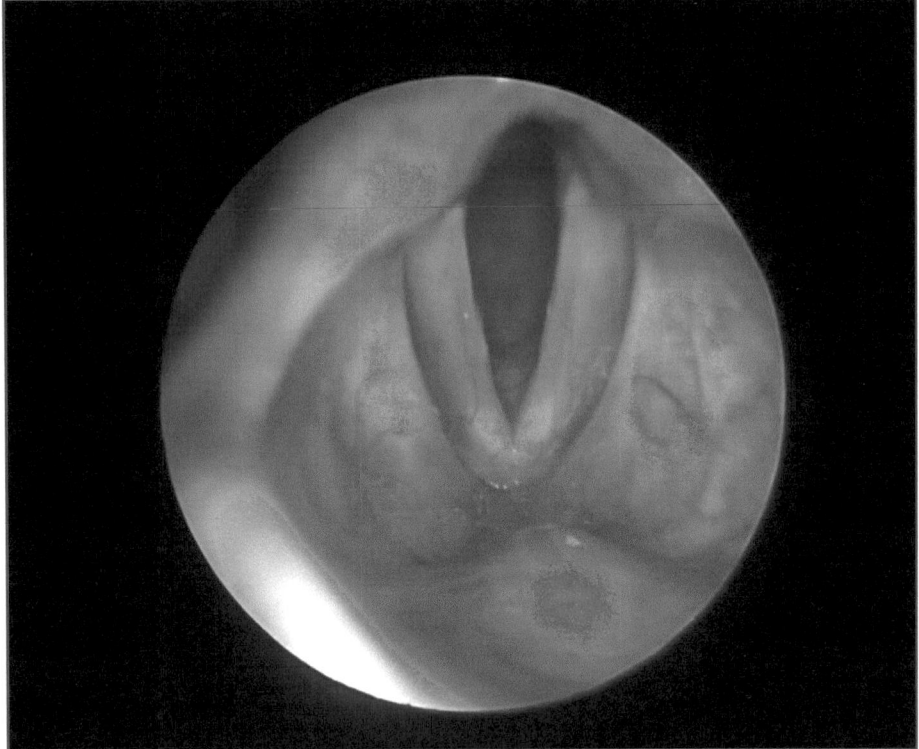

A

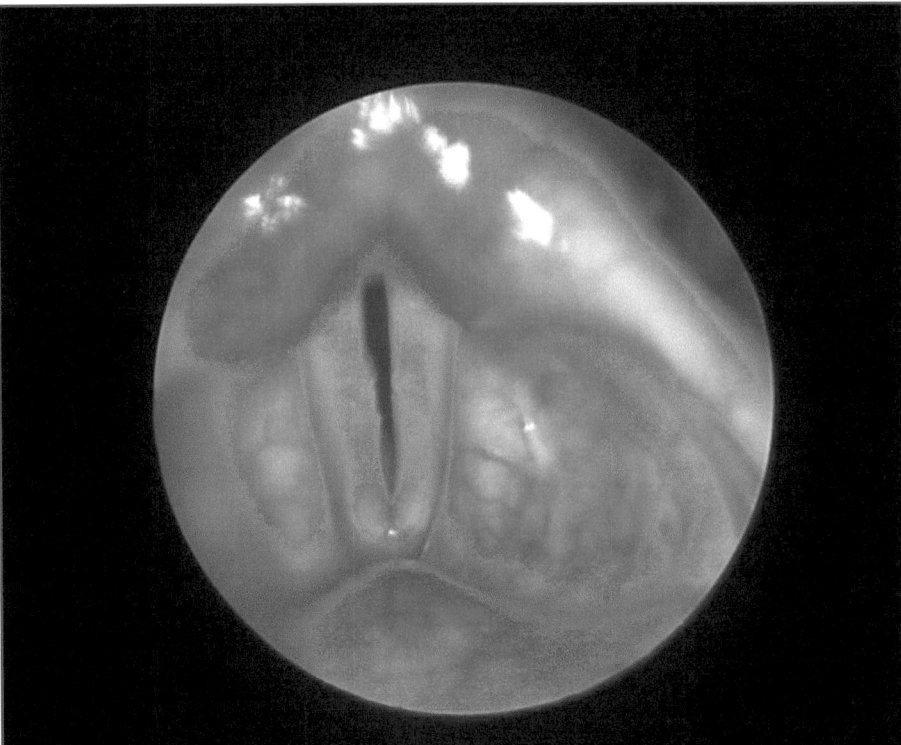

B

Figure 9–3. A 34-year-old male singer presenting with acute loss of the high notes and throat pain following a strenuous performance. Laryngeal videostroboscopic examination a few days after revealed right vocal fold mucosal tear. **A**. While breathing, **B**. while attempting phonation.

sinus surgery on asthma was evaluated by Senior et al using a questionnaire that was answered by 72 patients who underwent surgery.[20] The follow-up time ranged from 6 to 10.6 years. Of 30 patients who had asthma as a comorbid disease, 27 reported improvement in their asthma, and 74.1% reported a decline in the number of asthma attacks.[20] Similarly, a study by Ikeda et al in 15 patients who had endonasal endoscopic sinus surgery, both peak expiratory flow and total intake of glucocorticoid were compared 6 months prior to surgery and 6 months after surgery. There was a marked improvement in the peak expiratory flow in all patients and a reduced need for intake of glucocorticoid in almost half the patients.[21]

## Oral Cavity, Oropharyngeal Cavity, and Voice

The oral and oropharyngeal cavities are integral parts of the vocal tract, the shape of which can markedly impact voice quality. Anatomical and pathologic variations in these cavities carry important sequalae on the resonant characteristics of the vocal signal. A review of the literature supports the link between voice and variations in the dimensions of the oral and oropharyngeal cavities.[22–26] In a normal physiologic state, through the position and manipulation of the articulators such as lips, tongue, and jaw, one can tune his or her voice. Protruding the lips for instance can lower all the formants whereas lifting the larynx does the opposite. Similarly, moving the mandible affects mostly the position of the first formant whereas movement of the tongue affects mostly the position of the second formant. Modulating the shape of the laryngopharyngeal complex may also cluster the formants' energy for a better performance.[22] Today with the applicability of real time and dynamic magnetic resonance imaging (MRI) as emerging speech research tools, the interplay between the structures of the laryngopharyngeal complex and voice is better understood. There are more and more reports on the usage of radiologic imaging in the configuration of vocal tract dimensions at various registers. Recently high temporal fidelity with high spatiotemporal resolution in capturing the shape of the vocal tract during speech has been reported.[27] Another report by Echternach et al using dynamic MRI on 12 professional singers who were asked to sing the vowel /a/ using an ascending scale and at three different degrees of loudness, articulatory differences such as lip opening, pharyngeal width, and position of the larynx in the vertical dimension, were shown to vary with loudness and pitch. The pharyngeal width varied more with sound pressure rather than with vocal pitch.[28]

In addition to the length and configuration of the oropharyngeal complex as being determinants of formants' position and dispersion, the dimensions of the palate are also strongly linked to vocal classification. The study by Marunick et al on nine female singers demonstrated that palatal dimensions, in particular the depth and volume, can assist in stratifying a singer's voice as soprano, mezzo and alto.[23] Similarly, Macari et al reported that rapid maxillary expansion impacts the first two formants, F1 and F2 for the vowel /a/. The study was conducted on 14 patients who had maxillary constriction and underwent treatment.[24] See Figure 9–4. Along the same line of investigation, facial measurements, namely, length and projection of the upper and lower jaw, related to the fundamental frequency and habitual pitch. A significant negative moderate correlation between maxillary and mandibular width and F0 has been reported in a study on 50 subjects. Similarly there is a significant association between F3, F4, and the length of the mandible and maxilla for the vowels /a/, /i/, /o/, and /u/.[23]

That strong interplay between the oral cavity, pharyngeal dimensions, and voice is also clearly displayed in numerous reports that relate obesity to dysphonia in the context of variations in the oropharyngeal morphology. Da Cunha et al reported in their investigation of 45 obese patients, a higher prevalence of phonatory symptoms, namely, hoarseness and vocal strangulation compared to non-obese subjects.[29] Busetto et al demonstrated an inverse relationship between measurements of the upper airway and several obesity parameters. The cross-sectional area of the pharynx and oropharyngeal cavity correlated negatively with body mass index, waist, hip, and sagittal abdominal diameter.[30] Considering the intimate relationship between obesity and pharyngeal morphology, and given the role of this latter in voice production, it stands to reason that obesity as a morbid condition impacts significantly voice, at least at the oropharyngeal level.

Oropharyngeal variations may also cause phonatory changes thru their predisposition to snoring and/or obstructive sleep apnea. In a report on 30 patients who snore versus 30 controls, the prevalence of hoarseness was significantly higher in the snoring group.[6] This can be attributed to narrowing of the oropharyngeal lumen, thickening of the pharyngeal wall, and/or elongation of the epiglottis.[31,32] Shelton et al reported a direct relationship between the amount of adipose tissue in the vicinity of the pharyngeal airway and the severity of apnea. There was a direct correlation between the volume of adipose tissue and the apnea/hypopnea index.[33] In another study using magnetic resonance imaging, Mortimore et al demonstrated that even nonobese subjects with sleep apnea/hypopnea syndrome have more fat in

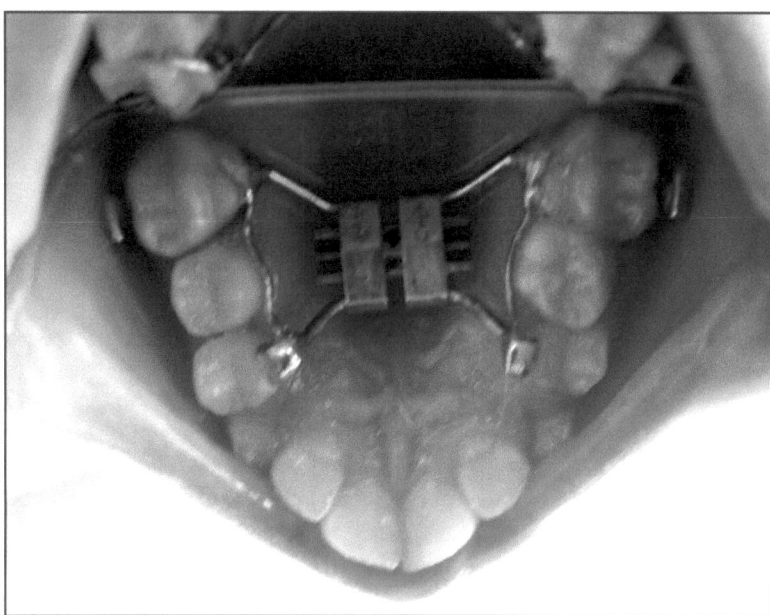

**Figure 9–4.** Rapid maxillary expansion device inserted in a patient with maxillary constriction. The patient had a decrease in F1/a/ and F2/a/ after treatment.

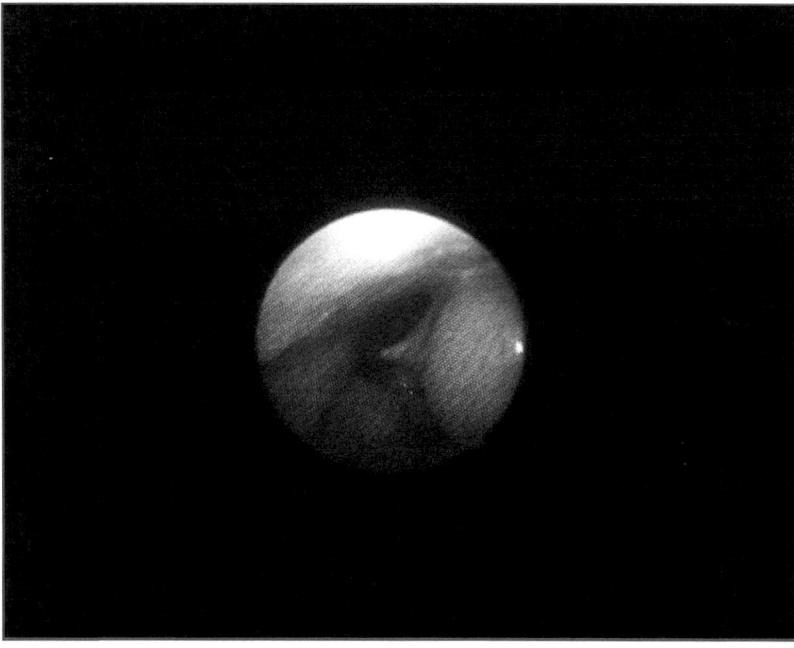

**Figure 9–5.** A 28-year-old man presenting with change in voice quality and mild shortness of breath. Fiberoptic laryngeal examination shows the presence of an epiglottic cyst.

the upper airway in comparison to subjects of same weight and no history of apnea.[34]

Similarly, masses of the oral cavity and oropharynx have an effect on voice quality. Affected patients may complain of change in their vocal characteristics, loss of vocal power and range, in addition to impairment in swallowing and breathing. Examples would include patients with enlarged tonsils, vallecular cysts, or hypertrophic lingual thyroid. See Figure 9–5. Orbelo et al reported the case of a 10-year-old boy who presented with dysphonia secondary a congenital lingual thyroid gland. Although the patient had concomitant vocal folds pathology, his voice quality improved following lingual thyroidectomy.[35] Similarly Erylimaz and Basal reported a 22-year-old man who presented with dysphonia and dysphagia secondary to a lingual thyroid. Using both the transoral and transhyoid approach, the gland was removed successfully and the patient's symptoms improved markedly.[36]

Surgeries that alter the shape and position of the mandible, maxilla, and hyoid bone have also been shown to impact voice and speech. This has been attributed to the subsequent changes in the resonance characteristics of these structures.[37–40] To name a few is the effect of tonsillectomy, or adenoidectomy on voice, exemplified by an increase in F2 /i/ and /a/. Similarly, extirpation of soft tissues such as partial glossectomy can result in a significant increase in F2 and F3.[39]

## Laryngeal Pathology and Voice

The configuration of the vocal tract has a strong impact on voice quality. By mechanism of reflection on its various walls, the vocal signal that originates at the level of the vocal folds is amplified carrying distinctive acoustic features, characterizing one's vocal identity. By altering the outline and thickness of the vocal tract wall, the position and dispersion of the formants, often referred to as preferred harmonics, are modulated. As a result, any change in the shape of the vocal tract can result in change in voice quality. Roers et al examined the vocal tract morphological changes or differences and their relation to voice classification. In their study on 132 radiologic images, they demonstrated that the length of the vocal tract significantly varied with different voice classification.[26]

Not only functional variations in the vocal tract configuration are causes of voice disorders, but also systemic and local diseases as well. This has been clearly demonstrated in the literature through the numerous reports on the change in voice quality in patients with inflammatory, benign, and neoplastic laryngeal lesions. The laryngeal manifestations of autoimmune diseases on voice have been thoroughly discussed in Chapter 12 of this book. Another example of laryngeal mass is false vocal fold bulk seen in a patient with laryngocele who may present with change in voice quality and possible airway symptoms. See Figure 9–6.

Laryngoceles are abnormal dilatation of the Morgani ventricle. Etiologies such as congenital malformation, increased intralaryngeal pressure, and/or laryngeal tissue laxity have been suggested.[41] Other causes such as neck surgeries and trauma must be ruled out. Affected patients may be asymptomatic;

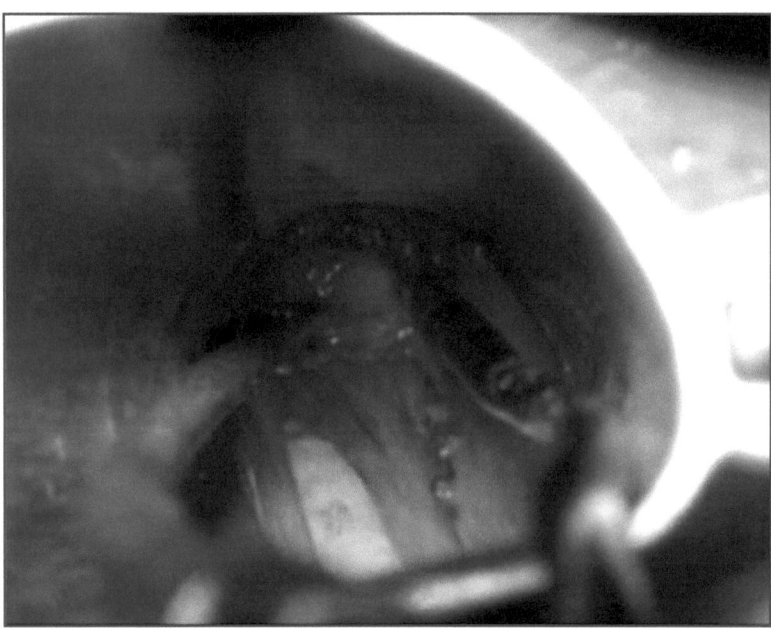

**Figure 9–6.** Case of internal laryngocele presenting with throat discomfort, foreign body sensation, and change in voice quality. Picture showing resection of the laryngocele using cold steel instruments and the Thulium laser.

however, symptoms such as dysphagia, or shortness of breath, in addition to change in voice quality may prevail. In a review by Luzzago et al of 18 cases, hoarseness, airway symptoms, and neck masses were the most common symptoms present in 44% of the cases.[42] The laryngopharyngeal symptoms are varied due to the extension of the laryngocele internally within the endolaryngeal lumen. Laryngoceles have also been seen in patients with chronic ventricular phonation as reported by Dray et al.[43]

Laryngeal surgery that results in soft tissue resection can also markedly affect voice quality. The impact of supraglottic laryngectomy on voice in 33 male patients revealed a reduction in the maximum phonation time and fundamental frequency with an increase in the perturbation parameters and noise to harmonics ratio.[44] Similarly following vertical hemilaryngectomy, there is also worsening of most of the acoustic parameters. In a study by Kim et al on 13 patients treated with vertical laryngectomy, there was a significant difference in the mean flow rate and perturbation parameters in comparison to controls. These phonatory changes were attributed to changes in the supraglottic and glottic configuration, namely, supraglottic voicing, incomplete closure, abnormalities in arytenoid adduction, and blunting of the anterior commissure.[45] When combined with radiation therapy, laryngeal surgery results generally in worse phonatory results. In a review of the voice and swallowing condition following laser endoscopic laryngeal excision, Jepsen et al has reported poorer outcome in patients who were irradiated.[46] Nevertheless with the introduction of robotic surgery, vocal dysfunction has been markedly reduced. In a prospective study by Roh et al on 21 patients with early glottic cancer who underwent partial supraglottic resection, the functional voice outcome was not affected.[47]

## Obstructive Airway Diseases

### Asthma and Voice

Asthma is a worldwide disease with a prevalence of around 8% in adults in the United States.[48] It is defined as "reversible obstructive airway disease in the absence of an alternative explanation such as heart failure."[49] It is characterized by narrowing of the airway with varying degrees of obstruction as a result of bronchial smooth muscle contractions in addition to mucosal inflammation and thickening of the airway secretions. Airflow measurements, namely, reduction in the peak expiratory flow, that is the maximum airflow in the beginning of a forced expiration, is commonly used to make the diagnosis and to follow up on the effect of therapy. An obstructive pattern is invariably observed and can be provoked with the administration of methacholine and reversed with bronchodilators. See Figure 9–7.

The reversible airway obstruction characteristic of asthma lead to a constellation of clinical symptoms of cough, paroxysms of dyspnea, chest tightness, and wheezing. As a result of this impairment in breathing, patients may complain of phonatory symptoms that can be ill defined and prevalent only after vocal loading. Professional voice users in particular, in view of their highly demanding vocal careers, are more susceptible than others to disturbances in their respiratory system. The phonatory symptoms may be more accentuated following prolonged performance, very similar to exercise-induced airway symptoms. This airway hyperreactivity often described as "airway reactivity–induced asthma "is being more and more diagnosed as a cause of vocal fatigue, shortness of breath, and abnormal laryngeal muscle tension patterns observed in singers. The cascade of events starts by hyperventilation while singing, followed by decreased airflow that leads to a compensatory hyperfunctional behavior, that manifests as excessive tension all along the vocal tract starting from the tongue and jaw to the level of the vocal folds.[50] In addition to the excessive vocal loading, singers are also exposed to occupational hazards such as stage smoke and allergens that may worsen their airway hyperreactivity and promote further the prevalence of phonatory symptoms.

There are quite a few reports in the literature on the phonatory changes and symptoms in patients with asthma. A large population study of 19,330 participants (which included asthmatics and nonasthmatics) were evaluated for subjective dysphonia and the presence of 12 types of organic vocal fold pathologies; out of 616 patients with asthma 7.8% had organic laryngeal lesions versus 7% in the control group. Moreover, 11.3% of those without vocal fold lesions had subjective dysphonia in the asthmatic group compared to 5.5% in the control group.[51] Similarly, in a prospective cross-sectional study by Bhalla et al on 46 asthmatic patients, they found that patients on inhaled corticosteroids had a higher prevalence of pharyngeal inflammation and worse vocal performance compared to those not on inhaled corticosteroids. They were also more likely to experience hoarseness, vocal weakness in addition to cough and throat irritation compared to controls.[52] Likewise in the study by Dogan et al on 40 patients with mild to moderate asthma, there were both subjective as well

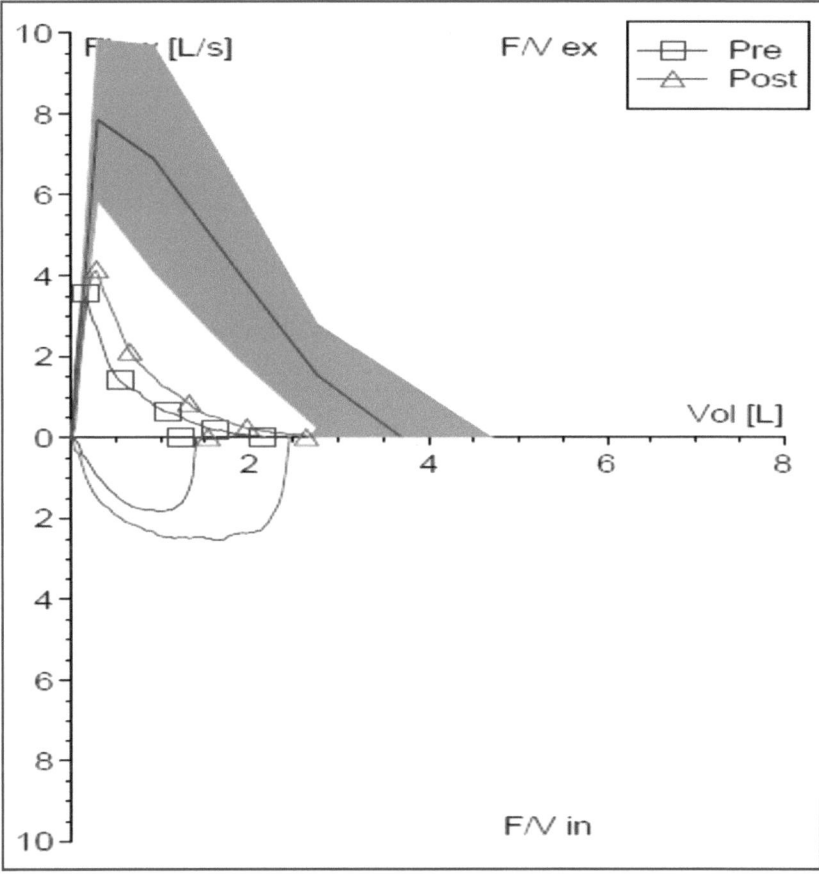

**Figure 9–7.** The flow volume curve of a 55-year-old male with asthma showing severe obstructive pulmonary impairment with significant response to bronchodilator challenge. Blue line: Before bronchodilator challenge; Red line: After bronchodilator challenge

as objective phonatory changes compared to age- and sex-matched controls. There was a significant difference in the self-assessment component using the VHI with 40% of asthmatic patients having above normal VHI scores.[53] Based on the retrospective study by Mirza et al, all patients who had started on inhaled corticosteroids and bronchodilators developed dysphonia 2 to 12 weeks following the initiation of treatment. The change in voice quality was described as rough with drop in vocal pitch.[54] In another study by Sellars et al using self-administered voice symptom score and perceptual evaluation in 43 patients with asthma, the median voice score was 26, and in 30% of the cases the (GRBAS) score was above one. It is worth noting that there was a significant association between the dose of inhaled corticosteroids and the GRBAS overall grading score.[55] In a cross-sectional controlled study by Hamdan et al on 50 subjects (31 asthmatic and 19 controls), the prevalence of dysphonia was significantly higher in asthmatic patients

compared to controls. On perceptual evaluation, the overall grade of dysphonia, asthenia, and straining were also significantly higher.[56]

The aforementioned subjective as well as self-perceived phonatory changes in asthmatic patients are invariably substantiated by abnormal findings on acoustic analysis. Dogan et al in his evaluation of voice quality in asthmatic patients, reported a significant difference in the acoustic parameters compared to controls. Asthmatic women had significantly higher perturbation parameters, namely, jitter and shimmer, and asthmatic men had significantly higher shimmer compared to controls of the same gender. There was also a significant difference in the noise-to-harmonic ratio value between female asthmatic patients and controls.[53] This increase in the intensity perturbation parameter has been corroborated in numerous other studies.[52,56,57] In a study by Lavy et al on 22 asthmatic patients using inhaled steroids, cycle-to-cycle irregularities were reported in almost

40% of the cases and maximum phonation time was reduced in more than two-thirds of the patients. In another prospective cross-sectional study by Bhalla on 46 patients with asthma, those on inhaled corticosteroids had significantly higher values for the acoustic perturbation parameters and higher closed-phase quotient scores.[52,57]

In addition to the phonatory and acoustic changes described above laryngeal abnormalities are seen as well. The prevalence of laryngeal movement disorders and vocal fold abnormalities is higher in patients with asthma compared to controls. In the study by Sellars et al on 43 asthmatic patients, 26 had either a functional or organic laryngeal abnormality. Mild and moderate laryngitis, defined as diffuse edema and redness of the glottis region, were the most common laryngeal findings. The most common functional laryngeal abnormalities observed were the presence of a glottic chink and false vocal fold phonation.[55] The laryngeal pathologies were mostly present in asthmatic patients receiving corticoid steroid inhalers. Based on a retrospective study by Mirza et al on 10 patients who were started on corticosteroids inhalers and bronchodilator therapy, vocal fold changes in the form of mucosal plaques, mucosal thickening, hyperemia, dilated vessels, capillary ectasias, and free vocal fold edge irregularities were reported.[54] In the study by Dogan et al, posterior laryngitis was present in 33 patients out of 40 asthmatic patients, a finding that was attributed to excessive throat clearing, cough, and possible irritation from refluxate material.[53] Similarly, in the study by Bhalla on 46 asthmatic patients, the pharyngitis scores were higher in the asthmatic group compared to controls, more often those on inhaled corticosteroids.[52]

The use of laryngeal video stroboscopic examination provided greater information on the vocal fold vibratory behavior in asthmatic patients. Based on the study by Dogan et al, abnormal laryngeal videostroboscopic findings were present in 97.5% of the 40 asthmatic patients enrolled in their study. The most common abnormalities were the degree of glottic closure (60%), irregularities in vibration (67.5%), phase, and amplitude asymmetry (30% and 40%, respectively). Additional findings included mucosal wave abnormalities and hyperadduction of the ventricular bands.[53] More so, one out of 4 patients had vocal fold bowing during phonation, a finding that was corroborated by the study of Lavy et al which showed apposition abnormalities in 43% of the cases, and mucosal changes and supraglottic muscle tension were present in 58% and 40% of the cases, respectively.[57] In the study by Mirza et al, eight out of nine patients receiving a combination of inhalers in the form of dry powder, had a decrease in vocal fold vibration, amplitude, and the extent that mucosal waves' propagation were attributed to various vocal fold pathologies.[54]

The phonatory symptoms experienced by asthmatic patients and the associated laryngeal findings seen on laryngeal examination may be the result of the inherent breathing impairment associated with asthma, the presence of allergy, the intake of corticosteroid inhalers, and last the presence of comorbidities such as sinonasal pathologies and gastroesophageal or laryngopharyngeal reflux disease. These four pathogenic mechanisms are briefly discussed below:

1. *Impaired breathing: Respiration* is an important component in voice production. As a power supply, the lungs energize the oscillator and set the vocal folds into vibration. Diseases of the respiratory system may alter the strength and consistency of subglottic pressure, and thus markedly affect vibratory behavior resulting in change in voice.[58] A recent study has shown the routine pulmonary function testing reveals unexpected pulmonary disease in many voice patients in whom pulmonary dysfunction is not suspected.[59]

   In asthmatic patients, breathing is impaired secondary to constriction of the bronchi smooth muscles, mucosal inflammation, and thickened secretions. The episodic airway obstruction leads to increased airway resistance manifested aerodynamically by a decrease in the expiratory peak flow and by reduction in maximum phonation time. Given the vital importance of breathing in phonation, voice is subsequently affected.[58] In addition to the aforementioned obstructive pattern, the increase in the amount and viscosity of the respiratory secretions exacerbates throat clearing and cough with subsequent irritation to the vocal folds. As a result, asthmatic patients may develop vocal fold pathologies such as exudative lesions of the lamina propria.[53,60,61]

2. *The high prevalence of allergy in patients with asthma*: Asthma can be triggered either by infectious diseases or by allergy. When allergy is the culprit, patients may also complain of dysphonia. Randhawa et al have investigated the impact of airborne allergies on voice and have demonstrated an increase in Voice Handicap Index in patients who were allergic to more than 4 allergens. The conclusion was that vocal dysfunction may be underdiagnosed in patients with allergy.[62] Brook et al in their investigation on the utility of allergy testing in patients with persistent laryngeal

symptoms, of 998 patients tested for allergy, 27 had primary complaints in the larynx and 51.8% percent of those were positive for one inhalant allergen at least. More so, based on these findings, the odds of having a positive allergy testing was similar in patients with laryngeal and nasal complaints.[63] Similarly, the study conducted by Turley et al on 134 patients revealed a higher prevalence of dysphonia in patients with allergic and non-allergic rhinitis compared to controls.[64] Other studies have demonstrated a prevalence of allergy in up to 76% of patients with dysphonia or laryngeal complaints.[63, 65] In a study by Randhawa et al on 15 patients with primary dysphonia, two-thirds had positive allergy testing. The authors alluded to the high prevalence of allergy in patients with atypical symptoms related to undiagnosed laryngopharyngeal diseases.[66] In another study conducted on singers using an allergy questionnaire, those with two or more vocal complaints were 25% more likely to have allergy compared to those with no vocal complaints.[67] Similarly, in the study by Simberg et al, subjects with allergy tended to have a higher prevalence of dysphonia compared to those with no allergy. The authors have used a questionnaire to solicit information on vocal symptoms in a group of 49 students with known allergy compared to another group of 54 students with no allergy.[68] In another study conducted on 30 subjects with known seasonal pollen allergy, Millqvist et al reported a higher prevalence of respiratory and phonatory symptoms in this group of patients compared to controls. This was also evident by the higher VHI scores in the functional and physical domains and in the overall score.[69] Krouse et al in another study examining the laryngeal manifestation of perennial allergy in 21 subjects with positive skin testing, again the VHI score was significantly higher in the allergic group compared to controls.[70]

Patients with allergy present with non-specific laryngopharyngeal symptoms such as cough, globus, throat clearing, and dysphagia, in addition to change in voice quality. Pathogenic mechanisms for these phonatory complaints include postnasal discharge reaching the glottis,[67] increased muscular activity of the posterior cricoarytenoid muscle via activation of negative pressure receptors in the nasal cavity, and the activation of the rhinolaryngeal reflex.[65] The phonatory symptoms when present are often substantiated by acoustic changes such as an increase in the perturbation parameters. In a study by Niedzielska et al the mean values of shimmer and Jitter were higher in patients with allergic rhinitis compared to controls.[71] Along the same line of investigation, Koc et al in his study on perennial allergic rhinitis, the mean VHI score and the mean s/z ratio were higher in patients with allergy compared to controls. The authors concluded that allergy may result in laryngeal dysfunction, the impact of which may be significant on quality of life.[72]

On examination, laryngopharyngeal signs of inflammation such as erythema and edema of the vocal folds and posterior glottis are commonly seen. Although these are non-specific, especially in the context of confounding diseases such as laryngopharyngeal reflux disease, when present, the diagnosis of allergy should be thoroughly investigated. In a large study by Hah et al looking at the prevalence of laryngeal diseases and associated factors in 19,000 patients, the authors reported a positive association between allergic rhinitis and vocal nodules, laryngitis, and epiglottic cyst. It is worth noting that laryngitis and vocal fold nodules were among the most common five laryngeal pathologies observed with a prevalence of 3.5% and 1.5%, respectively. The authors speculated that chronic throat clearing may precipitate laryngeal inflammation and thus lead to laryngitis.[73] These clinical observations were further substantiated by both human and animal studies supporting the causal relationship between allergen and vocal dysfunction. The study by Roth et al on five subjects challenged with an active allergic suspension revealed an increase in the phonatory threshold pressure after the allergen challenge. The authors concluded that vocal dysfunction can be secondary to the direct effect of the inhalant allergen on the vocal folds, and thus a causal relationship between the two is highly plausible.[74] More so, the animal study of Belafsky et al demonstrated a significant eosinophilic infiltration in the subglottis and trachea following sensitization to dust mite antigen and exposure to the same antigen and iron soot for 4 weeks.[75]

3. *Use of corticosteroid inhalers*: A third and probably most common cause of dysphonia in asthmatic patients is the use of inhalers as a treatment modality. Despite the usefulness and established role of steroid inhalers in controlling patients with chronic asthma, there are undesired side effects to these medications such as throat clearing and dysphonia.[76] Numerous studies have shown that the prevalence of change in voice

quality in patients treated with inhaled corticosteroids can be as high as 58% of the cases studied.[77-83] The meta-analysis by Rachelefsky et al on the adverse reactions to inhaled corticosteroids has shown that the potential to develop dysphonia, pharyngitis and or oropharyngeal fungal infection increases markedly with the use of any inhaled corticosteroid and depends heavily on the dosage and mode of usage.[84] In a study by Ihre et al looking at the prevalence of voice disturbances in asthmatic patients on steroid inhalers, a positive correlation between the use of inhaled cortisone and vocal symptoms was found. Based on the results of a questionnaire that consisted of 25 questions, some of which were related to voice, hoarseness was the most commonly reported symptom (52%) 2 weeks after the intake of the inhaled steroids. Other symptoms included lump sensation and excessive throat clearing.[60] Elderly subjects and those with voice-demanding professions had a higher prevalence of vocal disturbances compared to young subjects. More so there was a positive correlation between voice problems and the dosage of inhaled steroids, citing that those with more severe asthma had more voice problems compared to those with mild asthma. These results concur with the report by Kriz et al in 1977 on 23 asthmatic patients using triamcinolone acetonide aerosol. In his study, the most common side effects that occurred one to two weeks after initiation of the aerosol were hoarseness in 52% of the cases, followed by a coated tongue in 35% and sore throat in 26%.[85]

There are many reasons why phonatory symptoms in asthmatic patients may occur. These mechanisms include fungal infection (candidiasis), steroid-induced mucosal irritation and microtrauma, muscle-induced atrophy, and last is mucosal and mucous secreting glands atrophy. Based on a report by Vogt, the prevalence of oropharyngeal candidiasis in patients using corticosteroids inhalers can reach up to 77%.[79] See Figure 9–8. Several proposed mechanisms for the development of infection have been suggested. One is the development of the infection due to

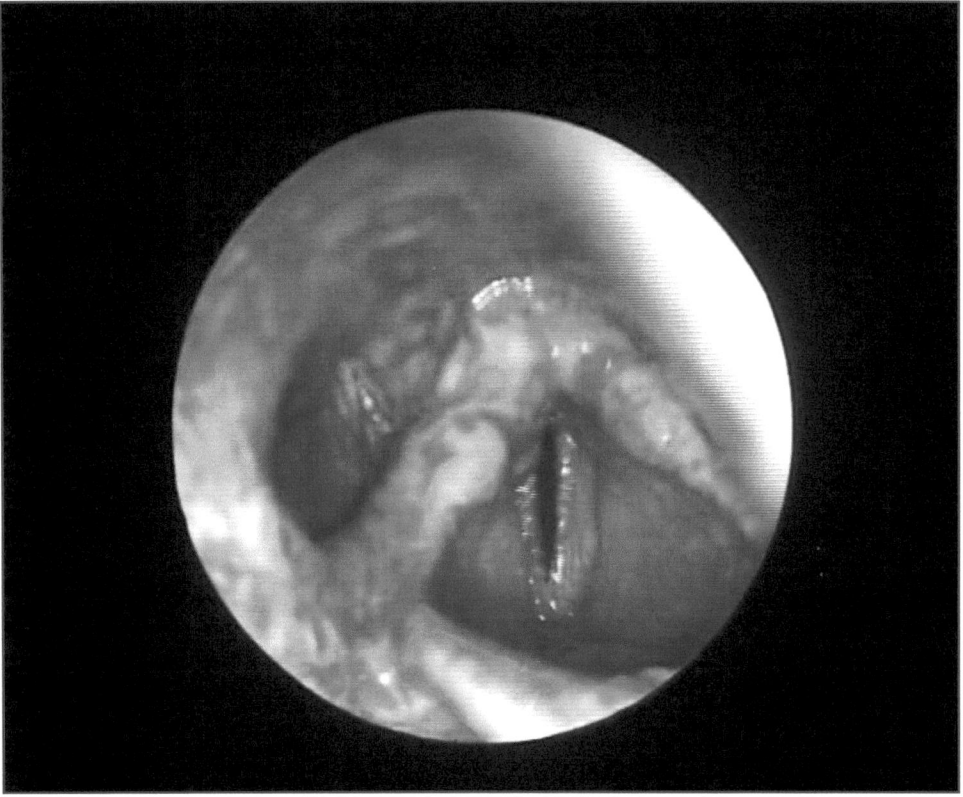

**Figure 9–8.** 46-year-old female known case of metastatic colon cancer to the lung treated with chemotherapy presented with dysphonia and throat discomfort. Laryngeal videoendoscopy showed fixed left vocal cord with whitish/yellowish debris on the pharyngeal and laryngeal mucosa suggestive of a fungal infection. Patient was treated with fluconazole successfully.

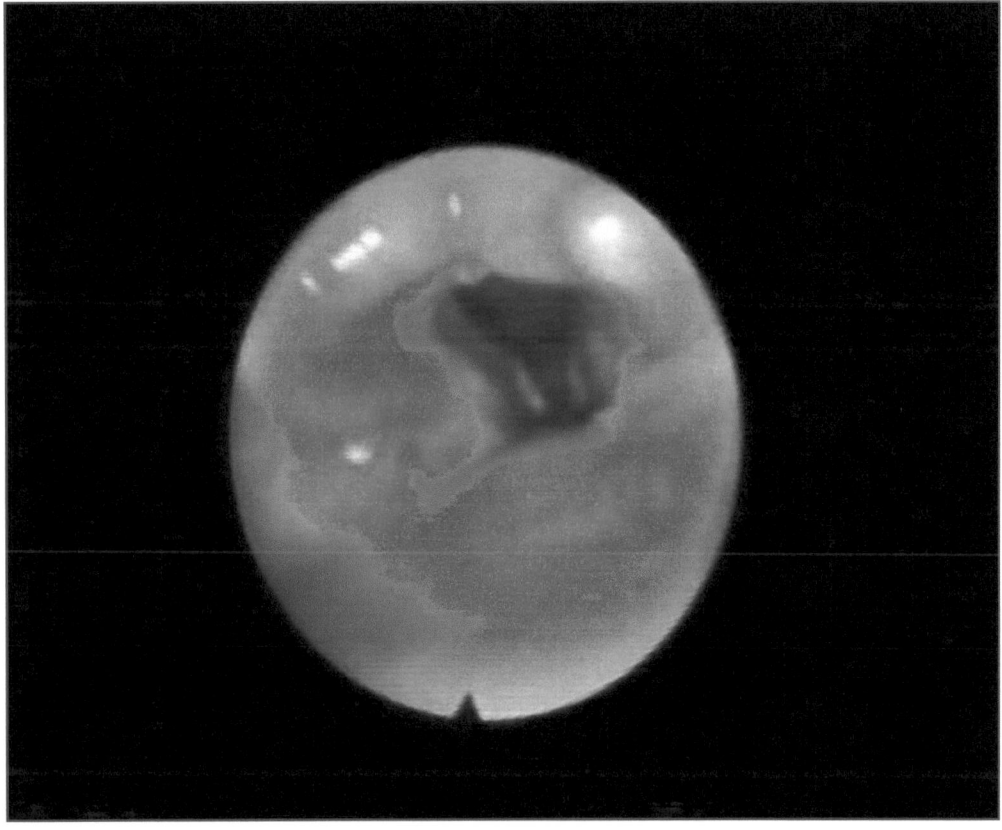

**Figure 9–9.** A 50-year-old physician presented with history of dysphonia following the intake of corticosteroid inhalers for the treatment of lower respiratory tract infection. The fiberoptic laryngeal endoscopy shows whitish plaques on both vocal folds mistaken for leukoplakia.

reduced immunity of the mucosal surface at the interface with the inhaled particles.[86] Fidel suggests that both local and systemic cell-mediated immunity are needed to protect against oropharyngeal candidiasis. Another suggested mechanism is elevated salivary glucose level.[86] In a study by Knight and Fletcher, the concentration of glucose within saliva withdrawn from three patients on steroids was elevated (mean of 32.8 mg/100 mL). The authors concluded that high glucose level in a bacterial flora medium allows fungi to grow and multiply.[87]

Fungal infection in patients on inhaled corticosteroids must be distinguished from steroid inhaler laryngitis, an entity described by DelGaudio in 2002. The author reported 20 patients who developed dysphonia following Fluticasone-inhaled therapy. Mucosal changes in the vocal folds such as edema, redness, and leukoplakia-like lesions were reported. These were attributed to a chemical form of laryngopharyngitis. Both vocal symptoms and laryngeal findings subsided

completely after the withdrawal of the inhaler.[88] See Figure 9–9.

Mirza et al has also reported vocal fold changes in 10 patient who were on asthma medications and had dysphonia. Vocal fold changes such as a hyperemia and plaque-like changes were described in parallel with decreased mucosal wave propagation.[55]

Steroid-induced myopathy is also a commonly proposed cause for the phonatory symptoms in patients on inhaled corticosteroids. In a study by Williams et al in 1983 on patients with persistent dysphonia while on inhaled steroids, vocal fold bowing was the most common finding in 9 out of 14 patients. It was attributed to local steroid myopathy which is both dose and potency dependent. To that end, the authors advocated early detection of laryngeal signs of myopathy given the reversibility of this pathology.[78] The adduction deficit reported by Williams et al was also observed in 4 patients out of 12 in the report by Acar et al.[89] Vocal fold adduction deficit was substantiated by the presence of myopathic potentials on electromyographic analysis of the thyroarytenoid and cricoarytenoid muscles in two out of the four affected patients. These were dose dependent similar to the phonatory symptoms and laryngeal findings in patients on inhaled corticosteroids.

To that end, three important factors affect the prevalence of the oropharyngeal and laryngeal symptoms: nature of the steroid and propellant used; the dosage and frequency of usage; and the delivery method of the inhaled corticosteroid. In a study by Watkin and Ewanowski, comparing the effect of triamcinolone acetonide and beclomethasone dipropionate on several acoustic and aerodynamic measures has shown that the use of the former reduces the vocal performance whereas the latter's effect was similar to that observed using oral steroids.[90] Ciclesonide, a non-halogenated inhaled corticosteroid, is gaining ground as an alternative to the conventional corticosteroid inhaler. Its added value lies in the reduced oropharyngeal side effects due to its small particle size.[91,92] Smaller particle size has superior lung efficacy, and yet less oropharyngeal deposition with subsequently less laryngeal and pharyngeal side effects. With respect to the methods used to deliver inhaled corticosteroids, two conventional ways are commonly prescribed, one is the pressurized metered-dose inhalers and second is the dry-powder inhalers.[93] The use of smaller particle size of less than 2 micrometers recently devised for pressurized metered-dose inhalers has enhanced the usage of the latter.

4. *Presence of co-morbidities*: The high prevalence of co-morbidities includes sinonasal pathologies and gastroesophageal or laryngopharyngeal reflux in asthmatic patients. Details on the pathogenic relationship between nasal and paranasal sinus diseases and asthma are discussed in the first section of this chapter. The relationship between gastroesophageal reflux disease and asthma is not new. One out of two patients with asthma have gastroesophageal reflux disease (GERD) based on a recent survey conducted by the German National Health.[94] More so, patients may also suffer from laryngopharyngeal reflux disease (LPRD) leading to a large spectrum of laryngeal and pharyngeal symptoms.bng factors for having LPR in asthmatic patients are many, most important of which are cough and abdominal distention. Kilic et al in their investigation on the prevalence of reflux in patients with asthma reported the prevalence of

LPRD and GERD in 70% and 46% respectively. The study was conducted on 50 patients using Reflux Symptom Index score. The prevalence was higher in uncontrolled asthmatic patients compared to controls.[95] The figures reported by Kilic et al were further corroborated by the study of Eryuksel et al where 75% of asthmatic patients had laryngeal findings of LPRD.[96] In the study conducted by Komatsu et al using intraluminal impedance resting on 27 asthmatic patients, 70% had hypophrayngeal reflux.[97] Similarly, Banaszkiewicz et al has reported a strong association between LPRD and the degree of asthma. The study was conducted in children using RSI and 24-hour pharyngeal pH monitoring. Hamdan et al has also reported a significantly higher mean of the RSI in 36 asthmatic patients compared to controls. More so, the prevalence of a positive RSI in the asthmatic group was higher compared to controls (15 cases vs 4).[98]

## Chronic Obstructive Pulmonary Disease

Chronic obstructive lung disease (COPD) is a common respiratory disease that affects millions every year. According to GOLD (Global initiative for chronic obstructive lung disease), it is defined as "—a common, preventable, and treatable disease that is characterized by persistent respiratory symptoms and airflow limitation that is due to airway and/or alveolar abnormalities usually caused by significant exposure to noxious particles or gases.[99] See Figure 9–10. It is classified into three different types: chronic bronchitis, emphysema, and asthma-COPD overlap syndrome. The literature on the association between COPD and voice is relatively scarce. Most of the reports highlight the importance of COPD as co-morbid disease in the presence of dysphonia and dysphagia in the elderly. In a cross-sectional study by Bassi et al on 32 male patients with oropharyngeal dysphagia, COPD was found to be one of the common co-morbidities in this subgroup of patients and as such was considered as a risk factor for oropharyngeal dysphagia.[100] In a review by Ryu et al of 3,791 elderly patients who underwent laryngoscopy, COPD in addition to other diseases such as asthma and thyroid diseases were found to be independently associated with dysphonia.[101]

Dysphonia has also been reported as an adverse effect of the usage of inhaled steroids, in the management of COPD patients. The importance of inhaled corticosteroid as an adjunctive medication to bronchodilators in the treatment of COPD cases has been

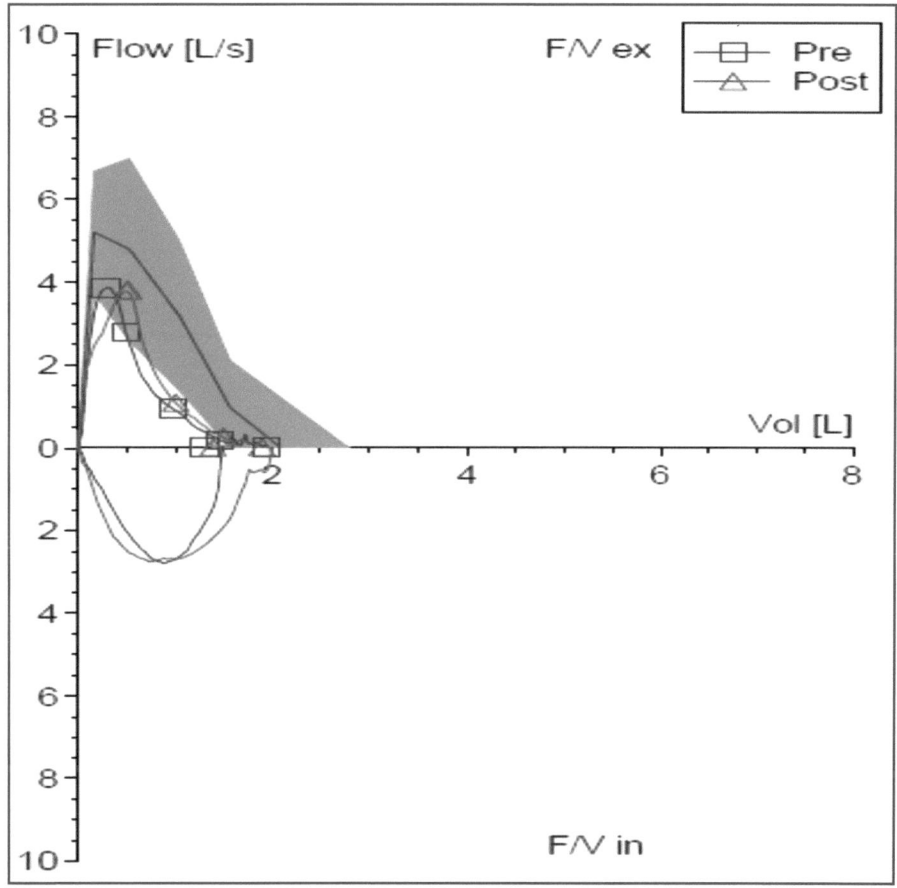

**Figure 9–10.** The flow volume curve of a 74-year-old female with COPD showing moderate obstructive pulmonary impairment with no significant response to bronchodilator challenge. Blue line: Before bronchodilator challenge; Red line: After bronchodilator challenge.

well substantiated in the literature. Their combined effect results in a decrease in the frequency of attacks, severity of breathlessness and a marked improvement in FEV1.[102] To that end, Kozak et al has reported the effect of chronic steroid inhalation on voice in a group of 22 patients with COPD. The only major finding was the decrease in the tonicity described as "increase of hypotonus" of the vocal folds" with no adverse fungal or bacterial infection.[103]

### Restrictive Lung Diseases

Given the intricate interplay between breathing and voice, pulmonary deficits are invariably associated with vocal disturbances.[104] In professional voice users, even a mild breathing impairment may jeopardize vocal performance and lead to phonatory symptoms. Restrictive lung diseases are among those respiratory diseases characterized by reduction

in lung volume and a decrease in forced vital capacity, FVC. See Figure 9–11. These can be stratified into parenchymal diseases, diseases that result in neuromuscular weakness, and diseases that restrict the movement of the chest wall such as morbid obesity and/or pleural diseases. Among the three, parenchymal diseases constitute the biggest subtype of restrictive lung diseases. These can be distinguished from other types of restrictive disease by measuring the diffusing lung capacity of carbon monoxide (DLCO). Diffuse lung capacity of carbon monoxide assesses gas exchange, the decrease of which in a restrictive pattern on spirometry suggests parenchymal disease. A normal DLCO on the other hand suggests an extrapulmonary cause of restriction. Parenchymal diseases are clustered into different categories that include idiopathic interstitial pneumonia, which is the most common idiopathic interstitial disease, pulmonary fibrosis, atelectasis, granulomatous diseases,

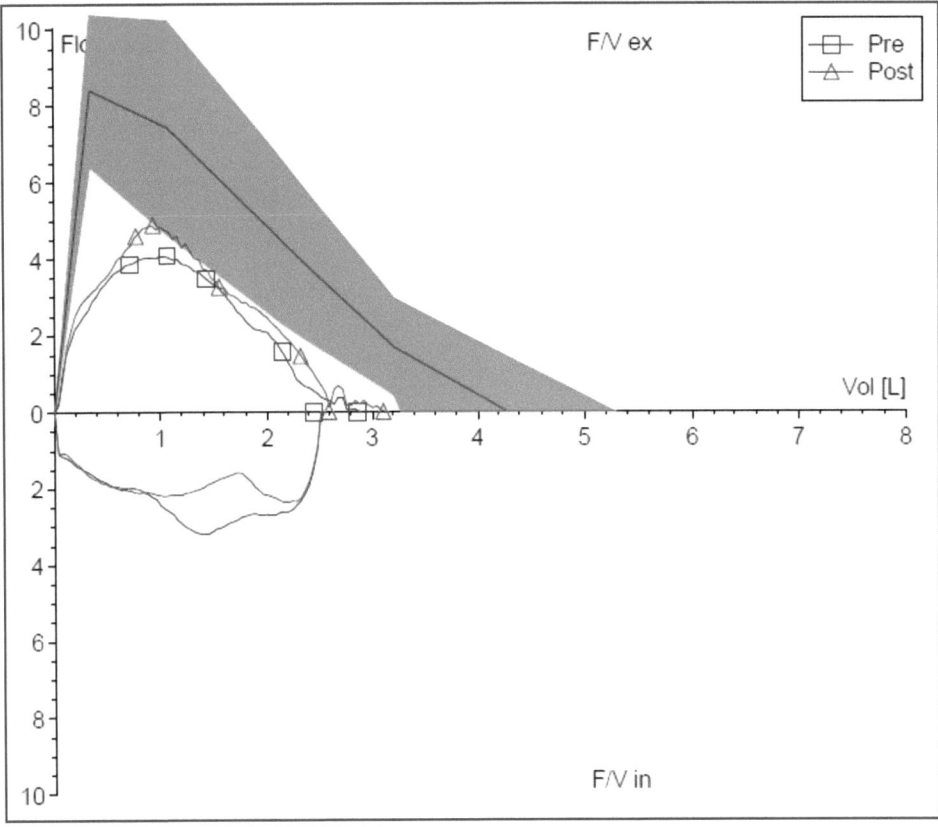

**Figure 9–11.** The flow volume curve of a 61-year-old male with coronary artery disease showing moderate restrictive pulmonary impairment. Blue line: Before bronchodilator challenge; Red line: After bronchodilator challenge.

hypersensitivity pneumonitis, neoplasms, drug-induced, and last but not least parenchymal diseases related to environmental exposure.

Despite the ubiquity of reports on systemic morbidities associated with parenchymal lung diseases, there are only a few reports in relation to phonatory disturbances. These are mostly related to environmentally induced parenchymal diseases such as asbestosis and silicosis.[105–107] *Asbestosis* has been thoroughly described as a parenchymal disease induced by the inhalation of asbestos, a fiber commonly found in industrial areas and mining fields. Inhaling these fibers can lead to severe inflammatory reactions that can result in permanent damage to the respiratory system with subsequent respiratory failure. The wide array of related pulmonary symptoms can develop up to 30 years after exposure and may be associated with phonatory changes. In a study by Gilbert on speech characteristics in patients with prolonged dust retention in the lungs, referred to as "black lung disease" (pneumoconiosis), several speech and pausal mea-sures were significantly different in affected patients compared to controls. Among these were the time needed to read the first paragraph of the Rainbow Passage (45.7 sec vs 33.9 sec), the mean of pauses between and within sentences, and the phonation time for a sustained vowel (10.6 sec vs 14.5 sec). The differences in speech parameters and airflow measurements were attributed to the respiratory symptoms often experienced by miners, such as dyspnea, breathlessness, and reduced breathing capacity. Other suggested mechanisms included reduced lung tissue elasticity secondary to the progressive inflammation and loss of parenchymal tissue. Affected subjects in that study also had an increase in vowel perturbation (14.96 vs 4.09) and a higher mean intensity variations compared to controls (8.85 dB vs 5 dB). These were ascribed to the deposition of the inhaled particles on the vocal folds resulting in inflammation, increase in mass, and cycle-to-cycle perturbation.[108]

Another environmentally induced parenchymal disease, is silicosis, a respiratory disease caused by inhalation of silica.[109] There are three case reports in the literature of silicosis associated with dysphonia, the last of which was described by Lardinois et al.[110–112] The authors reported a 76-year-old man who presented with left vocal fold paralysis secondary to compression of the recurrent laryngeal nerve. The diagnosis was made by video-mediastinoscopy which revealed a large fibrotic and granulomatous mediastinal lymph node.[112]

*Radiation therapy to chest, neck, and base of skull* is another etiology behind the development of parenchymal diseases often leading to dysphonia. The dysphonia may be secondary either to the restrictive lung disease and fibrotic changes induced by the radiation, or to injury to the recurrent laryngeal nerve. The neuropathy associated with radiation may be delayed even up to 34 years after treatment.[113,114] See Figure 9–12. Johanssn et al has reported 12 cases of vocal fold paralysis in a group of 150 patients with breast cancer who received radiation to the mediastinum.[115] Similarly, Crawley et al has also reported 10 cases of vocal fold paralysis following irradiation to the mediastinum, head, and neck, in patients diag-

nosed with Hodgkin's lymphoma, squamous cell carcinoma, and peripheral T-cell lymphoma. Patients had symptoms related to voice and swallowing that were treated by injection laryngoplasty in 40% of the cases.[116] The radiation-induced neuropathy is thought to be the result of direct injury to the nerve, and vascular insult, as well as to connective tissue changes with delayed fibrosis. This latter progresses in three stages, a prefibroptic phase, a fibrotic phase with altered fibroblast function, and a late stage characterized by atrophy and apoptosis.[117]

Neuromuscular weakness represents the second most common cause of restrictive lung diseases. Neurogenic and neuromuscular disorders such as amyotrophic lateral sclerosis (ALS) or Guillain-Barré syndrome can affect normal respiratory muscle function and severely restrict pulmonary volumes. There are many variants to GBS where multiple cranial muscles may be involved either early in the course of the disease or later. Neurologic signs include muscle weakness, ophthalmoplegia, ataxia, and loss of reflexes among other signs of cranial polyneuropathies. There are a few reports in the literature

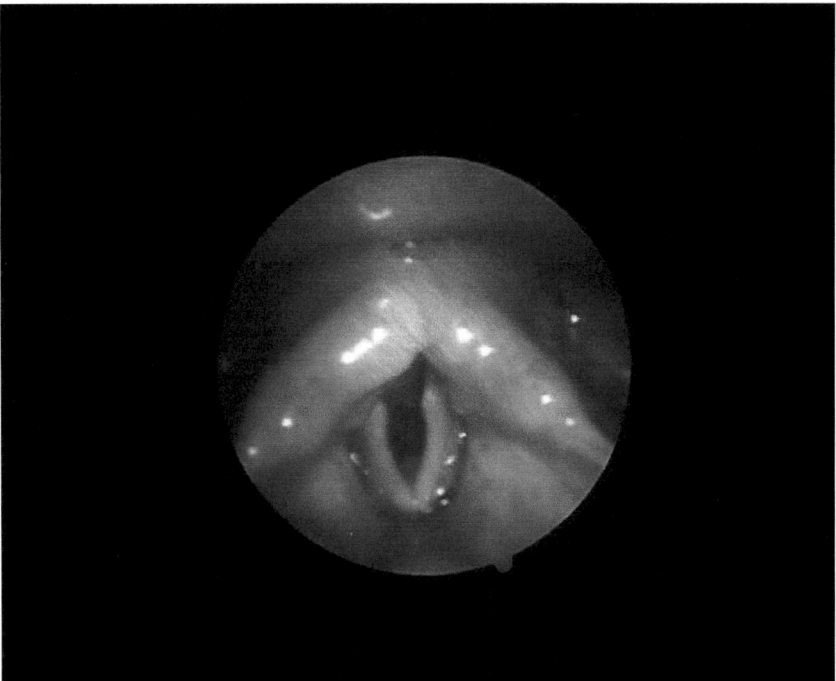

**Figure 9–12.** 40-year-old male, known case of optic nerve sheath meningioma and meningioma of the right tuberculum sellae treated by radiation therapy. Patient presented to the voice clinic 8 months after therapy with dysphonia and shortness of breath. Laryngeal videoendoscopy showed bilateral impaired mobility of the vocal folds with bowing. Patient denied any history of recent upper respiratory tract infection. The workup for myasthenia gravis including repetitive nerve stimulation was negative. Radiation-induced vagal neuropathy is suspected.

indicating that impaired swallowing, dysphonia secondary to vocal fold palsy, and altered nasality due to velopharyngeal incompetence, may be among the symptoms of this neuropathic disease. In the review by Holinger et al of 389 cases of abductor vocal fold paralysis, out of 240 adult cases 52 were of neurogenic origin that included Guillan-Barré syndrome.[118] Wada et al reported a case of oropharyngeal palsy in a 19-year-old women following enteritis. The patient had developed mild palatal muscle weakness with subsequent velopharyngeal incompetence, mainly to liquids, with increased nasality and spastic dysarthria. The symptoms gradually improved with time over the course of six to seven weeks.[119] Haug et al reported a case of hypernasality and dysphagia in addition to involvement of the abducens and glossopharyngeal nerve in a man following a sinus infection. The demyelinating neuropathy was confirmed by neurography and the patient recovered following plasmapheresis.[120] Other variants to GBS such as polyneuritis cranialis and Muller-Fisher syndrome have also been thoroughly discussed in the literature. Polo et al reported a 13-year-old boy who presented with dysphagia, dysphonia, and facial muscle weakness secondary to bilateral lower cranial nerve

involvement following a febrile illness. A demyelinating disease was highly suspected in view of the cerebrospinal fluid analysis and the close monitoring of the blink reflexes.[121] Similarly Howell et al described a rare case of Muller-Fisher syndrome who presented with respiratory, swallowing, and vocal symptoms in addition to perioral and acro-paresthesia. The authors advocate keeping a high index of suspicion in patients presenting with oropharyngeal and respiratory symptoms.[122]

*Restriction in chest wall* movement is the third category of restrictive lung disease caused by chest wall abnormalities. Common etiologies in that regard include kyphoscoliosis, ankylosing spondylitis, and chronic pleural effusion, all of which may cause extrinsic restriction on the lungs, limit their normal expansion, and thus decrease their overall volumes.[123–127] As a result of the restrictive chest expansion and impaired breathing, voice is naturally affected. See Figure 9–13. In a cross-sectional descriptive study by De Groot and De Witte investigating the physical impairment in patients with spinal muscular atrophy diagnosed before the age of 33 years, kyphoscoliosis was present in 36% to 90% of the cases. The authors have used both a structured medical interview and a

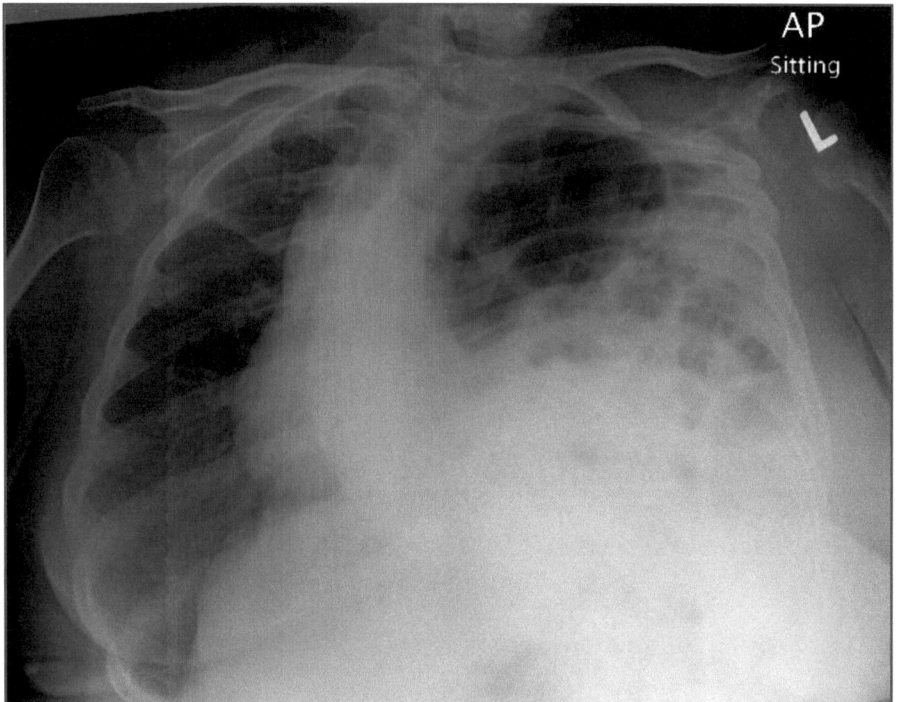

**Figure 9–13.** 52-year-old woman with severe S-shaped scoliotic deformity of the thoracolumbar spine with herniation of the stomach and bowel loops into the left hemi-thorax secondary to a left diaphragmatic hernia. Clear right lung. Maximum phonation time is 4.5 seconds.

questionnaire that included a section consisting of 51 questions regarding complaints/physical problems. Voice and speech problems were significantly prevalent in parallel with lung impairment and muscle weakness.[128] Ankylosing spondylitis (AS) can also affect voice by direct involvement of the cricoarytenoid joint.[129–134] Cricoarytenoid joint arthritis is a known complication of AS whereby there is destruction of the cartilage with evidence of diffuse synovitis. In a recent report by Desuter et al, these degenerative and inflammatory changes were successfully treated with subcutaneous injections of tumor necrosis factor-alpha.[135] The suggested mechanism for halting the erosive inflammatory changes is suppression of chondrocyte IL-1 activity.

*Obesity* is another cause of restrictive lung disease. It is a worldwide health issue that markedly impacts quality of life and is associated with numerous illnesses such as hypertension, diabetes, and cardiac diseases. Its negative effect on the respiratory system has been a subject of investigation for many decades with numerous reports indicating that obesity reduces the maximum inspiratory pressure and forced expiratory volume. As these two variables reflect respiratory muscle strength, their decrease alludes to ineffective diaphragmatic muscle biomechanics in obese subjects.[136,137] There is also reduction in the functional residual capacity and expiratory reserve volume secondary to an imbalance between lung inflation and deflation. Based on a study by Mafort et al, the reduction in ERV is an indicator of overweight and is primarily attributed to the accumulation of adipose tissue in the thoracoabdominal area.[138] To that end, two proposed mechanisms have been suggested: One is the mechanical effect due to the excess deposition of fat on the abdomen and chest wall. The downward movement of the diaphragm as well as the upward and forward pull of the ribs are limited by the excess fat in the thoracoabdominal area.[139] As a result of this impaired movement, patients feel the need to put more effort into breathing. The second is the state of systemic inflammation induced by the release of cytokines and bioactive mediators by the adipose tissue. Based on a report by Rasslan et al, this pro-inflammatory state, can further lead to pulmonary hypoplasia and respiratory distress.[140] The report by Wei et al on 94 patients undergoing bariatric surgery has shown an improvement in pulmonary function tests, namely, the forced expiratory volume during the first second of expiration.[141] Parreira et al in their longitudinal study on the effect of gastric bypass have shown an increase in the maximum inspiration pressure 36 months after surgery and a decrease in the maximum expiratory pressure after one month followed by an increase after 36 months.[142] On the other hand the study by Solomon et al on 8 obese and 8 non-obese subjects revealed no significant difference in any of the acoustic parameters, maximum phonation time, or laryngeal airway resistance, between the two groups. More so, no significant differences were observed postoperatively compared to preoperatively.[143]

## References

1. Sivasankar M, Fisher KV. Oral breathing increases PTH and vocal effort by superficial drying of vocal fold mucosa. *J Voice*. 2002;16(2): 172–181.
2. Verdolini-Marston K, Titze IR, Druker DG. Changes in phonation threshold pressure with induced conditions of hydration. *J Voice*. 1990;4(2):142–151.
3. Verdolini K, Min Y, Titze IR, et al. Biological mechanisms underlying voice changes due to dehydration. *J Speech Lang Hear Res*. 2002;45 (2):268–281.
4. Solomon NP, DiMattia MS. Effects of a vocally fatiguing task and systemic hydration on phonation threshold pressure. *J Voice*. 2000;14 (3):341–362.
5. Solomon NP, Glaze LE, Arnold RR, van Mersbergen M. Effects of a vocally fatiguing task and systemic hydration on men's voices. *J Voice*. 2003;17(1):31–46.
6. Hamdan AL, Al-barazi R, Kanaan A, Al-tamimi W, Sinno S, Husari A. The effect of snoring on voice: a controlled study of 30 subjects. *Ear Nose Throat J*. 2012;91(1):28–33.
7. Hamdan AL, Sabra O, Rifai H, Tabri D, Hussari A. Vocal changes in patients using nasal continuous positive airway pressure. *J Voice*. 2008;22(5):603–606.
8. Hemler RJ, Wieneke GH, Dejonckere PH. The effect of relative humidity of inhaled air on acoustic parameters of voice in normal subjects. *J Voice*. 1997;11(3):295–300.
9. Sataloff RT. Pollution and its effects on the voice. In: *Professional Voice: The Science and Art of Clinical Care*. Vol 2. 4th ed. San Diego, CA: Plural Publishing; 2017.
10. Benninger M, Murry T. Voice therapy for benign vocal fold lesions and scar in singers and actors. In: *The Performer's Voice*. San Diego, CA: Plural Publishing; 2015.
11. Dalston RM, Warren DW, Dalston ET. The identification of nasal obstruction through clinical judgments of hyponasality and nasometric assessment of speech acoustics. *Am J Orthodon Dentofac Orthoped*. 1991;100(1):59–65.
12. Fletcher SG. Cleft palate speech assessment through oral-nasal acoustic measures. *Comm Dis Rel Cleft Lip Palate*. 1989; pp. 246–257.
13. Seaver EJ, Dalston RM, Leeper HA, Adams LE. A study of nasometric values for normal nasal resonance. *J Speech Lang Hear Res*. 1991;34(4):715–721.
14. Dalston RM, Neiman GS, Gonzalez-Landa G. Nasometric sensitivity and specificity: a cross-dialect and cross-culture study. *Cleft Pal-Craniofac J*. 1993;30(3): 285–291.

15. Hosemann W, Göde U, Dunker JE, Eysholdt U. Influence of endoscopic sinus surgery on voice quality. *Eur Arc Oto-rhino-Laryngol.* 1998;255(10):499–503.

16. Chen MY, Metson R. Effects of sinus surgery on speech. *Arch Otolaryngol Head Neck Surg.* 1997;123(8):845–852.

17. Corren J, Rachelefsky GS. Inter-relationaship between sinusitis and asthma. *Immunol Allergy Clin North Am.* 1994;14:171–184.

18. Vining EM, Kennedy DW. Surgical management in adults. *Immunol Allergy Clin North Am.* 1994;14:97–111.

19. Bucca C, Rolla G, Scappaticci E, et al. Extrathoracic and intrathoracic airway responsiveness in sinusitis. *J Allergy Clin Immunol.* 1995; 95 (pt 1):52–59.

20. Senior BA, Kennedy DW, Tanabodee J, Kroger H, Hassab M, Lanza DC. Long-term impact of functional endoscopic sinus surgery on asthma. *Otolaryngol Head Neck Surg.* 1999;121(1):66–68.

21. Ikeda K, Tamura G, Shimomura A, et al. Endoscopic sinus surgery improves pulmonary function in patients with asthma associated with chronic sinusitis. *Ann Otol Rhinol Laryngol.* 1999;108(4):355–359.

22. Sundberg J, Rossing TD. The science of singing voice. *J Acoust Soc Am.* 1990;87(1):462–463.

23. Marunick MT, Menaldi CJ. Maxillary dental arch form related to voice classification: a pilot study. *J Voice.* 2000;14(1):82–91.

24. Macari AT, Ziade G, Khandakji M, Tamim H, Hamdan AL. Effect of rapid maxillary expansion on voice. *J Voice.* 2016;30(6):760–e1.

25. Macari AT, Karam IA, Tabri D, Sarieddine D, Hamdan AL. Correlation between the length and sagittal projection of the upper and lower jaw and the fundamental frequency. *J Voice.* 2014;28(3):291–296.

26. Roers F, Mürbe D, Sundberg J. Voice classification and vocal tract of singers: a study of x-ray images and morphology. *J Acoust Soc Am.* 2009;125(1):503–512.

27. Lingala SG, Zhu Y, Kim YC, Toutios A, Narayanan S, Nayak KS. A fast and flexible MRI system for the study of dynamic vocal tract shaping. *Mag Res Med.* 2017;77(1):112–125.

28. Echternach M, Burk F, Burdumy M, Traser L, Richter B. Morphometric differences of vocal tract articulators in different loudness conditions in singing. *PloS One.* 2016;11(4):e0153792.

29. Da Cunha MGB, Passerotti GH, Weber R, Zilberstein B, Cecconello I. Voice feature characteristic in morbid obese population. *Obes Surg.* 2011;21:340–344.

30. Busetto L, Mazza M, De Stefano F, Costa G, Negrin V, Enzi G. Upper airway size is related to obesity and body fat distribution in women. *Eur Arch Oto-Rhino-Laryngol.* 2009;266(4):559–563.

31. Ozturk E, Dalayman D, Sonmez G, et al. The effect of pharyngeal soft tissue components on snoring. *Clin Imaging.* 2007;31(4):259–263.

32. Maurer JT, Stuck BA, Hein G, Hörmann K. Videoendoscopic assessment of uncommon sites of upper airway obstruction during sleep. *Sleep Breath.* 2000;4(3):131–136.

33. Shelton KE, Woodson H, Gay S, Suratt PM. Pharyngeal fat in obstructive sleep apnea. *Am Rev Respir Dis.* 1993;148(2):462–466.

34. Mortimore IL, Marshall I, Wraith PK, Sellar RJ, Douglas NJ. Neck and total body fat deposition in non-obese and obese patients with sleep apnea compared with that in control subjects. *Am J Resp Crit Care Med.* 1998;157(1):280–283.

35. Orbelo D, Ekbom DC, Thompson DM. Dysphonia associated with lingual thyroid gland and hypothyroidism: improvement after lingual thyroidectomy. *Ann Otol Rhinol Laryngol* 2011;120(12):775–779.

36. Eryilmaz A, Basal Y. A large lingual thyroid extending to the epiglottis. *BMJ Case Rep.* 2015;2015:bcr2015212201.

37. Lundeborg I, Hultcrantz E, Ericsson E, et al. Acoustic and perceptual aspects of vocal function in children with adenotonsillar hypertrophy—effects of surgery. *J Voice.* 2012;26:480–487.

38. Heffernan CB, Rafferty MA. Effect of tonsillectomy on the adult voice. *J Voice.* 2011;25:e207–e210.

39. Kazi R, Prasad VM, Kanagalingam J, et al. Analysis of formant frequencies in patients with oral or oropharyngeal cancers treated by glossectomy. *Int J Lang Commun Disord.* 2007;42:521–532.

40. Chuma AV, Cacace AT, Rosen R, et al. Effects of tonsillectomy and/or adenoidectomy on vocal function: laryngeal, supralaryngeal and perceptual characteristics. *Int J Pediatr Otorhinolaryngol.* 1999;47:1–9.

41. Sataloff RT. Respiratory Behaviors and Vocal Tract Issues in Wind Instrumentalists. In: Sataloff RT. *Professional Voice: The Science and Art of Clinical Care.* 4th ed. San Diego, CA: Plural Publishing; 2017; 1017–1027.

42. Luzzago F, Nicolai P, Tomenzoli D, Maroldi R, Antonelli AR. Laryngocele: analysis of 18 cases and review of the literature. *Acta otorhinolaryngol Ital*: Organo ufficiale della Societa italiana di otorinolaringologia e chirurgia cervico-facciale. 1989;10(4):399–412.

43. Dray TG, Waugh PF, Hillel AD. The association of laryngoceles with ventricular phonation. *J Voice.* 2000;14(2):278–281.

44. Topaloğlu İ, Salturk Z, Atar Y, Berkiten G, Büyükkoç O, Çakır O. Evaluation of voice quality after supraglottic laryngectomy. *Otolaryngol Head Neck Surg.* 2014;151(6):1003–1007.

45. Chul-Ho Kim YC, Kim K, Kim YH, Choi HS, Kim KM, Choi EC. Vocal analysis after vertical partial laryngectomy. *Yonsei Med J.* 2003;44(6):1034–1039.

46. Jepsen MC, Gurushanthaiah D, Roy N, Smith ME, Gray SD, Davis RK. Voice, speech, and swallowing outcomes in laser-treated laryngeal cancer. *Laryngoscope.* 2003;113(6):923–928.

47. Roh JL, Kim DH, Park CI. Voice, swallowing and quality of life in patients after transoral laser surgery for supraglottic carcinoma. *J Surg Oncol.* 2008;98(3):184–189.

48. Centers for Disease Control and Prevention. Asthma Surveillance Data. Retrieved 20 Nov 2014, from: http://www.cdc.gov/asthma/asthmadata.htm.

49. Corrao WM, Braman SS, Irwin RS. Chronic cough as the sole presenting manifestation of bronchial asthma. *New Engl J Med.* 1979;300(12):633–637.

50. Cohn JR, Sataloff RT, Spiegel JR, Fish JE, Kennedy K. Airway reactivity-induced asthma in singers (ARIAS). *J Voice.* 1991 Jan 1;5(4):332–337.

51. Park B, Choi HG. Association between asthma and dysphonia: a population-based study. *J Asthma.* 2016; 53(7):679–683.

52. Bhalla RK, Watson G, Taylor W, Jones AS, Roland NJ. Acoustic analysis in asthmatics and the influence of inhaled corticosteroid therapy. *J Voice.* 2009; 23(4):505–511.

53. Dogan M, Eryuksel E, Kocak I, Celikel T, Sehitoglu MA. Subjective and objective evaluation of voice quality in patients with asthma. *J Voice.* 2007;21(2):224–230.

54. Mirza N, Kasper Schwartz S, Antin-Ozerkis D. Laryngeal findings in users of combination corticosteroid and bronchodilator therapy. *Laryngoscope.* 2004;114(9):1566–1569.

55. Sellars C, Stanton AE, McConnachie et al. Reliability of perceptions of voice quality: evidence from a problem asthma clinic population. *J Laryngol Otol.* 2009;123(7):755–763.

56. Hamdan AL, Ziade G, Kasti M, Akl L, Bawab I, Kanj N. Phonatory symptoms and acoustic findings in patients with asthma: a cross-sectional controlled study. *Indian J Otolaryngol Head Neck Surg.* 2017;69(1):42–46.

57. Lavy JA, Wood G, Rubin JS, Harries M. Dysphonia associated with inhaled steroids. *J Voice.* 2000; 14(4):581–558.

58. Spiegel JR, Sataloff RT, Chon JR, Hawkshaw M. *Respiratory dysfunction.* In: Sataloff RT ed. *The Professional Voice: The Science and Art of Clinical Care.* 2nd ed. San Diego, CA: Singular Publishing Group; 1997:375–386.

59. Meenan K, Catanoso L, Stephan S, Aoyama J, Chauvin R, Sataloff RT. The utility of pulmonary function testing in patients presenting with dysphonia. *J Voice.* In press.

60. Ihre E, Zetterstrom O, Ihre E, Hammarberg B. Voice problems as side effects of inhaled corticosteroids patients—a prevalence study. *J Voice.* 2004;18:403–414.

61. Phillips PS, Hirani SP, Epstein R. Peak flow and voice pathology. *J Voice.* 2009;23:521–528.

62. Randhawa PS, Nouraei S, Mansuri S, Rubin JS. Allergic laryngitis as a cause of dysphonia: a preliminary report. *Logoped Phoniatr Vocol.* 2010;35(4):169–174.

63. Brook CD, Platt MP, Reese S, Noordzij JP. Utility of allergy testing in patients with chronic laryngopharyngeal symptoms. Is it allergic laryngitis? *Otolaryngol Head Neck Surg.* 2016;154(1):41–45.

64. Turley R, Cohen SM, Becker A, Ebert Jr CS. Role of rhinitis in laryngitis: another dimension of the unified airway. *Ann Otol Rhinol Laryngol.* 2011;120(8):505–510.

65. Lauriello M, Angelone AM, Businco LD, Passali D, Bellussi LM, Passali FM. Correlation between female sex and allergy was significant in patients presenting with dysphonia. *Acta Otorhinolaryngol Ital.* 2011;31:161–166.

66. Randhawa PS, Mansuri S, Rubin JS. Is dysphonia due to allergic laryngitis being misdiagnosed as laryngopharyngeal reflux? *Logoped Phoniatr Vocol.* 2010;35(1):1–5.

67. Hamdan AL, Sibai A, Youssef M, Deeb R, Zaitoun F. The use of a screening questionnaire to determine the incidence of allergic rhinitis in singers with dysphonia. *Arch Otolaryngol Head Neck Surg.* 2006; 132(5):547–549.

68. Simberg S, Sala E, Tuomainen J, Rönnemaa AM. Vocal symptoms and allergy—a pilot study. *J Voice.* 2009;23(1):136–139.

69. Millqvist E, Bende M, Brynnel M, Johansson I, Kappel S, Ohlsson AC. Voice change in seasonal allergic rhinitis. *J Voice.* 2008;22(4):512–515.

70. Krouse JH, Dworkin JP, Carron MA, Stachler RJ. Baseline laryngeal effects among individuals with dust mite allergy. *Otolaryngol Head Neck Surg.* 2008; 139(1):149–151.

71. Niedzielska G. Acoustic estimation of voice when incorrect resonance function of the nose takes place. *Int J Ped Otorhinolaryngol.* 2005;69(8):1065–1069.

72. Koç E, Özbal A, Koç B, Erbek S. Comparison of acoustic and stroboscopic findings and Voice Handicap Index between allergic rhinitis patients and controls. *Balk Med J.* 2014;31(4):340.

73. Hah JH, Sim S, An SY, Sung MW, Choi HG. Evaluation of the prevalence of and factors associated with laryngeal diseases among the general population. *Laryngoscope.* 2015;125(11):2536–2542.

74. Roth DF, Abbott KV, Carroll TL, Ferguson BJ. Evidence for primary laryngeal inhalant allergy: a randomized, double-blinded crossover study. In: *Int Forum Allergy and Rhinol.* 2013;3(1):10–18.

75. Belafsky PC, Peake J, Smiley-Jewell SM, Verma SP, Dworkin-Valenti J, Pinkerton KE. Soot and house dust mite allergen cause eosinophilic laryngitis in an animal model. *Laryngoscope.* 2016;126(1):108–112.

76. Sant'Ambrogio G, Mathew OP, Fisher JT, Sant'Ambrogio FB. Laryngeal receptors responding to transmural pressure, airflow and local muscle activity. *Respir Physiol.* 1983;54:317–330.

77. Williamson IJ, Matusiewicz SP, Brown PH, Greening AP, Crompton GK. Frequency of voice problems and cough in patients using pressurized aerosol inhaled steroid preparations. *Eur Respir J.* 1995;8:590–592.

78. Williams AJ, Baghat MS, Stableforth DE, Cayton RM, Shenoi PM, Skinner C. Dysphonia caused by inhaled steroids: recognition of a characteristic laryngeal abnormality. *Thorax.* 1983;38:813–821.

79. Vogt FC. The incidence of oral candidiasis with use of inhaled corticosteroids. *Ann Allergy.* 1979;43(4):205–210.

80. Toogood JH, Jennings B, Greenway R, Chuang L. Candidiasis and dysphonia complicating beclometasone treatment of asthma. *J Allergy Clin Immunol.* 1980;65:145–153.

81. Williams SJ. Side effects of inhaled steroids. In: Haregreave FF, Hogg JC, Malo J, Toogood JH, Eds. *Experta Medica,* Amsterdam, The Netherlands; 1989:68–86.

82. FASS. Swedish Drug Compendium. LINFO, Läkeme-delsinformation AB.

83. Kass I, Nair SV, Patil KD. Beclometasone dipropio-nate aerosol in the treatment of steroid-dependent asthmatic patients. *Chest*. 1977;71:703.

84. Rachelefsky GS, Liao Y, Faruqi R. Impact of inhaled corticosteroid-induced oropharyngeal adverse events: results from a meta-analysis. *Ann Allergy Asthma Im-munol*. 2007;98(3):225–238.

85. Kriz RJ, Chmelik F, Do Pico G, Reed CE. A one-year trial of triamcinolone acetonide aerosol in severe steroid-dependent asthma. *Chest*. 1977;72(1):36–44.

86. Fidel Jr PL. Distinct protective host defenses against oral and vaginal candidiasis. *Med Mycol*. 2002;40(4):359–375.

87. Knight L, Fletcher J. Growth of Candida albicans in saliva: stimulation by glucose associated with anti-biotics, corticosteroids, and diabetes mellitus. *J Infect Dis*. 1971;vol:371–377.

88. DelGaudio JM. Steroid inhaler laryngitis: dysphonia caused by inhaled fluticasone therapy. *Arch Otolaryn-gol Head Neck Surg*. 2002;128:677–681.

89. Ozbilen Acar G, Uzun Adatepe N, Kaytaz A, et al. Evaluation of laryngeal findings in users of inhaled steroids. *Eur Arch Otorhinolaryngol*. 2010;267: 917–923.

90. Watkin KL, Ewanowski SJ. Effects of aerosol cor-ticosteroids on the voice: triamcinolone acetonide and beclomethasone dipropionate. *J Speech Hear Res*. 1985;28(2):301–304.

91. Engelstätter R, Banerji D, Steinijans VW, Wurst W. Low incidence of oropharyngeal adverse events in asthma patients treated with ciclesonide: results from a pooled analysis. *Am J Respir Crit Care Med*. 2004;169(7):A92.

92. Leach CL, Bethke TD, Boudreau RJ, et al. Two-dimensional and three-dimensional imaging show ciclesonide has high lung deposition and peripheral distribution: a nonrandomized study in healthy vol-unteers. *J Aeros Med*.

93. Chmielewska M, Akst LM. Dysphonia associated with the use of inhaled corticosteroids. *Curr Opin Otolaryngol Head Neck Surg*. 2015;23(3):255–259.

94. Steppuhn H, Langen U, Scheidt-Nave C, Keil T. Major comorbid conditions in asthma and association with asthma-related hospitalizations and emergency department admissions in adults: results from the German National Health telephone interview survey (GEDA) 2010. *BMC Pulmon Med*. 2013;13(1):46.

95. Kilic M, Ozturk F, Kirmemis O, et al. Impact of laryngopharyngeal and gastroesophageal reflux on asthma control in children. *Int J Ped Otorhinolaryngol*. 2013;77(3):341–345.

96. Eryuksel E, Dogan M, Golabi P, Sehitoglu MA, Celikel T. Treatment of laryngopharyngeal reflux improves asthma symptoms in asthmatics. *J Asthma*. 2006;43(7):539–542.

97. Komatsu Y, Hoppo T, Jobe BA. Proximal reflux as a cause of adult-onset asthma: the case for hypopha-ryngeal impedance testing to improve the sensitivity of diagnosis. *JAMA Surg*. 2013;148(1):50–58.

98. Hamdan AL, Jaffal H, Btaiche R, et al. Laryngopha-ryngeal symptoms in patients with asthma: a cross-sectional controlled study. *Clin Respir J*. 2016;10(1):40–47.

99. Global Strategy for the Diagnosis, Management and Pre-vention of COPD, Global Initiative for Chronic Obstruc-tive Lung Disease (GOLD) 2017 Report. Retrieved February 10, 2017, from: http://www.goldcopd.org.

100. Bassi D, Furkim AM, Silva CA et al. Identification of risk groups for oropharyngeal dysphagia in hospitalized pa-tients in a university hospital. *Codas*. 2014;26(1):17–27.

101. Ryu CH, Han S, Lee MS, et al. Voice changes in elderly adults: prevalence and the effect of social, behavioral, and health status on voice quality. *J Am Geriatr Soc*. 2015;63(8):1608–1614.

102. Claverley PM. The role of corticosteroids in chronic obstructive pulmonary disease. *Semin Respir Crit Care Med*. 2005;26(2):235–245.

103. Kozak E, Maniecka-Aleksandrowicz B, Frank-Pis-korska A, Witman D. Evaluation of the effect of chronic steroid inhalation therapy on the state of the upper airway in patients with chronic obstruc-tive pulmonary disease. *Pneumonolo Alergolog Polska*. 1991;59(9-10):33–137.

104. Hardy JC. Respiratory physiology: implications of current research. *Asha*. 1968;10(5):204.

105. Stell PM, McGill T. Exposure to asbestos and laryn-geal carcinoma. *J Laryngol Otology*. 1975;89(5):513–517.

106. Griffiths H, Malony NC. Does asbestos cause laryn-geal cancer?. *Clin Otolaryngol*. 2003;28(3):177–182.

107. Roggli VL, Greenberg SD, McLarty JL, Hurst GA, Spivey CG, Hieger LR. Asbestos body content of the larynx in asbestos workers: a study of five cases. *Arc Otolaryngol*. 1980;106(9):533–535.

108. Gilbert HR. Speech characteristics of miners with black lung disease (pneumoconiosis). *J Commun Dis*. 1975;8(2):129–140.

109. Hughes P, McGavin C. Recurrent laryngeal palsy and mediastinal lymphadenopathy. *Respir Med*. 1995; 89:584–585.

110. Sherani TM, Angelini GD, Passani SP, Butchart EG. Vocal cord paralysis associated with coalworkers' pneumoconiosis and progressive massive fibrosis. *Thorax*. 1984;39:683–684.

111. Capezzuto A. Silicosi e sindrome ricorrenziale. *Folia Med Napoli*. 1967;50:162–167.

112. Lardinois D, Gugger M, Balmer MC, Ris HB. Left recurrent laryngeal nerve palsy associated with sili-cosis. *Eur Respir J*. 1999;14(3):720–722.

113. Lin YS, Jen YM, Lin JC. Radiation-related cranial nerve palsy in patients with nasopharyngeal carci-noma. *Cancer*. 2002;95:404–409.

114. Stern Y, Marshak G, Shpitzer T, Segal K, Feinmesser R. Vocal cord palsy: possible late complication of radio-therapy for head and neck cancer. *Ann Otol Rhinol Laryngol*. 1995;104:294–296.

115. Johansson S, Löfroth PO, Denekamp J. Left-sided vocal cord paralysis: a newly recognized late com-

plication of mediastinal irradiation. *Radiother Oncol.* 2001;58(3):287–294.

116. Crawley BK, Sulica L. Vocal fold paralysis as a delayed consequence of neck and chest radiotherapy. *Otolaryngol Head Neck Surg.* 2015;153(2):239–243.

117. Pradat PF, Delanian S. Late radiation injury to peripheral nerves. *Hand Clin Neurol.* 2013;115:743–758.

118. Holinger LD, Holinger PC, Holinger PH. Etiology of bilateral abductor vocal cord paralysis: a review of 389 cases. *Ann Otol Rhinol Laryngol.* 1976;85(4):428–436.

119. Wada Y, Yanagihara C, Nishimura Y, Susuki K. A case of acute oropharyngeal palsy with nasal voice as main symptom. *Brain Nerve.* 2006;58(3):235–238.

120. Haug AK, Rothhammer V, Scherer EQ, Pickhard AC. Guillain-Barré syndrome with dysphagia after frontal sinusitis. *HNO.* 2013;61(1):52–54.

121. Polo A, Manganotti P, Zanette G, De Grandis D. Polyneuritis cranialis: clinical and electrophysiological findings. *J Neurol Neurosurg Psychiatry.* 1992;55(5):398–400.

122. Howell RJ, Davolos AG, Clary MS, Frake PC, Joshi AS, Chaboki H. Miller-Fisher syndrome presents as an acute voice change to hypernasal speech. *Laryngoscope.* 2010;120(5):978–980.

123. Kritek PA, Kasper DL, Choi A M K. *Harrison's Principles of Internal Medicine.* 19th ed. New York, NY: Mc Graw-Hill Education; 2015.

124. Judson MA, Boan AD, and Lackland DT. The clinical course of sarcoidosis: presentation, diagnosis, and treatment in a large white and black cohort in the United States. *Sarcoid Vasc Diff Lung Dis.* 2012; 29:119–127.

125. Martin L. 2004 Asbestos disease guidelines ignore mass screening abuse. *Am J Respir Crit Care Med.* 2005;171:665; author reply 666–667.

126. Schwaiblmair M, Behr W, Haeckel T, Markl B, Foerg W, Berghaus T. Drug-induced interstitial lung disease. *Open Respir Med J.* 2012;6:63–74.

127. Wells AU. The revised ATS/ERS/JRS/ALAT diagnostic criteria for idiopathic pulmonary fibrosis (IPF)—Practical implications. *Respir Res.* 2013;14(suppl 1):S2.

128. De Groot IJ, De Witte LP. Physical complaints in ageing persons with spinal muscular atrophy. 2005.

129. Miller FR, Wanamaker JR, Hicks DM, Tucker HM. Cricoarytenoid arthritis and ankylosing spondylitis. *Arch Orolaryngol Head Neck Surg.* 1994; 120:214–216.

130. Berendes J, Mielhke A. A rare ankylosis of the cricoarytenoid joints. *Arch Otolaryngol.* 1973;98:63–65.

131. Wojtulewski JA, Sturrock RD, Branfoot AC, Hart FD. Cricoarytenoid arthritis in ankylosing spondylitis. *Br Med J.* 1973;3:145–146.

132. Bienenstock H, Lanyi VF. Cricoaryntenoid arthritis in patient with ankylosing spondylitis. *Arch Otolaryngol.* 1977;103:738–739.

133. Libby DM, Schley WS, Smith JP. Cricoarytenoid arthritis in ankylosing spondylitis. A cause of acute respiratory failure and cor pulmonale. *Chest.* 1981;80:641–642.

134. Helfgott SM, Treseler PA. Cricoarytenoid synovitis in ankylosing spondylitis. *Arthritis Rheum.* 1990; 33:604–605.

135. Desuter G, Duprez T, Huart C, Gardiner Q, Verbruggen G. The use of adalimumab for cricoarytenoid arthritis in ankylosing spondylitis—an effective therapy. *Laryngoscope.* 2011;121(2):335–338.

136. Chlif M, Keochkerian D, Choquet D, Vaidie A, Ahmaidi S. Effects of obesity on breathing pattern, ventilatory neural drive and mechanics. *Respir Physiol Neurobiol.* 2009;168:198–202.

137. Arena R, Cahalin LP. Evaluation of cardiorespiratory fitness and respiratory muscle function in the obese population. *Prog Cardiovasc Dis.* 2014;56:457–464.

138. Mafort TT, Madeira E, Madeira M, et al. Intragastric balloon for the treatment of obesity: evaluation of pulmonary function over a 3-month period. *Lung.* 2012;190:671–676.

139. Brazzale DJ, Pretto JJ, Schachter LM. Optimizing respiratory function assessments to elucidate the impact of obesity on respiratory health. *Respirology.* 2015;20:715–721.

140. Rasslan Z, Stirbulov R, Lima CA, Saad JR. Lung function and obesity. *Rev Bras Clínica Médica.* 2009;7:36–39.

141. Wei YF, Tseng WK, Huang CK, Tai CM, Hsuan CF, Wu HD. Surgically induced weight loss, including reduction in waist circumference, is associated with improved pulmonary function in obese patients. *Surg Obes Relat Dis.* 2011;7:599–604.

142. Parreira VF, Matos CM, Athayde FT et al. Evolution of respiratory muscle strength in post-operative gastroplasty. *Rev Bras Fisoter.* 2012 Jun;16(3):225–230.

143. Solomon NP, Helou LB, Dietrich-Burns K, Stojadinovic A. Do obesity and weight loss affect vocal function? *Sem Speech Lang.* 2011;32 (1):31–42.

# 10

# Allergy

*John R. Cohn, Patricia A. Padams, Mary J. Hawkshaw, and Robert Thayer Sataloff*

About 1 of every 5 persons in the United States has an allergic disease. Allergy, in simple terms, is a specific, immunologically based adverse response to environmental substances that ordinarily do not adversely affect most people. In the most common usage, this refers to immediate hypersensitivity. An allergic reaction may occur in response to something an individual inhales, ingests, has contact with, or is injected with. Symptoms range from mild to severe (even fatal) and most commonly may include upper respiratory (allergic rhinitis) and lower respiratory (asthma) complaints. Individuals may suffer seasonal bouts of allergic symptoms or may be ill perennially, depending on what in their environment causes the symptoms. Allergic disease may be a particular problem for the professional voice user, who has little control of the work environment and is often travelling, resulting in further uncontrolled exposure. And, of course, optimal airway physiology is a key factor in maximizing the quality of spoken or sung vocal output.

The human immune response is based on a complex, interrelated system of cells and cell products. This system provides recognition and response to foreign substances (antigens) that contact the body, are ingested, or develop intrinsically. Ideally, these functions protect against harmful exposures to infectious organisms and even play a role in preventing cancer. Lymphocytes produce multiple classes of immunoglobulins that can be converted into specific antibodies targeting an antigen. After the immune response is initiated with the recognition of the antigen, the body's response is manifested by a growing list of cellular and intracellular mediators (complements, prostaglandins, leukotrienes, interleukins).[1]

Coombs and Gell[2] classified the mechanisms of hypersensitivity into 4 classes. Type I hypersensitivity is mediated primarily by immunoglobulin E (IgE) and is exemplified by the common allergic phenomena of allergic rhinitis, anaphylactic shock, urticaria, and asthma. Type II hypersensitivity is mediated by IgG or IgM directed toward cell-bound antigens. Hemolytic anemia in the newborn is an example. Type III hypersensitivity involves immune complex diseases such as found in serum sickness. Type IV reactions are characterized by delayed cellular-mediated immunity, such as contact dermatitis, of which poison ivy is a common but troublesome example. We now recognize that many reactions represent a combination of types.

Allergic individuals make abnormal amounts of antibodies of the IgE class, which are specific for the substances to which they are allergic.[3] Patients who have a genetic tendency to make specific IgE may react to a number of substances, and cross-reacting antibodies to related substances may be present, such as to pollens from various grasses and grass family foods.[4] In adults, most allergic reactions are to inhalant allergens, whereas food allergies are relatively rare. Allergic and certain nonallergic individuals may also be more sensitive to nonspecific irritants, such as strong odors, as well as to selected pharmacologic agents such as methacholine and histamine.[5] This chapter is limited to a discussion of the diagnosis and treatment of inhalant respiratory allergies, because they are most likely to adversely affect singers. Upper respiratory allergies will primarily be addressed here. Lower respiratory tract problems affecting singers, including the syndrome of airway reactivity-induced asthma in singers (ARIAS),[6] are discussed elsewhere in this text and in a review.[7] Nevertheless, it should be remembered that allergies to ingested substances (including foods) may affect singers by thickening secretions and causing congestion; similar reactions may also occur from skin contact and other allergic exposures.

The mechanism of the allergic reaction is more complex than initially believed. The traditional explanation, including release of mediators from mast cells and basophils, secondary to linkages between IgE on the cell surface and the allergen, has expanded to include a long list of intercellular messengers, cells, and mediators, all of which appear to play a role in the development of the allergic reaction.[8] Additionally, neurogenic factors may be involved.[9] The classic allergic reaction involves immediate hypersensitivity with symptoms resulting from exposure to the release of histamine and other cell mediators, noted within minutes. Of the 4 types of hypersensitivity reaction originally described by Coombs and Gell,[2] this is a type I hypersensitivity reaction. Late phase reactions, mediated by basophils and mast cells through other mediators such as prostaglandins and leukotrienes, can cause tissue inflammation for hours or days.[10]

Mild allergies are more incapacitating to professional voice users than to others because of their effect on the mucosal cover layer. If a singer has a short period of annual allergy and is able to control the symptoms well with medications that do not produce disturbing side effects, this approach is reasonable. When more sustained treatment is required, when medication side effects impair performance, or when relief is inadequate in the context of the voice user's increased demands, more extensive evaluation is required.

## Signs and Symptoms

The term *allergic rhinitis*, commonly referred to as hay fever or rose fever, describes an array of allergic symptoms involving the eyes, ears, nose, and throat. In effect, these terms are misnomers, because flowering plants do not have wind-borne pollen, and most fall allergic symptoms are brought on by weeds such as ragweed and not hay. Identical symptoms may occur in the summer and winter in response to exposures to common allergens such as animal dander and dust mites. Symptoms include nasal congestion, sneezing, and clear drainage from the nose; watery, itchy eyes; throat soreness and a sensation of the constant need for throat clearing (from postnasal drip); pain and/or pressure in the ears; and headache and fatigue. Professional voice users, especially singers,

with mild allergies may present with subtle vocal complaints such as occasional voice breaks or vocal fatigue that may be the result of relative drying in the vocal tract. These symptoms are most commonly seasonal, occurring when the grasses, trees, and weeds are pollinating. However, they may occur year round in some individuals. Pollinating seasons vary significantly across the United States, as do the allergens that are most problematic in each region.[11] This fact holds special importance for singers and actors who are commonly called on to travel often, sometimes weekly.

Allergies to dust and mold are aggravated commonly during rehearsals and performances in concert halls, especially older concert halls, because of the numerous curtains, backstage trappings, and dressing room facilities that are rarely cleaned thoroughly. Because many singers travel extensively, location is important to bear in mind when attempting to elicit an allergic history and when planning allergy treatment with regard to an upcoming performance schedule. Additionally, the history must include not only geographical location, but also details of recent working, living, and traveling environments.

Allergic rhinitis is one of the most common etiologies in the development of chronic sinusitis. Patients with chronic sinusitis suffer from nasal congestion, postnasal drainage, pressure headaches, and olfactory disturbances. Chronic sinusitis can also exacerbate asthma.

## Evaluation

Although the history may provide the best clues for the diagnosis of allergy, it can also be misleading.[12] Nasal examination classically reveals hypertrophied, boggy nasal mucosa with a pale bluish color. Clear rhinorrhea is often noted, but thicker secretions can be present if there is an element of chronic sinusitis or if there is relative dehydration. Allergic polyps are common in the nose and are usually found in the middle meatus or involving the middle turbinates. Polyps related to allergy are usually multiple, pale, yellowish, and firm. Most findings of allergic rhinitis can be seen on routine anterior rhinoscopy. However, when necessary, nasal endoscopy can be used for more detailed intranasal examination. Nasal examination performed before and after the application of topical mucosal decongestants (ie, phenylephrine, oxymetazoline) can help predict the patient's response to pharmacologic treatment. In addition to the findings on nasal examination, other head and neck signs of allergic rhinitis include conjunctival irritation and inflammation, periorbital ecchymosis ("allergic shiners"), serous otitis media, oral and pharyngeal drying, and lymphoid hypertrophy in Waldeyer's ring. On laryngeal examination, thick secretions with mucous stranding across the vocal folds, supraglottic edema, and vocal fold edema can be seen.

Radiologic testing is usually not necessary in the primary evaluation of allergic rhinitis. When sinusitis is suspected, a nonenhanced computed tomography (CT) scan is the best single study to evaluate the paranasal sinuses. Plain sinus X-rays have been used to screen children and patients with acute sinusitis, but the ready availability of computerized tomography has largely replaced plain films in most circumstances.

## Allergy Testing

As previously stated, allergy evaluation begins with a detailed history of the patient's symptoms and exposures. Appropriate testing can then be performed to look for demonstrated atopy. Prick skin testing can rapidly screen for reactions to a number of allergens. It is the quickest and least expensive means of confirming allergic sensitization. Patients must be off of most antihistamines for 5 days before skin testing can be performed. Tricyclic antidepressants, such as amitriptyline, have potent antihistamine activity and also interfere with allergy skin test results, as do a variety of other commonly used medications.[13] Skin testing is relatively contraindicated in patients on beta-blocker drugs because of the risk of exaggerated anaphylaxis if an adverse reaction to the skin testing occurs. Intradermal skin tests are the most sensitive way to look for signs of allergy.[14] They may also provide a rapid answer, but they carry a higher risk of adverse reaction. Extremely rare fatalities have been associated with skin testing, which should be reserved for experienced practitioners who are prepared to treat the rare allergic reactions that occur.

Laboratory testing for IgE antibodies has attracted increased interest.[15] The radioallergosorbent test (RAST) has been largely replaced by enzyme-linked methods that allow for measurement of specific antibody. It can measure antigen-specific IgE levels to multiple antigen classes from a single blood specimen. The ImmunoCAP assay is more expensive, but it is not altered by antihistamines. It is also not as sensitive as skin testing and usually requires a wait for results. It can be especially useful in patients with dermatologic conditions that make skin testing impossible or when patients cannot safely discontinue antihistamines or beta-blockers. The Immuno-

CAP also has been used as a screening technique[16,17] to confirm the diagnosis of allergy or as a basis for the development of immunotherapy, but there is inadequate evidence to justify its use as a substitute for conventional skin testing.

## Treatment

### Pharmacologic Treatment

A disadvantage of topical nasal medications is failure to control the ocular symptoms of seasonal and perennial rhinitis, which may accompany nasal complaints. Although less likely to impact negatively on the voice, ocular symptoms may produce considerable discomfort in the atopic singer whose nasal symptoms have been relieved by topical therapy. It may cause eye blinking, which gives an audience the false impression that the performer is nervous or uncomfortable. Eye irritation may also cause slight blurring of vision that may make it difficult to read music. A variety of topical anti-inflammatory medications that are generally safe and effective in the treatment of allergic conjunctive irritation have been introduced in recent years. These include azelastine hydrochloride (Optivar, Muro), ketotifen fumarate (Zaditor, Novartis), olopatadine (Patanol, Alcon), and pemirolast (Alamast, Santen). Vasoconstrictor topical ocular preparations are also available over the counter and may be used for transient relief. Almost all of these preparations are contraindicated in users of soft contact lenses, and care should be taken to exclude other causes of ocular discomfort, particularly when that is the sole complaint. The treatment of ocular allergy was recently reviewed.[19,20]

When topical preparations do not adequately control allergic rhinitis, oral antihistamines may be necessary. All antihistamines can potentially cause drying of the mucosal surfaces of the upper and lower airways. This can be a critical problem for a professional voice user, because even relatively mild drying may cause major problems affecting both vocal quality and vocal stamina. Additionally, most antihistamines potentially cause some level of sedation; although over the past few years, new drugs with minimal sedative and anticholinergic (drying) side effects have become available (Table 10–1).

Because antihistamines do not directly address the problem of nasal congestion, decongestants are commonly added to the medical regimen. Decongestants are often added to antihistamines to form combination preparations to both potentiate the mucosal drying effects and to take advantage of the stimulatory

**Table 10–1.** Antihistamines

| Drug | Strength/Dose | Recommended Dosing | Age Groups (in years) | Level of Sedation |
|------|---------------|--------------------|-----------------------|-------------------|
| **Allegra** (fexofenadine) | 180 mg tablet | 1 tablet daily | 12 and older | Nonsedating |
| | 60 mg tablet or capsule | 1 tablet twice daily | | |
| **Allegra-D** (fexofenadine/ pseudoephedrine) | 60 mg/120 mg Extended release tablet | 1 tablet twice daily | 12 and older | Nonsedating |
| **Claritin** (loratadine) | 10 mg tablet 10 mg RediTabs | 10 mg daily | 6 and older | Nonsedating |
| **Claritin-D 12 Hour** (loratadine/ pseudoephedrine) | 5 mg/120 mg Extended release tablet | 1 tablet twice daily | 12 and older | Nonsedating |
| **Zyrtec** (cetirizine) | 5 mg tablet | 5 mg or 10 mg once daily | 6 and older | Less sedating than first generation |
| | 10 mg tablet | once daily | 2 to 5 | |
| | 5 mg/5 mL syrup | 2.5 to 5 mg once daily (or 2.5 mg every 12 hours) | | |

side effects of decongestants to counteract the sedation from the antihistamine. Although the improved drying effects may control secretions more effectively, they may also interfere with singing or speaking by decreasing or thickening vocal fold lubrication. The newer, nonsedating antihistamines have also been combined with decongestants (fexofenadine/pseudoephedrine, loratadine/pseudoephedrine, Claritin-D). Decongestants can provide excellent control of allergic nasal congestion with no risk of central nervous system (CNS) sedation, but they can also cause mild stimulatory side effects such as insomnia and tachycardia. At present, these products are commonly available in the United States over the counter, although because pseudoephedrine can be used to manufacture illicit medications, restrictions on their sale are in effect. Montelukast, a leukotriene antagonist, may also have decongestant activity.[21,22] Combinations of this drug with antihistamines for the treatment of allergic rhinitis can be effective without the drying found with older decongestants.

The mucosal drying effects of both antihistamines and decongestants may be counteracted to some extent with mucolytic agents, which liquefy mucus and increase the output of thin respiratory tract secretions. Guaifenesin is an excellent mucolytic expectorant. It is available as a single agent or combined with a decongestant.

It is often necessary to experiment with several antihistamines, decongestants, or combinations in singers before finding a suitable balance between therapeutic effect and side effects. The clinician should be familiar with many different medications and drug classes, both to minimize side effects and because patients may develop tolerance to antihistamines with long-term use requiring changes in prescriptions. Professional voice users should generally avoid new medication shortly before a performance. Drugs are usually taken in small doses for short trial periods to determine both the level of allergy control and the effects on the vocal tract. If a singer obtains consistent control of allergic symptoms and does not suffer from excessive drying, sedation, or hyperstimulation, these medications can be used safely for both short- and long-term treatment.

Acute symptoms of allergic rhinitis are usually quite responsive to systemic steroids. Intramuscular or oral steroids can rapidly reverse allergic inflammation and can also result in mild mucosal drying and mild CNS stimulation. Steroids can be used to treat a singer or actor suffering an acute allergic "attack" or to rapidly initiate medical treatment because of a difficult upcoming performance schedule. In these instances, corticosteroids are usually administered as either a single intramuscular injection or a rapidly weaning course taken orally over 3 to 5 days. There is no evidence that inhaled steroids reduce vocal fold edema, whether it results from allergic or infectious etiologies. The use of long-term systemic steroids in the treatment of most patients with only allergic rhinitis is inappropriate due to the risk of serious side effects.

### Allergy-Directed Therapy

Singers may be particularly sensitive to both the effects of their underlying allergy and the medications prescribed to control their disorder. For this reason, specific allergy-directed treatment is virtually always indicated. Serious singers should be referred to a physician with specialized training and expertise in the treatment of allergic disorders. The American Boards of Pediatrics and Internal Medicine supervise 2-year fellowship training programs in the evaluation and treatment of allergic diseases. Physicians who complete the fellowship successfully may sit for the certifying examination. Although other medical specialties including otolaryngology also offer training in this area, medical allergists generally focus exclusively on allergic disease.

Appropriate testing is performed to look for demonstrated atopy. Once allergy is identified, avoidance measures provide a first step to limiting symptoms. It is well established that the less a patient is exposed to the allergens to which he or she is sensitized, the less difficulty he or she will have with unavoidable exposures. Environmental control may consist of measures such as providing air-conditioning in a performer's suite or dust control in the home environment. Alteration in props may also be helpful, as demonstrated by a singer who experienced difficulty in a new role that included a feather boa as part of the costume. After skin testing confirmed the presence of feather allergy, symptoms resolved with the substitution of a synthetic boa.[23]

Immunotherapy injections may provide the best possible therapeutic modality for many professional voice users.[24] They offer the opportunity for allergen-directed control of the allergic response with no worry about vocal tract side effects. Immunotherapy is based on the pattern of allergy and demonstrated specific sensitivity as determined by allergy testing. The patient receives injections of slowly increasing concentrations of various allergens at approximately weekly intervals. The mechanism by which allergen immunotherapy works is not known. It has been proposed that IgG antibodies develop and block the IgE molecules at the receptor sites on immune response cells, but a variety of physiologic responses have been demonstrated. Immunotherapy is effective in a majority of appropriately selected patients who complete the full dosing regimen.[25]

### Newer Treatments

A variety of newer treatments designed to block some of the mediators involved in the allergic process are under evaluation. Currently in the late phase of testing, and perhaps available by the time this is published, are a variety of interleukin blockers. Omalizumab is a monoclonal antibody to IgE. It may be highly effective in patients with allergic disease. Issues of cost and safety remain to be resolved for this medication, which must be given by injection. It may offer particular advantage to the travelling singer who has a suboptimal response to medication and who has a travel and performance schedule that makes conventional immunotherapy impractical.[26]

## Conclusion

Allergic disease is a common problem and must not be overlooked in the evaluation of professional voice users who seek medical attention for complaints of change in their voice. Even complaints of mild nasal congestion or dry scratchy throat, which may not alter the voice primarily, can cause chronic irritation that may impair vocal performance. It is important to remember that symptoms of allergy are generally chronic, but they may be acute with a new specific exposure. They may vary in severity and sometimes, but not always, have seasonal variation. Understanding the pathophysiology and immunology of allergy, as well as its diagnosis and treatment, is essential in providing comprehensive care to the professional voice user. An appreciation for allergy and its special implications for performers is important not only for physicians, but also for professional voice users and their teachers.

## References

1. Finkelman FD, Urban JF Jr. The other side of the coin: the protective role of the TH2 cytokines. *J Allergy Clin Immunol*. 2001;107:772–780.
2. Coombs RRA, Gell PGH. Classification of allergic reactions responsible for clinical hypersensitivity and disease. In: Gell PGH, Coombs RRA, eds. *Clinical Aspects of Immunology*. 2nd ed. Philadelphia, PA: FA Davis; 1968:575–596.

3. Ishizaka T. Mechanisms of IgE-mediated hypersensitivity. In: Middleton E Jr, Reed C, Ellis E, et al., eds. *Allergy Principles and Practice.* 3rd ed. St. Louis, MO: Mosby; 1988:71–93.

4. Kay AB. Allergy and allergic diseases. *N Engl J Med* 2001;344:30–37.

5. Cartier A, Bernstein IL, Burge PS, et al. Guidelines for bronchoprovocation in the investigation of occupational asthma: report of the Subcommittee on Bronchoprovocation for Occupational Asthma. *J Allergy Clin Immunol.* 1989;84(5, pt 2):823–829.

6. Cohn JR, Sataloff RT, Spiegel JR, Fish JE, Kennedy K. Airway reactivity-induced asthma in singers (ARIAS). *J Voice.* 1990;5:332–337.

7. Cohn JR, Spiegel JR, Sataloff RT. Vocal disorders and the professional voice user: the allergist's role. *Ann Allergy Asthma Immunol.* 1995;74:363–375.

8. Hayes JB, Hizawa N, Jenmalm M, et al. Developments in the field of allergy in 2014 through the eyes of Clinical and Experimental Allergy. *Clin Exp Allergy.* 2015; 45(12):1723–1745.

9. Kaliner M, Lemanske R. Rhinitis and asthma. *JAMA.* 1992;268(2):2807–2829.

10. Naclerio RM, Proud D, Togias AG, et al. Inflammatory mediators in late antigen-induced rhinitis. *N Eng J Med.* 1985;313:65–67.

11. Lewis WH, Vinay P, Zenger VE. *Airborne and Allergic Pollen of North America.* Baltimore, MD: Johns Hopkins University Press; 1983.

12. Wallace DV, Bahna SL, Goldstein S, et al. American Academy of Allergy, Asthma and Immunology Work Group Report: allergy diagnosis in clinical practice. *J Allergy Clin Immunol.* 2007;120:967–969.

13. Shah KM, Rank MA, Davé SA, Oslie CL, Butterfield JH. Predicting which medication classes interfere with allergy skin testing. *Allergy Asthma Proc.* 2010;31(6): 477–482.

14. Cohn JR, Padams P, Zwillenberg J. Intradermal Skin Test (IDST) results correlate with atopy. *Ear Nose Throat J.* 2011;90(4):E11–E16.

15. Hamilton RG, Franklin Adkinson N Jr. In vitro assays for the diagnosis of IgE-mediated disorders. *J Allergy Clin Immunol.* 2004;144(2):213–225.

16. King WP. Efficacy of a screening radioallergosorbent test. *Arch Otolaryngol.* 1982;108:781–786.

17. Nalebuff DJ. In vitro-based allergen immunotherapy. In: Krause HF, ed. *Otolaryngic Allergy and Immunology.* Philadelphia, PA: WB Saunders; 1989:163–168.

18. Mabry RL. Pharmacotherapy with immunotherapy of the treatment of otolaryngic allergic. *Ear Nose Throat J.* 1990;69:63–71.

19. Bielory L. Allergic and immunologic disorders of the eye. Part I: Immunology of the eye. Review. *J Allergy Clin Immunol.* 2000;106(5):805–816.

20. Bielory L. Allergic and immunologic disorders of the eye. Part II: Ocular allergy. Review. *J Allergy Clin Immunol.* 2000;106(6):1019–1032.

21. Malmstrom K, Hampel FC, Philip G, et al. Montelukast in the treatment of spring allergic rhinitis in a large, double-blind, randomized, placebo-controlled study. *J Allergy Clin Immunol.* 2001;107(2):S157.

22. Meltzer E, Malmstrom K, Lu S, et al. Concomitant montelukast and loratadine as treatment for seasonal allergic rhinitis: a randomized, placebo-controlled clinical trial. *J Allergy Clin Immunol.* 2000;105(5):917–922.

23. Cohn JR, Sataloff RT. Boa constrictor. *Chest.* 1993;103: 653.

24. Jutel M, Agache I, Bonini S, et al. International consensus on allergy immunotherapy. *J Allergy Clin Immunol.* 2015;136(3):556–568.

25. Creticos PS. Immunotherapy with allergens. *JAMA.* 1992;268:2834–2839.

26. Casale TB, Bernstein IL, Busse WW, et al. Use of anti-IgE humanized monoclonal antibody in ragweed-induced allergic rhinitis. *J Allergy Clin Immunol.* 1997; 100:110–121.

# Laryngeal Manifestations of Gastrointestinal Disorders

*Robert Thayer Sataloff, Donald O. Castell, Philip O. Katz, Dahlia M. Sataloff, and Mary J. Hawkshaw*

Laryngopharyngeal reflux (LPR) is gastroesophageal reflux disease (GERD) that affects the pharynx and larynx. Reflux laryngitis (RL) is a component of LPR. Laryngopharyngeal reflux and reflux laryngitis are diagnoses that remain a subject for debate because their symptomatology and clinical manifestations are not the same as those of GERD (gastroesophageal reflux disease). The otolaryngology literature prior to the 1970s and 1980s is almost nonexistent. However, during the 1970s and 1980s, several reports of LPR and GERD were published.[1–15] Usually, when RL is present, symptoms and signs of more generalized LPR are also present, although they are commonly missed if not elicited by specific questions during the medical history and meticulous physical examination.

Occult chronic gastroesophageal reflux is an etiologic factor in a high percentage of patients of all ages with laryngologic (ie, voice) complaints. In 1989, Wiener et al reported the results of double-probe pH monitoring in a series of 32 otolaryngology patients with clinical LPR; 78% of them had pH-documented LPR.[16] It has also been found to be a particularly common problem in professional voice users and singers. In 1991, Sataloff et al reported reflux laryngitis in 265 of 583 consecutive professional voice users (45%), including singers and others, who sought medical care during a 12-month period.[17] However, reflux laryngitis was often diagnosed incidentally and was not always responsible for the patient's primary voice complaint. The incidence of RL may be lower in patients with other vocations, but it is interesting to note that Koufman et al found gastro-esophageal reflux in 78% of patients with hoarseness and in about 50% of all patients with voice complaints.[18] Other reports have been published on the pathogenesis of voice disorders and other otolaryngologic manifestations of LPR and its prevalence.[19–32] Nevertheless, the prevalence of reflux laryngitis in all patients who seek evaluation for voice complaints remains unknown. Additional epidemiologic studies are needed to help clarify the clinical importance of this entity.

LPR involves multiple anatomical sites including the sphincter between the stomach and distal esophagus; the entire length of the esophagus; the upper esophageal sphincter; the structures of the larynx, pharynx, and oral cavity; and the trachea and lungs. Consequently, it should be evident that LPR is managed best through a multidisciplinary team approach. The team includes at least a laryngologist who is uniquely qualified to diagnose disorders of the larynx, an internist or primary care physician, a gastroenterologist and his or her laboratory personnel, a speech-language pathologist, and a pulmonologist. For voice professionals, a singing voice specialist and an acting-voice specialist should be included.[33] The availability of a knowledgeable psychologist and nutritionist is highly desirable, as well.[33,34] Although it is possible for one physician to manage most or all aspects of LPR, this approach does not provide comprehensive state-of-the-art care.

Laryngeal involvement by gastroesophageal reflux disease commonly results in dysphonia for which patients attempt to compensate through hyperfunctional voice use patterns (muscular tension dysphonia

[MTD]). The collaboration of a speech-language pathologist and other voice team members is invaluable in eliminating compensatory behaviors and optimizing phonatory technique. Although laryngologists can certainly purchase 24-hour pH monitoring equipment and may even perform manometry, they do not generally do so with the same level of expertise as a gastroenterologist whose entire career may be devoted to disorders of the esophagus. Just as certain laryngologists subspecialize in voice care, some gastroenterologists subspecialize in the management of reflux. This group of professionals and their ancillary staff may be best equipped to diagnose gastroesophageal reflux and its consequences.

Laryngopharyngeal reflux is almost always associated with some degree of aspiration. This may be clinically insignificant, or it may cause chronic cough, reactive airway disease, difficulties controlling asthma, pneumonia, or bronchiectasis. A knowledgeable pulmonologist is essential in recognizing and treating these conditions.

There are several issues of special concern in the management of otolaryngologic patients with reflux laryngitis, especially professional voice users. First, many of these patients are young and will require prolonged or lifetime use of high doses of $H_2$ antagonists or proton pump inhibitors. Despite being quite safe, the ultimate long-term effects of taking these medications over a long period of time are unknown, and they are expensive. The cost may be burdensome, and a financial strain often leads to poor compliance. Second, medications do not eliminate or cure reflux. They simply neutralize the refluxate and control the symptoms effectively in many patients. However, some patients may continue to aspirate pH-neutral fluid, bile salts, and other substances not appropriate for entry into the pharynx, larynx, and lungs. In professional singers and other high-performance voice users, this problem may continue to be symptomatic (throat clearing, excess phlegm, cough) even when acidity is controlled well, although no one has demonstrated that de-acidified gastric acid actually causes mucosal injury.

As stated above, medications do not cure reflux; however, surgery may actually eliminate reflux. Conveniently, surgical therapy for GERD has improved dramatically with the advent of laparoscopic Nissen fundoplication and endoscopic antireflux procedures that offer alternatives to chronic medical management. An increasing percentage of patients are being referred for surgical treatment.

It is essential for otolaryngologists to be familiar with the anatomy, physiology, pathology, diagnosis, and treatment options for LPR and GERD in general. Although much of this knowledge is outside traditional otolaryngology, familiarity with the latest concepts and techniques in the management of GERD and reflux laryngitis in voice patients helps the otolaryngologist assemble an appropriate voice team, interpret information from other colleagues on the voice care team, and ensure optimal patient care.

## Anatomy and Physiology of the Vocal Tract

Discussions of vocal fold physiology in previous chapters highlighted the importance of a complex, traveling mucosal wave with vertical phase differences. This complexity is necessary for normal phonation. Anything that interferes with it may result in voice dysfunction. Hence, it should be clear that gastric acid irritation of the vocal folds is capable not only of producing annoying, irritative symptoms (burning, lump in the throat), but moreover of actually interfering with phonation by causing edema of the vibratory margin and lamina propria that truly alters voice.

The anatomic and physiologic basis for many symptoms of LPR seems fairly obvious initially. Topical irritation, muscle spasm, bronchospasm in response to acidic aspiration, halitosis, sore throat, and other symptoms are easy to understand, although some have unexpectedly complex physiology. In addition, vagal reflexes triggered by distal esophageal acid irritation may cause events and responses that affect the voice even without acid contacting the larynx. Regardless of the mechanism, the effects of reflux laryngitis on voice function often seem greater than one might anticipate based on physical findings. To understand the impact of reflux disease on phonation, it is helpful to review current concepts in anatomy and physiology of the voice, as discussed elsewhere in this book.

## Anatomy and Physiology of the Esophagus and Its Sphincters

### Anatomy

The human esophagus is a muscular tube that has as its major function the transport of food from the mouth to the stomach[35] (Figure 11–1). It is bounded by a tonically contracted circular muscle sphincter at each end. The median length of the esophageal body,

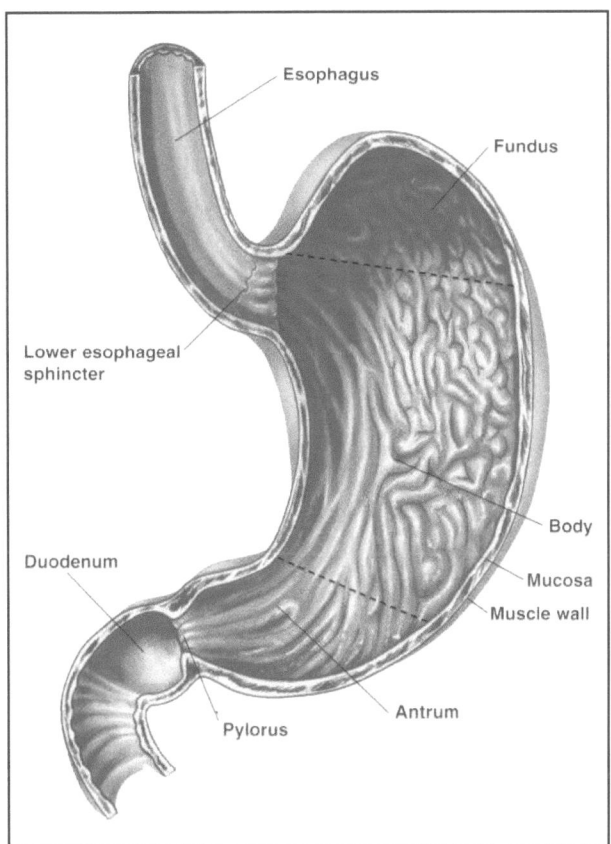

**Figure 11–1.** Normal stomach. (Republished from *Quick Reference to Upper GI Motility* with the permission of Janssen Pharmaceutica.)

between the 2 sphincters, is 22 centimeters (cm) in adult females and 24 cm in adult males. Individual variations in length are normally distributed in both genders[35] (Figure 11–2). The upper esophageal sphincter (UES) consists primarily of striated muscle of the cricopharyngeus muscle but is enhanced by the inferior pharyngeal constrictors and the circular muscles of the upper esophagus. The anterior attachment of the cricopharyngeus to the cricoid cartilage of the larynx results in the strongest contractile force of this sphincter occurring in the anterior-posterior direction, producing a slitlike configuration with the widest portion facing laterally.[36] The UES, like the striated musculature of the tongue, pharynx, and upper portion of the esophagus, is innervated like skeletal muscle, receiving motor input directly from the brainstem (nucleus ambiguus) to the motor endplates in the muscle. Tonicity is maintained by continuous stimulation, which is temporarily inhibited during a swallow.

The lower esophageal sphincter (LES), like most of the gastrointestinal (GI) tract, consists entirely of smooth muscle. This sphincter is much more rounded in its closure, yet still demonstrates some degree of radial asymmetry, having the higher pressures in the posterolateral direction.[37] Innervation of the LES originates from the dorsal motor nucleus of the brainstem, and the efferent fibers are carried through the vagus nerve and synapse in the myenteric plexus in the region of the LES.

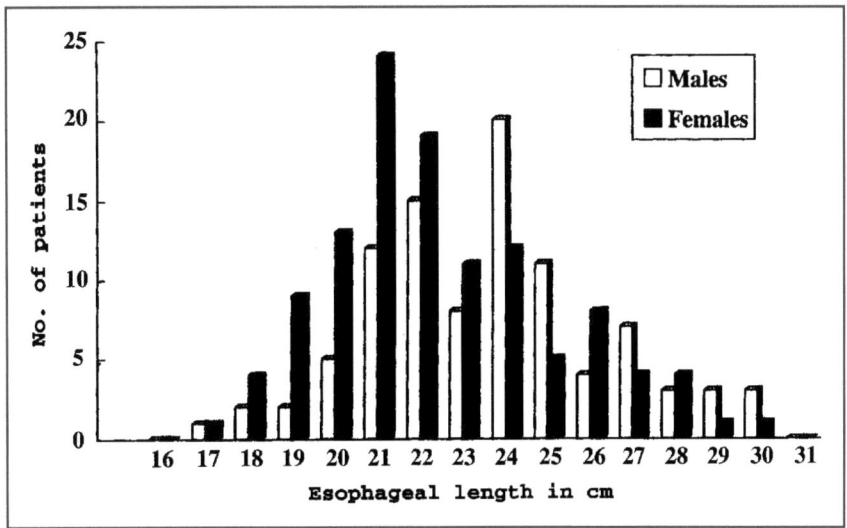

**Figure 11–2.** Distribution of esophageal length in 212 patients and normal volunteers. Males are shown in white, females in black. Approximation to a normal distribution is verified by similar means and medians (males: mean = 23.6 cm, median = 24 cm; females: mean = 22.4 cm, median = 22 cm).

The muscular wall of the esophagus is composed of an inner circular and an outer longitudinal layer, with no serosa overlying the muscle layers. The UES and the upper portion of the tubular esophagus are primarily striated muscle. Recent studies have indicated that smooth muscle occurs in the upper 4 to 5 cm of the human esophagus, although it is quite variable in different individuals and in the different muscle layers. Consistently, greater than the distal half of the human esophagus is entirely smooth muscle.[38] Like the LES, the smooth muscle portion of the tubular esophagus is innervated primarily via the vagus nerve from neurons arising in the dorsal motor nucleus connecting to the myenteric plexus.

## Physiology

Swallowing, or deglutition, has 3 stages: the oral (voluntary) stage, the pharyngeal (involuntary) stage, and the esophageal stage. These 3 closely coordinated and combined processes are regulated through the swallowing center in the medulla.[39]

### Oral Stage

This preparatory stage includes mechanical disruption of the food and mixing with salivary bicarbonate and enzymes (amylase, lipase). It is an essential process by which the swallowing mechanism is primed. Ingested food is voluntarily moved posteriorly by pistonlike movements of the tongue muscles, forcing the food bolus toward the pharynx and pushing it backward and upward against the palate. Once the food has been delivered to the pharynx, the process becomes involuntary. The oral, preparatory stage obviously requires proper functioning of the striated muscles of the tongue and pharynx and is the stage of swallowing that is likely to be abnormal in patients with neurologic or skeletal muscle disease. Appropriate mentation is also necessary.

### Pharyngeal Stage

During this stage of swallowing, the food is passed from the pharynx, through the UES, and into the proximal esophagus. This involuntary process requires the finely tuned coordinated sequences of contraction and relaxation, resulting in transfer of the ingested material, while protecting the airway. The presence of food in the pharynx stimulates sensory receptors, which send impulses to the swallowing center in the brainstem. The central nervous system (CNS) then initiates a series of involuntary responses that include the following:

1. The soft palate is pulled upward and closes the posterior nares.
2. The palatopharyngeal folds are pulled medially, limiting the opening through the pharynx.
3. The vocal folds are closed, and the epiglottis swings backward and down to close the larynx.
4. The larynx is pulled upward and forward by the muscles attached to the hyoid bone, stretching the opening of the esophagus and UES.
5. The UES relaxes. Active relaxation of the usually tonic cricopharyngeus is essential to permit the passive opening of the UES created by the movement of the larynx.
6. Peristaltic contraction of the constrictor muscles of the pharynx produces the force that propels food into the esophagus.

This sequence is a coordinated mechanism that includes impulses carried by 5 cranial nerves. Sensory information to the swallowing center is carried along cranial nerves V, VII, IX, and X. The motor responses from the swallowing center are carried along cranial nerves V, VII, IX, X, and XII and also the ansa cervicalis (C-1 and C-2). This intricate process takes just over 1 second from start to finish and requires coordination of pharyngeal contraction and UES relaxation (Figure 11–3). The UES is only open for approximately 500 milliseconds.

### Esophageal Stage

The main function of the esophagus is to transport ingested material from the mouth to the stomach. This active process requires contraction of both the longitudinal and circular muscles of the tubular esophagus and coordinated relaxation of the sphincters. At the onset of swallowing, the longitudinal muscle contracts and shortens the esophagus to provide a structural base for the circular muscle contraction that forms the peristaltic wave. The sequential contraction of esophageal circular smooth muscle from proximal to distal generates the peristaltic clearing wave. The neuromuscular control of this activity will be described below. As opposed to other GI tract smooth muscle, the esophageal smooth muscle has a unique electrical activity pattern, showing only spiked potentials without underlying slow waves. Circular muscle contractions can be characterized into 3 distinct patterns:

1. *Primary peristalsis.* This is the usual form of a contraction wave of circular muscle that progresses down the esophagus and is initiated by the central mechanisms that follow the voluntary

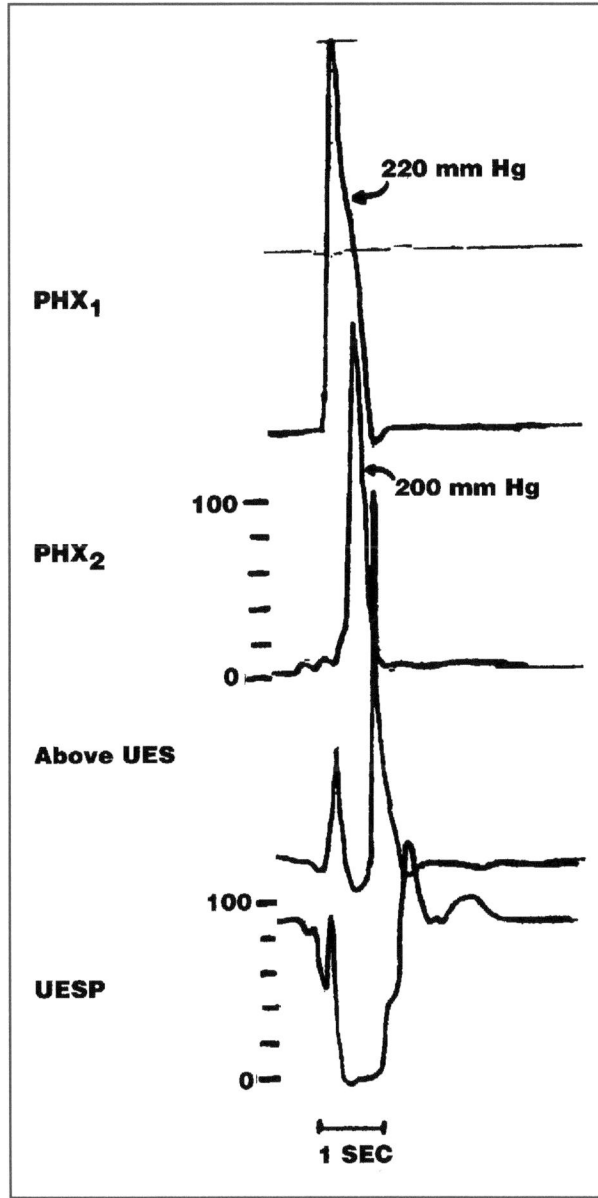

**Figure 11–3.** Motility tracing showing the coordinated sequence of contraction of the human pharynx and relaxation of the upper esophageal sphincter (UES). The 4 recording sites are spaced at 3 cm intervals, with the lowest in the UES high pressure zone (UESP), the second from bottom located just proximal to the UES, and the next 2 sites at 3 cm (PHX2) and 6 cm (PHX1) distances proximally. The sequential contraction in the pharynx is noted in the 2 proximal recording sites. Movement of the UES orad followed by UES relaxation and subsequent descent of the UES during the swallow generates the "M" configuration shown at the third recording site. The apparently longer UES "relaxation" seen in the distal sensor is an artifact produced by the movement of the sphincter orad away from the transducer during swallowing. The actual time of UES relaxation is approximately 0.5 seconds as shown in the recording located second from the bottom.

act of swallowing. It follows sequentially the pressure generated in the pharynx and requires approximately 8 to 10 seconds to reach the distal esophagus. The LES relaxes at the onset of the swallow and remains relaxed until it contracts as a continuation of the progressive peristaltic wave. These pressure relationships are shown in Figure 11–4.

2. *Secondary peristalsis.* This represents a peristaltic contraction of the circular esophageal muscle, which begins without central stimulation. That is to say, it originates in the esophagus as a result of distention and will usually continue until the esophagus is empty. Some food, particularly solid material, requires more than the single primary peristaltic wave for eventual clearance. This is accomplished by the secondary peristaltic waves. Thus, secondary peristalsis is the mechanism for clearing both ingested material and also material that is refluxed from the stomach. Experimentally, secondary peristalsis can be demonstrated by inflating a balloon in the mid-to-upper esophagus.

3. *Tertiary contractions.* This contraction pattern is identified primarily during barium x-ray studies of the esophagus. It represents a nonperistaltic series of contractile waves that appear as localized segmented indentations in the barium column. It has no known physiologic function.

One of the interesting phenomena seen in the esophagus occurs during the process of rapid sequential swallowing (10 seconds or less between successive voluntary swallows). This process results in inhibition of peristalsis, so-called "deglutitive inhibition." Peristalsis will be suspended during the continuation of a series of rapid swallows and a large "clearing wave" will occur at the completion of the swallows (Figure 11–5). This phenomenon occurs because of the inhibitory neural discharge that arises from the central swallowing center during swallowing, and also because the esophageal musculature shows a refractoriness, demonstrated to persist for up to 10 seconds.[40]

### Importance of the Sphincters

The esophagus is located in the thorax and has negative pressure relative to pressures in the pharynx proximally and the stomach distally. Therefore, the action of the sphincters must maintain constant closure to prevent abnormal movement of air or food into the esophagus. In the absence of a tonically contracted UES, air will flow freely into the esophagus

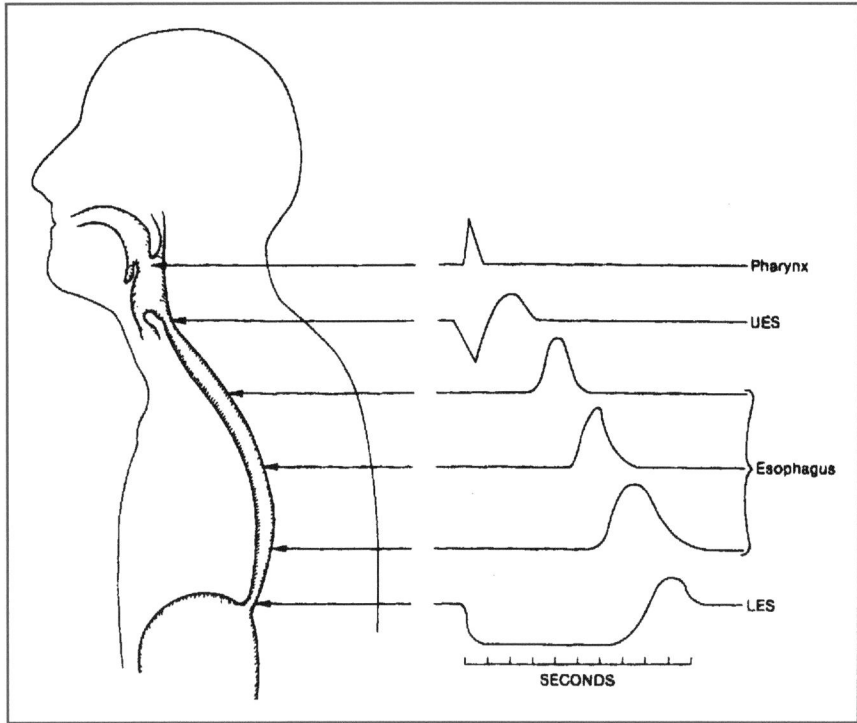

**Figure 11–4.** Schematic presentation of the pressure sequence of a normal primary peristaltic wave. Note the pressure complex that begins in the pharynx and progressively closes off the UES, then moves sequentially down the esophageal body and closes the LES. Also note that LES relaxation begins with the onset of the swallow and remains relaxed until the peristaltic wave reaches the distal esophagus (8–10 seconds).

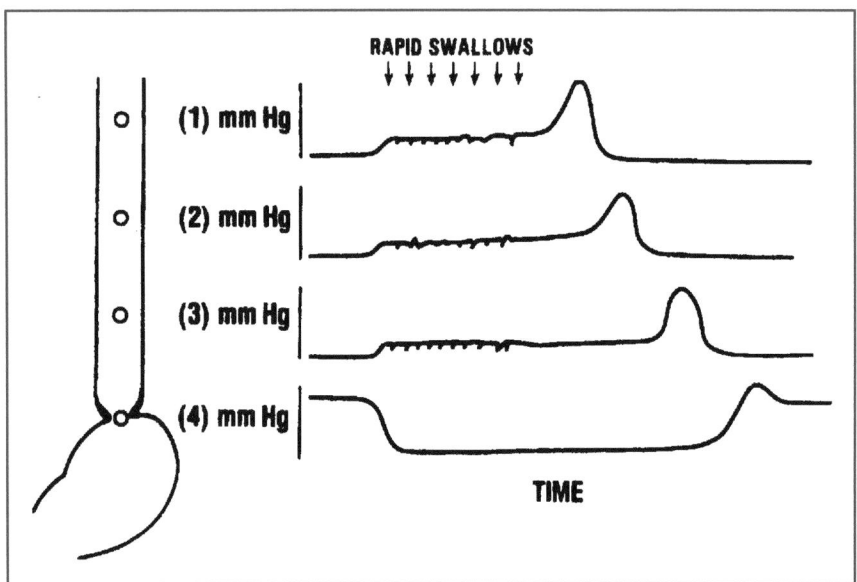

**Figure 11–5.** Demonstration of the phenomenon of deglutitive inhibition of the peristaltic sequence by rapid swallows separated by approximately 5-second intervals. The LES remains relaxed throughout the sequence as the esophageal body is inhibited from a peristaltic response until the termination of the swallows. At this point, the peristaltic clearing wave occurs.

during inspiration. In the presence of a weak LES, gastric contents are not inhibited from refluxing into the distal esophagus, particularly in the recumbent position. Pressure relationships, in and around the esophagus and its sphincters, are shown in Figure 11–6.

*Upper Esophageal Sphincter*

The UES maintains a constant closure with its strongest forces directed in the anterior-posterior orientation of the sling-shaped attachment of the cricopharyngeus to the cricoid cartilage. Normal pressures in the UES are approximately 100 mm Hg in

the anterior-posterior direction and approximately 50 mm Hg laterally.[36]

*Lower Esophageal Sphincter*

The tonically contracted LES normally maintains a closing pressure 10 to 45 mm Hg greater than the intragastric pressure below. By convention, LES pressure is measured as a gradient in mm Hg higher than intragastric pressure, which is used as a zero reference (Figures 11–7 and 11–8). At the time of swallowing, the LES relaxes promptly in response to the initial neural discharge from the swallowing center in the brain and stays relaxed until the

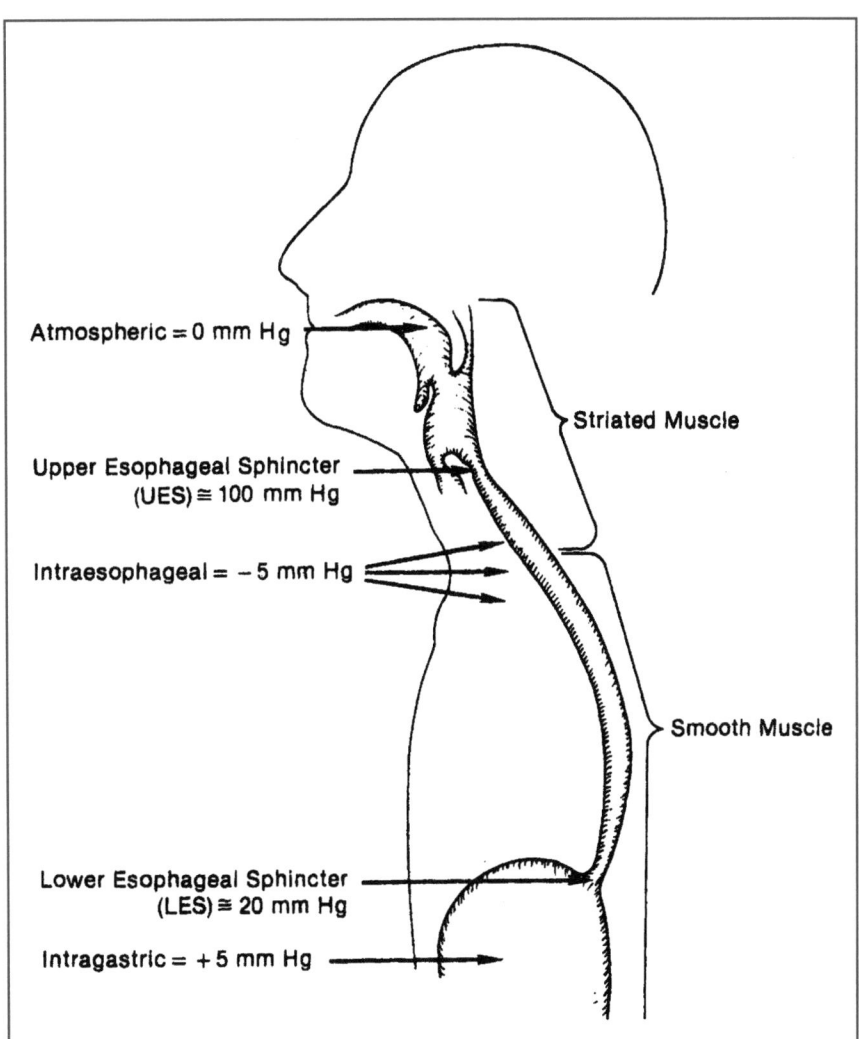

**Figure 11–6.** Schematic representation of the pressure relationships in the pharynx, esophagus, esophageal sphincter, and stomach. Note the negative intraesophageal pressure relative to both pharyngeal (atmospheric) pressure and intragastric pressure. Thus, the importance of the sphincters in prevention of abnormal movement of fluids and air is emphasized.

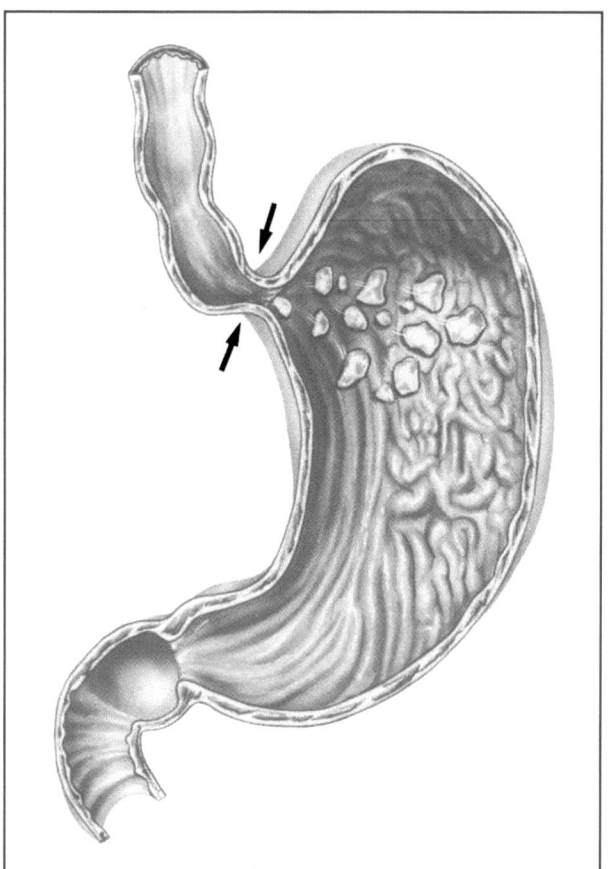

**Figure 11–7.** Normal lower esophageal sphincter (*arrows*) between the esophagus and the stomach. (Republished from *Quick Reference to Upper GI Motility* with the permission of Janssen Pharmaceutica.)

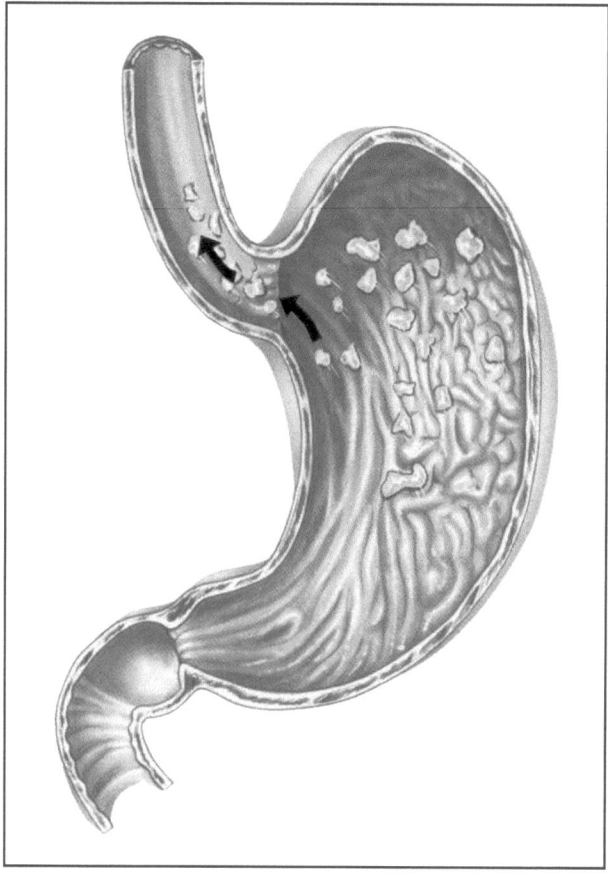

**Figure 11–8.** Incompetent lower esophageal sphincter. (Republished from *Quick Reference to Upper GI Motility* with the permission of Janssen Pharmaceutica.)

peristaltic wave reaches the end of the esophagus and produces sphincter closure. During relaxation, the pressure measured within the sphincter falls approximately to the level of gastric pressure; this is by definition "complete" relaxation. Although there has been much controversy over the years, it is now generally accepted that the LES does not have to be located within the diaphragmatic crus to maintain a constant closing pressure. Thus, the presence of a sliding hiatal hernia is not necessarily detrimental to the physiologic function of this sphincter.

The LES maintains 2 important physiologic functions; the first is its role in prevention of gastroesophageal reflux and the second is its ability to relax with swallowing to allow movement of ingested material into the stomach. The mechanism by which the circular smooth muscle of the LES maintains tonic closure has been a subject of considerable investigation over many years. At present, this is felt to be predominantly the result of intrinsic muscle activity, because investigations in animals have demonstrated that

resting LES tone persists even after the destruction of all neural input by the neurotoxin tetrodotoxin.[41] In addition, truncal vagotomy does not affect resting LES pressure in humans. Calcium-channel-blocking agents, which exert their effect directly on the circular smooth muscle, will produce decreases in LES pressures in animals and humans.[42,43] There also appears to be some cholinergic tone present in many animal species and in humans, as an injection of atropine or of botulinum toxin (Botox, Allergan) has been shown to produce marked decreases in resting LES pressure.[44,45]

The mechanism of relaxation of the LES in response to a swallow has also been a subject of considerable investigation and controversy. The precise neurotransmitter responsible for this response is not definitely known. It is clear that it is not a classic cholinergic or adrenergic agent, because specific pharmacologic blockade of these mechanisms does not inhibit LES relaxation. This is a neural event. It can be reproduced in animals by stimulation of the vagus nerve, and relaxation is inhibited by tetrodotoxin.[46] Their relationships are summarized in Figure 11–9. Recent studies indicate that the neurotransmitter might be a combination of vasoactive intestinal polypeptide (VIP) and nitric oxide.[46,47]

The resting pressure of the LES is dynamic. Pressures measured over long periods of time indicate that LES pressure will vary considerably, even from minute to minute. Much of this is due to the effect of a variety of factors that modulate pressure. These include foods ingested during meals and other events such as cigarette smoking and gastric distention. The normal LES will respond to transient increases in intraabdominal pressure by raising its resting pressure to a greater degree than the pressure increases in the abdomen below. This normal protec-

tive mechanism guards against gastroesophageal reflux. In addition, many hormones and other peptide substances produced in the GI tract and in other areas of the body have been shown to affect LES pressure. These are summarized in Table 11–1. Many of these likely represent pharmacologic responses that have been shown to occur after intravenous injection or infusions of these substances in man or animals. Whether they represent truly physiologic actions has not been clarified in most cases. The strongest candidates for physiologic hormonal control of the LES are cholecystokinin, which helps explain the decrease in LES pressure seen after fat ingestion, and progesterone, which explains the decrease in LES pressure that occurs during pregnancy. Finally, various neurotransmitters and pharmacologic agents have been shown to affect LES pressure. These are summarized in Table 11–2. The modulation of LES resting pressure is a complex mechanism that involves the interaction of the LES smooth muscle, neural control, and humoral factors.[48]

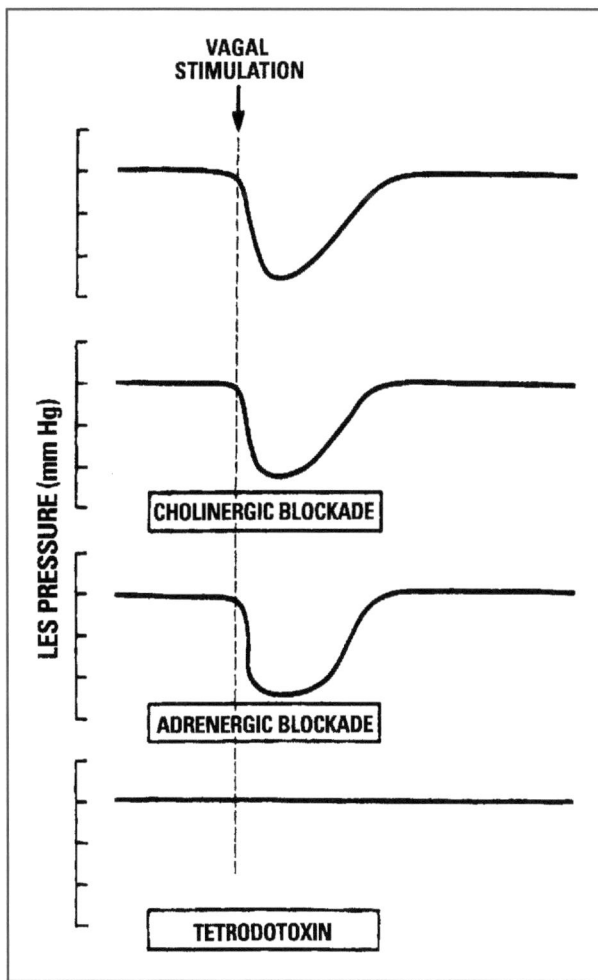

**Figure 11–9.** Summation of experiments in the opossum on the neural regulation of LES relaxation. Electrical stimulation of the vagus nerve produces relaxation, which is not inhibited by blocking either cholinergic or adrenergic pathways. However, the neural response is inhibited by the neurotoxin tetrodotoxin.

**Table 11–1.** Effects of Peptides and Hormones on LES Pressure

| Increases LES | Decreases LES |
| --- | --- |
| Gastrin | Secretin |
| Motilin | Cholecystokinin |
| Substance P | Glucagon |
| Pancreatic polypeptide | Gastric inhibitory polypeptide (GIP) |
| Bombesin | |
| Key-enkephalin | Vasoactive intestinal polypeptide (VIP) |
| Pitressin | Peptide histidine isoleucine |
| Angiotensin | Progesterone |

**Table 11–2.** Effects of Neurotransmitters and Pharmacologic Agents on LES Pressure

| Increases LES | Decreases LES |
| --- | --- |
| Cholinergic (bethanechol) | Nitric oxide |
| (α-adrenergic) | Dopamine (β-adrenergic) |
| Metoclopramide | Nitrates |
| Cisapride | Atropine |
| | Calcium channel blockers |
| | Morphine |
| | Diazepam |
| | Theophylline |

## Controls of Esophageal Peristalsis

As noted above, esophageal peristalsis is controlled via afferent and efferent neural connections through the swallowing center in the medulla. This central mechanism regulates the involuntary sequence of muscular events that occurs during swallowing (Figures 11–10 and 11–11) and simultaneously inhibits the respiratory center in the medulla so that respiration is stopped during the pharyngeal stage of swallowing.

The direct innervation to the striated muscle of the pharynx and upper esophagus is carried via fibers from the brainstem (nucleus ambiguus) through the vagus nerve. The innervation of the smooth muscle of the distal esophagus and LES arises from the dorsal motor nucleus of the vagus and is carried through cholinergic visceral motor nerves to ganglia in the myenteric plexus (also known as the Auerbach plexus). Noncholinergic, nonadrenergic inhibitory nerves also course within the vagus.

The myenteric plexus in the esophageal portion of the enteric nervous system (the "brain in the gut") receives efferent impulses from the central nervous system (CNS) and sensory afferents from the esophagus. Thus, impulses travel in 2 directions through this modulating area, which interconnects and regulates signals that result in normal peristalsis in the smooth muscle of the esophagus. One manifestation of the afferent control is the regulation of peristaltic squeezing pressures, to some degree, by the size of the ingested bolus. In addition, dry swallows often fail to provide adequate stimulation for the action of the myenteric plexus as the primary regulatory mechanism of esophageal peristalsis in the smooth muscle portion, as shown by observations that bilateral cervical vagotomy in animals does not abolish peristalsis in this area.

Interesting results have been obtained from in vitro studies of esophageal smooth-muscle preparations.[49] Using muscle from the opossum esophagus, it has

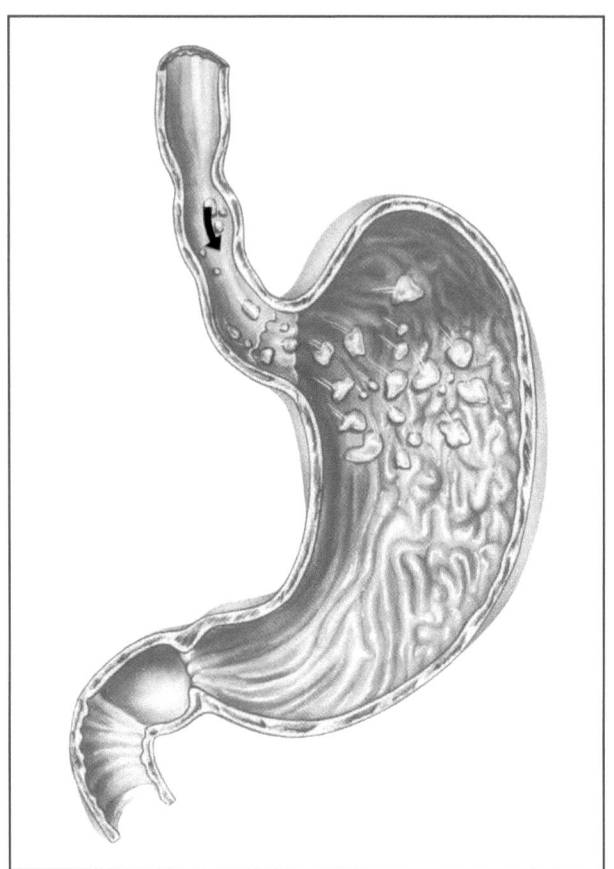

**Figure 11–10.** Normal esophageal peristalsis helping to move food from the esophagus to the stomach. (Republished from *Quick Reference to Upper GI Motility* with the permission of Janssen Pharmaceutica.)

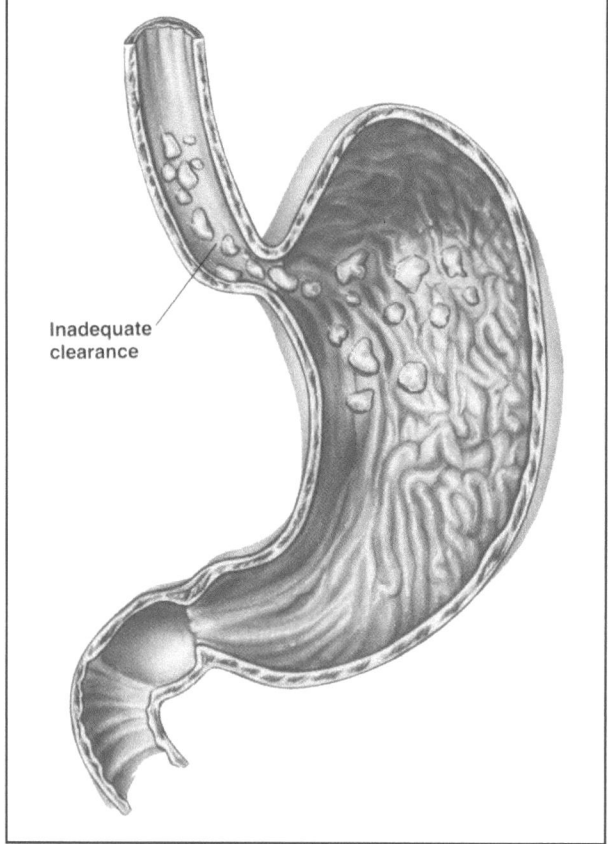

**Figure 11–11.** Mobility disorder with dysfunctional esophageal peristalsis. (Republished from *Quick Reference to Upper GI Motility* with the permission of Janssen Pharmaceutica.)

been shown that the longitudinal smooth muscle demonstrates a sustained contraction during electrical field stimulation; this is called the "duration response." This response is neural and cholinergic, because it can be blocked with both atropine and tetrodotoxin. The circular smooth muscle of the opossum esophagus shows a quite different response. With the onset of electrical stimulation, there is a brief, small contraction at the beginning of the stimulus, known as the "on-response." This response is quite variable and has no known physiologic role. The on-response is followed by a much larger contraction that occurs after the termination of the stimulus, known as the "off-response." This response is also neural in origin but is not cholinergic, because it is blocked only by tetrodotoxin and not atropine. Muscle strips taken from different segments of the smooth muscle portion of the esophageal body show progressively longer intervals for the off-response contraction following stimulation while moving distally in the esophagus. This phenomenon has been called the "latency gradient." These concepts are shown in Figure 11–12.

It has been proposed that these in vitro experiments from the opossum esophagus may help to explain some of the mechanisms of the development of normal peristalsis in the human smooth-muscle esophagus. With the initial swallowing event, an inhibitory neural discharge is sent to the circular smooth muscle of the entire esophagus. The LES relaxes from its resting tonic state. The remainder of the esophageal smooth muscle is already relaxed and shows no measurable change. Rebound contraction occurs following the end of the brief stimulus (the off-response). The latency of the gradient for this off-response, progressing distally down the esophagus, produces the peristaltic contraction wave. Although this concept does not entirely explain all of the phenomena that have been observed in human peristaltic activity, these in vitro observations are consistent with many aspects of normal human physiology. One example is the deglutitive inhibition referred to above. With repetitive swallowing at frequent intervals, the successive inhibitory neural impulses from the swallowing center prevent the contractions of the smooth-muscle portion of the esophagus until the last swallow occurs. The off-response and the latency gradient then allow the single peristaltic clearing wave that usually follows.

## Other Considerations

When gastric pressure becomes greater than LES pressure, reflux occurs. It must be remembered, however,

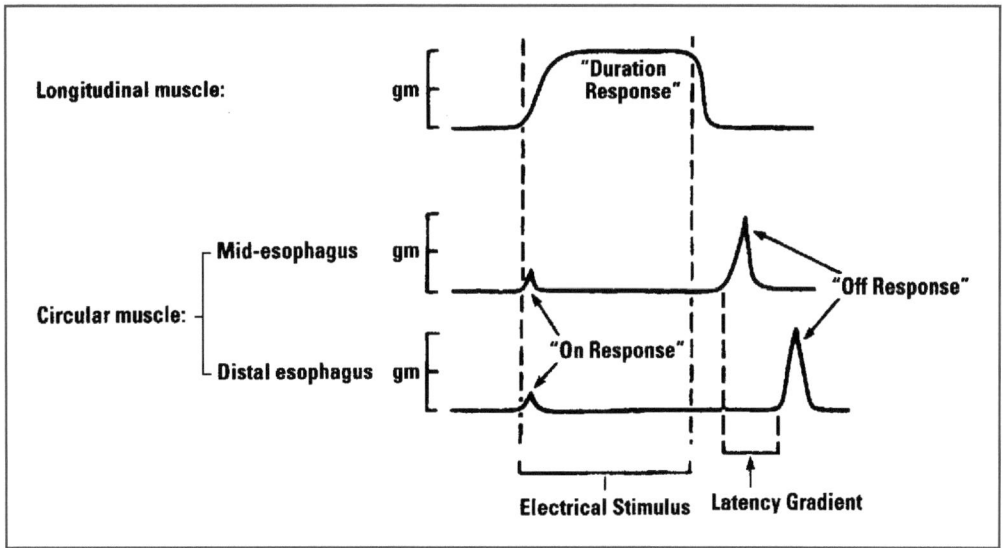

**Figure 11–12.** Summary of the in vitro esophageal smooth muscle responses shown in experiments in the opossum. During stimulation the longitudinal esophageal muscle contracts throughout the stimulus; this is known as the duration response. The circular muscle shows a brief positive impulse at the beginning of stimulation; this is known as the on response. This is followed by a much greater contraction following termination of the stimulus; this is known as the off response. Delay in the latter response, progressing daily in the esophagus, produces the so-called latency gradient (gm = contraction force in grams).

that mechanical sphincter dysfunction is not the only cause of reflux symptoms. Gastric pathology (ie, hypersecretion and alkaline gastroesophageal reflux), motility disorders, and other conditions such as impaired gastric emptying (Figures 11–13 and 11–14) must be considered.

## Clinical Presentation and Epidemiology of Gastroesophageal Reflux Disease: An Overview

Gastroesophageal reflux disease (GERD) is a spectrum of disease best defined as symptoms and/or signs of esophageal or adjacent organ injury secondary to the reflux of gastric contents into the esophagus or above into the oral cavity or airways. GERD is a common disorder often encountered in clinical practice and presents with a multitude of symptoms. Injury caused by GERD is defined based on symptoms or organ damage, which include esophagitis; inflammation of the larynx, pharynx, and oral cavity; or acute and/or chronic pulmonary injury. This section presents an overview of GERD including typical, atypical, and extraesophageal presentations.

### Typical Symptoms

The typical or classic symptoms of GERD are heartburn (pyrosis), defined as substernal burning occurring shortly after meals or on bending over that is relieved with antacids and regurgitation (the spontaneous return of gastric contents into the esophagus or mouth). When present together, heartburn and regurgitation establish the diagnosis with greater than 90% certainty. In clinical practice, heartburn is a daily complaint in 7 to 10% of the population in the United States and at least monthly in about 40 to 50%.[50-52] Over 20 million people in the United States have heartburn at least twice a week and use antacids or other over-the-counter (OTC) antireflux products on a regular basis. Regurgitation is experienced weekly by

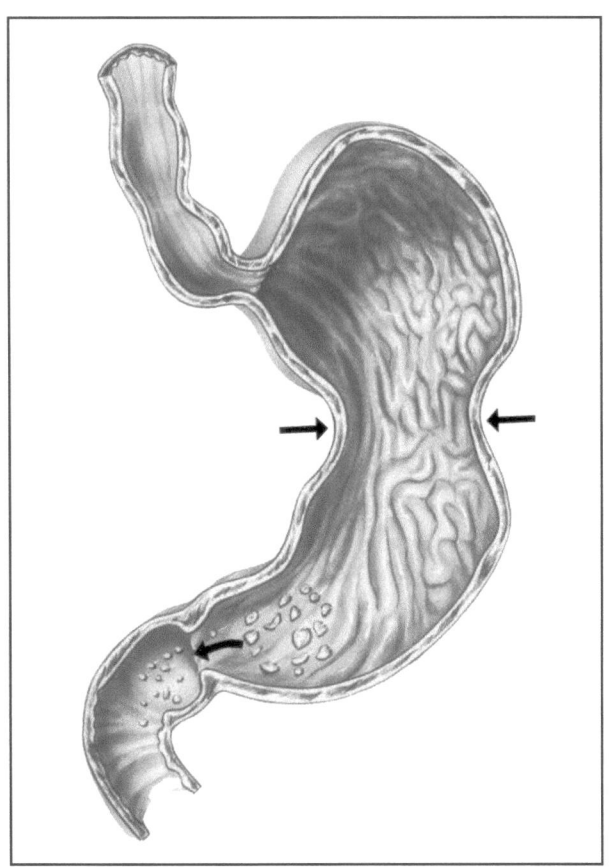

**Figure 11–13.** Normal gastric emptying. (Republished from *Quick Reference to Upper GI Motility* with the permission of Janssen Pharmaceutica.)

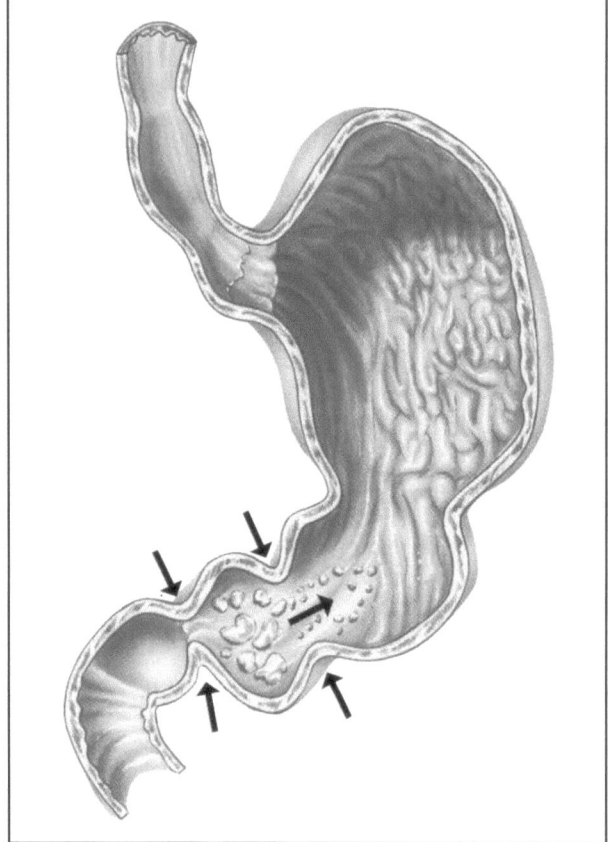

**Figure 11–14.** Abnormal, delayed gastric emptying. (Republished from *Quick Reference to Upper GI Motility* with the permission of Janssen Pharmaceutica.)

about 6% of the population according to one study.[51] In the same study, either heartburn or regurgitation was present weekly in 20% of patients surveyed and monthly in 59%. The prevalence of heartburn appears to decrease slightly with increasing age.

Classic heartburn is described typically by patients as a burning sensation under the breastbone with radiation upward toward the throat or mouth. Heartburn generally occurs 1 to 2 hours after meals, following heavy lifting or on bending over. Big meals, spicy foods, citrus products, such as a grapefruit and orange juice, and meals high in fat are more likely to produce heartburn. Colas, coffee, teas, and even beer may have an acidic pH and cause symptoms when ingested. Heartburn may also be caused by medications (Table 11–3). Meals eaten late in the evening, close to bedtime, or taken with alcohol make patients more prone to nighttime symptoms. Patients report often that their symptoms are relieved with an over-the-counter antacid preparation, $H_2$-receptor antagonists, or even by drinking water.

Although heartburn is often associated with the presence of regurgitation, the spontaneous experience of an acidic or bitter taste in the throat or mouth,

these are not synonymous symptoms. Heartburn should not be confused with dyspepsia or a more vague epigastric distress usually localized in the upper abdominal or lower substernal area and associated with nausea, bloating, or fullness after meals. Although dyspepsia (epigastric discomfort) may be a symptom of GERD, it is neither as sensitive nor as specific a symptom as heartburn. The generic terminology of "acid indigestion" used to encompass all symptoms related to GERD is inappropriate; these symptoms must be distinguished for accurate diagnosis and therapy. Waterbrash, the sudden filling of the mouth with a clear, salty fluid, should not be confused with heartburn. This symptom reflects the increase in salivary secretion seen as a reflex response to reflux or regurgitation of gastric acid into an inflamed distal esophagus.

Heartburn is a highly specific symptom of GERD, although GERD is not the only cause. For example, a heartburnlike symptom, suspected to be due to esophageal stasis from outflow obstruction, is described often in patients with achalasia. It is felt that fermentation of undigested food in the esophagus coupled with inflammation may create a heartburnlike sensation in the absence of true GERD. Functional heartburn may also be a component of irritable bowel syndrome. However, if heartburn is the only presenting esophageal symptom, it is likely due to GERD.

Despite the sensitivity and specificity of these two symptoms for the diagnosis of GERD, neither the presence of heartburn and/or regurgitation nor the frequency of these symptoms is predictive of the degree of endoscopic damage to the distal esophagus. Many patients with daily heartburn will have no endoscopic abnormalities. The frequency of heartburn usually does not correlate with the severity of GERD, although nocturnal heartburn suggests the possibility of erosive esophagitis. Only 50 to 60% of patients presenting to a physician with heartburn will have erosive esophagitis seen on a diagnostic endoscopic examination; the remainder will be diagnosed as having nonerosive GERD.[53] Severe disease, including Barrett's esophagus and peptic strictures, may present with infrequent or absent complaints of heartburn.

Most patients with esophagitis will not have progression of their disease beyond the severity of esophagitis seen at the time of initial endoscopy. In a series of 701 patients followed for up to 29 years, only 23% progressed to a more serious grade of esophagitis.[54] The patient with reflux symptoms and no evidence of esophagitis (nonerosive GERD) has even less likelihood of esophageal disease progression,

**Table 11–3.** Factors Causing Exacerbation of Heartburn

| Decreases LES Pressure | Mucosal Irritant |
|---|---|
| Food and beverages | Food and beverages |
|   Fats |   Citrus products |
|   Chocolate |   Tomato products |
|   Onions |   Spicy foods |
|   Carminatives |   Coffee, colas, tea, beer |
|   Coffee | |
| Alcohol | Medications |
| Smoking |   Aspirin |
| |   NSAIDs |
| Medications |   Tetracycline |
|   Progesterone |   Quinidine |
|   Theophylline |   Potassium tablets |
|   Anticholinergic agents |   Iron salts |
|   β-Adrenergic agonists |   Alendronate |
|   α-Adrenergic antagonists |   Zidovudine |
|   Diazepam | |
|   Meperidine | |
|   Nitrates | |
|   Calcium channel blockers | |

Abbreviations: LES = lower esophageal sphincter; NSAIDs = nonsteroidal anti-inflammatory drugs.

with less than 15% of patients progressing to a higher grade over 6 months.[55]

Regurgitation is often associated with heartburn and GERD. When the 2 symptoms are present together, the diagnosis of GERD is highly likely. Regurgitation without heartburn should raise suspicion of Barrett's esophagus (in which acid sensitivity is reduced), achalasia, or other esophageal abnormality. Regurgitation may also be seen as a more prominent symptom in extraesophageal manifestations of GERD, particularly in patients with pulmonary symptoms of reflux, and it may be an important prognostic factor in predicting outcome of therapy.[55-57] Regurgitation is often confused by patients as vomiting. The effortless return of food or fluid in the absence of nausea is an important distinction between these 2 symptoms. Esophageal and extraesophageal symptoms associated with GERD are outlined in Table 11-4.

### Extraesophageal (Atypical) Symptoms

A number of so-called atypical or extraesophageal symptoms have been associated with GERD, including unexplained substernal chest pain without evidence of coronary artery disease (noncardiac chest pain), asthma, bronchitis, chronic cough, recurrent pneumonia, hoarseness, chronic posterior laryngitis, globus sensation, otalgia, aphthous ulcers, hiccups, and erosion of dental enamel. In contrast to heartburn and regurgitation, the prevalence of these atypical or extraesophageal symptoms and their frequency in the general population have not been systematically studied until recently. In a large population-based

survey of Caucasians in Olmstead County, Minnesota,[51] designed to assess the prevalence of GERD in the general population, unexplained chest pain was seen in 23% of the population yearly and in 4% at least weekly. The frequency of unexplained chest pain surprisingly decreased with age. Forty percent had symptoms for more than 5 years, and 5% reported severe symptoms. Asthma was reported in approximately 9%, bronchitis in approximately 20%, and chronic hoarseness in 15% of patients who had atypical GERD symptoms.

The association of these atypical symptoms with heartburn and regurgitation is controversial. In the Minnesota study,[51] patients with heartburn and regurgitation had one or more atypical symptoms about 80% of the time. Atypical symptoms were more common in patients with frequent GERD symptoms compared to patients with no GERD symptoms. Heartburn or regurgitation was reported in more than 80% of the patients with unexplained chest pain and in 60% with globus sensation. The only exception was asthma. Approximately 60% of patients with asthma, bronchitis, hoarseness, and pneumonia had heartburn or regurgitation. The presence of heartburn is not predictive of otolaryngologic symptoms. However, in a case control study by the Veterans Administration, patients with a discharge diagnosis of erosive esophagitis had twice the prevalence of an associated otolaryngologic symptom as compared with control patients without esophagitis.[58] Observations in patients presenting with atypical GERD show that frequent heartburn and regurgitation are uncommon complaints; however, the absence of these typical symptoms should not preclude making a diagnosis. Prospective studies using endoscopy and ambulatory pH monitoring find GERD in as many as 75% of patients with chronic hoarseness,[32] between 70 and 80% of asthmatics,[59,60] and in 20% of patients with chronic cough.[61]

Reflux is a well-recognized cause of atypical chest pain and may be responsible for many (most) of the symptoms in the 75 000 to 150 000 patients who undergo normal coronary angiography in the United States annually.[62]

Approximately 45% of these patients with unexplained chest pain can be shown to have GERD.[63] Esophagitis in this population is less common, being seen in less than 10%.[64] Endoscopically, esophagitis is seen in 30 to 40% of patients with asthma[65,66] and about 20% of patients with reflux laryngitis. Distinguishing between cardiac and noncardiac chest pain due to GERD is difficult, and they may coexist in the same patient. All of the features of cardiac angina—

**Table 11-4.** Symptoms Associated With Gastroesophageal Reflux

| Esophageal | Extraesophageal |
|---|---|
| Chest pain | Asthma or respiratory problems (ie, wheezing, shortness of breath) |
| Dysphagia | |
| Heartburn | Chronic cough |
| Odynophagia (rare) | Dental hypersensitivity (from loss of dental enamel) |
| Regurgitation | |
| Waterbrash | Hoarseness |
| | Laryngitis or laryngospasm |
| | Nausea |
| | Otalgia |

tight, gripping, vicelike pain radiating to the neck, shoulder, or left arm and associated with exertion —may be seen with GERD also. Long episodes of pain (greater than 1 hour), pain relieved by eating, or pain awakening from sleep are more likely esophageal symptomatology. Antacids or $H_2$-blockers may relieve chest pain, later proven to be associated with coronary artery disease. It is therefore crucial to rule out cardiac disease before presuming GERD is the cause of chest pain. Omeprazole is an effective treatment for reflux-related, noncardiac chest pain[67]; in patients with infrequent (less than 3 times per week), noncardiac chest pain, high-dose proton pump inhibitor (PPI) therapy, such as omeprazole, may be a sensitive, specific, cost-effective strategy for diagnosing GERD.[68] However, it must be remembered that not all patients respond to PPI medications. Therefore, persistent chest pain during PPI therapy does not definitively rule out GERD as the etiology of the chest pain as the evaluation of patients with unexplained chest pain remains complex.[69] For example, the rare syndrome X is a condition involving anginal chest pain with objective signs of ischemia on exercise stress testing or myocardial scintigraphy, but with normal coronary arteries on angiogram. Esophageal hypersensitivity (as opposed to gross functional abnormality) may be an associated finding in these patients; and acid suppression may improve the condition in many patients.[70] The complex relationship between reflux and chest pain remains incompletely understood. Ambulatory pH monitoring, particularly during continued PPI therapy, remains the gold standard for diagnosis of GERD in this population.

Seventy to 80% of patients with asthma will have associated GERD. Whether there is a cause-and-effect relationship or the coincidental presence of 2 diseases is not clear. A careful history will reveal heartburn or regurgitation in only 50%. Onset of asthma late in life, the absence of a seasonal or allergic component, and onset after a big meal, alcohol consumption, or exercise suggest GERD-related asthma. Empiric treatment with acid reflux suppression followed by pH testing in nonresponders was suggested in one study as the most cost-effective means of determining whether GERD is aggravating a patient's asthma.[71] This approach seems reasonable, because it has been demonstrated that PPI therapy in asthmatics with gastroesophageal reflux improves peak expiratory flow rate and quality of life.[72]

Reflux is the third most common cause of chronic cough, after postnasal drip and bronchitis, and in many cases symptoms of postnasal drip may actually be associated with reflux. So the prevalence of reflux as an etiologic factor in chronic cough may be even higher than recognized previously. In the patient with cough, a normal chest x-ray, and no sinonasal postnasal drip, GERD should be considered as the most likely diagnosis.

Hoarseness is the most common otolaryngologic symptom of GERD. Most studies suggest that heartburn is present in only about 50% or less of otolaryngologic patients with extraesophageal manifestations (such as hoarseness) of GERD. However, some authors feel that a careful history may reveal heartburn to be present, at least occasionally, in as many as 75%.[73] Other associated symptoms of reflux laryngitis include halitosis, throat clearing, dry cough, coated tongue, globus sensation, tickle in the throat, chronic sore throat, postnasal drip, and others discussed later in this chapter. Difficulty in warming up the voice in the professional singer, voice fatigue, and intermittent laryngitis are associated symptoms. Erosion of the dental enamel may be due to GERD; however, its frequency is not known.

**Complications of GERD**

GERD may present with severe complications, including peptic stricture, ulceration, iron deficiency anemia, or more importantly Barrett's esophagus. Barrett's esophagus is a premalignant condition that involves a change from normal squamous epithelial lining to a metaplastic intestinal type epithelium with typical special staining characteristics. Estimates are that 2 to 10% of patients with GERD will have strictures,[74] and 10 to 15% will have Barrett's esophagus.[53,75] Dysphagia, odynophagia (painful swallowing), and upper gastrointestinal (GI) bleeding may occur with these complications of GERD. Slowly progressive dysphagia, particularly for solids, suggests peptic strictures. Liquid and solid dysphagia suggests a GERD-related motility disorder secondary to erosive esophagitis, Barrett's esophagus, or scleroderma. GERD-related motility disorders are seen with increased frequency in patients with otolaryngologic manifestations of GERD,[76] even though dysphagia is not usually a presenting symptom. Motility abnormalities pose important complications for the patient considering surgery (see Surgical Therapy for Gastroesophageal Reflux Disease). Odynophagia is uncommon in patients with reflux. Its presence suggests ulceration or inflammation, and it is seen most frequently in infectious or pill-induced esophagitis. Occasionally esophagitis may present with occult, upper gastrointestinal bleeding or iron deficiency anemia.[74] The frequency of these complications in patients with reflux laryngitis is not known.

## Anatomy and Pathophysiology of LPR

Findings highlight the important fact that gastric acid can reflux through the esophagus to the larynx without causing esophageal injury in transit. It has been assumed that this is because distal esophageal mucosa has specialization and defense mechanisms that help it tolerate acid exposure. Esophageal protective mechanisms include peristalsis, which clears acid from the esophagus; a mucosal structure that may be specialized to tolerate intermittent acid contact; the acid-neutralizing capacity of saliva that passes through the esophagus and bicarbonate production in the esophagus, which has been recognized since the 1980s.[77–79] Interestingly, however, if some patients stop reflux treatment after a few months, classic dyspepsia and pyrosis seem to be present commonly when symptoms recur, although this clinically observed phenomenon has not been studied formally. It should be noted that the larynx and pharynx do not have protective mechanisms, such as those found in the esophagus, to protect against mucosal injury. So, exposure to acid and pepsin that might be of no consequence in the distal esophagus may cause substantial symptoms and signs in the larynx and/or pharynx of some patients. Interestingly, preliminary data by Axford et al suggest that laryngeal mucosa has different cellular defenses from those of esophageal mucosa.[80] They also suggested that there may be specific differences in MUC gene expression and carbonic anhydrase that suggest a pattern of abnormality in patients with LPR.

In addition to prolonged vocal warm-up time, professional singers and actors may complain of vocal practice interference, manifested by frequent throat clearing and excessive phlegm, especially during the first 10 to 20 minutes of vocal exercises or singing. Hyperfunctional technique during speaking and especially singing is also associated with reflux laryngitis. This is probably due to the vocalist's unconscious tendency to guard against aspiration. Voice professionals can be helped somewhat in overcoming this secondary muscular tension dysphonia (MTD) through voice therapy with speech-language pathologists, singing voice specialists, and acting-voice specialists, but it is difficult to overcome completely until excellent reflux control has been achieved.

In addition to the paucity of typical GERD symptoms in patients with LPR, the tendency for under-diagnosis of LPR has been increased by 3 additional factors. First, the importance of various aspects of the physical examination is underappreciated. Posterior laryngitis and interarytenoid pachydermia are ignored frequently.[81] It is even more common to fail to recognize the causal relationship between reflux and edema with little or no erythema, especially if the edema is diffuse rather than most prominent on the arytenoids. Second, therapeutic medication trials may fail because patients are undermedicated (eg, a PPI only once daily), and assessed before signs of laryngopharyngeal reflux have had time to resolve (which may require a few months or more). Third, routine tests for gastroesophageal reflux disease can be falsely negative. This problem involves not only barium esophagrams, the Bernstein acid-hyperperfusion test, and radionucleotide scanning, but also esophagoscopy and 24-hour pH monitor studies (depending on the norms used). Consequently, laryngologists must maintain a high index of suspicion in the presence of symptoms consistent with LPR, evaluate such patients aggressively, and interpret test results knowledgeably and with awareness of their sensitivities, specificities, limitations, and controversies.

## Reflux Laryngitis and Other Otolaryngologic Manifestations of Laryngopharyngeal Reflux

Although the majority of otolaryngologists have recently acknowledged the importance of reflux in causing otolaryngologic disease, many authors have recognized the association for more than 2 decades.[1,3,4,11,12,14,16,32,82–102] Otolaryngologists are becoming increasingly diligent about looking for erythema and edema of the mucosa overlying the arytenoid cartilages, suspecting laryngopharyngeal reflux (LPR) as the underlying problem, and treating it as the primary approach to therapy for various reflux-related conditions. However, additional information has shown that the term "laryngopharyngeal reflux" describes a complex spectrum of abnormalities; and it is important for physicians to understand the latest concepts in basic science and clinical care of LPR. Symptoms and signs related to reflux have been identified in 4 to 10% of all patients seen by otolaryngologists,[18,28,32,103] and it is probable that these estimates are low. Among patients with laryngeal and voice disorders, laryngopharyngeal reflux appears to be strongly associated with, or a significant etiologic cofactor in, about 50% of these patients. Many of the current concepts regarding reflux laryngitis and related controversies have been reviewed recently in the otolaryngologic and gastroenterologic literature.[104–106]

## Other Clinical Practice Considerations

Treatment considerations in reflux patients are discussed in greater detail later in this chapter Research into appropriate treatment regimens is ongoing, and extensive additional investigation on the consequences of reflux on the larynx and all of the other mucosal surfaces above the cricopharyngeus muscle is needed.

LPR has been found in association with otitis media with effusion not only in the pediatric population, but also in adults.[107] Habesoglu et al studied the effects of LPR on tympanoplasty failure.[108] They reported the results of 147 patients who underwent tympanoplasty who had laryngoscopic evidence of LPR and positive reflux finding scores. The authors suggested that these findings should be considered as a factor in the failure of tympanoplasty, and they recommended that reflux evaluation and treatment should be considered in the treatment of patients with chronic otitis media and ear disease, including eustachian tube dysfunction.[108,109] Other studies have reported that LPR and obesity are risk factors associated with lingual hypertrophy and obstructive sleep apnea.[110,111] A study by Corvo et al reported significant LPR in association with patients known to have Sjögren's syndrome, confirmed by salivary analysis.[112]

Several studies have reported the presence of pepsin and amylase in oral and tracheal secretions.[113,114] Another report[115] suggested alterations in mucin gene expression in laryngeal mucosa and/or laryngeal mucosal metaplasia due to MUC3, 4, and 5 MucSAC expression being downregulated in LPR may predispose the larynx to mucosal damage from gastric refluxate. Eckley et al[116] studied salivary epidermal growth factor in adult patients with LPR pre- and post-treatment with PPIs. Saliva samples were obtained on 20 patients with LPR before and after a 16-week course of PPI therapy and compared to a control group of 12 healthy patients. Patients with LPR had lower salivary epidermal growth factor concentrations pre- and post-treatment compared with the healthy control group. The authors suggest that this finding indicates a defective mechanism of mucosal protection. Several recent studies have shown that scitintigraphic studies are useful as a screening tool for predicting aspiration in patients with LPR and GERD and in whom fundoplication surgery is being considered.[117,118] Endoscopy, olfactory function, and analysis of color and texture of laryngoscopic images also have been reported as part of the armamentarium in evaluating the presence of and/or predisposition to LPR.[119,120]

In treating LPR patients, the clinician is faced with management decisions centered on the entire aerodigestive tract. For example, the presence of pepsin in nasal lavage fluid has been documented in patients undergoing endoscopic sinus surgery.[121] LPR has been confirmed in these patients, suggesting a relationship between chronic rhinosinusitis and LPR. Nasal pepsin may prove to be an avenue of LPR screening.[121] Evidence also links LPR and chronic otitis media,[122] as discussed above, and surgical outcomes in laryngeal trauma surgery have proven better in patients with preoperative and postoperative PPI treatment.[123] Therefore, many different patient groups may benefit from reflux evaluation and treatment.

Pepsin has been found in tracheoesophageal puncture sites, as reported by Bock et al.[124] They performed tissue biopsy and collected secretions in 17 patients, 12 of whom had a history of GERD/LPR, and pepsin was detected in the majority of their patients. LPR also may play a role in the pathogenesis of dental disease and sleep disorders. Several studies have shown a relationship between LPR and dental erosion.[125,126] In an animal (rat) model study, Higo et al[127] identified microscopic dental erosion and loss of surface enamel secondary to regurgitation of acid, liquid, and gas, as well as destruction of teeth and supporting structures when they were exposed to gastric and duodenal contents. Ranjitkar et al[128] reported that casein phosphopeptide-amorphous calcium phosphate can protect teeth from erosion caused by acid and bile products.

Becker et al[129] studied the role of LPR in patients with complaints of intraoral burning sensations. They placed an oropharyngeal pH monitoring probe at the level of the uvula and found no causal relationship between LPR and intraoral burning. They suggested that PPI therapy is not indicated in this patient population.

Researchers and clinicians have examined a myriad of symptoms in patients with LPR and the relationships between LPR and voice disorders, benign and malignant lesions in the larynx, chronic cough, pulmonary disease, asthma and allergy, and obstructive sleep apnea in both adults and children. Chung et al[130] examined the relationship between LPR and benign vocal fold lesions. They reported LPR in 65% of their control group, 66% of the vocal nodules group, 75% of the vocal fold polyp group, and 95% of the patients with Reinke's edema. Saleh[131] suggested links among reflux, postnasal drip, and chronic cough. Randhawa et al[132] pointed out that it is sometimes difficult to determine the cause of dysphonia, noting that the laryngeal findings on nasopharyngolaryngoscopy may be similar in patients with LPR and in those with allergy. In their small sample population, they diagnosed allergy in 10 patients and LPR in only 3 patients, which they felt raised the question of LPR being overdiagnosed.

Recent studies suggest a relationship between LPR and obstructive sleep apnea. Eskiismir and Kezirian[133] suggested that the increased respiratory efforts used by patients with obstructive sleep apnea generate increased intrathoracic pressure, which contributes to increased reflux. Suzuki et al[134] suggested that relaxation of the LES might be the mechanism of reflux in patients with mild to moderate obstructive sleep apnea. They also found reflux-induced spontaneous arousals. Karkos and colleagues[135] reported that during sleep, UES pressures decrease significantly. However, they noted a lack of controlled trials and/or meta-analyses that address the correlation between reflux, snoring, and/or apnea. In 2010, Wang et al[136] examined the concentration of pepsin detected in oropharyngeal secretions in patients with LPR and obstructive sleep apnea. In the LPR population, they found higher levels of pepsin in sputum that correlated with a higher reflux symptom index and higher reflux finding score. In obstructive sleep apnea patients, they reported no relationship between pepsin levels and reflux symptom index.

Eryuksel et al[137] examined the relationship between LPR and chronic obstructive pulmonary disease. Before and following 2 months of PPI treatment, patients underwent laryngeal examinations and pulmonary function tests and were asked to complete questionnaires for LPR and chronic obstructive pulmonary disease. The authors reported significant improvement in chronic obstructive pulmonary disease symptom index and LPR symptoms and findings on laryngeal examination. De la Hoz and colleagues[138] studied reflux and pulmonary disease in 9-11 World Trade Center first responders. Their findings suggest that patients with reflux demonstrated reduced forced vital capacity, suggestive of air trapping and lower airway disease.

## Physical Examination

Physical examination of patients with throat and voice complaints must be comprehensive. A thorough head and neck examination is always included, with attention to the ears and hearing, nasal patency, signs of allergy, the oral cavity, temporomandibular joints, the larynx, and the neck. In some patients with LPR severe enough to involve the oral cavity, there is also loss of dental enamel. Hence, transparency of the lower portion of the central incisors may be seen occasionally in reflux patients, although it may

be more common in patients with bulimia and those who habitually eat lemons. At least a limited general physical examination is included to look for signs of systemic disease that may present as throat or voice complaints. More comprehensive, specialized physical examinations by medical consultants should be sought when indicated.

When the patient has complaints of vocal difficulties, laryngeal examination is mandatory. It should be performed initially using a mirror or flexible fiberoptic laryngoscope; but comprehensive laryngeal examination requires strobovideolaryngoscopy for slow motion evaluation of the vibratory margin of the vocal folds. Formal assessment of the speaking and singing voice also should be performed, when appropriate. Objective voice analysis quantifies voice quality, pulmonary function, valvular efficiency of the vocal folds, and harmonic spectral characteristics. Neuromuscular function can be measured by laryngeal electromyography (EMG). These aspects of the physical examination and tests of voice function are discussed elsewhere in the book and will not be reviewed in this chapter.

Most commonly, laryngoscopy in patients with LPR reveals erythema and edema. Classically, reflux laryngitis involves erythema of the arytenoid cartilages and frequently interarytenoid pachydermia (a knobbled or cobblestone appearance), as well as other signs[25,96,138-145] (Figures 11-15 and 11-16). However, many additional findings may be observed including edema of the false and true vocal folds; partial effacement or obliteration of the laryngeal ventricle; pseudosulcus (a longitudinal groove extending below the vibratory margin throughout the length of the vocal fold, including the cartilaginous portion); Reinke's edema; granulomas or ulcers (most commonly in the region of the vocal process); nodules and other masses; an interarytenoid bar; laryngeal stenosis; and other abnormalities. Koufman reported that edema was seen even more common than erythema, having been diagnosed in 89% of 46 patients, compared with 87% who had erythema; 19% with granuloma or granulation tissue; and 2% with ulceration.[146]

Belafsky et al[147] developed a reflux finding score (RFS) that rates signs and appears to correlate with the presence of LPR. They advocate use of this instrument in combination with the reflux symptom index (RSI).[148] The reflux finding score depends on observations of subglottic edema, ventricular obliteration, erythema/hyperemia, vocal fold edema, diffuse laryngeal edema, posterior laryngeal hypertrophy, granuloma/granulation tissue, and still, thick endolaryngeal mucus. Although additional research from other centers is needed to confirm the validity and reliability

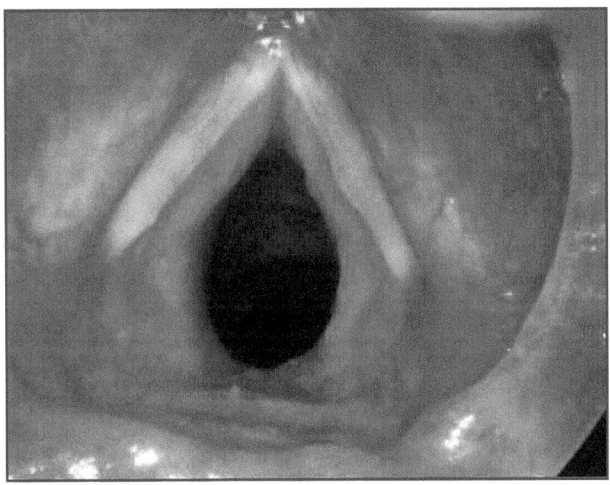 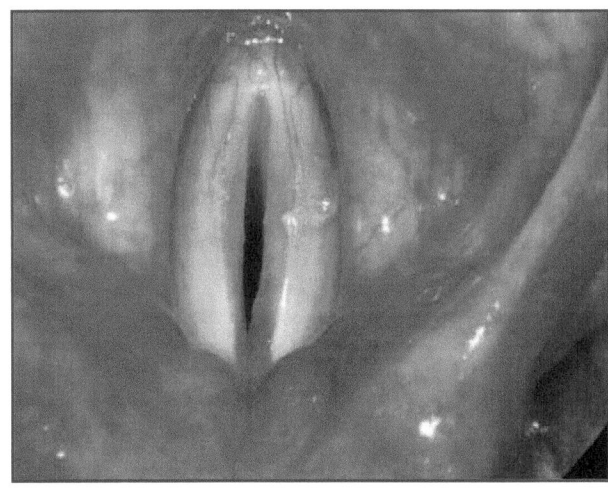

A                                                    B

**Figure 11–15.** Open (**A**) and closed (**B**) views of the vocal folds show the bilateral inferior glottic ridges that parallel the vocal folds and prevent closure of the musculomembranous vocal folds. There is posterior laryngeal cobblestoning and arytenoid erythema and edema.

of the RFS (which remains somewhat controversial), the authors found excellent inter- and intraobserver reproducibility (although all observers were practicing at the same medical center); they found the RFS to be an accurate instrument for documenting treatment efficacy in patients with LPR, and it is used widely (including by the authors of this chapter).

In patients with severe LPR, the finding of a hyperactive gag reflex is also common; of interest, they also may have decreased laryngeal sensation. One of us (RTS) has performed functional endoscopic evaluation of sensory threshold testing on patients with LPR and found that responses were diminished prior to treatment and were improved following treatment. These findings are consistent with preliminary observations by Jonathan Aviv, MD (personal communication, 2000).

It should be noted that controversy exists regarding the significance of laryngeal findings. Credible studies of the sensitivity and specificity of laryngoscopy for diagnosis of LPR are needed, although a few initial reports exist in the literature. Carr et al[149] studied 155 children retrospectively. In a chart review of direct laryngoscopy and bronchoscopy findings, they reported a positive predictive value of 100% for the combination of posterior chronic edema with any vocal fold or ventricular abnormality.

McMurray et al[150] evaluated 39 children prospectively with laryngoscopy, bronchoscopy, esophagoscopy, and pH monitoring prior to airway reconstruction. Full-thickness laryngeal mucosal biopsy specimens were obtained from the posterior cricoid area and the interarytenoid area, and esophageal biopsy specimens were obtained. These investigators were unable to demonstrate a correlation among pH probe data, laryngoscopic findings, and histologic findings. Hicks et al[151] studied 105 healthy, asymptomatic volunteers. On laryngoscopy, more than 80% had at least one "abnormal" finding, including (in order of frequency from most frequent to least) interarytenoid bar, medial arytenoid granularity, and true vocal fold erythema. This study did not perform 24-hour pH monitoring or any other tests to rule out the presence of "silent" reflux as a cause of the laryngoscopic abnormalities.

Despite many articles exploring signs and symptoms of reflux, including those cited above and other recent literature,[151–166] evidence confirming the diagnostic significance of various complaints and findings is scarce and contradictory. This is due to various problems, including the lack of a standard definition of "normal" in populations being studied. Continued interdisciplinary discourse and multicenter studies should be encouraged to answer important questions regarding the sensitivity and specificity of the many findings associated commonly with laryngopharyngeal reflux, as well as the impact of laryngopharyngeal reflux on quality of life and general health.[167]

### Pathophysiology

Laryngeal abnormalities may be caused by direct injury or by a secondary mechanism. Direct injury is due to contact of acid and pepsin with laryngeal

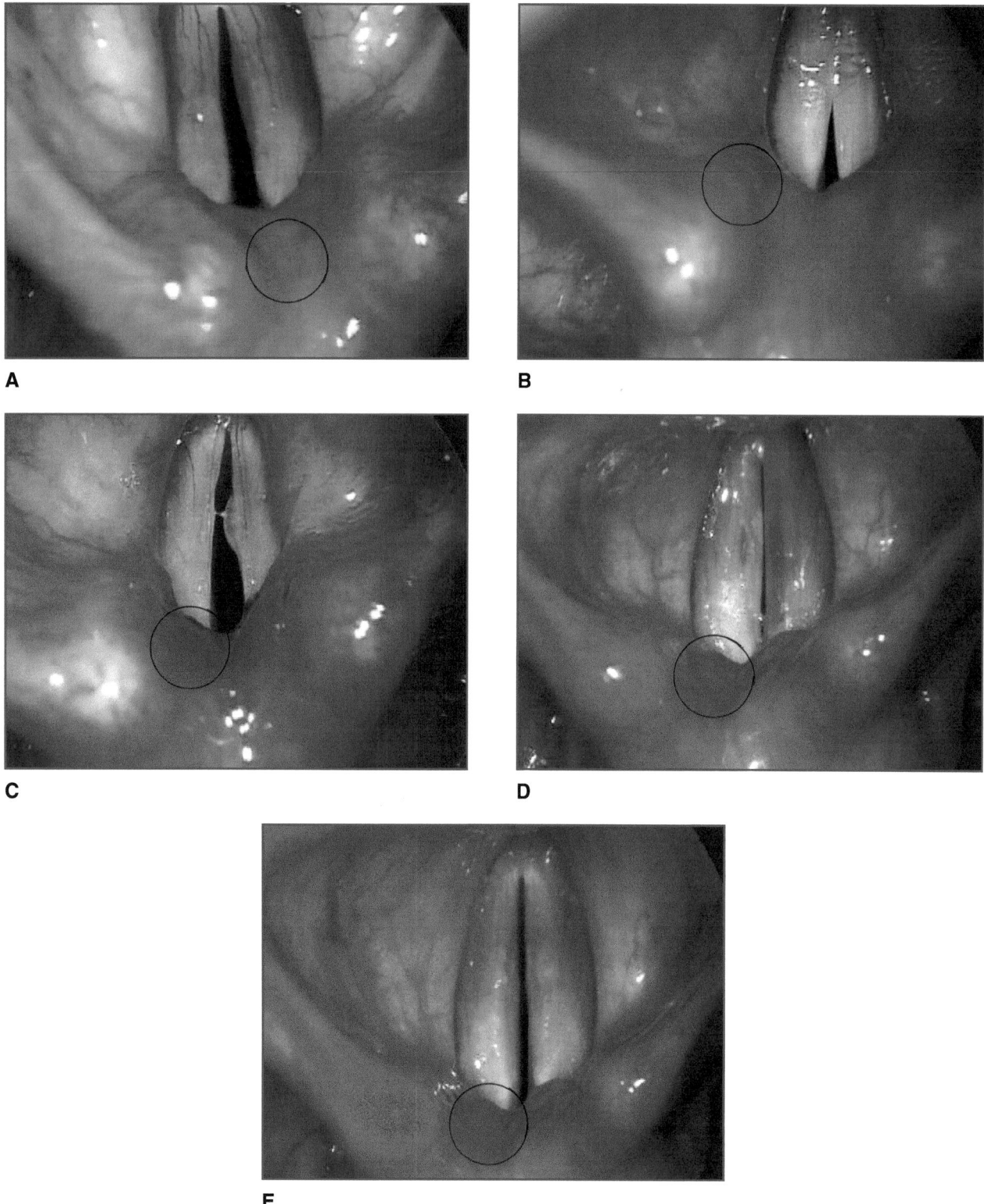

**Figure 11–16.** Assessing laryngeal erythema is one of the many and varied ways of evaluating laryngopharyngeal reflux (LPR). In the absence of the other irritants, acidic reflux is a major contributor to laryngeal erythema. In our center, the posterior larynx—including the medial face of the arytenoid complex, the interarytenoid area, and the posterior cricoid surface—is evaluated carefully. Erythema beyond the posterior larynx is also indicative of LPS, but our grading focuses on the posterior larynx. There are five categories of color: **A.** Normal, **B.** Mild, **C.** Moderate, **D.** Moderate-Severe, and **E.** Severe.

mucosa, resulting in mucosal damage.[3,95,96,168–171] Alternatively, irritation of the distal esophagus by acid may cause a reflex mediated by the vagus nerve, resulting in chronic cough and/or throat clearing, which may produce traumatic injury to the laryngeal mucosa.[83,96,172–176]

Researchers are attempting to delineate pathophysiology. To show LPR as an extra extraesophageal manifestation of GERD, Groome et al[177] hypothesized that GERD patients would have some LPR symptoms if the pathophysiology were truly common. Through a questionnaire administered to 1383 GERD patients, they determined that the prevalence of LPR increases with the severity of GERD.[177] Although based on nonstandard questionnaires, the finding suggests a relationship. A similar study sought to exclude other causes of laryngitis and found LPR in 24% of patients with reflux esophagitis. The presence of LPR was predicted best by age, hoarseness, and hiatal hernia.[178] A third study, strengthened by confirmed diagnoses of GERD and LPR with esophagogastro-duodenoscopy (EGD) and 24-hour pH monitoring, respectively, similarly showed that when both GERD and non-GERD patients were treated with PPIs, laryngitis symptoms and signs improved in the GERD group only.[179] These studies seem to point toward a common pathophysiology, suggesting that laryngeal symptoms are indeed caused by acid exposure.

Bile reflux also may cause laryngeal irritation.[180,181] In addition, recent findings raise many new questions about the pathophysiology of LPR. For example, Eckley et al[182,183] report that decreased salivary epidermal growth factor may be associated with LPR and warrants further study; Altman's discovery of a proton pump in laryngeal serous cells and ducts of submucosal glands is particularly intriguing.[184] It has been established that pepsin in the larynx results in depletion of carbonic anhydrase isoenzyme III (CAI III) and squamous epithelial stress protein (Sep70), 2 laryngeal protective proteins.[185,186] Pepsin is taken up by laryngeal cells and can be reactivated by a drop in pH, as seen in LPR. Pepsin is found in the esophageal mucosa of those with LPR.[187] Interestingly, pepsin irreversibly affects CAI III at pH below 4 only in laryngeal, not esophageal, epithelium.[188] These laryngeal receptors for pepsin may be another future target for intervention. They also might explain the presence of symptoms and signs of LPR with weakly acidic reflux, as pepsin may be active to some degree at any pH between 3 and 6.5,[189] although a longer exposure time may be necessary at pH 5 or above to produce damage.[190] Possible pepsin activity at pH much above 5 remains controversial. Mucin gene (muc) expression also is downregulated in the presence of pepsin.[190,191]

Animal studies have shown that acid combined with pepsin (acid-activated enzyme) compromises the integrity of the vocal fold epithelium. In 2010, Habesoglu et al[192] reported that rats exposed to an acidic pH in the presence of pepsin developed edema of the lamina propria, submucous gland hyperplasia, and muscular atrophy. Erickson and Sivansakar[193] reported that the epithelial barrier resistance of the vocal fold is compromised when exposed to acid and pepsin. They described transepithelial resistance as a marker of epithelial barrier resistance that measures the ability to restrict movement of solute and solvents. The authors pointed out that less than 3 episodes of reflux per week could injure vocal fold mucosa, in contrast to 0 to 50 reflux events daily that are considered normal exposure in the distal esophagus.

In 2009, Johnston et al[194] reported that pepsin invades the laryngeal epithelial cells by receptor-mediated endocytosis and that pepsin activity is maximal at a pH of 2. Bulmer et al[195] in 2010 showed that the effects of acid and pepsin exposure on porcine laryngeal mucosa were similar to the effects observed in the human larynx in patients diagnosed with LPR. Samuels and Johnston[196] reported that the presence of pepsin in the airway indicates reflux. However, they reported that there are only 2 methods used to identify pepsin in the airways: immunologic and enzymatic, both of which have advantages and disadvantages. Richter[197] stated that gastric acid combined with pepsin and bile salts is known to be causally related to the development of chronic esophagitis and Barrett's esophagus. In contrast, they reported that weak or non-acid refluxate has not been shown to cause damage to the esophageal or extraesophageal structures, including the larynx and the lungs.

Histopathologic inflammation and its association with the pathogenesis of esophageal and extraesophageal disease has been the subject of ongoing research. Some studies that have focused on histology have produced interesting findings. One found significantly increased CD8+ lymphocytes in the epithelium of patients with LPR, with proportionally more in the luminal epithelial layer. Additionally, nonclassical major histocompatibility complex (MHC) molecule expression was found to be involved in the response to refluxate, suggesting that relying upon classical markers may lead to erroneous conclusions about the response of laryngeal epithelium to reflux.[198] Wada et al[199] evaluated histopathologic inflammation of the upper esophagus in comparison with the lower esophagus. When compared with their control group, they found inflammation of the upper esophagus to be significantly greater in patients with abnormal laryngopharyngeal symptoms and significantly greater lower esophageal inflammatory histopathology in patients with classic reflux symptoms (ie, GERD).

Park et al[200] used transmission electron microscopy to examine cellular damage of the esophageal epithelium by gastric refluxate. They measured the intracellular space and quantified its dilatation. They compared 2 groups: patients who had LPR without GERD and patients who had LPR with GERD. They reported that the intracellular space of the esophageal epithelium was significantly more dilated in the LPR-with-GERD group. Amin and colleagues[201] reported that dilatation of intracellular spaces of esophageal epithelium is considered a specific marker in GERD. They studied a group of patients with LPR and sore throat in whom they found dilatation of intracellular spaces in oropharyngeal biopsy specimens. They also found dilatation of the intracellular spaces in the laryngeal mucosa in animal models exposed to pepsin.

There are important pathophysiologic differences between LPR patients and GERD patients. For example, combined upright and recumbent or nighttime reflux is typical for GI patients with GERD. Upright reflux and regurgitation also are the least common pattern in this population. However, patients with LPR are more likely to experience upright reflux commonly throughout the day,[16,28,32,202] often even in the absence of supine reflux.

We have observed some patients with LPR who experience reflux exclusively (and constantly) when they sing. Motility abnormalities have been demonstrated with higher frequency in patients with LPR, resulting in delayed acid clearance in one study.[203] In contrast, Postma et al[204] demonstrated that patients with GERD have significantly longer esophageal acid clearance times than those measured in patients with LPR. However, it is not unusual for LPR patients to have abnormal upper esophageal sphincter (UES) function. In 1978, Gerhardt et al[205] showed that experimental instillation of acid in the distal esophagus in patients with esophagitis and in normal controls produces increase in UES tone. This phenomenon does not occur normally in many patients with LPR,[103] although an increase in resting UES pressure has been demonstrated in patients with reflux laryngitis.[205] In 2010, based on their research, Szczesniak and colleagues[206] suggested upregulation of the esophago-UES relaxation as a possible mechanism in the pathophysiology of reflux laryngitis. They found that the UES relaxation reflex induced by rapid air insufflation of the esophagus is upregulated in patients with posterior laryngitis compared with healthy controls. They also found that this group of patients had a higher pharyngo-UES contractile reflex threshold, which is considered a mechanism of airway protection.

Vardouniotis et al[207] reported that a hypotensive lower esophageal sphincter (LES) is a significant pathophysiologic component of LPR, noting that complex molecular mechanisms involved in the function of the LES and genetic factors are involved in tissue protection from reflux. They reported that compared with the esophageal lining, laryngeal and pharyngeal mucosa is more susceptible to tissue damage from refluxate because the larynx is not protected by peristalsis or buffered by salivary bicarbonate. They reported that transforming growth factor-beta 1, which inhibits inflammatory response, has shown gene overexpression in postcricoid fibroblasts and that fibroblast growth factor 2 has shown decreased expression. Cheng et al[208] suggested that the microphage activation caused by gastric acid exposure should be considered also in the pathogenesis of GERD and aspiration-induced lung disease.

Chong and Jalihal[209] reported a greater percentage of LPR symptoms in patients with heterotrophic gastric mucosal patch (HGMP) of the distal esophagus. HGMP is ectopic gastric mucosa typically observed distal to the UES and thought to be congenital. Due to the fact that HGMP can produce acid, the authors suggested that this may be the etiology of LPR in some patients. In fact, in their study, patients with HGMP experienced LPR symptoms to a greater degree (73.1%) compared with their non-HGMP patients (25.9%).

Salminen et al and Basseri et al[210,211] have reported that the endoscopic prevalence of HGMP is low, ranging from 0.1 to 10% in reported patients 16 to 75 years old. Typical symptoms in patients with HGMP include dysphagia, globus pharyngeus, cough, hoarseness, and shortness of breath. They reported that the HGMP is a source of acid production, and this has been supported by pH monitor studies showing gastric acid in this area. Parietal cells with oxyntic mucosa are the most common histologic type reported.

Laryngopharyngeal reflux can affect anyone, but it appears to be particularly common and symptomatic in professional voice users, especially singers. This is true for several reasons. First, the technique of singing involves "support" by the forceful compression of the abdominal muscles designed to push the abdominal contents superiorly and pull the sternum down. This action compresses the air in the thorax, thereby generating force for the stream of expired air, but it also compresses the stomach and works against the LES. Singing is an athletic endeavor, and the mechanism responsible for reflux in singers is similar to that associated with reflux following other athletic activities, lifting, and other conditions that alter abdominal pressure, such as pregnancy (which is also influenced by hormonal factors). It has been established clearly by Clark et al[212] that reflux is induced by exercise even in asymptomatic, young volunteers (mean age, 28 years). They demonstrated that running induced reflux more often than did exercise with less bodily agitation, such as bicycling, but both forms of aerobic exercise caused reflux, as did weight lifting in some patients. Postprandial exercise-induced reflux has a similar pattern, but with a greater amount of refluxate. It may be that the effect of exercise on reflux is even more pronounced in patients with GERD or LPR than it is in research subjects with no history of reflux symptoms, although this question has not been studied.

Second, many singers do not eat before performing because a full stomach interferes with abdominal support and promotes reflux. Performances usually take place at night. Consequently, the singer returns home hungry and eats a large meal before going to bed.

Third, performance careers are particularly stressful. Psychological stress has been associated with esophageal motility disorders (which may be associated with reflux) and with other gastroenterologic conditions, such as irritable bowel syndrome.[213] Psychological stress alone acts to increase the amplitude of esophageal contractions.[214] Stress also may affect the production of gastric acid. If psychological stress increases LPR, it may create a vicious cycle. Pharyngeal stimulation may cause transient LES relaxation directly, or it may lower the threshold for triggering gastric distention.[215]

Fourth, many singers pay little attention to good nutrition, frequently consuming caffeine, fatty foods (including fast foods), spicy foods, citrus products (especially lemons), and tomatoes (including pizza and spaghetti sauce). In addition, because of the great demands that singers place on their voices, even slight alterations caused by peptic mucositis of the larynx produce symptoms that may impair performance. Thus, singers are more likely to seek medical care because of reflux symptoms than are individuals with fewer vocal demands. However, careful inquiry and physical examination reveal similar problems among many nonsinger patients. Most of the voice problems associated with reflux laryngitis appear to be due to direct mucosal damage from proximal reflux. The effects of distal reflux alone on laryngeal function have not been studied.

Voice abnormalities and vocal fold pathology may be due to reflux of gastric acid onto the vocal folds.

Severe coughing may cause vocal fold hemorrhage or mucosal tears, sometimes leading to permanent dysphonia by causing scar that obliterates the layers of the lamina propria and adheres the epithelium to deeper layers. Aspiration caused by reflux also makes reactive airway disease difficult to control. Even mild pulmonary obstruction impairs voice support. Consequently, afflicted patients subconsciously strain to compensate with muscles in the neck and throat, which are designed for delicate control, not for power source functions.[216,217] This behavior is typically responsible for the development of vocal fold nodules and other lesions related to voice abuse. Although it appears likely that some extraesophageal symptoms of reflux are due to stimulation of the vagus nerve rather than (or in addition) to topical irritation, the role of vagal reflexes in reflux laryngitis remains to be clarified.

## Posterior Laryngitis and Related Conditions

In addition to erythema and edema, more serious vocal fold pathology may be caused by reflux laryngitis. In 1968, Cherry and Margulies[96] recognized that reflux laryngitis might be a causative factor in contact ulcers and granulomas of the posterior portion of the vocal folds, conditions that are discussed in detail below. They also observed that treatment of peptic esophagitis resulted in resolution of vocal process granulomas. Delahunty and Cherry[97] followed up on this observation by applying gastric juice to the vocal processes of 2 dogs and applying saliva to the vocal processes of a third dog who was used as a control. The control dog's vocal folds remained normal; the other dogs developed granulomas at the sites of repeated acid application. The experiment by Delahunty and Cherry is particularly interesting. The posterior portion of the left vocal fold of 2 dogs was exposed to gastric acid for a total of only 20 minutes per day, 5 days out of every 7, for a total of 29 days of exposure in a 39-day period. A total of 20 minutes out of 24 hours may not seem like an extensive exposure period; however, erythema and edema were apparent in both dogs by the fourth day of the first week. At the beginning of the second week, the larynges appeared normal after the 2-day rest period. However, visible reaction was provoked within 2 days after application was resumed, and the vocal folds never regained normal appearance. Marked inflammation, thickening, and irregularities were apparent in both dogs by the fourth week, and epithelial slough at the site of acid contact occurred on day 29 in one dog and day 32 in the other. Granulation tissue appeared shortly thereafter. A similar procedure was performed on a control animal by applying saliva instead of gastric juice to the vocal fold, and the vocal fold remained normal. This research suggests that even relatively short periods of acid exposure may cause substantial abnormalities in laryngeal mucosa. Since then, numerous authors have recognized the importance of reflux laryngitis as a causative factor in laryngeal ulcers and granulomas, including intubation granuloma.[12,13,77,83,96,218–221] In addition to its etiological involvement in intubation granuloma, reflux laryngitis has long been recognized as a contributing factor to posterior glottic stenosis, especially following intubation.[222] Olson has suggested that it may also be a causative factor in cricoarytenoid joint arthritis through chronic inflammation and ulceration, beginning on the mucosa and involving the synovial cricoarytenoid joint.[7] We have encountered this problem, as well. In addition to posterior glottic and supraglottic stenosis, subglottic stenosis has been reported as a complication of reflux.[104,223]

### Laryngeal Granulomas

Laryngeal granulomas are a particularly vexing problem for patients and their physicians. Granulomas, like contact ulcers of the larynx, usually occur on the posterior aspect of the vocal folds, often on or above the cartilaginous portion. They may be unilateral, although it is also common to see a sizable granuloma on one side and a contact ulcer on the other. Patients with ulcers or granulomas may complain of pain (laryngeal or referred otalgia), a globus sensation, hoarseness, painful phonation, and occasionally hemoptysis. Surprisingly, even large granulomas are often asymptomatic. These benign lesions usually contain fibroblasts, collagenous fibers, proliferated capillaries, leukocysts, and sometimes ulceration. Although the term "granuloma" is universally accepted, these laryngeal lesions actually are not granulomas histopathologically, but rather chronic inflammatory lesions. However, granulomas and ulcers may mimic more serious lesions such as carcinoma, tuberculosis, and granular cell tumor. Consequently, the clinical diagnosis of laryngeal granuloma must always be made with caution and must be considered tentative until the patient has been followed over time and a good response to treatment has been observed.

Understanding the etiology of laryngeal ulcers and granulomas is essential to clinical evaluation and treatment. Traditionally, ulcers and granulomas in the region of the vocal processes have been associated with trauma, especially intubation injury. However, they are also seen in young, apparently healthy professional voice users with no history of intubation or obvious laryngeal injury. In fact, the vast majority of granulomas and ulcerations (probably even those from intubation) are caused or aggravated by laryngopharyngeal reflux disease. In some patients, muscular tension dysphonia producing forceful vocal process contact may be contributory or causal.

Evaluation of patients with laryngeal ulcers or granulomas begins with a comprehensive history and physical examination. In addition to elucidating specific voice complaints and their importance to the individual patient's life and profession, the history is designed to reveal otolaryngologic and systemic abnormalities that may have caused dysphonia. Special attention is paid to symptoms of voice abuse and of laryngopharyngeal reflux, as listed above. It must be remembered that reflux laryngitis is commonly not accompanied by pyrosis or dyspepsia in these patients. The history also seeks specifically symptoms consistent with asthma, including voice fatigue following extensive voice use. Exercise-induced asthma can be provoked by the exercise of voice use, and even mild reactive airway disease undermines the power source of the voice and may lead to compensatory muscular tension dysphonia and consequent laryngeal granuloma or ulcer. Inquiry also investigates systematically all body systems for evidence of other diseases that present with laryngeal pathology. It is important to include a psychological assessment. Excessive stress may lead to increased acid production, abnormal esophageal function, and symptomatic reflux and to muscular tension dysphonia. In such cases, it is important to identify and treat the underlying stressor, as well as the symptomatic expressions of the stress.

Mirror examination usually reveals the presence of a granuloma or ulcer, but more sophisticated evaluation is invaluable. In the presence of suspected laryngeal granuloma or ulcer, the author (RTS) routinely performs strobovideolaryngoscopy using both flexible and rigid endoscopes. Flexible endoscopic examination reveals patterns of phonation and is extremely helpful in identifying muscular tension dysphonia and determining phonatory behaviors associated with forceful adduction. Recent observations (Steven Zeitels, MD, personal communication, 1997, and the author's [RTS] experience) suggest that some granuloma patients have a vocal fold closure pattern with initial forceful vocal process contact. This implies an adduction strategy with lateral cricoarytenoid dominance, and this observation is important in the treatment of granulomas that are refractory to therapy (medical and/or surgical) or granulomas that recur. Rigid laryngeal stroboscopic examination provides magnified, detailed information of the lesions under slow-motion light, allowing analysis of their composition (solid granulomas versus fluid-filled cysts) and their effects on phonation. This examination also permits assessment of other areas of the vocal folds to rule out separate lesions (eg, vocal fold scar) that may be the real cause of the patient's voice complaint.

Evaluation also includes at least a formal assessment by a speech-language pathologist (SLP) skilled in voice evaluation and care. In the author's (RTS) center, we also include objective voice analysis and a vocal stress assessment with a singing voice specialist (even with nonsingers). In addition to a laryngologist, SLP, and singing voice specialist, other members of the voice team are often used, depending on the patient's problems. Additional team members include an acting-voice specialist, psychologist, psychiatrist, otolaryngologic nurse clinician, and consulting pulmonologist, neurologist, gastroenterologist, and others. The information provided by these evaluations helps establish the degree to which voice abuse/misuse is present, and it guides the design of an individualized therapy plan.

Reflux must be suspected in virtually all cases of granuloma. It can be evaluated by 24-hour pH monitor, barium swallow with water siphonage (routine barium swallows are not satisfactory for diagnosing reflux, and the accuracy of barium swallow even with water siphonage is debatable), other tests, and/or a therapeutic trial of medical management. If there is historical evidence of prolonged reflux symptoms, endoscopic evaluation to rule out Barrett's esophagus is often advisable. It may be appropriate to biopsy the presumed granuloma at the same time. If a therapeutic trial of medications without confirmatory tests is elected, marked improvement in symptoms and signs should occur following daily use of a PPI (before breakfast and dinner) within 2 to 3 months. Treatment for laryngopharyngeal reflux should be aggressive.

The efficacy of oral corticosteroids for treatment of laryngeal granulomas and ulcers has not been proven, but they are used commonly on the basis of anecdotal evidence, especially for small or medium-sized granulomas and ulcers that appear acutely inflamed. For these conditions, low doses of steroids for longer periods are usually given, such as triamcinolone 4 mg twice a day for 3 weeks. Steroid inhalers are not recommended. They may lead to laryngitis or laryngeal *Candida* infections, and prolonged use may cause vocal fold atrophy.

At the end of 2 months of therapy including anti-reflux measures, voice therapy, and possibly steroids, substantial improvement in the appearance of the larynx should be seen. Ulcers should be healed, and granulomas should be substantially smaller. Patients should be examined after 1 month to be certain that the lesions are not enlarging. If they appear worse, biopsy should be performed promptly. However, it should be noted that complete healing may take 8 months or more.[224,225] Repeated strobovideolaryngoscopic examinations allow comparison of lesion size over time. If improvements are noted, aggressive therapy and close follow-up can be continued until the mass lesion disappears or stabilizes. If the mass does not disappear, or if response to the first 2 months of aggressive therapy produces no substantial improvement, biopsy should be performed to rule out carcinoma and other diseases. If the surgeon is reasonably certain that the lesion is a granuloma, injection of an aqueous steroid preparation (such as dexamethasone) into the base of the lesion at the time of surgery may be helpful. As long as a good specimen is obtained, the laser may be used for resection of suspected granulomas because the lesions are usually not on the vibratory margin, and they often are friable. However, the author (RTS) usually uses traditional instruments to avoid the third-degree burn caused by the laser (even with a microspot) in the treatment of this chronic, irritative condition.

It is essential that causative factors, especially reflux and voice abuse, be treated preoperatively and controlled strictly following laryngeal surgery. The patient is kept on therapeutic doses of a PPI prior to surgery and for at least 6 weeks following surgery. Surgeons should not hesitate to use omeprazole (Prilosec) 20 mg as frequently as 4 times a day or the equivalent dose of another PPI under these circumstances and, if necessary, to add an $H_2$ blocker (ranitidine, 300 mg) at bedtime. Following surgery, absolute voice rest (writing pad) is prescribed until the surgical area has remucosalized. This is usually approximately 1 week and virtually never longer than 10 to 14 days. There are no indications for more prolonged absolute voice rest, although relative voice rest (limited voice use) is recommended routinely. Voice therapy is reinstituted on the day when phonation is resumed, and frequent short therapy sessions and close monitoring are maintained throughout the healing period.

As previously stated, granulomas recur in some patients. In all such cases, aggressive reevaluation of reflux with 24-hour pH monitor studies is warranted because granulomas are seen commonly in patients with reflux laryngitis. Often endoscopy and biopsy of esophageal and postcricoid mucosa is appropriate. Twenty-four-hour pH monitor studies should be conducted not only off all medications, but also when the patient is taking a PPI or $H_2$ blocker. A few patients are resistant to PPIs and will have normal acid secretions despite even 80 mg of omeprazole daily or the equivalent dose of another PPI; and some patients may respond to PPIs initially and then develop resistance. In such patients, $H_2$ blockers may be effective. When medical management of reflux is insufficient, laparoscopic fundoplication can be considered for patients with recurring granuloma. Voice use must also be optimized and monitored with the help of the SLP, always, and other members of the voice team when indicated. The laryngologist and voice therapists must be sure that good vocal technique is carried over outside the medical office into the patient's daily life.

Occasionally, even after excellent reflux control (including fundoplication), surgical removal including steroid injection into the base of the granulomas, and voice therapy, patients may develop multiply recurrent granulomas. Medical causes other than reflux and muscular tension dysphonia must be ruled out, particularly granulomatous diseases including sarcoidosis and tuberculosis, and neoplasm such as granular cell tumors. Pathology slides from previous surgical procedures should be reviewed. When it has been established that the recurrent lesions are typical laryngeal granulomas occurring in the absence of laryngopharyngeal reflux, the cause is almost always phonatory trauma. When voice therapy has been insufficient to permit adequate healing, some of these uncommonly difficult patient problems can be solved by temporary paresis of selected vocal fold adductor muscles (particularly the lateral cricoarytenoid) using botulinum toxin (Botox, Allergan, Irvine, California) injection. Although this treatment approach has been effective, it is not utilized ordinarily as initial therapy and is appropriate only for selected cases.

### Delayed Wound Healing

In addition to its possible carcinogenic potential, the chronic irritation of reflux laryngitis may be responsible for failure of wound healing. Reflux appears to delay the resolution not only of vocal process ulcers and granulomas, but also of healing following vocal fold surgery. For this reason, otolaryngologists are becoming increasingly aggressive about diagnosing and treating reflux before subjecting patients to vocal fold surgery, even for conditions unrelated to the reflux.

### Stenosis

As noted above, laryngeal stenosis has been associated with reflux.[32,84,104,105] Koufman has reported laryngopharyngeal reflux in 92% of his patients with laryngeal stenosis, all of whom were documented by 24-hour pH monitoring studies.[32] This is consistent with an earlier report by Little, Koufman, et al in which the authors were able to produce nonhealing ulcerations and subglottic stenosis experimentally in canines by applying gastric acid and pepsin to injured subglottic mucosa.[3] Long-term control of laryngopharyngeal reflux is essential to success in treating laryngeal stenosis.

### Globus Pharyngeus

The sensation of a lump in the throat or globus pharyngeus is associated commonly with laryngopharyngeal reflux. The literature on the association of globus with reflux does not provide definitive guidance.[15,16,89,90,225–229] However, reflux has been found in 23 to 90% of patients with globus.[32,90,225–228,230,231]

Smit et al studied 27 patients with globus pharyngeus alone, 20 patients with hoarseness alone (more than 3 months duration), and 25 patients with both globus and hoarseness.[231] Using dual-probe pH monitoring, pathologic reflux was diagnosed if patients had a pH below 4 for more than 0.1% of the total time, more than 0.2% of time in the upright position, and more than 0% of the time in the supine position in the proximal probe, or if they had more than 3 reflux episodes with pH below 4. The proximal probe was placed visually at the UES, and the distal probe was 15 cm from the proximal probe. Only 30% of patients with globus but without hoarseness had pathologic reflux. Similar findings were reported by Wilson et al (23%),[227] Curran et al (38%),[228] and Hill et al (30.8%).[230] Smit et al found that only 35% of patients with hoarseness alone had pathologic reflux. However, 72% (18 of 25) of patients with globus and hoarseness had pathologic reflux. Sixty-five percent of patients with pathologic GERD had abnormal findings during esophagoscopy, including 2 patients with Barrett's mucosa. The diagnosis of laryngopharyngeal reflux should be considered in patients with globus pharyngeus, and diagnostic evaluation and therapeutic trial with PPIs are warranted.[231–233]

### Laryngospasm

Laryngospasm is forceful, involuntary adduction of the vocal folds. It is associated with airway obstruction that is often severe enough to cause the patient to panic. Typically laryngospasm occurs suddenly and without warning. It may be precipitated by laughing or exercise, or it may occur with no apparent precipitating event. Nighttime attacks that awaken the patient are common. Reflux is a well-recognized cause of laryngospasm. The mechanism may be related to chemoreceptors on the epiglottis that respond to a pH of 2.5 or below by eliciting laryngospasm.[233] Loughlin et al also demonstrated that this reflex is dependent on a functioning superior laryngeal nerve.[234] In our experience, laryngopharyngeal reflux is the cause of paroxysmal laryngospasm in nearly all patients with this condition, and most respond to aggressive antireflux therapy.

## Muscle Tension Dysphonia

The relationship between laryngopharyngeal reflux and muscle tension dysphonia remains uncertain, but there is reason to consider an association possible. Koufman and coworkers found a 70% incidence of laryngopharyngeal reflux in patients with structural vocal fold lesions associated commonly with muscle tension dysphonia, including nodules, Reinke's edema, hematoma, ulcers, and granuloma.[32] Chronic reflux laryngitis causes irritation that leads not only to an inflammatory response, but also to laryngeal hyperirritability. Laryngospasm is the extreme manifestation of this condition. However, hyperfunctional posturing of the laryngeal muscles in response to chronic irritation, or as a defense against unpredictably timed episodes of laryngeal aspiration of acid, conceivably could lead to hyperfunctional patterns of voice use. Alternatively, in some patients, laryngopharyngeal reflux and muscle tension dysphonia may occur coincidentally, but injury to the vocal fold mucosa by acid and pepsin may make the vocal folds more prone to injury and to the development of structural lesions associated with phonotrauma. Traditionally, otolaryngologists and speech-language pathologists have viewed muscle tension dysphonia as a primary condition in the majority of cases. In the author's (RTS) opinion, a high percentage of patients with muscle tension dysphonia have an underlying disorder such as reflux laryngitis or superior laryngeal nerve paresis that may have been responsible for the patient's hyperfunctional voice disorder. In all patients with voice abnormalities, including muscle tension dysphonia, it is essential to seek out and treat the primary etiological condition.

Paroxysmal vocal fold movement disorder is a laryngeal dystonia characterized by intermittent glottic obstruction by adduction of the vocal folds on inspiration. It is also called paradoxical vocal fold adduction, respiratory dysphonia, and other names, including paradoxical vocal fold movement disorder (PVFMD). Yelken et al[235] point out that PVFMD "mimics asthma," and patients are often diagnosed incorrectly initially. In their patients, they reported no relationship between asthma attacks and severity and PVFMD. However, they found LPR and allergy to be prevalent in their patients with PVFMD.

Cough associated with PVFMD was studied by Murry and colleagues.[236] They suggested that chronic cough associated with PVFMD might be due to laryngeal sensory deficits secondary to chronic acid exposure in the laryngopharynx, which triggers the cough reflex. They suggested also that the cough reflex could be an adaptive mechanism to clear particulate matter from the laryngopharynx.

## Reinke's Edema

Prolonged acid/pepsin irritation of the laryngeal mucosa can result in significant alterations in laryngeal tissues including carcinoma, as discussed below. Reinke's edema appears to be one such tissue alteration. Koufman demonstrated abnormal 24-hour pH monitoring results in a majority of their patients with Reinke's edema,[32] and this is consistent with our experience. In the author's (RTS) opinion, in many cases, it is unclear whether reflux is the primary cause of Reinke's edema or is a cofactor with other laryngeal mucosal irritants such as smoking, hyperfunctional voice use, or hypothyroidism. However, we evaluate all patients with Reinke's edema for reflux and treat LPR aggressively. Many patients seeking optimal restoration of voice quality require surgical treatment despite good reflux control, voice therapy, smoking cessation, and correction of any thyroid abnormalities. Good reflux control should be maintained long term, but it is especially critical in the immediate postoperative period, as discussed previously in the section on delayed wound healing.

## Carcinoma

The association of gastroesophageal reflux disease with Barrett's esophagus and esophageal carcinoma has been well established. It is now thought possible that LPR is associated with laryngeal malignancy, as well.[237-241] Delahunty biopsied the posterior laryngeal mucosa in a patient with reflux laryngitis and reported epithelial hyperplasia with parakeratosis and papillary down-growth.[78] In the 1980s, Olson and others reported on patients (including young, nonsmokers, nondrinkers) with posterior laryngeal carcinoma in whom he believed reflux to be a cofactor.[1] This issue was addressed also by Morrison.[242] He reported 6 cases of vocal fold carcinoma in patients who had severe reflux but had never smoked. In 1997, Olson reaffirmed that the relationship between reflux and cancer is not conclusive.[243]

The mechanisms by which reflux may cause laryngeal cancer remains speculative. Both smoking and alcohol consumption promote reflux by lowering lower esophageal sphincter pressure, impairing esophageal motility and mucosal integrity, increasing gastric acid secretion, and delaying gastric emptying. So, a high incidence of reflux in laryngeal cancer patients who smoke and drink is not surprising. However, the association does not explain how LPR may act as a cofactor in these patients or as a primary factory in patients who do not smoke and drink. Richtsmeier et al[244] have suggested that a deficiency in T-cell mediated immunity is causally related to immunodeficiency in cancer patients. There is a subgroup of suppressor T cells with histamine-type 2 receptors. Cimetadine, a histamine-type 2 receptor antagonist, inhibits the expression of suppressor T cells and enhances immune responses. Richtsmeier and Eisele found that skin test anergy in laryngeal cancer can be reversed by cimetadine.[245] This led Richtsmeier et al to recommend the use of an $H_2$ blocker not only to treat reflux in laryngeal cancer patients, but also to address their underlying immune dysfunction,[246] although this thinking is not accepted widely.

Although some questions remain regarding the relationship between LPR and laryngeal carcinoma, the studies cited above, as well as more recent evidence,[246] suggest that the 2 conditions are probably associated. At present, patients with laryngeal cancer, or those at risk to develop laryngeal cancer, should be screened for reflux; antireflux therapy should be instituted when it is present. Cancer surveillance is reasonable even in patients without known risk factors other than chronic LPR. The long-term efficacy of such treatment with regard to prevention of malignancy remains unknown, but we have seen resolution of laryngeal structural abnormalities, including suspicious leukoplakia, in patients with LPR alone, and even in patients who continue smoking and consuming alcohol. Koufman has had similar experiences.[247]

In 1988, Ward and Hanson recognized reflux as a potential cofactor for the development of laryngeal cancer, particularly in nonsmokers.[248] In 1991, Koufman documented LPR in 84% of 31 consecutive patients with laryngeal carcinoma, only 58% of whom were active smokers.[32] Frieje et al reviewed retrospectively 23 patients with T1 and T2 carcinomas of the larynx, and they concluded that GERD plays a role in the etiology of carcinoma of the larynx particularly in patients who lack typical risk factors (14 of their patients had quit smoking more than 15 years prior

to developing laryngeal carcinoma) and may act as a co-carcinogen in smokers and drinkers.[249] In 1997, Koufman and Burke felt that the causal relationship between LPR and laryngeal malignancy remained unproven, but noted that most patients who develop laryngeal malignancy have LPR in addition to being smokers.[247] Until more definitive data are available, we believe that long-term antireflux therapy in these patients should be considered.

Research has shown that GERD is a factor in the development of esophageal cancer.[249] Studies also have examined the potential carcinogenic role of LPR. Conflicting data exist, complicated recently by published stories that show no carcinogenic effects but that were limited by short periods of acid injury.[250,251] Although some studies have shown LPR as a risk factor in animal models, others have not, and the true relationship between LPR and laryngeal malignancy remains uncertain. However, there are enough data indicating a possible link to suggest that at present, known reflux patients should be screened for laryngeal cancer and be made aware of this risk.[252]

Given the risk of esophageal adenocarcinoma in reflux patients, the value of EGD screening has been assessed. It has been argued that LPR symptoms are better indicators of esophageal adenocarcinoma than are gastroesophageal symptoms.[253] Studies have shown esophagitis in 12 to 18% of LPR patients, and of 3 to 7% Barrett's metaplasia patients.[254,255] Additionally, in patients on long-term PPI's, *Helicobacter pylori* is known to accelerate the loss of specialized gastric glands, causing atrophic gastritis and gastric cancer.[256] *H pylori*, breath, or fecal testing or biopsy may screen for this infection. Diagnosis of hiatal hernia would also potentially affect treatment and is facilitated by EGD. Some have suggested routine EGD for patients complaining of heartburn; others suggest it for all LPR patients.[254]

Until the true relationship is defined, screening with either transnasal esophagoscopy or EGD (which may be performed at the time of routine colonoscopy in appropriate patients) is advisable. Many gastroenterologists are now advising visualization of the larynx during EGD. This has led to the diagnosis of LPR in up to 4.6% of patients undergoing EGD for GERD.[257]

Current literature reflects ongoing research on the causal effects of gastric refluxate (pepsin) and the carcinogenic effects on the larynx, pharynx, and upper airway epithelium.[258–262]

Laryngopharyngeal (LPR) has been considered a risk factor in the development of squamous cell carcinoma of the larynx, but it remains unproven.

## Sudden Infant Death Syndrome and Other Pediatric Considerations

Laryngopharyngeal reflux is important in the pediatric population, although it has been studied much less extensively than has reflux in adults. Unlike adults, infants and young children are unable to complain of symptoms associated with LPR. Nevertheless, LPR has been associated with various problems in infants and children including halitosis, dysphonia, laryngospasm, laryngomalacia, asthma, pneumonia, sleep apnea, and sudden infant death syndrome (SIDS).[6,24,263–285] The diagnosis can be established by laryngoscopy and bronchoscopy, and 24-hour pH monitor studies. Children can be treated with $H_2$ blockers and/or PPIs, and fundoplication is appropriate in selected cases, particularly in patients with life-threatening complications of reflux.

Evidence suggests that SIDS may be causally related to acid reflux into the larynx. Hence, SIDS must join laryngeal and esophageal cancer at the top of the list of serious otolaryngologic consequences of reflux laryngitis. Wetmore investigated the effects of acid on the larynges of maturing rabbits by applying solutions of acid or saline at 15-day intervals up to 60 days of age.[264] Because the larynx is not only a site of resistance in the airway, but also contains the afferent limb for reflexes that regulate respiration, he discovered that acid exposure resulted in significant obstructive, central, and mixed apnea. Gasping respirations and frequent swallowing were observed as associated symptoms. Central apnea occurred in all age groups but had a peak incidence at 45 days. Acid-induced obstructive apnea in rabbits is similar to obstructive apnea previously recognized in human infants with gastroesophageal disease. However, the demonstration of acid-induced central apnea produced by acid stimulation of the larynx is more ominous. Central apnea has been demonstrated in other animal models as a result of different forms of laryngeal stimulation. Central apnea resulting in fatal asphyxia has also been described in several animal models. Wetmore's study[264] suggests that gastroesophageal reflux alone is capable of triggering fatal central apnea. This is particularly compelling when one recognizes that the peak incidence of central apnea occurring at 45 days in the rabbit corresponds well within the peak incidence of SIDS in humans, which occurs between 2 and 4 months of age.

Otolaryngologists should be aware of the prevalence of LPR/GERD in children and infants. Studies have shown that reflux is associated commonly with regurgitation and vomiting, disturbed sleep patterns, colic, gastrointestinal pain, croup, and hoarseness in the pediatric population.[265–288]

Monitoring of pH is valuable to infants with laryngitis, including pharyngeal monitoring, which may diagnose undertreated LPR or LPR missed on esophageal monitoring.[289] LPR is a known common cause of hoarseness in children and should be in the differential diagnosis of dysphonia.[290] It may be misdiagnosed as recurrent croup when reflux triggers intermittent airway obstruction.[291] The diagnosis of LPR is still often missed in children with hoarseness or frequent respiratory disorders.

Barreto et al[292] examined the laryngeal and phonatory effects associated with untreated growth hormone deficiencies. Values for roughness, breathiness, and strain were higher, and LPR signs were also more common in this population. More research is needed. Otolaryngologists should be familiar with this association.

Ongoing research continues to examine the relationship between LPR and otitis media in children. Several studies have confirmed the presence of pepsin and pepsinogen in children with otitis media with effusion.[293,294] One study reported positive *H pylori* results in 6 of 31 children (19%) with middle ear effusion.[295] Miura et al[296] suggested that reflux disease in children with chronic otitis media with effusion appears to be factorial, but the "cause-effect" relationship is unclear. They suggested that, based on current research, "anti-reflux therapy for otitis media cannot be endorsed." Other studies have identified increased presence of reflux in children with upper respiratory infections associated with cough, runny nose, otitis media, and chronic rhinosinusitis.[297–299] Another study reported the presence of pepsin in the tears of children with LPR.[300] Andrews and Orobello[301] compared biopsies of the posterior cricoid region and nasopharyngeal pH results in diagnosing LPR in children. They reported their retrospective review of 63 patients ages 6 months to 17 years, and found 80% of patients tested positive for reflux by both methodologies. Katra et al[295] investigated the relationship between *H pylori* in hyperplasia of the adenoids and reflux episodes in children detected by impedance and pH monitoring. Their study population was small, 30 children with a mean age of 5.34 years. The children underwent adenoidectomy and pH/impedance monitoring with a proximal impedance sensor 1 cm above the UES. Their results confirmed their hypothesis that reflux episodes that reached the UES could have a significant role in *H pylori* reaching lymphoid tissue in the nasopharynx and the development of adenoid hyperplasia in children.

## Diagnostic Tests for Reflux

The approach to diagnosis of laryngopharyngeal reflux (LPR) in a general or otolaryngologic practice includes careful physical examination and diagnostic testing. This section discusses the use of each of these modalities in the management of GERD in general, with specific reference to the otolaryngologic patient (Table 11–5).

### Therapeutic Trial

When a patient presents with typical heartburn and regurgitation, diagnostic studies may not be needed. Relief of symptoms after a therapeutic trial with $H_2$-antagonists, prokinetic agents, or PPIs for 8 to 12 weeks can confirm that the symptoms are secondary to GERD. Because heartburn generally is absent in the otolaryngologic patient, the endpoint of the therapeutic trial is dependent on other presenting symptoms, and diagnostic tests are often necessary to confirm the diagnosis. Historical clues that otolaryngologic symptoms may be due to GERD, specifically LPR, include morning hoarseness, halitosis, excess phlegm, dry mouth, throat clearing, and others.

If a therapeutic trial is used in a patient with suspected GERD and otolaryngologic symptoms, higher doses of antireflux therapy, usually with a PPI, for longer periods of time are needed. However, neither the cost-effectiveness nor clinical efficacy of any medical regimen in patients with LPR has been tested. We

**Table 11–5.** Diagnostic Tests for Gastroesophageal Reflux

**Is reflux present?**
  Barium swallow
  pH monitoring

**Is there mucosal injury?**
  Barium swallow (air contrast) study
  Endoscopy
  Mucosal biopsy

**Are symptoms due to reflux?**
  Therapeutic trial
  pH monitoring (with symptom index)

**Can prognostic or preoperative information be obtained?**
  Esophageal manometry
  pH monitoring

currently use a PPI twice a day initially for a minimum of 8 to 12 weeks as a therapeutic trial for laryngeal symptoms suspected to be due to reflux.

It should be emphasized that patients with reflux laryngitis frequently require more intensive therapy with higher doses of $H_2$ blockers or earlier use of PPIs than patients with dyspepsia in the absence of laryngeal symptoms and signs. In addition to monitoring symptoms and signs of reflux laryngitis, response to treatment is best judged by combined intraesophageal and intragastric pH monitoring of patients while they are receiving treatment. Such studies are worthwhile even when patients are taking PPIs, because some patients are omeprazole-resistant,[168,169] and resistance to other protein pump inhibitors may occur, as well. Our recent observations suggest that omeprazole resistance also can develop in patients who respond well initially to the medication. Moreover, it must be recognized that a normal pH 24-hour monitor study does not indicate the absence of reflux. Rather, it demonstrates the absence of *acid* reflux. Regurgitation of pH-neutral liquid may still be present and may produce symptoms, especially in singers and actors. Study of this phenomenon and its optimal management is needed badly. At the present time, although there are no data to support the superiority of surgery over medical therapy for LPR patients, it appears that selected patients may benefit from surgery over medicine, especially considering the efficacy and decreased morbidity associated with laparoscopic fundoplication and the potential costs and risks associated with the use of $H_2$ blockers or PPIs for periods of many years. If endoscopic suturing and Stretta techniques prove efficacious, one or both of these techniques may be useful, but at present, they have not been studied in LPR or compared to surgery or medical therapy.

### Barium Radiographs

Barium studies are relatively inexpensive and widely available for use in the diagnosis of esophageal disease. When evaluating the esophagus, a double-contrast barium swallow is needed for optimal assessment. An upper GI (gastrointestinal) series usually results in insufficient evaluation of esophageal function, concentrates excessively on the stomach and duodenum, and does not give enough attention to potential mucosal or motility abnormalities in the esophagus. A hiatal hernia is the most common abnormality seen on barium swallow. However, up to 60% of the adult population will have a hiatal hernia,[302] making this a nonspecific finding and not diagnostic of GERD. Free reflux is seen in up to 30% of "normal" patients and may be absent in up to 60% of patients with GERD established by pH monitoring,[303] making the barium study an insensitive and nonspecific study for GERD. It has been suggested that reflux of barium to or above the carina or to the thoracic inlet is indicative of the potential for aspiration and is useful as an aid in the diagnosis of GERD-associated laryngitis. There are no prospective or controlled studies to substantiate this clinical impression. This finding is reported usually with the patient in the supine position, making this observation of relatively little use. The so-called "high" reflux on a barium study has not been well correlated with proximal acid exposure on ambulatory pH monitoring. Barium swallow with water siphonage has been used to aid in the diagnosis of reflux in otolaryngology patients. Patients may show abnormalities on barium swallow with water siphonage, which may be interpreted as confirming a diagnosis of pathologic reflux, although interpretations should be made with caution as the true positive predictive value has not been confirmed. However, barium swallow with water siphonage has more value than recognized by many radiologists. The literature on this subject was reviewed in 1994 by Ott.[302] Because early reports revealed a wide discrepancy in reflux detection rates, barium esophagrams were considered insensitive, and provocative tests (ie, water siphonage) were believed to increase the sensitivity at the expense of specificity. Thompson et al found that a reflux detection rate increased to 70% when using the water siphonage test, as compared with 26% for spontaneous reflux.[303] However, this gain in sensitivity may be counterbalanced by the low specificity of this test.

In professional singers and actors especially, barium swallow with water siphonage seems to provide a good clinical approximation of daily reflux episodes. To optimize mucosal function, it is essential for singers and actors to remain well hydrated. Consequently they drink large amounts of water, routinely carry water bottles with them, and drink substantial quantities shortly before they sing. This routine behavior is similar to the water siphon portion of the barium swallow, which raises the question of whether positive water siphonage tests may provide useful information, at least in professional voice users, even when a 24-hour pH monitor study is normal. Specific mucosal abnormalities on double-contrast barium studies, such as thickening of esophageal mucosal folds, erosions, or esophageal ulcers, are seen in a minority of patients with GERD, making this study relatively insensitive for this diagnosis.

The diagnosis of Barrett's esophagus is conclusive also by a barium swallow.

The optimal use of the barium study is to evaluate patients with suspected complications of GERD, such as motility abnormalities or peptic stricture that are commonly seen in patients with solid and/ or liquid dysphagia. A barium swallow can identify rings, webs, or other obstructive lesions including carcinoma that are seen in patients with dysphagia, but these are unusual complications of GERD. A solid bolus such as a marshmallow or a barium cookie can be given to help localize the site of obstruction in a patient with solid dysphagia.

Although the barium swallow allows demonstration that reflux is occurring and can demonstrate mucosal injury, it is of inconsistent value in establishing a diagnosis of GERD. Its best use is in evaluation of the patient with dysphagia, and it should be performed in conjunction with endoscopy in these patients. Nevertheless, in some patients, barium esophagram provides important additional information that may be missed without radiologic imaging or esophagoscopy.[28,303,304] In a series of 128 patients, for example, barium studies showed esophagitis in 18%, a lower esophageal ring in 14%, and peptic stricture in 3% of patients.[305,306] Consequently, if endoscopy is not planned, patients with LPR should be considered for further evaluation by barium swallow.

**Radionucleotide Studies**

Scintigraphic studies have been suggested as valuable in diagnosis of GERD.[307] A radioisotope (Technetium 99m-sulfur colloid) marker is mixed with a measured quantity of liquid (usually $H_2O$), and graded abdominal compression is used to unmask reflux. Originally proposed as a sensitive test, its reliability has been questioned, and it is no longer considered a useful investigation.[308]

**Endoscopy**

Endoscopy is used to document mucosal disease and establish a diagnosis of erosive esophagitis or Barrett's metaplasia. When patients with frequent heartburn and regurgitation are studied prospectively, erosive esophagitis is seen in 45 to 60% of patients.[309] The others will have nonerosive disease (mucosal edema, hyperemia, or a normal-appearing esophagus). Erosive esophagitis suggests a serious form of GERD in which patients require continuous medical therapy with a PPI or antireflux surgery for effective symptom relief and healing. Barrett's esophagus is seen in 10 to 15% of reflux patients undergoing endoscopy.[94] Unfortunately, there is no classic presentation of Barrett's esophagus, but it is most common in white males over 50 years of age.[75]

Erosive esophagitis is uncommon in patients with extraesophageal symptoms. Although 50% of patients with unexplained chest pain and normal coronary arteries have GERD, the prevalence of erosive esophagitis is 10% or less.[64] GERD-associated asthma and evidence of esophagitis on endoscopy have been reported in 30 to 40% of adult patients.[59,60] In patients with reflux laryngitis, erosive esophagitis is seen in only 20 to 30%, making this study of low diagnostic yield in GERD.[16]

There are no absolute indications for endoscopy in the patient with suspected GERD. In general, endoscopy is performed in patients who do not respond to a therapeutic trial of medical therapy, patients with symptoms for greater than 5 years to rule out Barrett's metaplasia, and patients with the "alarm" symptoms of dysphagia—odynophagia, weight loss, anemia, or gastrointestinal bleeding.[310]

Endoscopic findings may help predict the prognosis and outcome of medical therapy. Patients with erosive esophagitis will almost always require long-term PPI therapy for healing and symptom relief. Recurrence of erosive esophagitis is seen in up to 80% of patients within 3 to 6 months following the discontinuation of medications[311]; these patients usually require continuous pharmacologic therapy for effective long-term control. Because patients with non-erosive esophagitis seldom progress to more severe forms of esophagitis, they can be managed with a range of pharmacologic treatments. Endoscopy is useful for long-term treatment planning in difficult-to-manage cases.

Given the rarity of erosive esophagitis, we do not use endoscopy routinely as the initial study in patients with suspected GERD-related otolaryngologic disease, chest pain, asthma, or cough, preferring ambulatory dual-probe pH monitoring or a therapeutic trial of antireflux medications as the initial diagnostic test.

## Esophageal Biopsy

Biopsy and cytology are of limited value in evaluation of the patient with GERD unless Barrett's esophagus or malignancy is suspected, and the author (POK) biopsies only the esophagus in these patients. The light microscopic signs of GERD—elongation of rete pegs and hyperplasia of the basal cell layer do not distinguish between acute and chronic disease and do not help predict response to therapy.

The microscopic signs of active esophagitis, polymorphonuclear leukocytes and eosinophils, are seen in a minority of adult patients, so they are insensitive diagnostic findings. Biopsy may be more useful in the pediatric population where the frequency of these findings is higher.

If Barrett's metaplasia is suspected, a systematic biopsy protocol should be followed to confirm the diagnosis and rule out dysplasia or carcinoma. Endoscopic surveillance with biopsies to rule out dysplasia every 1 to 2 years is the current standard of practice for management of patients with Barrett's metaplasia.[74]

## Prolonged Ambulatory pH Monitoring

Prolonged (16–24 hour) pH monitoring is the most important study to quantify esophageal reflux and determine whether symptoms are related to GERD. The study is performed by placing an antimony catheter (2 mm diameter) transnasally into the distal esophagus with an electrode placed 5 cm above the lower esophageal sphincter, which is identified by esophageal manometry (Figure 11–17). Precise positioning is important for accuracy in the interpretation of results. The probe is connected to a small microcomputer that is worn on a belt or clipped to the waist so that the patient can be monitored in an ambulatory setting. Activity can be tailored to provoke reflux in the setting in which symptoms are typically produced. For example, a patient with chronic hoarseness who sings professionally will be reminded to sing during the study. We have found some patients who reflux constantly during singing, and rarely at other times (see Figure 11–17).

Multiple electrodes can be placed on a single catheter to monitor intragastric and intraesophageal pH, distal esophageal, and proximal esophageal acid exposure, or all 3 simultaneously. Abnormal acid exposure in the proximal esophagus, just below the upper esophageal sphincter, predicts the potential for aspiration in patients with otolaryngologic symptoms. An intragastric electrode allows monitoring of the gastric acid response to antireflux therapy. Several investigators have placed probes above the upper esophageal sphincter in the hypopharynx[312,313] to document reflux above the UES, thus being more certain of aspiration as the cause of symptoms. Unfortunately, this placement creates difficulty in standardizing the distance between the proximal and distal probes and causes difficulty in placement of the distal esophageal probe 5 cm above the LES, the standard used in developing normal values. Probes in the hypopharynx can be uncomfortable; normal

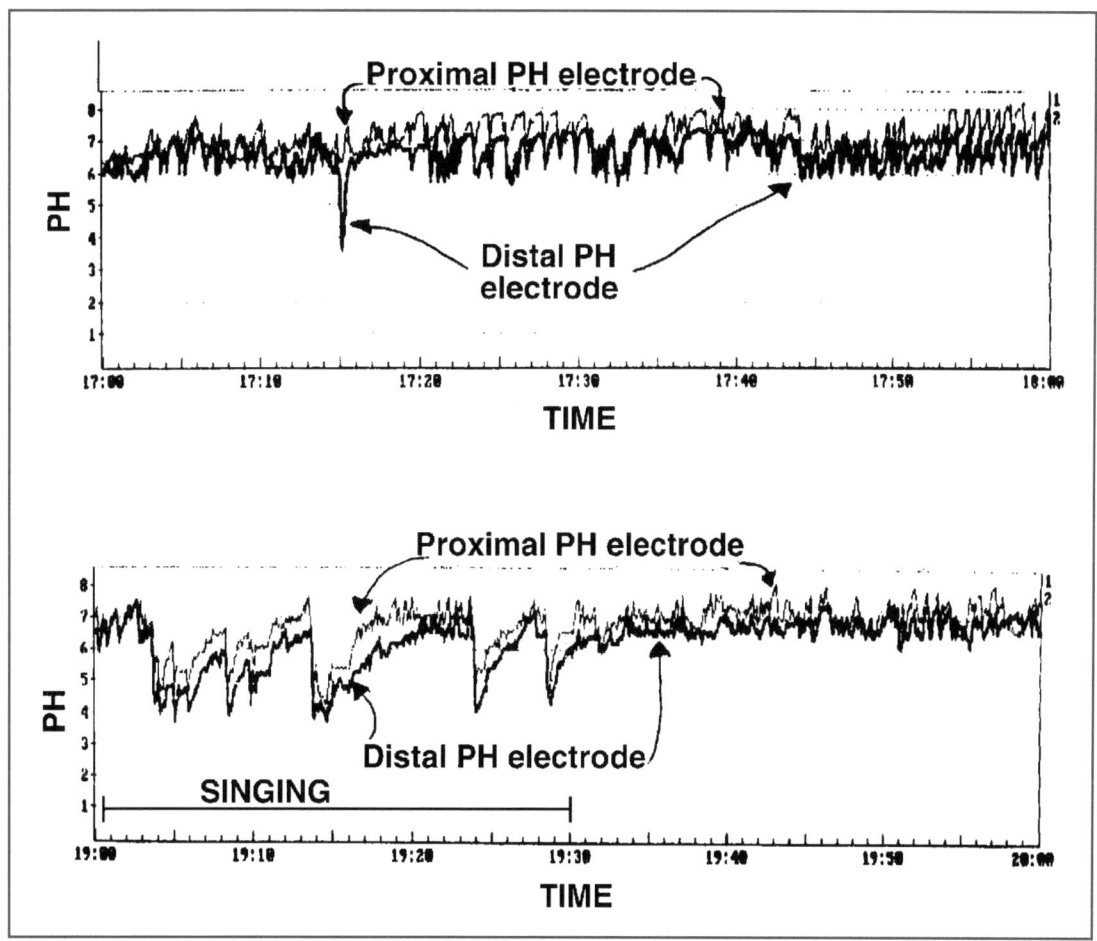

**Figure 11–17.** Dual-electrode pH probe monitoring while singing for a 30-minute period of the 1 hour shown. The patient experienced typical heartburn, and increased proximal and distal acid exposure was prominent during singing.

values are not available; and pharyngeal probe data are occasionally subject to interpretation error, including incorrect diagnosis of reflux due to probe drying and acidic food or liquid ingestion, both artifacts resulting in a drop of pH to less than 4 that is not a true reflux episode. Some investigators who believe that pharyngeal probe placement is important and that data are valid and reliable, for example, Koufman and colleagues,[312] place the proximal probe immediately above the cricopharyngeus, posterior to the larynx. This position prevents drying of the probe and reportedly produces valid data. They consider any pharyngeal acid exposure (even one episode) abnormal. Although placement of the proximal probe (just above the cricopharyngeus or just below it) remains controversial, the need for dual-probe pH monitoring is clear. Without a proximal probe, the sensitivity of single-probe esophageal pH monitoring has been shown to be only 62% for LPR190; that

is, 38% of patients had pharyngeal reflux with distal esophageal parameters that were considered within normal limits. At present normal values for distal reflux at 5 cm above the lower esophageal sphincter and for proximal reflux 20 cm above the sphincter are available, making this a more useful protocol.[95,313] Normal values vary slightly between laboratories and should be included with reports from the laboratory performing the procedure.

The microcomputer (data logger) has a symptom button that allows recording of up to 6 symptoms during a single study. The patient is asked to push the symptom button as well as to record symptoms on a diary card. This allows correlation of reflux events with symptoms in order to determine a symptom index,[314] which is especially valuable in patients with asthma, cough, and chest pain and allows correlation between symptoms and reflux in patients who have continued symptoms on medical therapy.

Symptom correlation in the otolaryngologic patient may be more difficult on a single study, particularly when symptoms are continuous and not produced by a single reflux episode. This scenario is more likely in patients with laryngitis or chronic sore throat. Other symptoms such as throat clearing, cough, or symptoms provoked by singing may be correlated with single reflux episodes.

Prolonged pH monitoring is used in patients with heartburn to establish a diagnosis when symptoms have not responded to a trial of antireflux therapy and endoscopy is negative. In this case, a single-channel pH probe can be placed with the distal probe 5 cm above the lower esophageal sphincter. Symptoms are correlated with reflux, and reflux frequency is assessed. Patients with known GERD who have heartburn and regurgitation not responding to medical therapy can be monitored while still on therapy with a dual-channel intragastric and distal esophageal probe to assess the adequacy of gastric acid suppression, to assess esophageal reflux frequency, and to correlate symptoms with reflux events. Patients with continued esophageal acid exposure and/or symptoms may require additional therapy.

Patients with otolaryngologic symptoms, or other upper airway symptoms suggestive of GERD, are ideal candidates for prolonged ambulatory pH monitoring. We prefer performing monitoring early in the clinical course to establish a diagnosis and symptom correlation when possible. Dual-channel pH monitoring with one electrode 5 cm above the LES and a second probe 20 cm above in the proximal esophagus just below the UES (Figure 11–18) is our procedure of choice. Abnormal distal esophageal acid exposure can be documented, establishing a diagnosis of GERD. Abnormal proximal reflux can be demonstrated, suggesting the potential for aspiration and lending stronger probability that the otolaryngologic symptom is due to GERD. If symptom correlation can be demonstrated, this will establish the diagnosis. The presence of proximal reflux appears to predict the response to medical therapy in patients with pulmonary disease.[315–317] This is less clear in the otolaryngologic patient. A small percentage of patients will have normal percent time of distal esophageal acid exposure, but demonstrable increased frequency of proximal reflux or reflux into the hypopharynx. This is seen in up to 30% of patients with otolaryngologic symptoms. In one study of 10 patients with reflux laryngitis, 3 of 10 (30%) demonstrated hypopharyngeal reflux with normal distal acid exposure.[318] In a larger, retrospective series of patients with pulmonary disease, 12% of patients reviewed had only abnormal proximal reflux[317]—a group that would have been

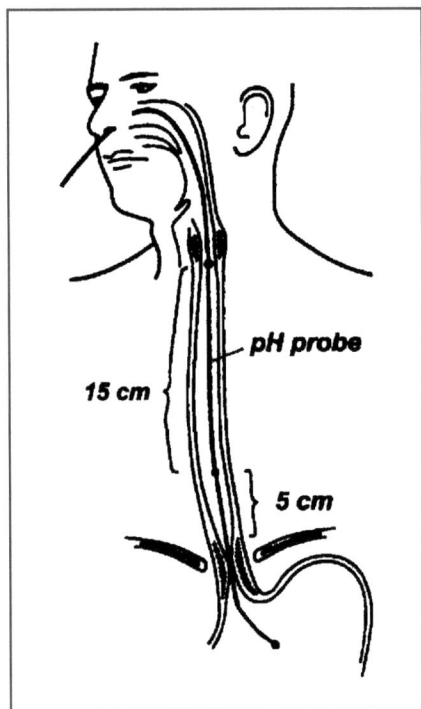

**Figure 11–18.** A dual-channel antimony pH probe with electrodes 15 cm apart. Distal electrode is placed 5 cm above the lower esophageal sphincter. Proximal electrode is 20 cm above the lower sphincter just below the upper esophageal sphincter.

diagnosed incorrectly as normal had only a single-channel study been performed. These patients should be considered abnormal and treated aggressively. Studies in our laboratory have shown that dual-electrode pH recording can document abnormal distal and proximal esophageal reflux induced by singing. A singing challenge (shown in Figure 11–17) can also unmask significant reflux in patients with otherwise normal 24-hour pH monitor studies.

Studies in adults with a variety of otolaryngologic symptoms demonstrate abnormal amounts of acid in reflux in up to 75% of patients.[16] Abnormal acid exposure has been documented in upright and supine positions, although upright reflux seems more common. Ambulatory pH monitoring is most useful in assessing response to antireflux therapy, particularly in the patient who has failed to respond to a therapeutic trial of a PPI twice daily for 8 to 12 weeks. Intragastric, distal esophageal, and proximal esophageal pH can be monitored while therapy is continued. Adequacy of intragastric acid suppression can be assessed, as can the presence of esophageal acid exposure and correlation between reflux events and symptoms. This study is particularly valuable in patients who do not respond (or are resistant) to PPIs. If acid reflux is still present, treatment can be increased or modified. If adequate acid suppression is achieved and symptoms persist, alternative diagnosis can be sought. However, the definition of "adequate acid suppression" is more complex than it might appear. For example, Shi et al[317] reviewed 771 consecutive patients who had undergone 24-hour pH monitoring studies. Statistically significant association was found between symptoms during reflux episodes in 96 patients (12.5%) with esophageal acid exposures that were within the laboratory's normal values. In these patients, the duration of reflux episodes was shorter and the pH of reflux episodes was higher than in patients who were diagnosed with GERD. The authors hypothesized that the underlying pathological feature in these patients was hypersensitivity to acid. However, there are other possible explanations. For example, it is possible that normative values have been established at levels higher than desirable.

An area of some controversy is the evaluation of the patient with continued symptoms but no esophageal acid exposure on 24-hour pH monitoring. This is when a question of alkaline or pH-neutral reflux may be raised. Current pH monitoring technology makes it possible to detect bilirubin pigment (bile) by use of a bilitec probe in addition to standard probes used for 24-hour pH monitoring. However, current data using this technique suggest that esophageal bile reflux rarely, if ever, occurs in the absence of acid reflux, making the bilitec probe useful only in select patients (see Approach to the Patient with GERD, below). The diagnosis of alkaline reflux should not be made based solely on the rise in pH above 7; careful analysis of pH rises above 7 coupled with symptom correlation may suggest alkaline reflux; but it is rarely, if ever, diagnosed conclusively by pH testing. A new approach to detecting pH-neutral reflux utilizes measurements of electrical impedance at numerous points along an esophageal probe. This device detects the presence of liquid in the esophagus regardless of pH, and sequential measurements along the chain of sensors indicate whether the liquid is traveling from proximal to distal or is refluxing from distal to proximal. This technology is now available commercially and has proven useful. However, the decision to proceed with surgical management for the suspicion of alkaline or pH-neutral reflux is a clinical one and must be made after careful consultation among the health care team, including the patient. Current pH technology cannot confirm this diagnosis definitively.

Although prolonged pH monitoring is used extensively in the evaluation of patients with suspected LPR, controversy exists as to its overall sensitivity and specificity. This is particularly important when addressing the issue of hypopharyngeal reflux. A recent study by Shaker and colleagues[318] found a similar number and duration of hypopharyngeal reflux events in control subjects and patients with suspected LPR. Another study[319] revealed no major difference between hypopharyngeal acid exposure in 36 patients with LPR signs and symptoms and healthy controls. Using a newer methodology for triple-probe monitoring, Maldonado et al[320] found a 10% prevalence of abnormal pH in normal controls. These data remind us of the importance of standardization of measurement of hypopharyngeal reflux to optimally understand the causal relationship between this phenomenon and LPR.

Sato et al[321] described their experience using a tetra-probe 24-hour pH monitoring system. The proximal probe is placed in the hypopharynx; a second probe is placed in the mid-esophagus; the third probe is placed a few centimeters above the LES (but not specifically 5 cm); and the distal sensor in placed in the stomach. This system is advantageous in that it measures pH simultaneously at all 4 sites, providing information regarding the relationship of these values. However, in our opinion, there are significant disadvantages associated with failure to have a sensor 5 cm above the LES, a standard site that permits comparison with other literature. In a separate report,[322] the authors described their results using the tetra-probe 24-hour pH monitoring system to evaluate patterns of LPR and GERD and to determine the validity of using pH 5 as an indicator of LPR. The data suggest that pH levels less than 4 and less than 5 are indicative of significant LPR events. An interesting study was reported in 2010 by Zelenik et al.[323] They performed a prospective dual-probe pH monitoring study in 46 patients with complaints of globus pharyngeus for more than 3 months. They collected data from this group using a pH less than 4 and from a second data group using pH both less than 4 and less than 5. Extraesophageal reflux was found in 23.9% of their patients using analysis of pH less than 4. When data were calculated using pH both less than 4 and less than 5, they found extraesophageal reflux in an additional 4 (8.7%) patients whose reflux had not been detected when pH less than 4 alone was used.

In addition, abnormal findings on pH monitoring do not necessarily predict patient response to therapy. Similarly, a recent placebo-controlled study[324] of 145 patients treated with either esomeprazole or placebo found that symptomatic or laryngeal improvement was independent of pretherapy pH-monitoring results. The apparent dichotomy in the clinical usefulness of hypopharyngeal pH monitoring is likely due to several key factors:

1. Lack of consensus on the duration and amount of reflux that constitute abnormal pharyngeal acid exposure.
2. High operator dependence and variability of probe positioning (eg, use of manometry vs direct visualization)
3. Variable sensitivity of pH monitoring in detecting reflux, which may vary from day to day.[325]

All these variables have been reported to result in a diagnostic yield from 14 to 83%.[326] The yield may improve with better data evaluation parameters. Reichel and Issing[327] suggest the use of reflux area indices of 4 and 5, which would include time at pH 5. The data regarding pepsin activity at pH 5 have generated somewhat less controversy than the data on activity at higher pH. The reflux area index is calculated from the number and duration of proximal reflux events and the degree to which the pH drops below a given value.[327] Incorporating several data points and including a reflux area index of 5 may increase the sensitivity of pH monitoring.

As such, 24-hour pH monitoring cannot be used to conclusively establish or rule out reflux as the cause of suspected LPR. Until the value of other tests such as wireless esophageal pH monitoring and/or impedance monitoring (see later section) has been established, an empiric trial with an effective dose of PPI remains the most important determinant of the relationship between reflux and LPR symptoms.

Ongoing research continues to examine the value of pH impedance monitoring in the diagnosis and treatment of patients with LPR.[328–333] In 2015, Gooi et al[334] reported the findings of the American Bronchoesophageal Association (ABBA) evaluation of the changes in the management and evaluation of patients with LPR over a 10-year period between 2002 and 2012. 426 ABBA members were e-mailed questionnaires to be completed online, of whom 63 (14.8%) responded. Their responses showed that dual pH probe testing remained highly regarded for sensitivity and specificity in the evaluation of LPR but was being used less often in 2012 compared to 2002 (63.8% vs 78.3%, respectively). Empirical medical management of LPR was more common in 2012 (82.6% compared to 56.3% in 2002).

### Telemetry Capsule pH Monitoring

The development of telemetry capsule-based (tubeless) pH monitoring has added to laryngologists'

armamentarium and ability to monitor patients with suspected reflux disease. The system is safe, well tolerated, and reliable, allowing 48-hour assessment of esophageal acid exposure. It is unobtrusive, comfortable, and allows longer duration of acid monitoring. Its use in LPR has not been studied, and the technology is limited by current inability to place the capsule proximally due to discomfort and bulk. Further refinements in methodology, recording protocols, and diagnostic accuracy have made this an extremely useful test in typical GERD patients. One of us (POK) uses the telemetry capsule to perform off-therapy monitoring in patients prior to antireflux surgery to be certain that abnormal acid exposure is present prior to an operation. This new technology will likely become valuable in assessing patients with LPR.[335]

### Role of Combined Multichannel Intraluminal Impedance pH

Combined multichannel intraluminal impedance (MII) and pH monitoring is a promising technique that identifies gas, liquid, and mixed gastroesophageal reflux and allows differentiation of them into acid (pH <4), weak acid (pH 4.1–7) and nonacid (pH > 7) types. The current catheter allows simultaneous monitoring of intragastric and distal esophageal pH with the ability to assess the height of refluxate from 3 to 17 cm above the LES. Early data suggest that a number of patients with so-called extraesophageal disease may have symptoms associated with weak acid or nonacid reflux, although the clear relationship of this type of reflux to LPR remains to be studied. Wu[336] reported that combining MII and dual-channel pH monitoring increased the diagnostic yield by ~10% compared with combined MII and single-channel pH monitoring systems. Lee and colleagues[337] reported a 2-fold increase in diagnosing reflux in patients with LPR symptoms, using combined dual-channel impedance/pH-metry. Loots et al[338] reported that the addition of MII to standard pH monitoring increased the yield of symptom association in children and infants with confirmed reflux. Combined MII/pH monitoring is a useful tool in evaluating all patients with persistent symptoms of acid-suppressive therapy, particularly those with LPR.[339]

### Pharyngeal Monitoring

Although the gold standard for diagnosis always has been pH testing, many physicians rely on the reflux finding score (RFS) and reflux symptom index (RSI) as means to diagnose laryngopharyngeal reflux (LPR) and indications to begin treatment with PPI or $H_2$-blockers. In addition, many believe that a reduction in RSI/RSF scores reflects improvement or resolution of LPR. However, numerous studies have raised questions about the utility or validity of these indicators, and over the safety and effectiveness of empiric prescription of antireflux medications. In a 2011 prospective study of 82 participants (72 patients and 10 controls), Musser et al[340] studied the agreement between RSI, RFS, and pH probe findings at pH levels of 4 and 5. Regardless of which pH criterion was used, RSI and RFS failed to identify the LPR patients from controls, and failed to correlate with severity of disease. In addition, in 2005, Park et al[341] evaluated 57 patients with globus sensation with 24-hour pH probe, RSI and RFS scores. In this study, RFS and RSI showed low specificity, and there was no significant difference between test and control groups. These findings suggest that both RSI and RFS should not be used as the sole diagnostic test for initiating PPI therapy.

Routine, long-term use of PPI in patients with elevated RSI/RFS, without proven LPR, may be ill-advised because of potential complications of therapy discussed elsewhere in this chapter. In addition, while PPIs are widely prescribed, resolution of LPR symptoms has been equivocal and often incomplete. Patients presenting with symptoms consistent with LPR are difficult to diagnose definitively, with most technologies providing no solid evidence on which a diagnosis or treatment can be based.[342]

Borrowing from the standards of gastroesophageal reflux disorder (GERD), the suggested definition of LPR has been a single episode of pH <4 or 1% total time below a pH of 4 on dual lumen probe.[343-345] Although standard 24-hour monitor technique has good diagnostic utility for the presence of LPR, it often causes significant patient discomfort, both in placement and throughout the monitoring period.[346,347] Other studies have reported lack of sleep and dysphagia with a dual lumen probe.[348] Hence, patients who alter their eating and sleeping habits may have tests that are not representative of their disease state. A new probe has been developed for monitoring the oropharyngeal pH and for the diagnosis of at least severe LPR. Multiple studies have demonstrated the ability of this device to detect reflux events compared to a traditional pH probe.

In 2009, Golub et al[348] studied 15 patients with symptoms of LPR by simultaneously placing a dual lumen pH probe and the Restech (Houston, Texas) oropharyngeal probe. This study revealed that the correlation between the 2 probes for reflux events was 0.95 (P < .001). In a separate study, Wiener et al[346] compared the Restech probe to 3 traditional pH probes (2 esophageal, 1 pharyngeal), in 15 patients

with symptoms of LPR. In this study, all events detected by the Restech probe were preceded by events in the distal esophagus. This study revealed the Restech probe to be a sensitive device that can detect pH events that originate in the distal esophagus and migrate toward the oropharynx.

In addition to the high correlation with traditional pH, the Restech probe offers some significant advantages. First, sensors in conventional pH probe require a liquid environment to function properly. Traditional probes placed in the oropharynx have a tendency to dry out and lead to "false-positive" readings (pseudo-reflux). The Restech probe does not require a liquid environment to provide real-time pH readings. Second, the sensors for traditional probes are located on the side of the catheter, which leads to the possibility of masking by the mucosal wall and "false-negative" readings. The sensor on the Restech probe is located on the teardrop-shaped tip, which decreases the possibility of mucosal masking. Furthermore, the placement of a traditional probe requires manometric (radiographic in infants) confirmation of placement. The placement of the Restech probe can be confirmed visually with simple oropharyngeal examination by localizing the red LED light in the catheter tip.

Currently, multiple studies have addressed the utility of the Restech probe in a clinical setting. A recent study by Friedman et al[349] revealed that in a group of 163 patients with suspected LPR, there was no correlation between RSI and the oropharyngeal environment. In addition, the calculated positive and negative predictive values for RSI and severe reflux (positive Ryan Score) were 44.3 and 58.7%, respectively. The authors recommend that diagnosis and treatment decisions regarding LPR should be on the basis of symptoms (RSI), signs (RSF or oropharyngeal findings), and a confirmatory test (pH testing). In a recent prospective study[350] of 18 patients with symptoms of LPR, 100% of patients with positive Ryan Scores (by Restech) responded to PPI therapy, while less than half of those with a negative study responded. While the specific pH profile of Ryan-negative PPI responders needs to be elucidated, these results suggest that the Restech probe may be useful in determining which patients will respond to PPI therapy. In a separate 2011 study by Friedman et al,[351] 143 patients were offered either empiric PPI treatment (70 patients) or Restech-based treatment (73 patients) for symptoms of LPR. This study revealed that patients tested with the Restech probe had significantly greater compliance with medication (68.5 vs 50%, P = .019) and lifestyle modification (82.2 vs 25.7%, P < .01) as well as significantly greater reduction in RSI (36.6 vs 24%, P = .023). Collectively, these studies suggest Restech has utility in the diagnosis of LPR and selection of patients who might benefit from treatment, as well as in improving patient compliance.

Based on current literature and the side effect profile of antireflux medication, questions must be considered about whether to treat all symptomatic patients empirically without first determining their oropharyngeal pH profile. More research is needed (and is in progress). If the Restech probe is really as reliable and valid as traditional dual lumen probes and offers some advantages over dual lumen probes placed below the UES or in the oropharynx, it may become a standard diagnostic tool. While often associated with GERD, LPR is a different disease state that presents its own set of problems in terms of diagnosis and treatment protocols. This becomes especially true with patients in the "gray zone" presenting with mild to moderate reflux. Currently, multiple groups are using the Restech probe to help better determine disease state/severity. This determination should lead to improved ability to predict those who will respond well to standard antireflux therapy versus those who need more aggressive management. Equally important is the elimination of empiric treatment for those who do not have LPR and faster work-up to identify the true etiology of their symptoms and signs.

### Esophageal Manometry

Manometry will establish abnormal LES pressure or esophageal motility and is necessary preoperatively to evaluate contraction amplitude in the esophageal body. A single measurement of LES pressure is rarely low in patients with GERD. In the author's (POK) experience, only 4% of patients with GERD have a low LES pressure.[352] Esophageal motility abnormalities are found more frequently. The most common finding appears to be ineffective esophageal motility (IEM) (amplitude of contraction in the distal esophagus less than 30 mm Hg occurring with 30% or more of water swallows). In our experience, this is the most common abnormality in patients with GERD, seen in approximately 35% of patients with esophagitis.[352] IEM appears even more common in GERD-related laryngitis, asthma, and cough.[57] Esophageal manometry is performed prior to antireflux surgery to establish the presence or absence of ineffective esophageal motility. The surgeon will usually perform a Nissen fundoplication (360° wrap) in patients with normal peristalsis and a Toupet procedure (240° wrap) in patients with significant IEM. Patients with IEM and respiratory symptoms do not appear to respond as well to antireflux surgery if respiratory complaints are the presenting symptom.

Esophageal manometry is important also for proper placement of probes for pH monitoring. Although the proximal probe can be positioned accurately by direct vision using a flexible fiberoptic laryngoscope, mirror, or telescope, without manometry there is no way to position the distal probe precisely. However, when compared to manometry, even proximal probe placement was accurate in only 70% of cases in the study by Johnson et al.[353] Distal probe placement was accurate in just 40% of cases using estimated interprobe distance. Using fixed interprobe distances of 15 cm and 20 cm, distal probe placement was accurate in only 3% (for 15 cm) or 40% (for 20 cm) of cases. These errors are critical because the normative values for distal esophageal acid exposure were established with the distal probe positioned 5 cm above the LES.[354–357] Even slight modifications in the distance between the distal probe and the lower esophageal sphincter cause substantial changes in acid exposure data.[358–361]

### Hiatal Hernia

A hiatal hernia is not predictive of reflux as a cause of the patients' symptoms.[362] Up to 60% of patients over the age of 60 will demonstrate a hiatal hernia identified on barium swallow examination. One study suggested that only 9% of patients with a radiographically demonstrated hernia have typical reflux symptoms.[77]

Hernias do change the relationship of the LES and crural diaphragm. The LES is displaced above the diaphragm. The low pressure in the hernia can act as a reservoir for acid, allowing earlier reflux during LES relaxations, and may delay esophageal clearance.[363] Patients with large hernias who also have low LES pressure may be more prone to reflux[364] if changes occur in intraabdominal pressure.

### Evaluation for *Helicobacter pylori*

*Helicobacter pylori* (H pylori) appears to play a role in the development of chronic type B gastritis, gastroduodenal ulcer disease, and gastric carcinoma.[365,366] Its significance in gastroesophageal reflux disease remains uncertain, and it is unclear whether it is necessary to treat *H pylori* in reflux patients, or even advisable to do so. *H pylori* can be detected through serologic determination of immunoglobin (IgG) antibodies to the organism. This blood test is performed using an enzyme-linked immunosorbent assay (ELISA)/2-step indirect sandwich assay on directly coated microtiter plates.[367] This test is believed to have a sensitivity of 94% and specificity of 85%.[367]

Researchers continue to examine the relationship between *H pylori* infection, LPR, and laryngeal diseases.[368,369] Suipsinskiene et al[370] performed a prospective case control study to examine the presence of *H pylori* through biopsy of the larynx in patients with laryngeal cancer and patients with benign laryngeal disease, including LPR and vocal fold polyps. They examined the biopsy results from 67 adult patients with benign and malignant laryngeal disease and compared them with a control group of 11 patients. They reported *H pylori* infection in greater than one-third of the patients studied, with the majority found in patients with laryngeal cancer (46.2%) and in those with chronic laryngitis (45.5%). The authors reported that these findings differed significantly from the control group (9.1%) ($p < 0.05$), adding that they found no significant relationship between LPR-related symptoms and *H pylori* detected in the larynx. They stated that *H pylori* can colonize in patients with benign laryngeal disease and laryngeal cancer, but that further research is needed. Another study by Islam et al[371] also examined the presence of *H pylori* in patients with benign and malignant laryngeal disease. They performed a prospective study of 50 patients who underwent microlaryngoscopy over a 2-year period. Their patient population was diagnosed as having LPR based on a reflux symptom index (RSI) greater than 12, and a reflux finding score (RFS) greater than 6. The patients were diagnosed with *H pylori* based on a positive urea breath test, HP citotoxin-associated gene A(CAGA)-IgG and HP-IGG test results. Intraoperatively, 2 surgical specimens were obtained, one from the interarytenoid area, and one from the primary vocal fold lesion. The authors reported that *H pylori* was not found in any interarytenoid specimen, and they found no histologic evidence of *H pylori* in the vocal fold pathology specimens. They also reported "there was no difference between RSS-positive and RSS-negative patients in terms of HP-IGG and UBT," adding that, "the presence of HP in the gastric mucosa does not have an effect on the RSS and RSI." Their study conclusions disagree with other reports in the literature and with the author's (RTS) experience.

## Approach to the Patient With GERD-Related Otolaryngologic Abnormalities

In patients with GERD-related otolaryngologic complaints, a thorough history, physical examination, and laryngoscopy should be performed (Figure 11–19). If dysphagia is present, a functional endoscopic evaluation of swallowing (FEES) or videoendoscopic swallowing evaluation should be considered, and a barium swallow should be obtained to rule out stricture or motility abnormalities. The clinician's dilemma revolves around the choice of early diagnostic testing with prolonged pH monitoring or institution of a therapeutic trial of medication. The "best" approach is not clear. Although diagnostic testing with ambulatory pH monitoring would be ideal, there are several limitations: (1) pH monitoring is not always available; (2) the sensitivity and specificity are clearly not 100%; (3) patients do not reflux with the same frequency every day; and (4) variability in both distal and proximal esophageal acid exposure time in patients with extraesophageal GERD is common, increasing the possibility of a false-negative pH study if physiologic acid exposure is seen on a single study.

If the history and laryngoscopic examination raise a high clinical suspicion of GERD or LPR, if prolonged monitoring is not available, if frequent heartburn and regurgitation are present, or if there is endoscopic documentation of GERD or LPR, a therapeutic trial of antireflux therapy is a reasonable initial choice. An early study with empiric omeprazole, 40 mg at bedtime, in patients with suspected reflux laryngitis found a 67% response in patients with laryngeal symptoms suggestive of GERD.[372] Another study found 70% success with empiric omeprazole 20 mg BID for a similar time period.[373] We use a trial of a PPI twice daily in combination with dietary and behavior modification initially for 8 to 12 weeks. If the patient does not respond, pH monitoring should be performed while PPI therapy is continued. A dual-channel probe with intragastric and distal esophageal electrodes should be placed to ascertain adequate gastric acid suppression and to assess the presence of esophageal acid exposure. If distal esophageal acid exposure is seen more than 1.2% of the time, this is definitely abnormal and additional medical therapy is indicated.[374] "Normal" esophageal acid exposure, particularly when any proximal esophageal acid exposure is documented, may not always be a negative study. A positive symptom index may be seen even in patients with "normal" distal acid exposure, and this, too, is abnormal and warrants additional therapy. The *absence* of any esophageal acid exposure and presence of adequate gastric acid suppression (pH >4, 50% of total time) suggests adequate medical therapy in most patients, and an alternative diagnosis should be considered. If GERD-associated otolaryngologic disease is documented, endoscopy is indicated in many cases to rule out Barrett's esophagus prior to initiating long-term medical therapy or surgery.

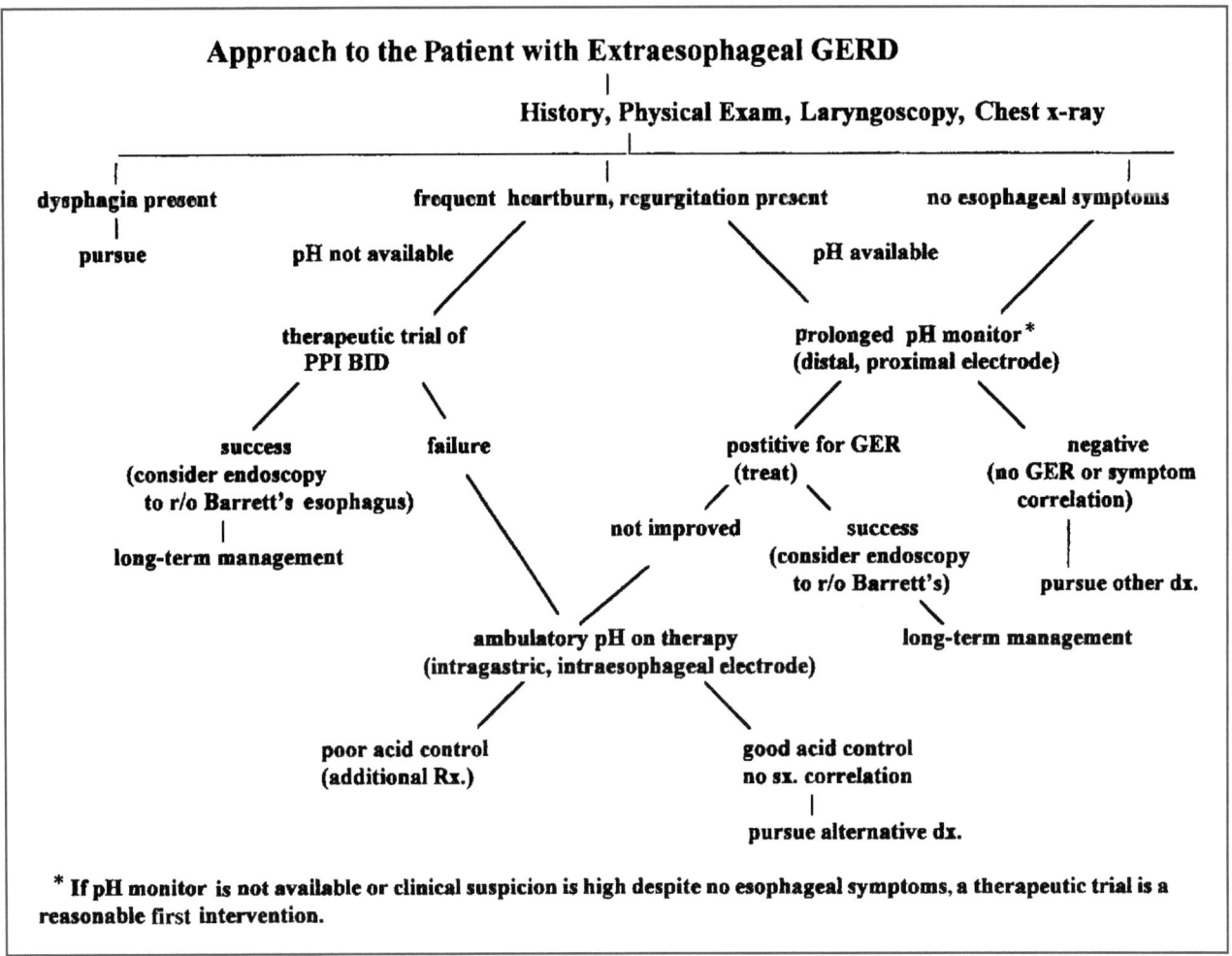

**Figure 11–19.** Outline of approach to the patient with gastroesophageal reflux disease and otolaryngologic disease. (PPI = proton pump inhibitor; GER = gastroesophageal reflux; BID = twice daily.)

## Outcomes Measures

In addition to using instruments discussed elsewhere such as the Voice Handicap Index (VHI)[375] that were designed to measures outcomes of voice disorders, Belafsky, Postma, and Koufman have introduced "The Reflux Finding Score (RFS)."[376] The RFS depends on observations of subglottic edema, ventricular obliteration, erythema/hyperemia, vocal fold edema, diffuse laryngeal edema, posterior laryngeal hypertrophy, granuloma/granulation tissue, and thick endolaryngeal mucus. Although additional research from other centers is needed to confirm the validity and reliability of the RFS, the authors found excellent inter- and intraobserver reproducibility (although all observers were practicing at the same medical center); they found the RFS to be an accurate instrument for documenting treatment efficacy in patients with LPR. Other quality-of-life evaluations have highlighted the impact of GERD and LPR on patient function.[377,378] The Pharyngeal Reflux Symptom Questionnaire was developed by Andersson et al.[379] It is a self-administered questionnaire specific for LPR patients. They compared this tool with the LPR-Health Related Quality of Life and the reflux symptom index and reported strong correlation. The authors also reported that the questionnaire discriminated between patients without and with LPR. Several reports[380,381] have suggested that anxiety, depression, and depression symptoms can impact subjective responses to quality-of-life tools and symptom indices and thus diminish the predictive value of symptom assessment, which raises concern about the usefulness of these tools. Researchers in China[382] reported significantly higher Voice Handicap Index scores and higher depression scores in their patients with LPR.

Nishumura et al[383] evaluated postoperative LPR in patients who had undergone surgery for esophageal cancer. They proposed a classification system for grading findings on endoscopy to facilitate more accurate diagnosis of LPR in this patient population.

## Behavioral and Medical Management of Gastroesophageal Reflux Disease

Treatment of the patient with GERD requires careful consideration of the primary symptom presentation, degree of mucosal injury, and the presence or absence of complications. Treatment focuses on 4 goals: elimination of symptoms, healing of mucosal injury if present, management of complications, and maintenance of symptomatic remission. Treatment should combine lifestyle modifications, pharmacologic therapy, and appropriate use of antireflux surgery. GERD is a chronic condition that may recur quickly if therapy is stopped or medication dosage is decreased; therefore, long-term therapy is the key to effective management and often requires continuous full prescription doses of appropriate medications. Symptom relief and mucosal healing in GERD are directly related to control of intragastric acid secretion (the time during which gastric pH is less than 4) and reduction of esophageal acid exposure.[384] Clinical trials in patients with symptomatic erosive esophagitis suggest that a careful and systematic stepwise approach to medical therapy will result in satisfactory symptom relief in over 90% of patients.[385]

In contrast, there have been relatively few clinical trials of treatment involving patients with asthma, cough, laryngopharyngeal reflux (LPR), and other extraesophageal manifestations of GERD. Most trials have been uncontrolled, and maintenance trials are lacking. Treatment is based on the principles for treating patients with heartburn and erosive esophagitis and observations from available clinical trials and clinical experience. As a general rule, patients with LPR and the other extraesophageal manifestations of GERD require higher doses of pharmacologic therapy, usually with PPIs twice daily, with longer periods of treatment needed to achieve complete relief of symptoms compared to patients with heartburn and erosive esophagitis. Although relief of symptoms, healing of mucosal injury, and maintenance of remission are still the primary goals, assessing these endpoints is somewhat more difficult as the "gold standard" for diagnosis is not always clear. The principles of the medical treatment of GERD with specific emphasis on LPR and other extraesophageal manifestations of GERD are discussed below.

**Lifestyle Modification and Patient Education**

Simple and effective changes in lifestyle are crucial in controlling symptoms of GERD. Educating patients about the recurring nature and chronicity of GERD and LPR is crucial to compliance with long-term medical management. Studies with overnight pH monitoring have shown a significant decrease in total esophageal acid exposure after elevation of the head of the bed 6 inches compared to sleeping flat.[385] Recent studies continue to support the critical importance of head of bed elevation in the management of LPR.[386,387] A similar effect can be produced by placing a foam rubber wedge under the patient's mattress. A long (full length) wedge is preferable to tilt the whole mattress rather than bending it at the waist level. The use of pillows in lieu of a wedge or head-of-the-bed elevation cannot be recommended, because bending of the waist and change in body position may paradoxically increase intraabdominal pressure and increase reflux. In addition, if patients roll over on their stomachs while sleeping on pillows, bending backward may result in lower back pain, which may lead them to stop complying with instructions to elevate their torsos. An effective alternative approach is to instruct patients to preferentially sleep lying on their left side. This will place the esophagogastric junction in an advantageous position above the gastric contents and has been shown to significantly decrease recumbent reflux.[388]

Elimination or decreasing of gastric irritants from the diet will reduce symptoms. These agents include citrus juices, tomato products, coffee (both caffeinated and decaffeinated), and alcohol. Colas, tea, and other acidic fluids are often overlooked as potential gastric and esophageal irritants.[389] A meal high in fat will increase postprandial reflux episodes in patients with GERD,[390] so a low-fat diet is recommended. Chocolate and other carminatives will decrease lower esophageal pressure (LES) and increase reflux frequency,[391] as will onions, and should be eliminated from the diet (Table 11–6). Koufman[392] evaluated the clinical impact of a low-acid diet on therapeutic outcome in patients treated for LPR. She studied a group of 20 patients with persistent signs and symptoms of LPR despite twice-daily use of a PPI and a histamine-2 (H$_2$) blocker at bedtime. The low-acid diet described by Koufman eliminated all foods and beverages with a pH less than 5. The patients were placed on this diet for a minimum of 2 weeks, and both the reflux symptom index and the reflux finding score were determined before and after the diet. Koufman's findings show that both the clinical signs and symptoms in these patients who had had

**Table 11–6.** Lifestyle Modifications for Treatment of Gastroesophageal Reflux

Elevation of head of bed (6 inches)—avoid waterbed

Dietary modifications

1. Lower fat, higher protein
2. Avoid specific irritants
   a. Citrus juices
   b. Tomato products
   c. Coffee, tea
   d. Alcohol
   e. Colas
   f. Onions
3. No eating prior to sleeping (allow at least 2 hours)
4. Avoid chocolate, carminatives (lower LES pressure)

Decrease or stop smoking

Avoid potentially harmful medications

1. Affect LES pressure
   a. Anticholinergics
   b. Sedatives/tranquilizers
   c. Theophylline
   d. Prostaglandins
   e. Calcium-channel blockers
2. Potentially cause esophageal injury
   a. Potassium tablets
   b. Ferrous sulfate
   c. Antibiotics (gelatin capsules), eg, tetracycline
   d. NSAIDs, aspirin
   e. Alendronate

Abbreviation: LES = Lower esophageal sphincter.

persistent symptoms despite PPI treatment improved following an acid-free diet.

Gastric distention provides the major stimulus for transient lower esophageal sphincter relaxation (TLESR), the most common abnormality responsible for individual reflux episodes. Eating large, high-fat meals increases gastric distention and slows gastric emptying, probably increasing TLESRs. Going to sleep on a full stomach or lying down after a meal also creates a stimulus for TLESR and is likely to increase reflux. It is therefore critical to remind patients to avoid eating within 2 to 3 hours of sleep and to avoid recumbency after a meal, especially if reflux occurs when they are supine (which is not always the case with LPR).[391] An interesting study by Hamdan et al[393] studied the effects of fasting vs nonfasting (12 hours) on LPR findings in 22 males and reported no significant effects on LPR symptoms in this population (RSI scores), or in RFSs of laryngeal examinations.

Smoking may decrease LES pressure and delay esophageal clearance, increasing reflux frequency and potentially mucosal injury. This is likely due to the effects of nicotine. Smoking may decrease the effectiveness of $H_2$-receptor antagonists, especially at night (when reflux injury is more severe due to delayed esophageal clearance of refluxate); however, the effect of smoking on the action of PPIs is not known. Clearly smoking can be detrimental to overall health—exacerbation of GERD is no exception. One study examined the effects of lifestyle modifications including raising the head of the bed 6 inches, eliminating meals before bedtime, and using antacids in the treatment of patients with respiratory symptoms and GERD. Outcomes were compared to patients not using antireflux measures for 2-month periods. In this study, both esophageal and respiratory symptoms were reported to improve with lifestyle modifications compared to no antireflux therapy. However, no objective changes were noted in pulmonary function and endoscopy was not performed.[386] This suggests that the addition of the conservative measures outlined in Table 11–6 is useful in treatment of extra-esophageal GERD. No studies have specifically examined lifestyle modifications in patients with LPR. However, we routinely recommend the use of these conservative measures as patients often reflux during the postprandial period, even when they are upright.

The importance of including lifestyle modifications as part of a treatment program at a time when very efficacious drug therapy, such as PPIs, is available has been debated. All clinical trials have included these lifestyle changes as part of treatment, so the effect of eliminating them is not known. These lifestyle modifications are easy to explain and implement and are of low economic cost. Based on symptom severity and control, patients can decide for themselves how diligent they should be. Some patients with mild, infrequent symptoms may avoid regular prescription medications by following these modifications as recommended. They appear somewhat less likely to be sufficient in many voice professionals, especially in singers who experience upright reflux when they sing due to increased intraabdominal pressure that occurs with proper voice support. However, if 24-hour pH monitor studies show that these patients do not experience supine and/or nocturnal reflux, it may be unnecessary for them to elevate the head of the bed. Head of bed elevation can be a substantial inconvenience for performers who may spend 200 nights per year or more in hotel rooms. Therapies for such patients should be rational and individualized on the basis of symptoms, signs, and test results.[82]

The diagnoses represented within the gluten sensitivity spectrum are as diverse and nebulous as are its presenting symptoms, as we have discussed elsewhere[394] and are reviewing here. One of the best categorizations found in the recent literature subdivides gluten sensitivity into allergic, autoimmune, and nonallergic/nonautoimmune, or simply immune.[395] The allergy category includes wheat allergy (WA) or food allergy, wheat-dependent exercise-induced anaphylaxis (WDEIA), occupational or Baker's asthma, and contact urticaria. The autoimmune category includes celiac disease (CD), dermatitis herpetiformis, and gluten ataxia. Nonceliac gluten sensitivity (NCGS) belongs to the third category, which is the newest and least studied but also the most intriguing. The scientific community is just beginning to recognize the existence of NCGS as a disease with distinct pathophysiologic and epidemiologic characteristics. While the prevalence of CD in the United States is between 0.5% and 1%,[396] epidemiologic studies place NCGS prevalence in the United States slightly higher, with best estimates ranging from 0.55 to 6%.[397,398]

Gluten sensitivity including CD and NCGS presents with gastrointestinal and extraintestinal symptoms. The most common GI complaints include irritable bowel syndrome (IBS)–like symptoms (eg, bloating, abdominal pain, bowel habit abnormalities such as diarrhea and/or constipation) and even symptoms of GERD (heartburn and regurgitation).[399] For example, between 2004 and 2010, 5896 patients were seen at the Center for Celiac Research, University of Maryland.[400] The criteria for gluten sensitivity were fulfilled by 347 (6%) of the patients seen. Their symptoms included abdominal pain (68%); eczema and/or rash (40%); headache (35%); "foggy mind" (34%); fatigue (33%); diarrhea (33%); depression (22%); anemia (20%); numbness in the legs, arms, or fingers (20%); and joint pain (11%). Other studies have confirmed these symptoms in this population.[401,402] Gluten sensitivity, particularly CD, also has been associated with an increased risk of other autoimmune disorders such as autoimmune thyroiditis, type I diabetes mellitus, Addison disease, Crohn's and ulcerative colitis, myasthenia gravis, and psoriasis.[400] It is equally important to recognize that some of these patients have minimal or no symptoms, making it even more difficult to select those who would benefit from a diagnostic workup. Fasano et al found that 41% of patients with positive serology for CD were asymptomatic.[401] This problem is compounded further by the nonspecific nature of extraintestinal

symptoms, the variable effect of gluten on an individual's immune system, the observation that many patients are already on a gluten-free diet (GFD) or a low fermentable oligo-di-monosaccharides and polyols (FODMAP) diet at the time of presentation, and the possibility that other extra-intestinal symptoms may be linked but not yet identified. It is conceivable, given the current evidence linking gluten sensitivity with GERD, that the signs and symptoms attributed to LPR also might be linked to gluten sensitivity in this population, but this possibility has not been studied.

At the present time, there are insufficient data linking CD and NCGS with LPR. Conversely, studies have identified that the esophagus is not spared in patients with gluten sensitivity. Consistent data are now available on the presence of disturbed motility of the esophagus, along with the stomach, small intestine, gallbladder, and colon of untreated patients with CD.[403–410] Using esophageal manometry, Usai et al studied the presence of specific esophageal motor disorders in this population.[408] They reported motor abnormalities in 67% of 18 patients with CD. They consisted of nutcracker esophagus (50%), low pressure in LES associated with simultaneous contractions (11%), and frequent repetitive contractions (22%). No subjects in the control group (34 patients) and the ulcerative colitis group (9 patients) had these manometric abnormalities. Additional interesting findings in the study group were the presence of dysphagia in 50% (vs 9% of controls) and odynophagia in 14% (vs 0% of controls) of 36 patients with CD.

There have been studies exploring GERD in the gluten sensitive population, primarily those with CD. The findings show that GERD symptoms are more common in patients with CD than in the general population. In a study by Nachman et al, 30% of patients complained of moderate-to-severe GERD symptoms at the time of CD diagnosis (defined as score >3 in the Gastrointestinal Symptoms Rating Scale),[410] a rate 6-fold higher than the rate seen in healthy controls (5.7%). A GFD has been shown to improve symptoms of GERD in patients with CD, irrespective of PPI therapy.[408–411] Because GERD-like symptoms can be a presentation of active celiac disease and nonceliac gluten sensitivity, some studies have concluded that celiac disease should be considered, and investigated, by means of serology or with duodenal biopsies during EGD, in patients with refractory GERD, especially if these patients exhibit other signs or symptoms suggestive of CD.[412] Although Collin et al argued against screening for CD in patients with reflux esophagitis concluding that GERD is not a major manifestation of CD, they also commented that a GFD may result in symptomatic relief of reflux symptoms in patients with CD.[413] The study also did not explore this question in patients with NCGS.

A study by Lamanda et al documented esophageal erosive lesions in 23% of 65 adult patients diagnosed with CD over a year, a prevalence far above that which was established for the general population.[410] Cuomo et al monitored esophageal pH in 15 out of the 39 celiac patients included in their case series; 14 out of 15 showed pathologic pH levels. Furthermore, lower esophageal sphincter (LES) pressure values trended lower than those observed in healthy controls, although the differences did not reach statistical significance.[414]

There is interesting literature illustrating the relationship that exists between GERD and GFD in patients with CD. A GFD alone reduces severity of both heartburn and regurgitation significantly in adults with CD.[415,416] In patients with CD treated with PPI, a GFD also reduced the risk of recurrence of GERD-related symptoms after discontinuation of antisecretory treatment. Nachman et al found that after 3 months from the start of the GFD, GERD-related symptom scores had decreased significantly in their series of adult patients with CD, reaching values similar to those of healthy controls.[409] Lamanda et al showed that GERD symptoms had remitted in 91% of adult patients with CD after 4 weeks of treatment with PPI at standard doses, with no relapse in any case after 12 months of follow-up on GFD.[410] A GFD also has been shown to prevent recurrence of GERD-related symptoms in patients with CD who have both erosive and nonerosive esophatitis.[402,403] Long-term benefits of a GFD on GERD symptoms still persist in the event of partial compliance.[412]

The potential association between LPR and gluten sensitivity was not investigated until our (RTS) preliminary study. In our practice, this connection has become more apparent after a growing number of patients have reported improvement in symptoms usually associated with LPR while following a GFD.

Numerous mechanisms have been proposed to explain the association of gluten sensitivity and GERD. In summary, they have included nutrient malabsorption affecting gastroesophageal motility, GI hormonal derangements causing decreased LES pressures and dysmotility, and the inflammatory reaction to gluten resulting in increased mucosal permeability.[393,394] Wex et al report that zonulin, a protein involved in the regulation of interepithelial permeability in the intestines of CD patients, may be implicated because it was found to be expressed in esophageal epithelial cells, as well.[415] In addition to these potential mechanisms, Tursi has proposed the possible involvement of neurotransmitters and the direct toxic effect of gluten on muscular tissues.[402] In a similar manner, one or more of these potential mechanisms could contribute to the presence of LPR in these patients.

Tursi reported on 3 patients with GERD refactory to antisecretory treatment who were diagnosed with CD after duodenal biopsies and who had rapid and long-lasting remission of symptoms after starting a GFD.[402] In one example, a 24-year-old woman had persistent GERD symptoms despite esomeprazole 80 mg/day. Twenty days after starting PPI therapy, celiac disease was diagnosed based on histologic evaluation, and the patient was started immediately on a GFD. Symptoms improved within 7 days and disappeared completely within 2 weeks of GFD despite cessation of PPI therapy, and she remained symptom-free 6 months later.

Lucendo acknowledged this observation by stating that the lack of response to PPI therapy to improve GERD symptoms, even after increasing the doses, could be the key for suspecting and actively excluding CD.[403] Regardless of the pathophysiology of GERD symptoms in patients with CD, the question arises whether GFD should be added to antisecretory treatment, because it appears that symptom improvement may be more related in these patients to gluten suppression than to medication. In his editorial, Tursi proposed avoiding antisecretory medications altogether and instead using antacids such as sodium alginate to treat nonerosive GERD in patients with CD until gluten elimination reversed clinical symptoms.[412]

The current literature has shown that GERD is more prevalent in patients with CD and that it responds favorably to GFD. Pending future studies, a similar observation is likely to be established between GERD and NCGS. The impact of gluten sensitivity on LPR, however, represents a new frontier of untapped research potential. From our clinical observations and identifications of current gaps in existing knowledge, it can be concluded that further research investigating this potential relationship is warranted. We have incorporated consideration for possible gluten sensitivity into our routine assessment of patients with suspected LPR (Figure 11–20). At a minimum, the knowledge presented here should prove useful for laboratory screening and referring patients to our gastroenterology colleagues if suspicion for gluten sensitivity arises. Following the most recent literature and national guidelines on CD and NCGS including the American College of Gastroenterology (ACG),[417,418] our practice has initiated laboratory testing for patients with LPR, particularly

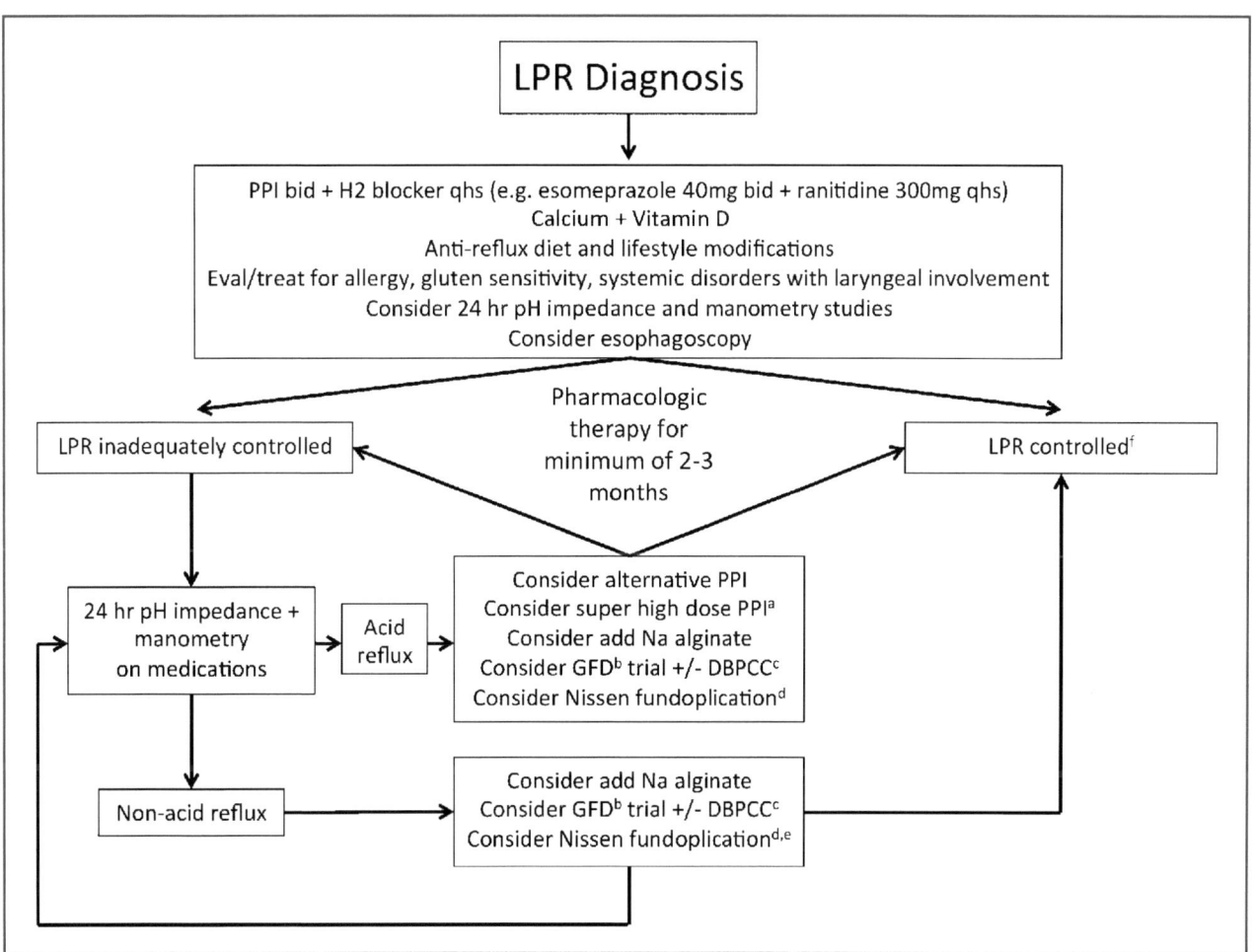

**Figure 11–20.** Laryngopharyngeal reflux algorithm incorporating gluten sensitivity evaluation and management. **A.** Portnoy JE, Gregory ND, Cerull CE, et al. Efficacy of super high dose proton pump inhibitor administration in refractory laryngopharyngeal reflux: a pilot study. *J Voice.* 2014;28(3):369–377. **B.** Gluten-free diet may be considered at any step in the pathway with serologic testing recommended prior to initiation. **C.** DBPCC = double-blind placebo controlled (gluten) challenge. **D.** Repeat 24 hr pH impedance with manometry off anti-secretory medications is recommended 3 months post-Nissen fundoplication. **E.** Nissen fundoplication is likely to be therapeutic for non-acid reflux laryngitis, especially if a positive symptom index during 24-hour pH impedance testing. **F.** Nissen fundoplication should be considered for patients who do not want to use anti-secretory medications long term.

when refractory to antisecretory reflux therapy or when indicated by the patient's history. This laboratory panel includes the following:

- Tissue transglutaminase (TTG) IgA, IgG
- Deamidated gliadin peptide (DGP) IgA, IgG
- Antigliadin antibody (AGA) IgA, IgG
- Total IgA
- Wheat-specific IgE
- HLA-DQ genotyping

Some laboratories have incorporated reflex testing into their celiac disease panels to look for tissue transglutaminase IgG if total IgA is low, for example,

because 2 to 3% of patients with celiac disease also have IgA deficiency. HLA DQ2 or DQ8 is present in nearly 100% of patients with celiac disease, while it is present in 50% of patients with NCGS and 30 to 40% of the general population. This test, along with AGA IgG (positive in 56% of patients with NCGS) presently are the only 2 commercially available laboratory tests that have been shown to be positive more often in NCGS patients than in the general population. Algorithms have been developed to help guide evaluation and workup,[419–421] and our approach is summarized in Table 11–7. If CD is diagnosed or if NCGS is suspected, a GFD trial may be recommended, along with referrals to a gastroenterologist and a nutritionist.

**Table 11–7.** Laboratory Evaluation of Gluten Sensitivity

| Lab Test | Can Test on Gluten-Free Diet? | Indication | Sensitivity | Specificity |
|---|---|---|---|---|
| Tissue transglutaminase (TTG) | | | | |
|    TTG IgA | No | Celiac disease | 98% | 98% |
|    TTG IgG | No | Celiac disease | 70% | 95% |
| Deamidated gliadin peptide (DGP) | | | | |
|    DGP IgA | No | Celiac disease | 88% | 95% |
|    DGP IgG | No | Celiac disease | 80% | 98% |
| Anti-gliadin antibody (AGA) | | | | |
|    AGA IgA | No | Celiac disease | 85% | 90% |
|    AGA IgG | No | Celiac disease/**NCGS** | 85% (CD) | 80% (CD) |
| Endomysial Antibody IgA | No | Celiac disease | 95% | 99% |
| Wheat specific IgE | No | Wheat allergy (IgE) | 83% | 43% |
| HLA DQ2 and DQ8 | Yes | Celiac disease/**NCGS** | ~100% (CD) | Low; varies depending on population |

Abbreviations: CD = celiac disease; NCGS = nonceliac gluten sensitivity.

Medications that decrease esophageal pressures and promote reflux include anticholinergics, sedatives or tranquilizers, tricyclic antidepressants, theophylline, nitrates, and calcium-channel blocking agents. Many other drugs are known to cause direct esophageal injury (pill-induced esophagitis).[422] The most common are KCl (potassium chloride) tablets, iron sulfate, gelatin capsule antibiotics, nonsteroidal antiinflammatory drugs (NSAIDs), and alendronate (Fosamax).[423] These should be used with caution in patients with GERD. Although there is no direct evidence that these agents cause GERD, they can cause esophageal injury and may make mucosal injury from reflux more severe (see Table 11–6). The effects of these agents vary from patient to patient. Experience suggests that none of these drugs greatly exacerbates GERD, so discontinuing a needed agent is usually not necessary, especially with concomitant use of PPIs.

### Over-the-Counter Agents

Numerous antacids and over-the-counter H$_2$-receptor antagonists are available to treat patients with symptomatic reflux. These agents should be used exclusively to treat symptoms such as heartburn that is intermittent and as adjuncts to prescription therapy for breakthrough symptoms. Symptom relief is similar with equipotent antacids and all of the H$_2$-antagonists available over the counter. Because patients with LPR often require long-term (or lifetime) therapy with high doses of PPIs or H$_2$-blockers in full prescription doses, management with over-the-counter (low-dose) H$_2$-blockers is rarely adequate.

The use of antacids remains controversial. Experts agree that they should be superfluous if *sufficient* doses of acid suppression medication therapy are used. However, there are differences of opinion regarding the level of control achieved in most patients on the customary doses of PPIs (omeprazole 40 mg daily, or the equivalent), and on the importance of occasional episodes of breakthrough reflux. It is well known that reflux may still occur on daily 40 mg doses of omeprazole or 60 mg of lansoprazole. This has been confirmed by pH monitor studies often in clinical settings, and some patients require higher doses for complete acid suppression. The occasional reflux episodes experienced by many patients on

40 mg of omeprazole per day may be "normal" and not significant; however, in patients with LPR, especially voice professionals, any laryngeal acid exposure is detrimental. Rather than doing 24-hour pH studies on medication for every patient with LPR or prescribing even higher doses of PPIs routinely, some physicians use antacids, $H_2$ blockers, and/or lifestyle modifications in addition to PPIs. The antacids are used at bedtime and before strenuous exercise (such as singing). This regimen may be useful for singers whose laryngeal appearance improves, but incompletely, on PPIs.

More recently, in treating patients with laryngopharyngeal reflux, PPIs have been combined with an $H_2$ blocker at bedtime, for reasons discussed below. Clearly, research into optimal treatment regimens is needed.

Baclofen relaxes skeletal muscle and is used primarily to treat spasticity. It is a GABA receptor agonist. Recently, it has been used effectively to treat reflux.[424] In 2012 Constantino et al[425] published the results of a randomized clinical trial that showed that baclofen was associated with a significant decrease in upright reflux. Upright reflux is common in patients with LPR. Abasinazari et al compared omeprazole with a combination of omeprazole and sustained-release baclofen (SR baclofen) and demonstrated that the combination therapy works better than omeprazole alone for treatment of regurgitation and heartburn (although they used only 20 mg per day of omeprazole in both arms of the study).[426] Scarpellini et al showed that baclofen does not alter the intragastric acid pocket but limits its extension into the esophagus by an increase in postprandial LES pressure.[427] In 2014, a meta-analysis found that there was good evidence to suggest that baclofen is useful for treatment of reflux, but the authors recommended a large, well-designed study.[428] Baclofen has been shown to be effective in the treatment of children with refractory reflux.[429] It may also be helpful for treatment of chronic cough,[430,431] ruminaton, and supragastric belching/aerophagia,[432] and reflux-induced sleep disturbances.[433] Baclofen comes as 10 mg and 20 mg pills. It is given in divided doses (3 times daily or 4 times daily), and daily total doses range from 20 to 80 mg per day. It can be started at 5 mg 3 times daily and increased by 15 mg per day every 3 days. When discountinued, the dose should be tapered gradually, not stopped abruptly.

## $H_2$-Receptor Antagonists

Since their introduction in the late 1970s, $H_2$-receptor antagonists have been the mainstay of the treatment of GERD. The only mechanism of action of these drugs is to inhibit gastric acid secretion; they have no effect on LES pressure or esophageal clearance. The 4 $H_2$ blockers (cimetidine, ranitidine, famotidine, and nizatidine) are equal in efficacy when used in equivalent doses. These agents are extremely well tolerated in all age groups and have been shown to relieve heartburn completely in 60% of patients treated.[434] Healing of mucosal abnormalities in the esophagus is less frequent and often overestimated, being seen in 0 to 82% (mean = 48%) of patients.[435] The best results are seen in patients with nonerosive esophagitis where success rates are as high as 75%.[436,437] Higher doses of $H_2$ antagonists, up to 4 times daily, are usually needed to treat erosive esophagitis;[437] however, the cost of this double-dose therapy is greater and therapy is not as clinically effective as using a single daily dose of PPIs. Maintenance of heartburn relief and healing of esophageal mucosal injury is seen in only 25 to 50% of patients treated with continuous therapy of traditional doses of $H_2$-antagonists (eg, ranitidine 150 mg twice daily) for 1 year.[437]

$H_2$-receptor antagonists are remarkably safe agents. Side effects are rarely seen with greater frequency than placebo in clinical trials. Rare cases of hepatitis, qualitative platelet defects, and mental confusion with intravenous administration have been reported. Drug interactions are extremely rare, although they seem to be slightly more prevalent with cimetidine. Caution should be exercised in patients on Dilantin, warfarin, and theophylline, although clinically problems are rare.[435]

Cimetidine has also been associated with male infertility. Although the cause-and-effect relationship has not been proven, impotence and gynecomastia have also been reported as possible complications. An uncontrolled study by Van Thiel et al[438] reported that the concentration of sperm in 7 males was reduced during treatment with cimetidine (Tagamet) 300 mg qid for 9 weeks. In only one patient did the count fall below the lower limit of normal of 50 000 000/mL (ie, 45 000 000/mL). After the treatment period, the concentrations returned to pretreatment levels. In contrast, a controlled double-blind study by Enzmann et al[439] on spermatogenesis in 30 normal males who received cimetidine (300 mg qid or 400 mg hs) or placebo for 6 months did not demonstrate any effects of cimetidine on spermatogenesis, sperm count, sperm motility and morphology, or on fertilizing capacity in vitro; and the blood levels of androgen and gonadotropin were unchanged in this study population.

Carlson et al[440] studied the endocrine effects of cimetidine after acute and chronic administration in both men and women. These investigators noted the rise in prolactin levels after the acute intravenous administration of cimetidine (Tagamet). However, no acute change in the prolactin levels was noted after oral administration (300 mg cimetidine) or intravenous injection (50 mg cimetidine). The patients taking cimetidine on a chronic oral basis experienced no significant changes in serum prolactin, testosterone, free testosterone, estradiol, LH (leuteinizing hormone), or FSH (follicle stimulating hormone). The authors concluded that it is likely that the impotence and breast changes occasionally seen during cimetidine therapy are due to peripheral antagonism of androgen action rather than to alterations in circulating hormone levels.

Winters et al[441] analyzed the effects of cimetidine on androgen binding to the human prostate, testes, and semen. They found that cimetidine competed for dihydrotestosterone (DHT) binding sites in the human prostate and no apparent binding to the testes or semen. In agreement with Carlson et al, these authors postulate that androgen antagonism may be the mechanism of the endocrine side effects of cimetidine in men.

Jensen and coworkers[442] studied the use of cimetidine to determine the long-term efficacy of medical management in 22 patients with gastric hypersecretory states (20 patients had Zollinger-Ellison syndrome and 2 had idiopathic hypersecretions). Of the 22 patients followed, 11 reported impotence, breast tenderness, gynecomastia, or some combination of these symptoms. The remaining 11 patients were asymptomatic. The mean dose of cimetidine in the patients with impotence or breast changes tended to be higher than those in patients without these side effects ($5.3 \pm 3.5$ vs $3 \pm 1.3$ grams per day). This dosage is more than 4 times that used in the therapy of uncomplicated gastric or duodenal ulcers where impotence and gynecomastia have been reported extremely rarely.

Malagelada et al[443] also studied the long-term use of cimetidine in 18 patients with Zollinger-Ellison syndrome. The patients received an average cimetidine dose of 2 g/day and were followed for an average of 28.9 months (range: 7–59 months). Unlike Jensen's findings, none of these patients presented with major side effects. There were no reports of impotence among this group; however, one patient developed tender gynecomastia.

These problems have not been reported prominently with other $H_2$ antagonists (which have not been studied as extensively), but complications can occur with all of the medications in this class, and physicians should be familiar with them. It is also helpful to warn patients that $H_2$ receptor antagonists may result in increased blood alcohol levels and functional impairments after consumption of amounts of alcohol that would be considered safe in the absence of $H_2$ receptor antagonist therapy. This problem is particularly prominent with cimetidine.[444]

There are few trials in which $H_2$-receptor antagonists have been evaluated systematically in the treatment of extraesophageal GERD; and all of the reported trials have been in patients with either asthma or chronic cough. The largest study by Larrain et al[65] randomized patients to placebo, cimetidine 300 mg 4 times a day, or antireflux surgery in a 6-month treatment trial. Most of the patients had mild GERD. Before treatment, heartburn was seen less than once a week in all patients, and 66% had no evidence of esophagitis by endoscopic examination. All patients had abnormal esophageal acid exposure during prolonged pH monitoring. Both pulmonary and esophageal symptoms were improved in the cimetidine and surgery groups compared to placebo. However, the response to surgical therapy was statistically superior to medical therapy. Response was slower in patients with extraesophageal reflux than in typical patients with heartburn, with many patients achieving optimal response only after 4 to 6 months of treatment.[66]

Another study comparing ranitidine, 150 mg 3 times daily, with antireflux surgery showed a statistical advantage for antireflux surgery.[443] These studies reinforce that the superior control of esophageal acid exposure seen after antireflux surgery compared to that of $H_2$ blockers may be needed for optimal relief of pulmonary (and other extraesophageal) symptoms. Several other short-term studies using $H_2$-receptor antagonists in doses from 150 mg ranitidine at bedtime up to 150 mg 3 times a day for periods of 1 to 8 weeks have consistently demonstrated improvement in heartburn. However, they demonstrate limited improvement in objective changes of pulmonary function and symptoms at the end of these 8-week trials.[445–448] Improvements in respiratory symptoms, if they occurred, lagged weeks behind esophageal symptoms. Clinical experience confirms these findings.

Cimetidine has been used successfully in unblinded and uncontrolled trials of patients with chronic cough associated with GERD. Improvement of cough has been reported in 70% to 100%.[449–452] Time to symptom improvement was quite prolonged, usually about 161 to 179 days. Patients with heartburn as the primary GERD symptom usually improved in 1 to 3 weeks. Despite reports of clinical improvement, no correlation was seen between clinical response and reduction in esophageal acid exposure by prolonged pH monitoring, which was performed at the end of the study. Although they were used extensively before the introduction of PPIs, there are no definitive studies in which $H_2$-receptor antagonists have been used to treat LPR. Currently we use them in patients who are unable to tolerate PPIs, and in those who have symptoms from nocturnal acid secretion despite the use of PPIs. If they are to be used, high-dose therapy is required, using as a minimum the equivalent dose of ranitidine, 150 mg 4 times a day (Table 11–8).

### Prokinetic Agents

Drugs that increase LES pressure and accelerate esophageal clearance and gastric emptying are ideal agents to "correct" one of the pathogenic problems underlying GERD. Unfortunately, the results seen with the 2 most commonly prescribed prokinetic agents, metoclopramide and cisapride, have been somewhat disappointing in treating GERD. Equal efficacy is seen with either agent. Heartburn relief can be achieved with cisapride in close to 60% of

patients when 10 mg is given 4 times a day and is equal in efficacy compared with $H_2$-receptor antagonists.[453] Studies suggest that comparable heartburn relief can be achieved with 20 mg twice a day, a dose that will increase compliance.[454] Cisapride has been withdrawn from the US market because of concerns over cardiac side effects. Limited access through the manufacturer is still possible but difficult.

The central nervous system side effects of metoclopramide (drowsiness, irritability, extrapyramidal effects) make its use problematic, particularly in the elderly and in voice professionals. Because cisapride does not cross the blood-brain barrier, these side effects are not seen, so it has largely replaced metoclopramide as the prokinetic agent of choice. The major side effects of cisapride are diarrhea (about 10%) and nausea. Prolongation of the QT interval and development of ventricular arrhythmias may be seen in patients on cisapride who are treated concomitantly with macrolide antibiotics (eg, erythromycin) or antifungal agents.[455] Use of these drugs in combination

**Table 11–8.** Standard Medical Therapy for Gastroesophageal Reflux

| Agents | Dosage |
| --- | --- |
| **Promotility agents** | |
| Metoclopramide | 5–10 mg 4 times a day |
| Cisapride | 10 mg 4 times a day (available only for "Compassionate use" |
| **Acid suppressive agents** | |
| $H_2$-receptor antagonists[a] | |
| Cimetidine | 400 mg 2 times a day (nonerosive symptomatic disease) |
| | 800 mg 2 times a day (erosive esophagitis) |
| Ranitidine | 150 mg 4 times a day (nonerosive symptomatic disease) |
| | 150 mg 4 times a day (erosive esophagitis) |
| Famotidine | 20 mg 2 times a day (nonerosive symptomatic disease) |
| | 40 mg 2 times a day (erosive esophagitis) |
| Nizatidine | 150 mg 2 times a day (all forms of reflux disease) |
| **Proton pump inhibitors[b]** | |
| Omeprazole | 20 mg a day (AM) acute maintenance therapy |
| Lansoprazole | 30 mg a day (acute) |
| | 15 mg a day (maintenance) |
| Pantoprazole | 40 mg a day (acute and maintenance) |
| Esomeprazole | 20–40 mg once a day (healing) |
| Rabeprazole | 20 mg a day (acute and maintenance) |

[a]Also available over-the-counter in reduced dose for medication as needed.
[b]Higher doses are required for treatment of extraesophageal disease. See text.

should be avoided. Metoclopramide is available in the United States for routine use.

Cisapride's major use was in patients with mild or nonerosive esophagitis who have nocturnal heartburn. Superior symptom relief and healing in combination with $H_2$-receptor antagonists are seen when compared to either drug alone. However, cost and compliance issues with this combination offer no advantage over PPIs.

Prokinetic agents have been used alone or in combination therapy with $H_2$ antagonists for treatment of cough, predominantly in children, but they have not been extensively studied in the treatment of cough-related asthma and/or LPR. Improvement in cough was seen in 64.5 to 100% of patients in two uncontrolled studies.[456–459] Cisapride was studied in 22 infants aged 4 to 26 weeks with abnormal sleep patterns characterized by apneic episodes and associated GERD by pH monitoring,[456] as well as in a group of 19 children aged 3 months to 10 years (mean: 7 years) with either nocturnal cough, wheezing, or bronchitis, all of whom also had GERD by pH monitoring.[456] Apnea, night cough, and asthma symptoms were improved in 70% to 90%. Objectively, GERD was decreased by pH monitoring after treatment. A third study evaluating the use of cisapride in 27 children (mean age 6 years) with refractory asthma and GERD confirmed by pH monitoring reported partial or complete improvement in respiratory symptoms in 80% after 3 months of treatment.[460]

A recent preliminary study by Khoury et al,[461] a double-blind controlled trial in 16 adult patients with pulmonary symptoms and GERD documented by ambulatory pH monitoring, compared cisapride, 10 mg 4 times a day, with placebo and showed significant improvement in FEV1 and FVC in patients on cisapride compared to placebo. No improvement in objective assessment of esophageal acid exposure by ambulatory pH monitoring or in esophageal symptoms could be documented. Prokinetic agents have not been studied for efficacy in patients with LPR.[462]

## Proton Pump Inhibitors Are the Most Effective Nonsurgical Treatment for GERD

Treatment of GERD with extraesophageal manifestations, including LPR, remains a topic of much debate. However, otolaryngologists and laryngologists prescribe PPI therapy, often in combination with an $H_2$ antagonist (typically before bedtime), but the daily dosages of PPIs prescribed vary among treating physicians.[463,464]

Proton pump inhibitors (omeprazole, lansoprazole, rabeprazole, pantoprazole, and esomeprazole)

inhibit the H+K+ATPase enzyme that catalyzes the terminal step of acid secretion in the parietal cells. Profound acid inhibition is possible with these agents, resulting in improved symptom relief and healing of erosive disease. Several studies have shown increasing evidence that PPI treatment is effective in controlling the symptoms of LPR such as dysphonia and hoarseness.[465–473] A single daily dose of either omeprazole or rabeprazole will produce a 67 to 95% (mean 83%) rate of symptom relief and healing of erosive esophagitis.[463] A large trial comparing omeprazole 20 mg daily to lansoprazole 30 mg daily showed comparable healing rates of over 85% after 8 weeks of therapy.[465] Successful, complete symptom relief and healing of erosive esophagitis is seen in 85% of patients when continuous therapy is given over 1 year.[465] Continuous therapy is significantly superior to alternative day or weekend therapy and to $H_2$-receptor antagonists in the long-term treatment of GERD. Continuous therapy with omeprazole 20 to 60 mg a day has been shown to maintain complete symptom relief and healing for up to 5 years even in patients refractory to $H_2$ antagonists.[467] This study illustrates several key points: long-term remission is possible in up to 100% of patients if adequate doses of PPIs are used, up to 30% of patients refractory to $H_2$ antagonists will require either twice daily or more frequent dosing of PPIs, and most patients respond to stable doses of omeprazole long term without the development of tolerance. A preliminary report of continued follow-up of the same patient group shows continued success of omeprazole for 11 years. Relapse occurred in one patient per 9 years of treatment, with minimal side effects.[468]

Combination therapy with PPIs and prokinetics is used commonly in patients whose reflux is difficult to manage. Unfortunately, no studies have shown a statistical advantage for combination therapy compared to increasing the dose of PPIs. Proton pump inhibitors appear to have their best effect when given before a meal; if more than a single dose is required, they should be given in divided doses twice daily before breakfast and dinner,[471] or more frequently. Omission of breakfast will reduce the efficacy of the PPIs.[470] If PPIs are used in combination with antacids, the medications should be separated by about an hour with the antacids being taken about one-half hour after meals. If an $H_2$ antagonist is added, it should be given at bedtime. Recent data suggest that combining a PPI twice daily with an $H_2$ antagonist at bedtime may be particularly helpful. Peghini et al demonstrated nocturnal gastric acid breakthrough between 2 AM and 5 AM in a majority of patients and normal volunteers taking PPI twice daily.[471] In a follow-up study, Peghini et al suggested that this nocturnal acid breakthrough is histamine related, and they demonstrated that an $H_2$ blocker (ranitidine 300 mg) at bedtime is more effective than bedtime omeprazole for controlling residual nocturnal acid secretion.[472]

There are clinical situations in which difficulty swallowing mandates alternative methods of administrating proton pump inhibitors. Multiple studies with omeprazole and two studies with lansoprazole have shown that these proton pump inhibitors can be given to patients who are unable to ingest intact capsules by opening the capsule and mixing the intact granules with water, preparing a bicarbonate-based suspension, administering the capsules in apple or orange juice, or sprinkling the granules on applesauce or yogurt. The capsules should not be crushed.[473] Adequate control of intragastric pH has been demonstrated when omeprazole suspension is given via percutaneous gastrostomy, jejunostomy, or nasogastric tube. This is particularly useful in postoperative patients prone to aspiration, patients at risk for stress ulceration, or the patient on chronic enteral feeding via gastrostomy tube.

Since omeprazole and lansoprazole were introduced, additional PPIs have become available. Rabeprazole, pantoprazole, and esomeprazole have slightly different pharmaconetic profiles, and they have been studied less extensively than omeprazole and lansoprazole, but all 5 PPIs appear effective for GERD and probably for LPR. Omeprazole has been studied for treatment of posterior laryngitis and was found to improve symptoms and signs of LPR.[474] It is important to recognize that symptoms improve before signs in most cases. A recent study by Belafsky et al[475] supports this common clinical observation. They noted that symptoms improved maximally during the first 2 months of therapy, but laryngeal findings improved slightly during the first 2 months, and continued improving for at least the first 6 months of therapy.

Proton pump inhibitors have an excellent safety profile with no side effects greater than placebo seen in clinical trials. The major side effects, headache and diarrhea, are quite rare. There has been concern about long-term safety of PPIs because of their profound acid suppression. Current evidence suggests this fear is unjustified, as ample gastric acid is produced in a 24-hour period to allow for normal protein digestion, iron and calcium absorption, and to prevent bacterial overgrowth and maintain $B_{12}$ absorption. The most important concern with long-term use of PPIs is hyperplasia of enterochromaffin-like (ECL) cells and development of gastric carcinoid tumors because of hypersecretion of gastrin. As of this writing, there have been no reports of gastric carcinoid or any gastric malignancy with up to 11 years of omeprazole.[468] Hyperplasia of ECL cells is seen in 4% or less of patients on PPIs. A recent study suggested that patients on long-term omeprazole who were infected with H pylori developed atrophic gastritis (a proposed precursor of gastric adenocarcinoma) at a more rapid rate than patients who were not infected, prompting these authors to recommend screening and treatment of H pylori in patients on long-term proton pump inhibitors.[476] A US Food and Drug Administration (FDA) panel determined that these data are insufficient to support this recommendation.[477] No specific laboratory monitoring—in particular serum gastrin—is required for patients on long-term PPIs.

Several clinical trials have been conducted using PPIs in patients with extraesophageal symptoms, principally asthma and LPR. All of the trials were conducted with omeprazole. Two short-term studies, one with omeprazole 20 mg once a day for 4 weeks[478] and the other with 20 mg twice daily for 6 weeks, showed an improvement in pulmonary function tests on omeprazole compared to placebo. However, little change in bronchodilator use or asthma scores could be demonstrated. A longer trial by Boeree et al,[479] a randomized double-blind controlled trial in 36 patients comparing omeprazole 40 mg twice daily to placebo for 3 months, showed a reduction in nocturnal cough during treatment with omeprazole compared to placebo. However, objective changes in FEV1 and other pulmonary function tests were not seen. The study by Meier et al[480] using omeprazole 20 mg twice daily found that 6 of 11 patients who failed to improve on omeprazole also did not heal their esophagitis. This suggests that acid suppression was inadequate in these patients. The patients who did have control of their asthma also had healed their esophagitis, reinforcing the fact that adequate acid control can relieve pulmonary symptoms.

Important insights into the treatment of patients with extraesophageal GERD come from a well-designed study by Harding et al[57] in which 30 patients with documented asthma and proven GERD by prolonged pH monitoring were treated with increasing doses of omeprazole beginning with 20 mg a day, increasing by 20 mg daily after every 8 weeks of treatment for 3 months or until esophageal acid exposure was reduced to "normal." Normalization of esophageal acid exposure resulted in improvement in pulmonary symptoms in 70% of patients. There are several important observations from this trial: 8 of 30 patients (28%) required more than 20 mg of omeprazole daily to normalize esophageal acid exposure; many patients required the entire 3-month period of treatment to achieve optimal symptom relief with improvement progressing continuously over the 3-month period; a favorable response to omeprazole was seen in patients who presented with frequent regurgitation (more often than once a week) and/or abnormal proximal acid exposure demonstrated by ambulatory pH monitoring (see Reflux Laryngitis and Other Otolaryngologic Manifestations of Laryngopharyngeal Reflux). The study emphasizes the importance of adequate esophageal acid control to achieve improvement in patients with extraesophageal symptoms. Complete elimination of esophageal acid exposure is often necessary in patients with extraesophageal disease (including LPR) to effectively relieve symptoms. The author (DOC) requires that esophageal pH be greater than 4 for 99% of the time during prolonged pH monitoring while on proton pump inhibitor therapy before accepting that acid suppression is optimal. In selected cases, even that is not adequate in patients with LPR if the 1% period of reflux includes proximal acid exposure with persistent laryngeal symptoms and signs.

Hanson et al evaluated 16 patients with posterior laryngitis (LPR) who had failed to respond to initial treatment with conservative, lifestyle measures for a 6-week period, with omeprazole 40 mg daily for at least 6 weeks.[481] Laryngeal and esophageal symptom scores improved significantly at the end of 6 weeks compared to pre-omeprazole scores. Objective improvement compared to pretreatment values was also seen when the larynx was evaluated by a blinded investigator using videolaryngoscopy. Six patients had improvement in their laryngoscopic scores but not in laryngeal symptom scores. Symptoms relapsed within 6 weeks in all patients after therapy was stopped. Poorer response was seen in patients with abnormal proximal esophageal acid exposure on ambulatory pH monitoring. It is reasonable to speculate that 40 mg a day of omeprazole was inadequate therapy for these patients and that they might have responded to higher doses or to a regimen combining other medications.

The same authors studied 182 patients with posterior laryngitis and at least one of the following symptoms: postnasal drip, persistent or recurrent sore throat, cough, or hoarseness.[481] Patients were treated sequentially with conservative lifestyle modifications for an initial period of 6 to 12 weeks followed by famotidine 20 mg at bedtime for 6 weeks. Omeprazole 20 mg at bedtime was given to nonresponders. Omeprazole was then increased in 20 mg increments every 6 weeks until 80 mg a day was reached. Laryn-

gitis was characterized as mild if posterior laryngeal erythema was seen; moderate if marked erythema, secretions, and mucosal granularity were present; and severe if ulceration, granulation tissue, or hyperkeratosis were seen. Patients with mild symptoms and minimal laryngeal changes responded to conservative doses of famotidine, whereas patients with severe laryngitis required PPIs.[481] These studies emphasize variability in response of patients with LPR, the need to treat for longer periods before seeing a response when disease is severe, the need for higher doses of PPIs, and the rapid relapse of symptoms when therapy is discontinued, emphasizing that long-term treatment is often needed in patients with LPR.

Wo et al[482] studied 22 patients with posterior laryngitis felt to be secondary to GERD and diagnosed by indirect laryngoscopy, using an 8-week trial of omeprazole 40 mg at bedtime. Laryngeal symptoms improved in 67% of these patients. Increasing omeprazole to 40 mg twice a day in nonresponders did not improve response. Relapse was seen in 40% when omeprazole was stopped. There were no predictors of response, although nocturnal symptoms were more common in nonresponders. Perhaps this group had nocturnal acid breakthrough and continued to reflux despite high-dose PPI therapy. It is likely that results would have been improved if omeprazole were given twice daily (before breakfast and dinner), a treatment regimen that produces superior acid suppression to other modes of administration of this drug. The response rate to omeprazole in this trial does, however, support empiric therapy for LPR.

Metz and colleagues[483] studied 10 patients with laryngitis documented by endoscopy who also had GERD diagnosed by abnormal ambulatory pH monitoring. They used 40 mg omeprazole as a single daily dose and found improvement in 7 of 10 (70%) patients at the end of 8 weeks. Jaspersen and colleagues studied 34 patients with laryngeal symptoms, laryngoscopic changes of LPR and erosive esophagitis treated with omeprazole 20 mg a day for 4 weeks, reporting improvement in esophagitis and laryngeal symptoms in 32 of 34 patients (92%).[484] No comment was made about laryngeal examinations. These studies were uncontrolled but showed excellent results with omeprazole. Although lansoprazole has not been studied in this patient population, comparable healing rates for omeprazole 20 mg and lansoprazole 30 mg a day, respectively, are seen in erosive esophagitis,[484] suggesting that this PPI should be equally effective in patients with LPR and other extraesophageal disease.

El-Serag and colleagues performed a randomized controlled trial in 20 patients with LPR comparing lansoprazole 30 mg bid to placebo.[485] After 16 weeks, 50% of the treated patients had complete relief of LPR symptoms compared to 10% with placebo. Laryngeal findings were not highlighted.

Clinicians must be cognizant of the fact that PPI therapy is not universally effective. Failure rates are high in patients receiving a PPI only once daily.[486] In addition, a morning dose of omeprazole has been shown to last an average of only 13.8 hours.[487] The problem of nocturnal acid breakthrough has been discussed above and may be viewed as effectively limiting the duration of the evening dose of PPI to a period of 7½ hours.[488] In addition, a few patients produce substantial (or normal) acid levels even when receiving high doses of PPIs. Amin et al[486] studied LPR patients receiving PPIs up to 4 times a day and reported a medical treatment failure rate of 10%. At the author's (RTS) voice center,[488] we evaluated the use of super high-dose PPI administration in a group of patients that appeared refractory to standard twice daily PPI dosing in controlling their LPR. A restrospective review of 35 medical records of patients (ages 20–76 years) who were treated with high-dose PPI therapy was conducted. Three blinded raters compared RSS scores and 24-hour pH impedance scores on standard and super high-dose PPI therapy. RSS scores revealed some improvement in reports of laryngeal symptom pathology, with the most significant changes noted on standard high-dose therapy. The authors concluded that neither RSS nor 24-hour impedance scores appeared to be sufficient enough to detect improvement in LPR with these results, given a relatively small sample population. Lee et al examined the effects of PPI therapy for LPR related to age.[489] They conducted a prospective study at 3 medical centers of 264 patients diagnosed with LPR between 2010 and 2012. Thirty-five patients were lost to follow-up, so results are reported on 135 males and 94 females. The patients were grouped according to age. There were 111 patients in the oldest group (ages 60–79); 83 patients aged 40 to 59 years; and 35 patients aged 18 to 39 years. All patients receive lansoprazole 15 mg twice daily for 3 months. RSI, RSS, and LPR-HRQLL (health-related quality of life) data were recorded pretreatment, at 1 month on treatment and at 3 months post-PPI treatment. Based on the scores at all 3 intervals, the older patients' results reflected less response to PPI therapy in regard to their symptoms and quality of life as compared to the younger patients.

A prospective, placebo-controlled study of PPI therapy for patients with LPR was published by El-Serag et al[490] in which 22 patients from a Veteran's Administration hospital population were treated with lansoprazole 30 mg twice daily or placebo for 3 months. Subjects underwent esophagoscopy, 24-hour pH monitor studies, and indirect laryngoscopy using a laryngeal telescope. The lower sensor was 5 cm above the LES, and the sensors were separated by 15 cm. Their primary outcome criterion was complete resolution of laryngeal symptoms. Of the 20 patients (out of 22) who finished the study and had all information available, 11 received lansoprazole and 9 received placebo. Seven patients were complete responders, 6 of whom received lansoprazole and 1 of whom received placebo. The difference was statistically significant. At the end of this study, 58% of the patients treated with lansoprazole had complete ($n = 2$) or partial ($n = 5$) resolution of laryngeal signs of reflux (posterior laryngitis), and 30% of the placebo-treated group had partial resolution of laryngeal signs (none had complete resolution). The authors concluded that lansoprazole is effective in the treatment of LPR. The study was well designed, but the population was fairly small, and a VA hospital population is not necessarily comparable with the general population (21/22 subjects were male; mean age was 59 years in the lansoprazole group and 65 years in the placebo group).

In 2001, Noordzij et al[491] reported on 53 patients with reflux laryngitis. Of these, 30 subjects were enrolled, who had more than 4 episodes of proximal reflux during their 24-hour monitor study. Fifteen received omeprazole 40 mg twice daily, and the other 15 received placebo. The study lasted for 2 months. They assessed symptoms and laryngeal signs of LPR. During 24-hour pH monitor studies, the upper sensor was placed under flexible laryngoscopic guidance 1 cm above the UES, and the distal sensor was 18 cm from the proximal sensor. The patients were instructed to avoid behavioral activities known to have an effect on gastroesophageal reflux. The mean age (years) in the treatment group was 51.7 and in the placebo group, 45.3. Subjects were fairly evenly divided by gender. There were large differences in initial symptom severity between the omeprazole and placebo groups for some symptoms. The authors reported that most symptom scores improved for both groups, although mild hoarseness and throat clearing may be treated effectively by omeprazole, but they also concluded that there was a placebo effect. It is interesting that laryngoscopic findings showed no improvement in either group. Although complete resolution of laryngeal signs commonly takes many months, improvement in erythema usually is seen in less than 2 months, and improvements in edema often are seen during this time, as well. Their results may have been due to the fact that abnormalities in laryngeal signs were very mild in the entire study population (in blind subjective assessments, the 5 laryngeal signs were all rated in the 0–1 range). Hence, very little change in laryngeal findings could be expected. Findings might be different in a population with more severe disease.

In 2003, Eherer et al[492] reported a placebo-controlled, double-blind crossover study of the effects of pantoprazole on LPR. They assessed 62 patients. Twenty-four showed reflux on 24-hour pH monitoring, and 21 were entered into the study. The proximal sensor was located 1 to 3 cm above the UES, and the distal sensor was placed 15, 18, or 21 cm below the upper sensor. Studies monitoring pH were performed for each subject prior to entry into the study and between its 3-month arms. The requirement for 2 pH monitoring studies, and the duration of the study (>6 months) may be responsible for the fact that only 14 patients completed all portions of the research protocol. All subjects were nonsmokers. However, the methodology makes no mention of preventing patients from adopting behavioral changes that might have contributed to improvements in both groups. The authors reported that both pantoprazole and placebo were associated with "marked improvement" in laryngitis scores and that there was no significant difference between the 2 groups after 3 months. After a 2-week washout period, a second pH monitoring study confirmed persistence of reflux in most subjects. Switching the placebo group to pantoprazole resulted in further improvement of laryngitis scores. In the pantoprazole group switched to placebo, a minority of patients had recurrence of symptoms and signs. Changes in symptom scores were not significantly different between the 2 groups. After reversal of treatments, there was also no significant change in symptoms, although one patient who switched from pantoprazole to placebo had a severe recurrence of symptoms. Like the study by Noordzij et al,[491] these results are somewhat difficult to interpret because of the fairly mild severity of LPR in both groups. For example, the maximum possible score for esophageal symptoms was 48 (the higher, the worse). The esophageal score prior to treatment in the placebo/pantoprazole group was 11, and in the pantoprazole/placebo group 3.3.

Similarly, the maximum laryngeal symptom score was 72. The pretreatment placebo/pantoprazole score was 17.4, and the pantoprazole/placebo score was 14.6. Hence, there was not much room for improvement, and these patients had mild disease, in which spontaneous fluctuations in severity are common. This problem, combined with the small number of subjects, raises questions about the conclusions of this otherwise well-designed study from which the authors deduced that pantoprazole may be helpful in relieving acute symptoms but that the advantage of long-term treatment has been overestimated. Substantially larger numbers and inclusion of patients with long-term, moderate-to-severe symptoms and signs will be needed to assess these concerns definitively.

Other recent studies of LPR also have failed to provide incontestable answers to questions about diagnostic accuracy and treatment efficiency.[493,494]

Bruley des Varannes et al[495] reported that the superiority of PPIs over other drugs has been well established for both short- and long-term treatment of GERD. Patients with erosive esophagitis are more responsive to PPIs than patients with nonerosive reflux disease. PPIs also have become widely used and have been proven to be safe and effective in the management of GERD in children, although to date, only omeprazole, lansoprazole, and esomeprazole are approvd for use in children.[496,497]

A randomized placebo-controlled study revealed improved LPR symptoms compared with placebo after 12 weeks of treatment with rabeprazole 20 mg twice daily.[498] The authors reported a relapse of symptoms 6 weeks after stopping PPI therapy, suggesting that LPR requires longer duration of treatment. Many clinicians still advocate the use of empiric therapy with twice-daily PPI dosing for 6 to 12 weeks (on average) as a diagnostic tool in patients with suspected LPR.[499,500] However, we believe that this is not an adequate approach, particularly for nonresponders, as some patients may produce acid even when taking 2 or more PPIs daily. Monitoring of pH while on medications is invaluable in detecting these patients, and for many patients, PPI treatment must be continued indefinitely.

Dadabhai and Friedenberg[501] reported that rabeprazole has a faster onset of action in comparison with other PPIs. They cited rabeprazole's high pKa of 5, which facilitates activation at a higher pH, as a possible reason for its faster onset. They described rabeprazole's pathway of metabolism as nonenzymatic, thus making it less affected by the genetic polymorphisms of the CYP2C19 on which the other PPIs depend.

In 2010, Fass et al[502] reported the results of a randomized, placebo-controlled study that evaluated the effectiveness of esomeprazole twice daily in their patients with LPR, all of whom had undergone endoscopy and pH monitor testing. Following the 3-month trial, the results revealed no significant difference in videostroboscopic reflux finding score and no significant difference in acoustic measures after treatment, comparing the esomeprazole group and the placebo group. The patients completed a voice use and quality diary and a symptom diary pretreatment and at the end of the study, and no significant differences were found in these between the 2 groups.

Recognizing that PPI therapy is not universally effective, caution must be exercised in interpretation of available literature. An insightful analysis Lby Johnston et al[503] revealed that in a recent meta-analysis, all but 2 studies fell within a funnel plot. The only 2 that did not show PPI effect were flawed by publication bias. Meta-analyses commonly magnify inherent flaws in the included studies, and more rigorous studies need to be performed. A randomized, double-blind, placebo-controlled study[504] revealed improvement in reflux finding score and reflux symptom index after treatment with esomeprazole in both placebo and PPI groups for 6 weeks. However, diffuse laryngeal edema showed significantly greater improvement in the PPI group, and ventricular obliteration and laryngeal erythema trended toward greater improvement in the PPI group. Posterior laryngeal hypertrophy improved significantly in the PPI group only. Lifestyle modifications were not instituted, so improvement was probably from medical intervention. Whereas a placebo effect has been shown repeatedly, including in this study, improvements were greater in the PPI group in several parameters.

Belafsky et al[505] describe the presence of esophagopharyngeal reflux—as distinct from LPR—which should also be considered as a possible cause for treatment failures. This disorder is characterized by regurgitation of proximal esophageal contents into the laryngopharynx secondary to inadequate volume clearance and dysmotility, rather than acid and peptic injury. Further studies are needed to elucidate this process, as treatment with antireflux medications, prokinetics, dilatation, and diet modification ameliorate symptoms in 50% of affected individuals.[505] We also have noted substantial problems associated with intraesophageal (or esophagopharyngeal) reflux in some patients after fundoplication, as well as in other patients who have not undergone surgery.

## Side Effects of PPIs

Clinical experience suggests that most patients with LPR have chronic gastroesophageal reflux and require long-term medical therapy or antireflux surgery, or both. Of note, it is common for laryngeal reflux findings and symptoms to take longer to

resolve than esophageal symptoms. Also, symptoms often improve before clinical findings, which may take 6 months or longer to reverse.[506] Reichel et al[507] noted control of LPR symptoms on daily PPI after an average of 4 weeks when combined with lifestyle modifications. Resistant cases could be treated with twice-daily medication at higher doses. Improvement can be seen not only in symptoms and signs but also in objective assessments, such as acoustic parameters. Jin et al[508] reported that jitter, shimmer, and harmonic-to-noise ratio improved significantly after 1 to 2 months of treatment. The dose of PPIs and other medications and the decision to perform antireflux surgery should be individualized to maintain symptom relief and mucosal healing. Current evidence suggests that long-term medical therapy is safe and that tolerance or tachyphylaxis is extremely rare.

A recent review article[509] and editorial[510] (from which the following 9 paragraphs are adapted) highlight many of the potential problems encountered in patients who receive PPI treatment for many months or years. PPIs are fairly safe, especially compared with many other prescription drugs, but adverse effects occur and should be known to physicians who prescribe PPIs. In 2008, Davies et al[511] studied almost 12 000 patients treated with esomeprazole over an 8-month period, with an average treatment duration of 26 weeks. Only 119 events were reported as possibly related to the medication. The few serious adverse effects were hypersensitivity reactions, including 3 cases of angioedema and 2 cases of anaphylaxis that were possibly related to the medication. This study did not examine long-term effects of PPI treatment.

PPIs are designed to cause hypochlorhydria. Therefore, they may interfere with calcium absorption. Numerous studies have confirmed that PPIs impair calcium absorption, and perhaps the best-known study showed an association between PPI use and hip fracture. Interestingly, Yang's study[512] showed that with long-term PPI use, risk for hip fracture was greater in men than in women. It has been speculated that this was due to the fact that many women use calcium replacement after menopause, and most men do not. At present, many of us are counseling our patients on long-term PPIs to take calcium and vitamin D supplementation while more is being learned about this problem. Since then, there have been more than 30 studies investigating the effects of PPIs on bone density, and it is now uncertain that the risk exists. For example, data from the study of women's health across the nation (SWAN) was analyzed.[513] This was a multiethnic, multicenter, community-based cohort report related to menopause. The association of bone mineral density changes associated with PPI and $H_2$-antagonist users was examined. The subjects included 207 new users of PPIs, 185 new users of $H_2$-antagonists, and 1676 nonusers. Subjects were followed for a period of approximately 10 years, and their median age was 50. The results of the study showed no difference in annual measurements of bone mineral density changes in any of the 3 groups.

Calcium absorption is not the only potential nutritional problem associated with long-term PPI use. It is also possible that vitamin $B_{12}$ and iron levels may be affected in some patients taking PPIs for long periods of time.[514]

Diarrhea caused by *Clostridium difficile* has been associated with virtually all antibiotics. Recently, Aseeri et al[515] suggested that the use of PPIs may increase the risk for diarrhea under some circumstances. They felt that the inhibition of gastric acidity impaired the body's defenses against ingested bacteria. However, this study was performed in hospitalized patients, and the implications for the general healthy population remain uncertain. This is a problem that has not been encountered widely in outpatient clinical practice.

Similarly, there has been a suggestion that PPIs may be associated with an increased risk of community-acquired pneumonia. However, there are shortcomings in the papers that have studied this issue, and the conclusions of some of the studies suggesting an association remain controversial.

One of the most striking adverse effects described recently is the interaction between at least some PPIs and clopidogrel. Well-executed studies have pointed out that some PPIs reduce the biological action of clopidogrel, decreasing its effect and increasing the risk for serious cardiovascular problems, including myocardial infarction.[516,517] Clearly there is a problem with concomitant use of omeprazole and clopidogrel. This is of particular concern, not only because omeprazole is readily available over the counter, but also because many insurance companies require patients to use omeprazole (because it is inexpensive) before permitting use of a later-generation PPI. Interactions between other PPIs and clopidogrel remain under study.

Other potential adverse effects may be associated with long-term PPI use, including atrophic gastritis, possibly progressing to metaplasia and adenocarcinoma,[518] hypergastrinemia (an increase in circulating gastrin hormone that has been associated with the development of carcinoid tumors of the gastric mucosa in rats),[519] and other problems.

Potential side effects associated with PPI therapy include headache, diarrhea, and dyspepsia in less than 2% of users. Switching to another PPI can be considered if this occurs. Chapman et al reviewed complications of PPI treatment.[509] More recently, new discussions have been raised regarding associations with vitamin and mineral deficiencies, new data on infections including community-acquired pneumonia and *C difficile*, associations of PPI use with long bone fractures, and cardiovascular events in patients receiving concomitant therapy with clodipogrel (Plavix). Clopidogrel is a platelet activation inhibitor used as a "blood thinner" in many patients with cardiovascular disorders, often in association with aspirin. The FDA issued warnings regarding the potential for adverse cardiovascular events among clopidogrel users taking PPI therapy in 2009 and regarding the potential for wrist, hip, and spine fractures among PPI users in 2010. In late 2012, the FDA issued a class warning for *C difficile* infections.

In an editorial published in *ENT Journal*, the authors provided a summary review of adverse side effects associated with PPI use, widely prescribed in the United States.[510] They and others have cited the research of several reporters and their discussions. Further studies reported that chronic PPI use was associated with chronic and acute kidney disease and with interstitial nephritis.[520,521] The author reported that in 2011, the FDA issued a warning that prolonged use of PPIs may not be beneficial.[522] Cheungpasitporn et al[523] reported that meta-analysis of multiple observational studies revealed a 40% increased risk of low magnesium levels in patients using PPIs compared to participants not using PPIs. They also cited an increased incidence of *C difficile* infections; increased risk of bone fractures secondary to decreased calcium absorption and subsequent decrease in bone density; increased rates of pneumonia, and an increase in myocardial events in patients taking PPIs and clopidrogrel has been reported.[524–530]

In 2014, Shin et al[531] stated that recent reports have suggested that PPI therapy may worsen vitiligo, but the effects on the melanocytes are yet to be determined. They performed an in vivo study of the effects of PPIs on the melanogenesis. They examined zebra fish embryos to investigate the effects of PPIs on pigmentation. They measured TIR (tirosinate) activity and tirosinase-related protein-1 (PRP-1) by Western blot technique. The results suggested that functional inhibition of melanization may cause or aggravate vitiligo in predisposed patients on PPI therapy.

Two recent studies examined the association between PPI usage and the risk of myocardial infarction.[531,532]

Both studies' results showed that the data support an association of PPI use with the increased risk of myocardial infarction. Shah et al reported, however, that they did not find an associated risk of cardiovascular events with the use of $H_2$-blockers.[531] Chia-Jen et al pointed out that despite the increased risk of myocardial infarction, the benefits of PPIs "may outweigh the risk of adverse cardiovascular effects, with the number needed to detect harm of 400 per 1357" in their study.[533] Their study utilized the propensity score-matching analysis and a second using case-crossover analysis that included 126 367 PPI users and 126 367 propensity score match for PPI nonusers.

Two recent reviews demonstrated evidence that PPI therapy reduces the absorption of protein-bound vitamin $B_{12}$, but did not generate enough clinical evidence to document $B_{12}$ deficiency in chronic PPI users or the need to check $B_{12}$ levels. Recent studies have suggested that in elderly, institutionalized, long-term PPI users, $B_{12}$ deficiency is more likely to develop and should be considered.[513] Researchers at Kaiser Permanente in Oakland, California, performed a case-control study over a period of 14 years to see if there is an association between vitamin D deficiency and use of acid-suppressing drugs, and reported that both PPIs and $H_2$-receptor antagonists may lead to malabsorption of vitamin $B_{12}$ due to suppression of gastric acid.[514]

Gastric acid is needed to allow absorption of non-heme iron and enhance iron salt dissociation from ingested food. Iron deficiency anemia has been reported in patients with atrophic gastritis, gastric resection, or vagotomy. To date, no data are available demonstrating the development of iron deficiency anemia in normal subjects on PPI therapy.

By their effects in increasing gastric pH levels, PPIs may encourage growth of gut microflora and increase susceptibility to organisms such as *Salmonella, Campylobacter jejuni, Escherichia coli, C difficile, Vibrio cholera,* and *Listeria*. An increased susceptibility in PPI users for *Salmonella, Campylobacter,* and *C difficile* infections was found in a systematic review.[524,525] Current recommendations are to carefully evaluate the need for PPI therapy in hospitalized patients who need intravenous antibiotics to reduce risk for *C difficile*.

An increased risk for community-acquired pneumonia is difficult to demonstrate in association with PPI therapy. A meta-analysis showed that the overall risk for pneumonia was higher among users of PPIs. If only randomized controlled trial data are analyzed, $H_2$-receptor antagonists rather than PPIs have been associated with an elevated risk for hospital-acquired pneumonia.[527] A more recent meta-analysis did find an increased risk for pneumonia associated with PPI use, but the results were confounded by methodologic issues. Paradoxically, short duration of use was associated with increased odds of community-acquired pneumonia but chronic use was not.[528] No definite recommendation can be given in this complex area.

Clinical studies in patients taking PPI therapy have shown mixed results regarding fracture. The study with the longest clinical follow-up matched cases with abnormal bone mineral density (osteoporosis) at the hip or lumbar vertebrae (T-score $\leq -2.5$) to controls with normal bone mineral density (T-score $\geq 1$). PPI use was not associated with having osteoporosis in either the hip or the lumbar spine for PPI use more than 1500 doses over the previous 5 years. In the longitudinal study, no significant decrease was observed in bone mineral density at either site attributable to PPI use. This suggests that the association between PPI use and hip fracture was probably related to factors independent of osteoporosis.[534]

In a recent meta-analysis, the pooled odds ratio (OR) for fracture was 1.29 (95% confidence interval [CI], 1.18–1.41) with PPIs and 1.10 (95% CI, 0.99–1.23) with $H_2$-receptor antagonist use compared with nonuse. Another study showed that the hip fracture risk among PPI users was seen only in persons with at least one other fracture-risk factor.[535] A meta-analysis covering 1 521 062 patients showed significant risk for spine fractures (OR, 1.50; 95% CI, 1.32–1.72; $p < .001$). For hip fractures, there was an increased risk for fractures with PPIs (OR, 1.23; 95% CI, 1.11–1.36; $p < .001$). Overall, an OR of 1.2 is seen for PPIs, and an OR of 1.08 is seen for $H_2$-receptor antagonists (95% CI, 1–1.18; $p + .06$). Again, short duration of PPI use may be associated with increased risk for developing hip fracture (OR, 1.24; 95% CI, 1.19–1.28), but not in long-term PPI users (OR, 1.3; 95% CI, 0.98–1.7).[536] No change in bone mineral density was seen in patients using PPIs continuously for 5 to 10 years in a Canadian study[537] despite the finding of a lower baseline bone mineral density in those same patients.

In 2009, the FDA issued a warning regarding the potential for increased adverse cardiovascular events in concomitant users of PPIs and clodipogrel, particularly users of omeprazole, lansoprazole, and esomeprazole. In vitro, the antiplatelet activity of clopidogrel requires activation by cytochrome (CY) P2C19, which is the same pathway through which PPIs are metabolized. Although overall studies have been conflicting, the newest data suggest that dexlansoprazole does not inhibit platelets in vitro to the same degree as do the 3 former PPIs. Pantoprazole appears to have less inhibition as well. A recent meta-analysis (23 studies) focused on primary myocardial infarction, stroke, stent occlusion, death, and secondary outcomes (rehospitalization for cardiac symptoms or revascularization procedures).[538] Outcomes from the 2 randomized controlled trials did not show an increased risk for adverse outcomes. Meta-analysis of primary and secondary outcomes showed an increased risk difference for all studies. Essentially, the risk for adverse cardiac outcomes was 0% based on data from well-controlled randomized trials.[539] Data from retrospective studies and the addition of probable vascular events slightly but significantly increased the risk estimates, likely due to lack of adjustment for potential co-founders. Recent consensus is that PPIs can be used with clopidogrel if they are clinically indicated.

The most comprehensive paper investigating the possible association of PPI use with the risk of dementia appeared in print during the week when final revisions on this chapter were completed. It is a large study that includes a comprehensive review of references on the subject. While the study does not provide definitive answers and contains weaknesses (many of which are acknowledged by the authors), Gomm et al provide data that raise serious questions about the possible association of PPI use and dementia,[540] and the study warrants increased consideration of this possible risk, as well as additional research. The study reviewed insurance data from 73 679 participants in the German health system. They were 75 years of age or older and free of dementia at the beginning of the study according to the records. The study revealed a significantly increased risk of incident dementia in patients receiving PPI medication, in comparison with those not receiving PPIs (hazard ratio of 1.44; $p < .001$). The risk was slightly higher in males than in females. Potential confounding factors were controlled as well as possible in a study of this design, and this included analysis of depression (the condition with the highest risk associated with incident dementia), age (also associated), diabetes, polypharmacy, and others. Use of anticholinergic medications (a known risk factor for dementia) also was considered. The 3 most common PPIs used were omeprazole, pantoprazole, and esomeprazole. The risk was slightly greater with esomeprazole than with the other 2 more common medications. Patients on rabprazole were included in the study, as well. The association between PPI use and dementia was clear, although causation could not be established in this study. The authors offered several speculations regarding mechanism. Lansoprazole and omeprazole cross the blood-brain barrier and have the potential to affect the brain directly. PPI use appears to increase beta-amyloid levels in the brain in mice, a substance associated with Alzheimer's disease, and it is possible that PPIs may alter degradation of brain substances, some of which is pH dependent. Unfortunately, the authors did not have information on vitamin $B_{12}$ levels in their cohort. Vitamin $B_{12}$ deficiency has been associated with PPI use and can cause dementia. If this is the primary mechanism, then it is possible that the dementia risk can be mitigated or eliminated by maintaining $B_{12}$ levels. However, substantial further research will be required to determine causation. The authors also mentioned that antihypertensive drugs such as calcium channel blockers and renin-angiotensin system blockers may prevent dementia, but there are no data on whether simultaneous use of these medications with PPIs would alter the dementia risk. Interestingly, Gomm et al also found that the risk of incident dementia associated with PPIs decreased gradually with age, with the highest risk occurring between 75 and 79 years of age. This is also true of potential confounding factors associated with dementia such as depression and stroke. Despite numerous strengths, the study was limited by the inability to completely rule out affects of confounding factors (eg, educational level and ApoE4 allele status were unknown). The authors also were unable to differentiate between different causes of dementia, such as vascular dementia vs Alzheimer's disease. In addition, although not mentioned in their article it is possible (unlikely) that there is an association between reflux and dementia (as opposed to between reflux treatment with PPIs and dementia). This could be studied by comparing a group of treated reflux patients with a group of untreated reflux patients, but such data were not available in Gomm's study and were also not available in any other research, so far. The statistical association between PPI use and the risk of dementia warrant further research and careful consideration of the risks of treatment with PPIs vs nontreatment in each individual patient. If it is shown eventually that there is a causal relationship between PPIs and dementia, then clearly alternative treatment approaches will need to be considered, possibly including increased referral for antireflux surgery to minimize or avoid use of all antireflux medication.

## Other Treatment Options

A novel approach to the treatment of pharyngolaryngeal reflux was introduced by Smoak and Koufman.[541] They studied the effects of chewing regular sugarless gum or sugarless gum containing bicarbonate on pharyngeal and esophageal pH. They demonstrated significant increases in mean pharyngeal and esophageal pH for both types of gum, but the improvements were more pronounced with sugarless gum containing bicarbonate. The beneficial effects of chewing bicarbonate gum lasted twice as long as the actual gum-chewing periods (25 minutes vs 49 minutes), and the beneficial effects of gum chewing were significantly greater than the buffering effect in control subjects obtained by eating a meal. In some patients, gum chewing completely abolished reflux episodes on 24-hour pH monitor study. Additional study is needed, but it appears as if gum chewing may be useful adjunctive antireflux therapy.

Durkes and Sivansakar[542] examined bicarbonate effects on vocal fold mucosal epithelium exposed to acid in 32 viable porcine vocal folds. Their findings suggest that bicarbonate has potential therapeutic effects in reducing acidic pH abnormalities associated with laryngeal pathology, including reflux, inflammation, and carcinogenesis.

Koufman has shown the potential value of using alkaline water.[543] Our experience suggests that this has value for some patients. She also has suggested using atomized alkaline water (pH 11) through a handheld sprayer as an inhalant (personal communication, 2015). Koufman has found that inhaling a topical spray of alkaline water resolves arytenoid erythema and improves symptoms of LPR, although formal confirmation by Koufman and others is pending.

### Helicobactor pylori

If a decision is made to treat *H pylori* after its presence has been proven, a combination of agents are used. Triple therapy with clarithromycin, metronidazole, and a PPI has been reported as efficacious, and there are few side effects.[544] At present, our therapy consists of a PPI twice daily, clarithromycin 500 mg twice daily and amoxicillin 1 g twice daily for 1 week.

## Surgical Therapy for Gastroesophageal Reflux Disease

Although comparison studies are inconclusive, it is likely that long-term medical therapy with PPIs and antireflux surgery are equal options for most patients with regard to acid injury, and the choice can be left to the patients in consultation with their treating physicians. Acid suppression does not always provide adequate control of symptoms in patients who note symptoms from suspected pH-neutral or alkaline reflux, especially singers; although this has not been

demonstrated by clinical trials, such patients may be considered for surgical therapy.[545–547]

The history of surgical therapy for the treatment of gastroesophageal reflux began with Phillip Allison who was the first to correlate the symptoms of hiatal hernia with gastroesophageal reflux.[548] His repair, described in 1951, emphasized the need to place the gastroesophageal junction intraabdominally to improve its function. This maneuver alone, however, was found to be associated with a high rate of symptom recurrence. More sophisticated attempts at securing the gastroesophageal junction below the diaphragm culminated with the posterior gastropexy described by Hill in 1967.[549] This operation is still in use, although it has largely been replaced by fundoplication.

Rudolph Nissen described his gastric fundic wrap in 1956.[550] His innovations were followed by a flurry of interest in surgical management for this disease. However, over the past 2 decades, surgical treatment for reflux has become much less commonly utilized, owing to the introduction of more effective medical therapy, specifically H$_2$ blockers and PPIs.

In 1991, the first reports of laparoscopic antireflux surgery (Nissen fundoplication) were published.[551] Minimally invasive approaches to this disease made operations more acceptable to gastroenterologists and patients, leading to a resurgence in interest for surgical correction of gastroesophageal reflux disease (GERD). Since the initial clinical reports in 1991, numerous studies have been published on the laparoscopic approach to antireflux surgery.[552–555]

Medical therapy is effective in controlling acid reflux in the majority of patients with GERD. However, while usually effective in controlling symptoms, medical therapy does not correct the mechanical abnormality that causes reflux. Patients often require long-term or indefinite courses of medications, as discontinuation frequently leads to recurrence of symptoms. In a series of 196 patients with severe esophagitis responsive to omeprazole, 82% developed recurrent erosions within 6 months after cessation of therapy.[185] Moreover, the consequences of long-term acid-suppression are unknown.

In 1992, Spechler[556] compared the outcome of medical vs surgical therapy for complicated GERD. Surgery was significantly more effective, resulting in greater patient satisfaction, higher lower esophageal sphincter (LES) pressures, lower grades of esophagitis, and lower levels of esophageal acid exposure. This study had an average 2-year follow-up, but was done without the use of PPIs.

However, in the follow-up study in 2001, Spechler et al found no significant long-term differences between the groups in terms of grade of esophagitis, frequency of treatment of esophageal stricture and subsequent antireflux operations, SF-36 standardized physical and mental component scale scores, and overall satisfaction with antireflux therapy.[557] They suggested that antireflux surgery should not be advised with the expectation that patients with GERD will no longer need to take antisecretory medications or that the procedure will prevent esophageal cancer among those with GERD and Barrett's esophagus. So et al compared laparoscopic fundoplication results in patients complaining of atypical symptoms with results in patients who had typical GERD symptoms (heartburn and regurgitation).[558] They found that postoperative relief of atypical symptoms was less satisfactory and more difficult to predict than relief of heartburn and regurgitation. The only predictors of relief of atypical symptoms were preoperative response to pharmacologic acid suppression and dual-probe pH testing (only in patients with laryngeal symptoms). Preoperative relief of atypical symptoms with use of a PPI or $H_2$ blocker was associated significantly with successful surgical outcome. Findings of other authors who have assessed the effects of antireflux surgery on atypical symptoms have been variable.[559-572] For example, Larrain et al found that antireflux surgery produced symptomatic improvement in GERD-related asthma and reduced the need for bronchodilators.[65] However, Pitcher et al found that antireflux surgery did not correct reflux-related asthma reliably.[573] In 1996, Hunter et al reported atypical symptom improvement rates of 80 to 91% in patients undergoing laparoscopic fundoplication, with particularly good results in the subset of patients with laryngopharyngeal symptoms.[574] Although the role of antireflux surgery remains controversial, in our experience it has proven valuable in appropriately selected voice patients.

Proton pump inhibitors continue to be the primary treatment for symptoms of LPR by most otolaryngologists. However, some patients' symptoms appear refractory to medical management with PPIs (twice or more daily dosing), and another subset of symptomatic patients are not willing to take daily medications for an extended period of time. At our voice center (RTS et al),[575] we performed a retrospective review of the patients' medical records to examine the effectiveness of antireflux surgery on LPR symptoms refractive to medical treatment in 25 professional voice users ranging in age from 14 to 75 years, most of whom did not meet traditional surgical criteria. Twenty-four-hour pH impedance studies were performed pre- and postoperatively. Reflux finding scores were graded (blind raters) pre- and postoperatively; these scores revealed no significant differ-

ences pre- and postoperatively with good inter- and intrarater reliability. This was not a great surprise, since most patients were on 2, 3, or 4 doses of PPI at the time of the pre-op study. Postoperative 24-hour pH impedance studies postlaprascopic Nissen fundoplication revealed a significant decrease in reflux episode. Approximately 60% of patients were on no medication postoperatively, and 76% of patients who had been on BID PPI dosing, and 86% who had been on super-high dose PPI (3 or 4) administration reported satisfaction with the results of Nissen fundoplication in managing their symptoms. DeMeester scores also were normal before and after surgery and not helpful for outcomes assessments. Our findings also suggest the reflux finding score may lack sensitivity as a tool for monitoring the severity of LPR symptoms.

A study by Trad et al[576] examined the long-term outcomes of patient satisfaction and symptom resolution in a group of patients who underwent transoral incision-less fundoplication (TIF) for GERD and/or LPR symptoms. Thirty-four patients had a confirmed diagnosis of GERD that was not controlled medically with antisecretory drugs (PPIs) and reported unwillingness to continue taking medications. All 34 patients underwent TIF surgery using the esophX. Follow-up data were obtained on 28 of 34 patients: 50% of the study population was female, 50% male, with a mean age of 57 years. The authors reported that "standard TIF-2 protocol was used and resulted in reduction of hiatal hernia and restored GE junction anatomy (heal grade 1)." They reported no postoperative complication in any patient. Follow-up at 14 months found 82% (23 of 28) patients were off daily PPIs and 68% (19 of 28) reported improvement in their symptoms compared to preoperatively. They utilized the RSI to evaluate LPR symptoms including throat clearing, cough, and hoarseness, and reported that these symptoms were eliminated in 63% (17 of 28) patients.

Fahin et al[577] also examined the effect of laprascopic antireflux surgery on laryngeal symptoms, physical findings, and voice analysis. They performed a prospective analysis on 2 groups of patients preoperatively and 2 years after laparoscopic antireflux surgery (LARS). Group 1 included 41 patients (24 men) with GERD and LPR symptoms. Group 2 included 26 patients (16 men) with GERD and no LPR symptoms. All patients underwent EGD, 24-hour pH or M11-pH monitoring. Patients completed RSI and VHI-10 questionnaires. Laryngeal findings were evaluated by blinded otolaryngologists utilizing the RFS and the GRBS scale. The Multi-Dimensional Voice Program (MDVP) was used for objective voice measurements. Follow-up for both groups was at approximately

25 months following surgery. The authors reported that group 1 had significantly lower RSI and RF scores following surgery. They stated further that "LARS substantially improved RFS, RSI, and VH1 in carefully selected patients with GERD, especially the signs and symptoms related to the larynx and voice." The authors pointed out that "indications for LARS are limited in patients with LPR" but suggested that their findings support consideration of the procedure in the management of patients LPR.

Hoppo et al[578] studied the role of hypopharyngeal multichannel intraluminal impedance (HM11) testing in patients undergoing antireflux surgery for reflux disease associated with chronic cough. The authors defined cough as lasting greater than or equal to 8 weeks and of undetermined etiology. They performed HM11 testing on 314 symptomatic patients, looking for high esophageal reflux (2 cm distal to the upper esophageal sphincter). Forty-nine patients were identified as having chronic cough, and 36 of the 49 patients (73%) were found to have abnormal proximal exposure. Sixteen of the 36 patients underwent antireflux surgery, and 81% (13 patients) reported resolution of cough. The authors suggest that HM11 aids in the diagnosis of LPR and potentially in identifying those patients who might benefit from antireflux surgery.

Another study by Mazzoleni et al[579] suggests that 24-hour pH impedance (pH-M11) is not reliable for the diagnosis of LPR and that oropharyngeal (OP) pH monitoring with the Dx-pH probe is a better diagnostic tool. They studied 36 patients with both tests concommitantly and reported weak correlations between results of both tests. They suggest that the etiology of pH alteration is uncertain, thus making determination of the best test for diagnosing LPR problematic.

Toomey et al[580] compared the results of patients with GERD who underwent transoral incision-less fundoplication (TIF) with those patients who underwent Toupet or Nissen fundoplication between 2010 and 2013. They performed a case-controlled study of 20 patients in the 3 cohorts; those undergoing TIF, those undergoing laprascopic Nissen fundoplication, and those undergoing Toupet fundoplication. Their case-control data included age, preoperative DeMeester scores, and body mass index. They found that the patients undergoing TIF procedures had shorter operative times and shorter hospitalization time. In all 3 procedures, patients reported "dramatic and similar reduction in symptom frequency and severity." Patients reported experiencing symptoms less than once a month included 83% following TIF, 80% after Nissen fundoplication, and 92% after Toupet fundoplication. They concluded that TIF is safe and effective as compared to Nissen and Toupet procedures and recommended they continue use.

## Indications for Surgical Therapy

Indications for surgery include persistent symptomatology despite reasonable medical management and patient intolerance to medications. Surgery may also be an option for patients who are concerned about the costs and consequences of long-term medical therapy. In patients whose symptom control requires continuous medical therapy, surgery is an important option. Patients with complicated gastroesophageal reflux disease, manifesting Barrett's metaplasia, stricture, or ulceration and those who require long-term therapy should also be considered for surgery.

In the past, surgery for GERD was recommended infrequently due to the risks associated with abdominal surgery under general anesthesia, significant postoperative discomfort, and the recognition of substantial long-term complications such as dysphagia, "gas bloat," and others. Since the initial description of the operation by Rudolph Nissen in 1956, the operation has undergone significant modifications that have lessened the incidence of postoperative complications.[550] In addition, the introduction of the laparoscopic approach to antireflux surgery has minimized the postoperative discomfort and many of the risks. It has also shortened postoperative recuperation from 6 to 8 weeks to 2 to 3 weeks, allowing patients to return to normal activities in an acceptable period of time.

## Preoperative Evaluation

Thorough preoperative evaluation is essential to successful surgical management of GERD. Although the typical patient with this disorder has well-recognized gastrointestinal symptoms, GERD may underlie certain cases of asthma and other respiratory diseases, laryngitis, chronic cough, and chest pain. In addition, other upper gastrointestinal conditions may present with symptoms similar to those seen with GERD. Thus, it is critical to firmly establish the diagnosis and to exclude other conditions.

Further goals of preoperative evaluation are to assess the anatomy and physiology of the swallowing mechanism and stomach. Adequacy of esophageal motility and gastric emptying are important preoperative considerations, because disorders in either of these areas will affect the choice of a surgical procedure. It is also important to document complications of reflux, specifically the presence or absence of Barrett's metaplasia, ulceration, or stricture.

The preoperative evaluation should include the following:

1. A complete history and physical examination is especially important both to determine symptoms related to reflux and to exclude other conditions. Evaluation of the general medical status is also crucial.

2. Upper gastrointestinal endoscopy is important to exclude other lesions and to assess for the presence or absence of Barrett's metaplasia. Stricture and ulceration may also be seen. The presence or absence of *H pylori* may be determined.

3. Roentgenographic barium contrast study of the upper gastrointestinal tract defines the anatomy of the esophagus and stomach, as well as the relationship of the gastroesophageal junction of the hiatus. The length of the esophagus is easily assessed. A foreshortened esophagus would alter surgical management significantly, as discussed below. The presence of a sliding or paraesophageal hernia can be assessed. In addition, other anatomic abnormalities of the esophagus and stomach can be identified, such as strictures, webs, masses, or diverticula. Furthermore, this is a dynamic study allowing the radiologist to assess the motility of the esophagus and the emptying function of the stomach. Although reflux of barium is not always identified, the absence of this finding does not rule out the presence of reflux; demonstration of significant reflux of barium during this radiographic procedure is almost always considered abnormal. An assessment of gastric emptying also can be performed. This information can be obtained from the upper GI series or from a gastric emptying study. It is important to document the status of gastric emptying prior to surgical intervention that occurs in the area of the vagal trunks, as there have been occasional reports of postoperative gastroparesis.

4. Twenty-four-hour pH monitoring is considered the most accurate test for documenting the presence of abnormal acid reflux. This is particularly useful in patients who present with atypical symptoms such as asthma, chronic cough, hoarseness, chest pain, and others. This study quantifies the amount of abnormal reflux, its relationship to symptomatology, its presence in upright or supine positions, and the relationship of reflux episodes to time of day and specific activities. Although it is not strictly obligatory to obtain this study in patients with typical symptoms of reflux and evidence of reflux by other means (eg, endoscopic evidence of ulcerative esophagitis or Barrett's metaplasia), having this study is a useful baseline to help objectively assess postoperative results.

5. Esophageal manometry is obligatory in the preoperative evaluation of the patient with GERD. This essential study provides information regarding lower esophageal sphincter (LES) pressure, length, and relaxation. It also provides vital information regarding esophageal motility. Major motility abnormalities of the esophagus alter the choice of surgical procedure.

6. Other studies and evaluations include pulmonary function testing and comprehensive voice evaluations in selected patients. These are particularly valuable in patients presenting with atypical symptoms.

Although definitive information on the incidence, true causal relationship, and importance (relative to the risk of untreated LPR) of many of these adverse effects remains unknown, it is important for otolaryngologists to be aware of the potential problems associated with all of the medications we prescribe frequently.

Review of these potential problems is not intended to suggest that PPI therapy is overprescribed or should not be prescribed. The consequences of untreated LPR can be substantial and potentially life threatening. However, much of the research on adverse events of PPIs is known widely by otolaryngologists. Otolaryngologists need to make an extra effort to remain current on new findings so that we can counsel and treat our patients optimally. Caution should be exercised particularly when using PPIs in patients with acute coronary syndromes, and cardiology consultation should be considered when PPIs are necessary in patients taking clopidogrel.

Refractory cases may be particularly challenging. Inadequate medication dosage, resistance to medication, reactivity to nonacid reflux in adequately controlled patients, and misdiagnosis are all potential factors. Medication dosages can be increased as discussed above, as can the frequency of administration, although such modifications are "off label." Promotility agents and histamine receptor antagonists can be added. Monitoring of pH during medication use can be useful in determining the cause of persistent signs and symptoms in patients receiving treatment for LPR.

Reimer et al[581] described symptom-producing rebound acid hypersecretion following withdrawal of PPI therapy after 2 months. Acid-related symptoms occurred in a group of healthy volunteers after treatment was stopped, which the authors interpreted as suggesting that rebound acid hypersecretion may result in PPI dependency. We believe that it is also possible because of healing of sensors that were not functional due to long-term acid exposure but recover on PPIs. Hence, it is not uncommon for LPR patients who have never had heartburn to develop heartburn during treatments with PPIs (especially at low doses) or after PPIs are stopped. Patients who choose long-term medical therapy can be reasonably expected to avoid acid-induced mucosal injury, without risk for serious complications. Although comparison studies are inconclusive, it is likely that in most patients, long-term medical therapy with PPIs and antireflux surgery are equivalent options for minimizing acid injury, and the choice can be left to the patient in consultation with the treating physician. Acid suppression does not always provide adequate control of symptoms in patients who note symptoms from suspected pH-neutral or alkaline reflux, especially singers; although this has not been demonstrated by clinical trials, such patients may be considered for surgical therapy.

## Current Operations for Correction of Gastroesophageal Reflux Disease

Antireflux procedures can be classified into 2 groups: those that involve some form of fundoplication and those that do not. They can also be classified by surgical approach, specifically whether performed through the abdomen or through the chest. Additionally, all of these operations can be done open or with minimally invasive techniques (laparoscopic and thoracoscopic approaches).

In selecting an antireflux operation, all preoperative information needs to be considered. Esophageal function and motility affect the choice of operation. When motility is normal, the Nissen fundoplication with a full 360° wrap is the operation of choice. Conversely, with major motility abnormalities, a partial fundoplication is usually preferable.

Second, the length of the esophagus is important. Esophageal shortening should be treated with the addition of a gastroplasty. Third, the presence or absence of hypersecretions of gastric acid may play a role in choice of surgical procedure. An acid-reducing procedure such as a selective vagotomy may be considered in addition to the antireflux procedure. Fourth, the finding of a significant gastroparesis preoperatively may prompt consideration of an additional gastric procedure such as a pyloroplasty at the time of antireflux repair.

## Surgical Repairs Involving Fundoplication

**Nissen Fundoplication.** In 1956, Rudolph Nissen described his 360° gastric fundic wrap.[550] Since that time, modifications regarding the length and looseness of the wrap have been made, allowing the most effective antireflux procedure with minimal morbidity. Currently, this is the most popular antireflux procedure. The steps in performing fundoplication, which are similar whether the approach is open or laparoscopic, include

1. Incision of the gastrohepatic omentum at the gastroesophageal junction to expose the esophagus and the diaphragmatic crura (Figures 11–21 and 11–22).
2. Identification and preservation of the anterior and posterior vagus nerves (Figure 11–23).
3. Circumferential dissection of the esophagus (Figure 11–24).
4. Assessment of mobility of the fundus.
   a. Mobilization of the fundus by division of the short gastric vessels if the fundus is not sufficiently floppy (Figure 11–25).
   b. With a sufficiently floppy fundus, mobilization of the short gastric vessels can occasionally be omitted, creating a Rossetti modification of the Nissen fundoplication.
5. Closure of the crura (Figure 11–26).
6. Construction of a loose fundoplication around the distal esophagus just proximal to the gastroesophageal junction. This is performed over a large (54–56 Fr) dilator and is created 2 cm in length (Figure 11–27).

**The Laparoscopic Approach.** In the 1990s, the first reports of laparoscopic antireflux surgery were published.[551] They described a minimally invasive surgical approach to treatment of this disease with low mortality and morbidity. The laparoscopic approach can be used in most patients undergoing antireflux surgery and has become the approach of choice. Contraindications to a laparoscopic antireflux operation include major coagulopathy, severe obstructive pulmonary disease, and possibly pregnancy. Prior abdominal surgery is not a contraindication. Reoperative antireflux surgery usually cannot be performed laparoscopically. Occasionally, a laparoscopic approach may be attempted but generally, conversion to an open procedure is necessary. This is usually due to severe central obesity or a large left lobe of the liver, both of which preclude adequate visualization of the relevant anatomy.

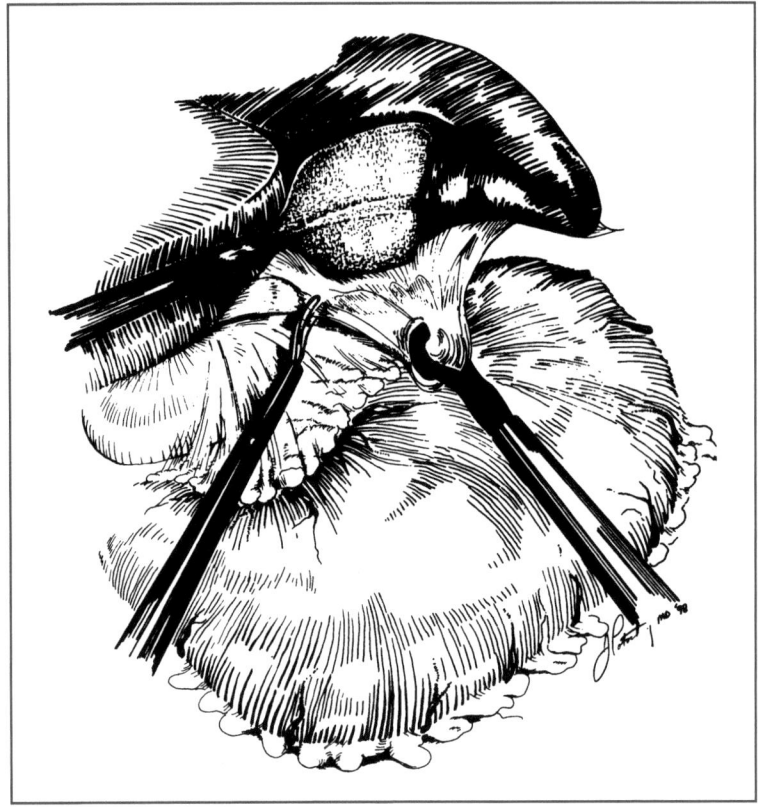

**Figure 11–21.** Incision of gastrohepatic omentum.

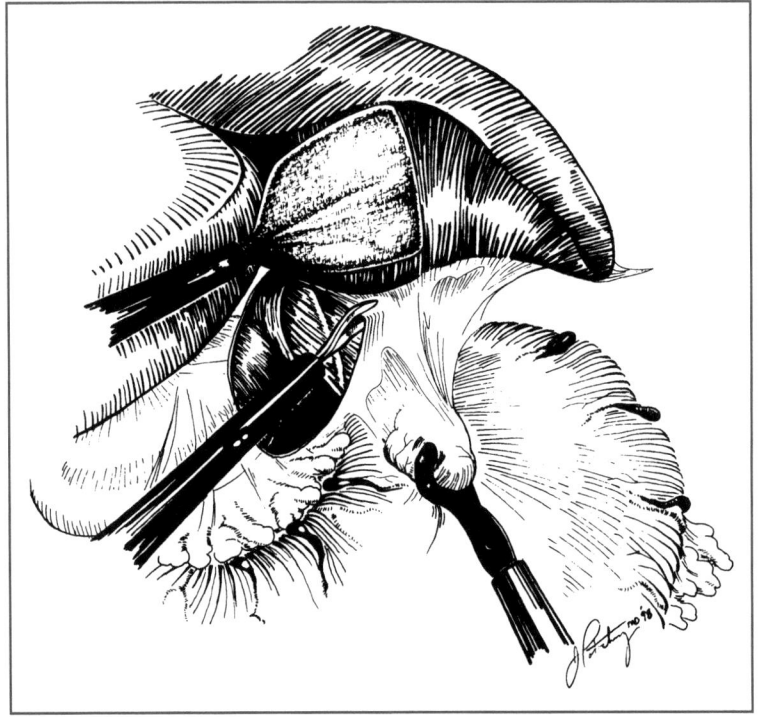

**Figure 11–22.** Exposure of esophagus and diaphragmatic crura.

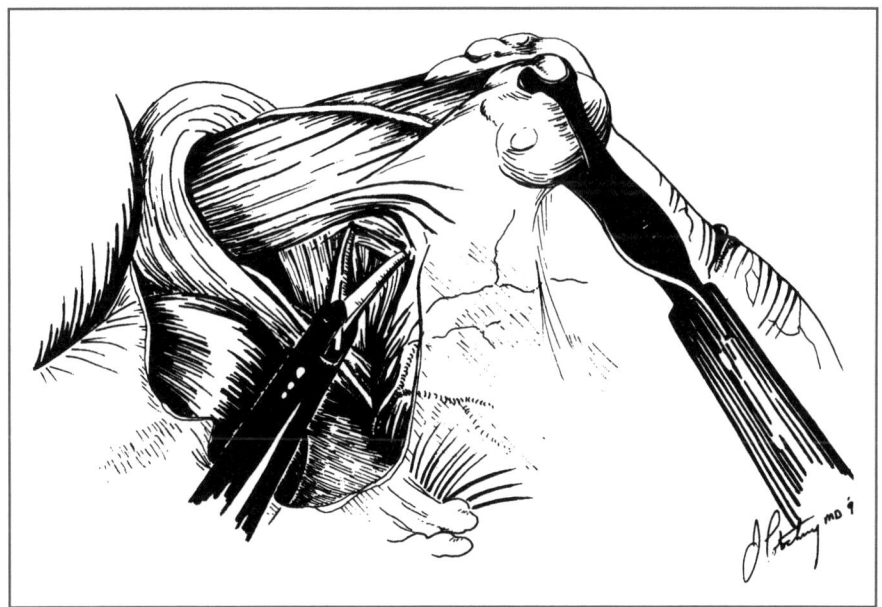

**Figure 11–23.** Identification of vagus nerves.

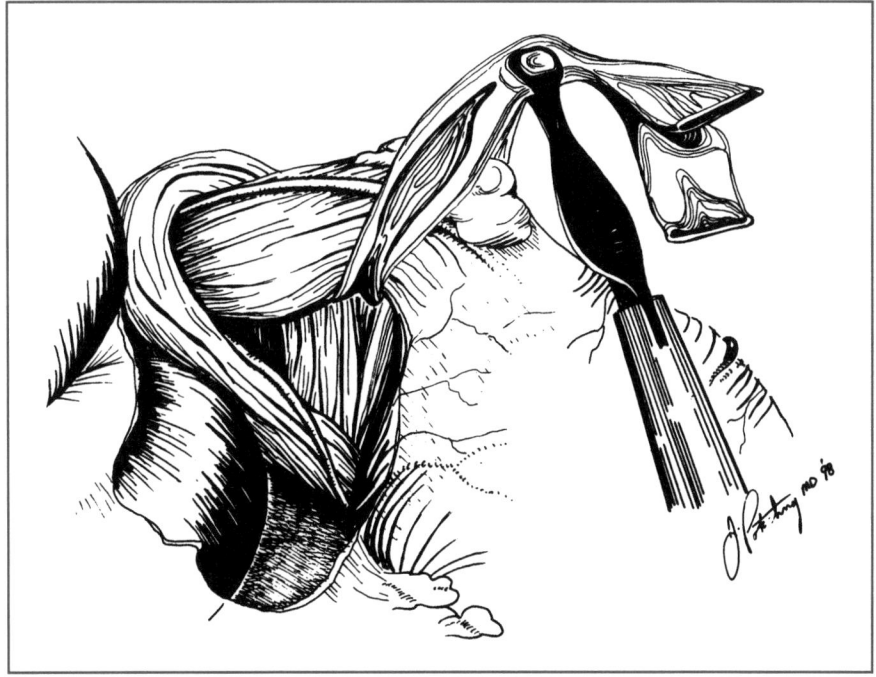

**Figure 11–24.** Circumferential dissection of the esophagus.

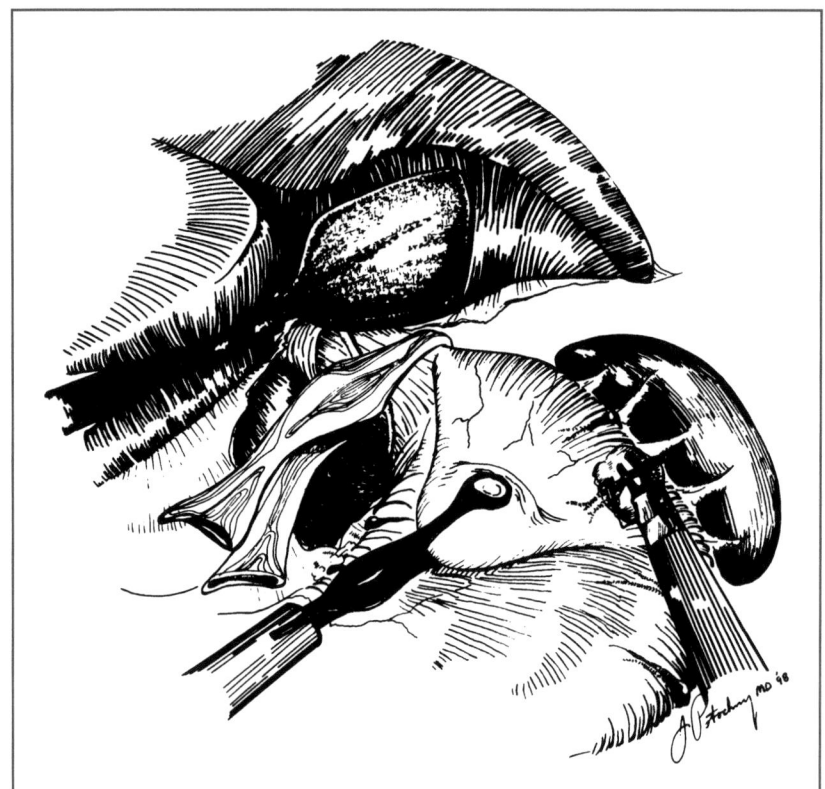

**Figure 11–25.** Mobilization of the proximal greater curvature.

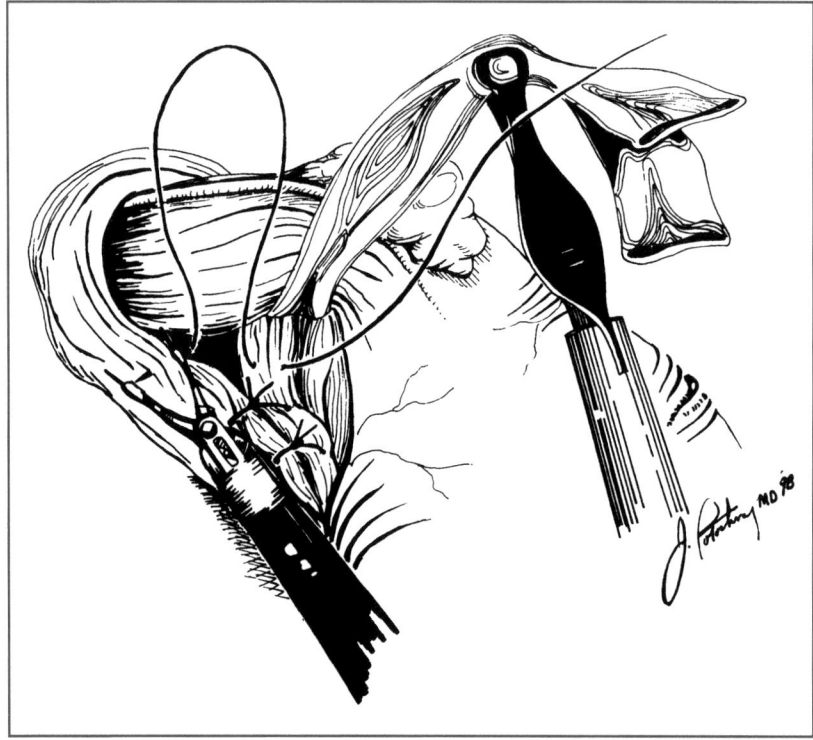

**Figure 11–26.** Closure of the crura.

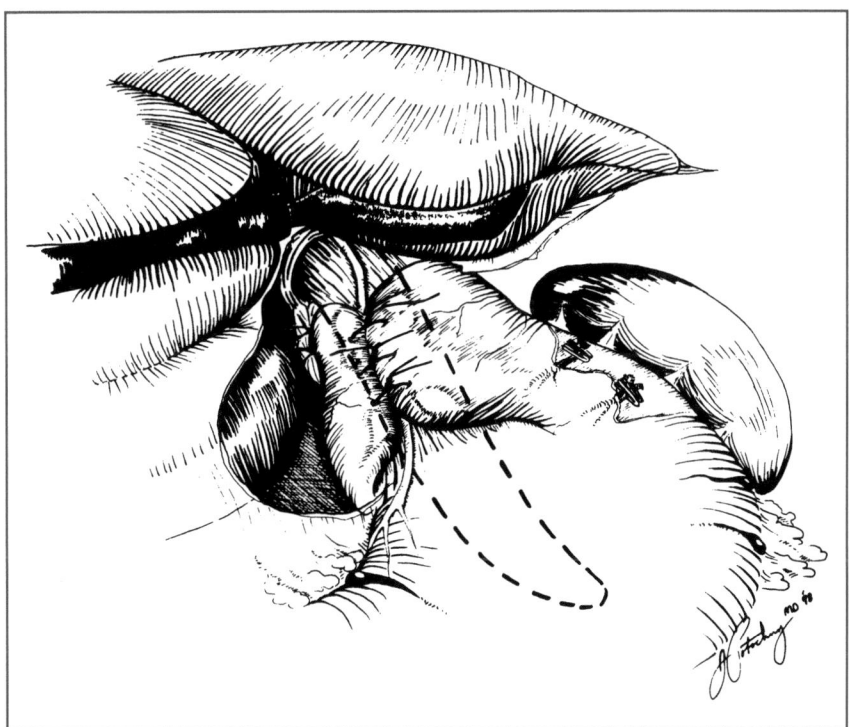

**Figure 11–27.** Construction of fundoplication.

The patient is placed on the operating table in lithotomy and reverse Trendelenburg positions. This allows the surgeon to be positioned between the patient's legs which facilitates 2-handed dissection essential to satisfactory performance of this procedure. However, the 2-handed technique also can be used effectively with the patient in the supine position, having the surgeon on the left side of the table and modifying port placement somewhat (Figure 11–28).

A 12 mm port is positioned to the right of the xiphoid for the liver retractor. Right upper quadrant and left upper quadrant 10 mm ports are positioned, functioning as dissecting ports. An additional 10 mm port is placed in the midline for placement of the camera, and a 10 mm port is placed in the left mid-abdomen for retraction of the stomach. The left lobe of the liver is retracted upward, exposing the gastroesophageal junction. A laparoscopic Babcock clamp is utilized to pull down the fundus, exposing the hiatus.

The gastrohepatic omentum overlying the gastroesophageal junction is incised, and the right crus is identified. The right crus is then dissected away from the right lateral wall of the esophagus. The left crus is then identified and dissected away from the left side of the esophagus. The esophagus is then retracted upward, and the posterior aspect of the esophagus is

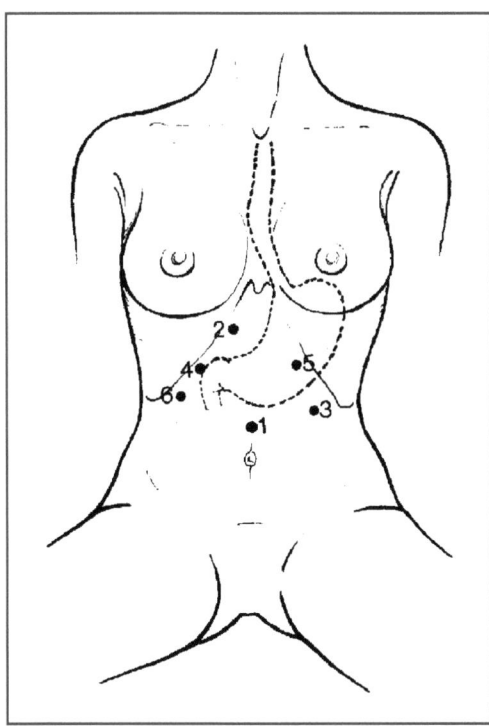

**Figure 11–28.** Port placement for laparoscopic fundoplication: (1) 30° laparoscope; (2) liver retractor; (3) stomach retractor; (4) dissecting port; (5) dissecting port; (6) optional dissecting port.

dissected under direct vision. To avoid perforation, it is important to perform the esophageal dissection under direct vision at all times. Furthermore, dissection should not stray from the esophagus, because dissection in the pleural space can occur, causing pneumothorax. Once the esophagus is circumferentially dissected, a Penrose drain is placed around it, and the Babcock clamp previously used to retract the fundus is repositioned on the Penrose drain. The anterior (left) and posterior (right) vagus nerves are identified. The posterior nerve is excluded from the Penrose drain.

The fundus is then inspected to assess its mobility. In most cases, it is advisable to divide the short gastric vessels to allow for a loose, tension-free wrap. This can be accomplished using the harmonic scalpel or using clips. The proximal third of the greater curvature is mobilized in this manner.

The diaphragmatic opening is made appropriately snug. This is performed with a 54 to 56 Fr dilator within the esophagus to avoid making the closure too tight. Once the diaphragmatic closure is completed, the dilator is retracted into the mid-esophagus by the anesthesiologist or an assistant. The fundus is then drawn around the posterior surface of the esophagus. The wrap is accomplished over the 54 to 56 Fr dilator by placing three 2-0 silk sutures. These sutures are placed from the fundus to the esophagus to the other side of the fundus in each instance. The abdomen is then irrigated and hemostasis is ensured. All trocars are removed under direct vision, and port sites are closed.

**The Transthoracic Approach.** Indications for performing an antireflux procedure via the thorax are

1. Reoperative antireflux surgery
2. Patients who require concomitant procedures on the intrathoracic esophagus
3. Patients with coexistent left pulmonary pathology that requires surgery
4. Patients with a foreshortened esophagus
5. Obese patients in whom an abdominal approach may afford poor visualization
6. Surgeon preference

**Partial Fundoplication.** In the presence of esophageal dysmotility, partial fundoplication is the operation of choice. This can be performed through a thoracic approach such as a Belsey Mark IV partial fundoplication, which creates a 240° anterior partial fundoplication. Alternatively, the Toupet partial fundoplication can be performed transabdominally as an open or laparoscopic procedure. The technical aspects of this procedure are similar to those for

a Nissen fundoplication with the exception of the wrap. After mobilization of the fundus and pulling it around posterior to the esophagus, the fundus is sutured to the right crus using three 2-0 silk sutures.

The anterior aspect of the fundus is then sutured to the esophagus. The fundus is similarly sutured to the left crus and anteriorly along the left side of the esophagus. This wrap necessitates placement of 12 sutures in the 4 rows (Figure 11–29).

### Collis Gastroplasty

In patients with a foreshortened esophagus, a Collis gastroplasty is utilized to lengthen the esophagus. This is followed by a partial or complete fundoplication around the gastric tube with placement of the repair intraabdominally (Figure 11–30).

### Nonfundoplication Repairs (Gastropexy)

In 1967, Lucius Hill[549] described his experience with posterior gastropexy. After his initial series, approximately 20% of his patients had recurrence of reflux symptoms with long-term follow-up. This led to modifications of the technique to include calibration of the lower esophageal sphincter pressure intraoperatively. The physiologic basis of the current Hill operation is that the lower esophageal sphincter segment is restored to the high-pressure environment of the ab domen and secured in that position by anchoring the gastroesophageal junction to the median actuate ligament posteriorly. The hiatal hernia defect is corrected, and the lower esophageal sphincter pressure is restored using intraoperative manometry (Figure 11–31).

The Hill repair has been described utilizing an open or laparoscopic technique.[549] The following steps are common to both:

1. The crura are dissected.
2. The anterior and posterior vagus nerves are identified and preserved.
3. The esophagus is dissected circumferentially.
4. The medial aspect of the gastric fundus is mobilized from its adhesions to the diaphragm, which occasionally also includes division of several short gastric vessels.
5. The preaortic fascia is dissected down to the area of the median actuate ligament.
6. The esophageal hiatus is loosely closed around the esophagus.
7. Sutures are placed in the anterior and posterior phreno-esophageal bundles, avoiding the esophagus. Three such sutures are placed.

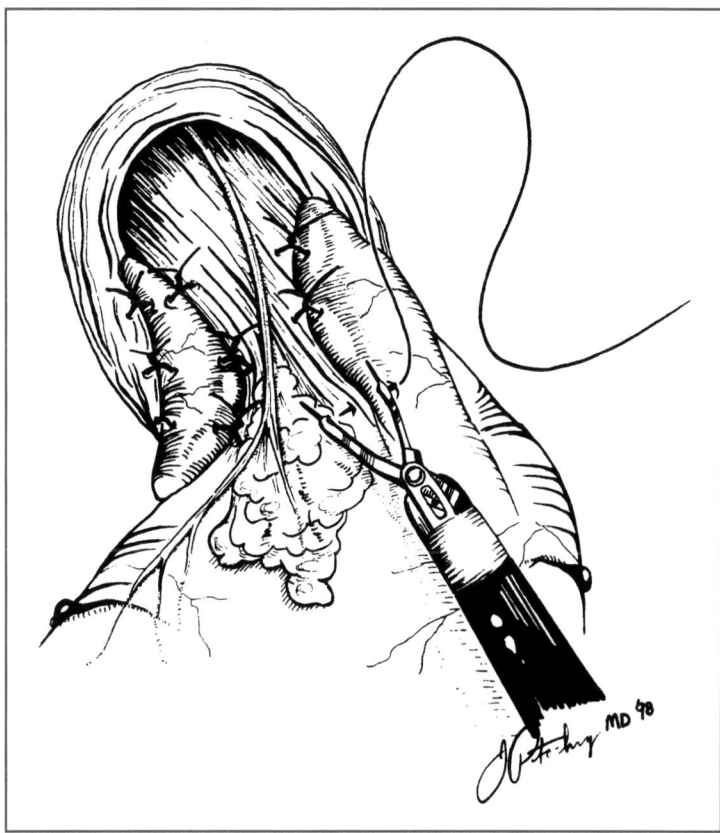

**Figure 11–29.** Partial fundoplication (Toupet).

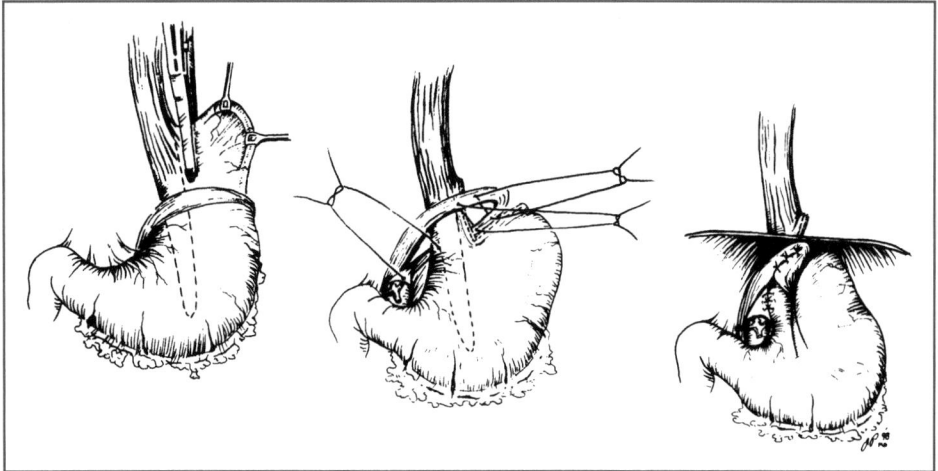

**Figure 11–30.** Collis gastroplasty.

8. Intraoperative manometry is performed. Sutures are placed through the imbricated bundles and carried through the preaortic fascia.
9. Additional sutures are placed from the fundus through the diaphragm to further reinforce the GE valve.

**Postoperative Care**

Patients are admitted to the hospital preoperatively. A nasogastric tube is not used routinely. Antireflux medications are not restarted. On the first postoperative day, patients undergo an upper gastrointestinal

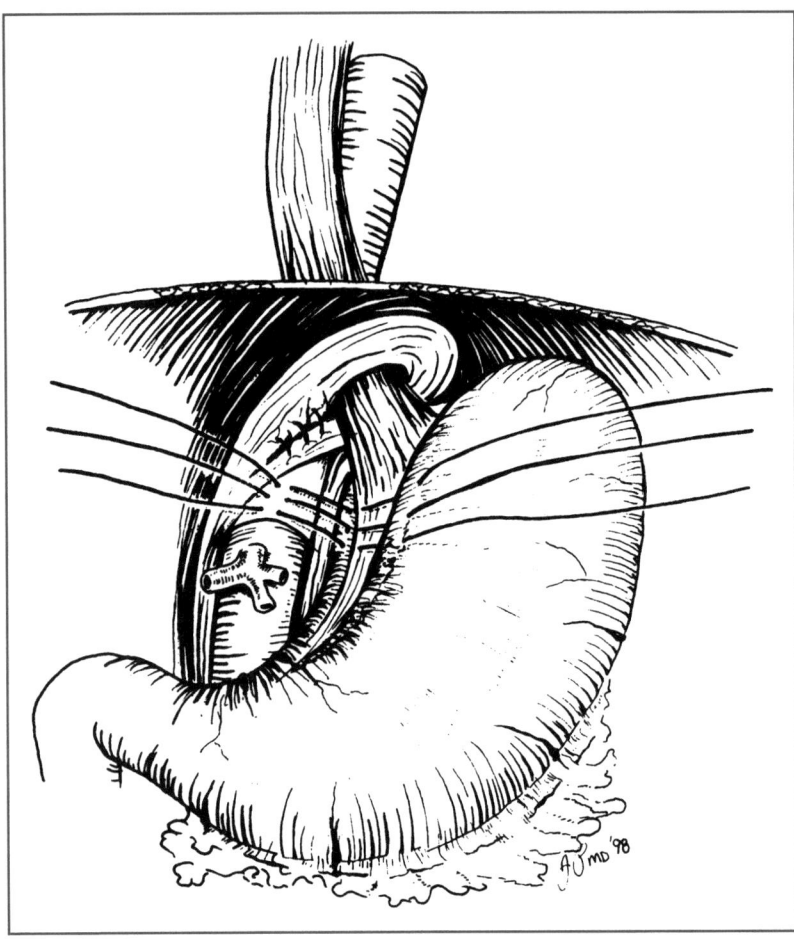

**Figure 11–31.** Hill posterior gastropexy.

contrast study using water-soluble contrast to rule out the presence of a leak. If no leak is identified, the patient is asked to swallow a small amount of barium to better delineate the postoperative anatomy and to assess emptying function of the esophagus and stomach. Clear liquids are started on the first postoperative day, and diet is advanced as tolerated. With laparoscopic surgery, patients are generally discharged on the second postoperative day. Some degree of minor transient dysphagia is common, but in nearly all cases this resolves within 8 to 12 weeks.

Patients are seen in follow-up at 2 weeks. At 3 and 12 months, patients are asked to undergo repeat 24-hour pH monitoring and esophageal manometry.

### Operative Complications

In general, antireflux surgery, whether performed open or closed, is safe. In several large series, mortality rates are essentially zero.[548–567] Wound complications such as infection and herniation are seen slightly more often with the open technique. In addi-

tion, splenic injury is reported as occurring in 1 to 2% of open fundoplications; but it is very rarely, if ever, seen with the laparoscopic approach.

Complications following laparoscopic antireflux surgery include those common to all operations, those specific to laparoscopy, and those related to the specific surgical procedure. Operative complications common to all procedures include bleeding and infection. Bleeding complications are rarely, if ever, seen with laparoscopic antireflux surgery. It is virtually never necessary to transfuse patients. Wound infection is also extremely uncommon. Another complication common to many operations performed under general anesthesia is pulmonary emboli. In our series of 70 laparoscopic antireflux procedures, this complication occurred in 2.8% of patients. In no instance was it fatal.[557]

Complications specific to laparoscopy include trocar injuries, hypercapnea requiring ventilation, pneumothorax, and pneumomediastinum. Trocar injures are rare. We utilize an open technique for inserting the initial trocar and have not had any injuries. Many patients have pneumothorax. As part of the author's (DMS) original protocol, all patients underwent routine chest x-ray in the recovery room, and this finding was incidentally noted commonly. In all instances, patients were asymptomatic, and the pneumothorax resolved on follow-up chest x-ray the next day. In addition, pneumomediastinum with air occasionally tracking into the subcutaneous tissues of the neck and chest was also seen. In all instances, these findings resolved within 24 hours.

Complications specific to the operation include persistent dysphagia, defined as dysphagia still present more than 3 months after surgery. In the literature, patients have required reoperation for this complication, although we have not had that experience in our series to date.

Occasionally, persistent dysphagia can be corrected with endoscopic dilatation. Postoperative gastroparesis is occasionally seen and thought to be due to edema around the vagus nerves secondary to the operative dissection. This complication is rare and is effectively treated with prokinetic agents such as cisapride or metoclopramide. This phenomenon is generally transient, and these medications can be discontinued several weeks after surgery.

Esophageal or gastric perforation occurring intraoperatively has also been described. Should these complications be recognized intraoperatively, they can be repaired laparoscopically. However, this requires an experienced surgeon well versed in advanced laparoscopic techniques. Failure to recognize these complications may lead to septic complications, which frequently requires a return to the operating room. Fortunately, these are also rare.

## Results

Many studies report the efficacy of antireflux surgery with 90% of patients demonstrating symptom control. The laparoscopic approach achieves similar outcomes to open antireflux surgery, although follow-up is shorter.

Professional voice users often will demonstrate reflux during singing. This reflux may be acidic or pH neutral. This subgroup of patients does well following surgery with improved vocal quality and strength, although some of these patients will still require antireflux medication, at least occasionally.

## Endoscopic Antireflux Therapy

Although medical and surgical therapies for GERD are extremely successful, well-studied, and effective alternatives for patients with need for long-term therapy, many patients would prefer a nonsurgical, nonpharmacologic option for treatment of their symptoms. This has led to extensive research and development of endoscopic procedures designed to treat GERD. Four of these procedures are approved by the Food and Drug Administration (FDA) for treatment of GERD: radiofrequency energy delivery to the gastroesophageal junction (Stretta, Curon Medical, Fremont, California), transoral flexible endoscopic suturing (EndoCinch, Bard, Murray Hill, New Jersey), injection of a biocompatible, nonbiodegradable copolymer to reinforce the muscular layer of the LES (Enteryx, Boston Scientific, Natick, Massachusetts), and an endoscopic, full-thickness plicator device (NDO plicator). All attempt to reduce reflux by mechanically altering the LES. The exact mechanism for their efficacy is unknown.

Several key generalizations can be made. To date, a relatively small number of patients have been studied, follow-up time is relatively short (≤3 years), and a few major side effects have been reported. Studies have been performed in patients with heartburn and regurgitation.

All patients treated have had good response to PPIs. Only patients with mild erosive esophagitis (grade 2 or less) and small hiatal hernias have been evaluated. Therefore, patients with severe erosive esophagitis, Barrett's esophagus, and other manifestations of GERD (cough, asthma, laryngopharyngeal reflux [LPR]) have not been studied. Although long-term side effects are few, chest pain, dysphagia, and fever are seen immediately after the procedure in most patients. Unfortunately, several deaths have been associated with the procedures (Stretta and Enteryx); other rare major complications such as pleural effusion, esophageal perforation, and aspiration have also been reported.

### Stretta

Six months after therapy, patients in an open-label study in the United States who were treated with radiofrequency energy showed an improvement in heartburn score, regurgitation, quality of life, and patient satisfaction compared with baseline without any changes in esophageal motility.[582]

The initial study reported no major complications. At 6 months, 70% were not on any antisecretory therapy and 87% were able to discontinue PPIs. At 1-year follow-up, more than 60% continued to be off antisecretory therapy and had sustained improvement in heartburn. Unfortunately, serious side effects have been reported to the FDA, including aspiration, pleural effusion, atrial fibrillation, and deaths in the first 1000 procedures performed.

Stretta has been studied in a prospective, sham-controlled study.[583] Sixty-four patients were randomly assigned to radiofrequency energy delivery to the gastroesophageal junction (35 patients) or to a sham procedure (29 patients). Radiofrequency energy delivery significantly improved GERD symptoms and quality of life compared with the sham procedure (61% of patients in the treatment group compared with 33% of patients who received a sham procedure ceased to have daily heartburn symptoms), but it did not decrease esophageal acid exposure or medication use at 6 months. Symptom improvement persisted 12 months after treatment, and no perforations or deaths were reported.

## EndoCinch

The second approved procedure, endoluminal gastroplication (EndoCinch), was reported initially in a multicenter trial of 64 patients with heartburn more often than 3 times a week, dependence on antisecretory medication, mild erosive esophagitis, and abnormal 24-hour pH monitoring. They were treated with EndoCinch, an endoscopic suturing system designed to create an "internal placation" of the stomach.[584]

In this uncontrolled trial, improvement in the number of reflux episodes was seen. No change in upright, recumbent, or total esophageal acid exposure was seen at 3 and 6 months. Sixty-two percent of patients were able to decrease drugs to less than 4 doses of antisecretory medications per month. Improvement was seen in patient satisfaction, heartburn severity, and heartburn score compared with the initial measurements. With the exception of a "stitch" perforation that required short-term hospitalization, no major complications were reported. To date, no sham trial has been reported in full manuscript form using this method.

Most recently, a 2-year follow-up study in 33 patients originally treated with this endoscopic device was reported.[585] After a mean follow-up of 25 months, heartburn severity and score and frequency of regurgitation showed continued improvement compared with baseline measurements. However, only 8 patients (25%) initially on PPIs were completely off antisecretory medications, with 9% taking half or less of their initial dose. Forty percent required full-dose medications, and 6% had undergone a laparoscopic Nissen fundoplication because of the therapeutic failure.

In an open-label, multicenter US trial,[586] 85 patients with GERD were treated with endoluminal gastroplication. At 12 and 24 months postoperatively, 59 and 52%, respectively, showed heartburn symptom resolution, and 73 and 69% decreased their PPI use by at least 50%. Eleven patients had adverse events, only 2 of which were serious: one patient had severe dysphagia necessitating removal of the plications, and one had severe bronchospasm requiring intubation to allow completion of the procedure. These data are disappointing and suggest that long-term efficacy of this procedure as designed originally will not be forthcoming.

## Enteryx

The Enteryx procedure was granted approval by the FDA in April 2003. The procedure is performed by injecting a biopolymer (ethylene vinyl alcohol, EVA) into the muscular layer of the LES under fluoroscopic guidance. The proposed mechanism of action is based on enhancing the gastroesophageal barrier against reflux via a space-occupying effect, inducing fibrosis in the area of injection, and altering the compliance of the sphincter during gastric distention.[586,587]

In the expanded, multicenter, open-label, international clinical trial of Enteryx implantation for GERD,[588] promising results at 12 and 24 months were reported: 78 and 72%, respectively, of patients were able to reduce their previous PPI dose by at least 50%, and 78 and 80% reported significant improvements of their heartburn-related quality of life symptoms during the same time periods. None of the patients had what was considered a potentially life-threatening adverse event. The most common adverse event was transient retrosternal chest pain in 85% of patients, which resolved with prescription pain medications in 84% of affected patients. One of the 144 enrolled patients developed a paraesophageal fluid collection diagnosed at 6 weeks after the procedure, which resolved completely with intravenous antibiotics.

In a recent randomized, single-blind, prospective, multicenter clinical trial in Europe,[589,590] 64 patients with classic heartburn symptoms controlled on PPI therapy were randomized into 2 groups of equal sizes to receive either the Enteryx procedure or a sham procedure consisting of a standard upper endoscopy and were followed before allowing for crossover for 3 months. 81% of patients in the Enteryx group achieved ≥50% reduction of their PPI use compared with 53% of those in the sham group, and 68% of patients in the Enteryx group vs 41% of patients in the sham group ceased PPIs completely. More Enteryx-treated (81%) than sham-treated (19%) patients did not undergo retreatment. Pain, odynophagia/dysphagia, and fever were the most common adverse events in the Enteryx group. An esophageal ulcer with extrusion of the copolymer was noted in one patient. Preliminary results of the US multicenter trial were recently reported with results similar to the European trial. Overall, although pH studies have shown statistical improvement from baseline, normalization is seen in less than one-third of patients.

Although few major side effects have been reported in the organized clinical trials, at least one procedure-related death has been reported, as well as case reports of mediastinitis and pleural effusion.

**Endoscopic Full-Thickness Plicator**

This system creates a transmural plication 1 cm distal to the esophageal-gastric junction, reinforcing the competency of the gastroesophageal barrier. It was granted premarket approval by the FDA in April 2003.

Data on the intermediate-term safety and efficacy of this device were published recently in a multicenter North American trial[591]; 64 patients requiring maintenance antisecretory therapy for chronic heartburn received a single endoscopic full-thickness plication in the gastric cardia 1 cm distal to the gastroesophageal junction. Of the 57 patients who completed the 12-month follow-up by the time of publication, 70% were off PPI therapy. Median heartburn-related quality of life scores improved significantly compared with baseline both while not taking PPIs and while taking such medication. Normal pH scores were observed in 30% of patients. Common procedure-related adverse events included sore throat (41%) and abdominal pain (20%), resolving spontaneously after several days. The same group had reported 6 serious adverse events during the initial follow-up at 6 months[589]: 2 patients experienced severe dyspnea, 1 developed pneumothorax, 1 pneumoperitonum, 1 gastric perforation, and 1 fundic mucosal abrasion. None resulted in long-term patient injury.

In 2010, Velanovich[592] reported his experience using Esophyx, a device for endoscopic fundoplication. Esophyx was used in 24 patients; 20 had symptoms and signs of GERD and 4 had been diagnosed with LPR. Four of the 24 patients had recurrent symptoms following Nissen procedures. He suggested that much research is still needed and that endoscopic fundoplication is most effective in patients with mild-to-moderate symptoms of GERD and those with small hiatal hernias. Its value for patients with LPR has not been established.

**Summary and Role in LPR**

The concept of endoscopic therapy is excellent, and its potential is exciting. Nonetheless, we are early in our evaluation of these evolving techniques. No organized clinical trials have been done or are in process in LPR. Therefore, efficacy in these difficult-to-treat patients cannot be predicted. Based on the current outcomes in patients with heartburn, the best that one might expect is the opportunity to reduce PPI dosage. More data on efficacy and safety are needed before we can recommend these techniques widely. Patients should be reminded that medical therapy is safe and surgery a reasonable alternative when performed by an experienced surgeon. Francis et al[593] examined the role of antireflux surgery in patients with signs and symptoms of LPR refractory to medical management with PPIs. They pointed out the controversy regarding the role of fundoplication in patients with PPI-refractory symptoms and abnormal nonacid reflux by pH impedance monitoring. In their patients, 59% reported symptom improvement postsurgery. They defined preoperative refractory symptoms as <50% improvement following at least 12 weeks of twice-daily PPI therapy. Their patients underwent esophagogastroduodenoscopy, wireless 48-hour pH monitoring, and esophageal motility testing off acid suppression to determine their baseline acid exposure. The patients also underwent 24-hour impedance pH monitoring while on twice-daily PPI therapy. The authors could not confirm that the impedance of pH parameter measured while on therapy was a predictor of symptom response following fundoplication.

If endoscopic antireflux therapy is considered, patients should have it only after careful consideration of the alternatives and with clear understanding of the absence of long-term data and the small but real risk for major complications. At present, these procedures should not be considered as indicated for those who have failed medical therapy.

## Conclusion

Antireflux surgery is a safe, effective therapeutic alternative in the management of gastroesophageal reflux disease. In expert hands, laparoscopic antireflux surgery is safe, effective, and corrects the underlying cause of reflux with minimal morbidity and high patient satisfaction. It eliminates the problems of pH-neutral reflux and the need for prolonged use of acid-suppressing medications. Surgery should be considered as an appropriate option in the treatment of reflux disease. Newer endoscopic approaches to improve the function of the LES require further refinement and study. They have potential to be less invasive and less morbid than even laparoscopic surgery. If they prove to be safe and effective, if they do not affect adversely the results of subsequent laparo-scopic fundoplication for patients in whom they fail, and if they are not associated with an excessive number of serious complications, then they may become desirable therapeutic options for patients with LPR, especially professional voice users. However, at present, preliminary data do not justify their routine use for patients with LPR.

# References

1. Olson NR. The problem of gastroesophageal reflux. *Otolaryngol Clin North Am.* 1986;19:119–133.

2. Menon AP, Schefft GL, Thach BT. Apnea associated with regurgitation in infants. *J Pediatr.* 1985;106: 625–629.

3. Little FB, Koufman JA, Kohut RI, Marshall RB. Effect of gastric acid on the pathogenesis of subglottic stenosis. *Ann Otol Rhinol Laryngol.* 1985;94:516–519.

4. Kambic V, Radsel Z. Acid posterior laryngitis. Aetiology, histology, diagnosis and treatment. *J Laryngol Otol.* 1984;98:1237–1240.

5. Feder RJ, Michell MJ. Hyperfunctional, hyperacidic, and intubation granulomas. *Arch Otolaryngol.* 1984; 110:582–584.

6. Belmont JR, Grundfast K. Congenital laryngeal stridor (laryngomalacia): etiologic factors and associated disorders. *Ann Otol Rhinol Laryngol.* 1984;39:430–437.

7. Olson NR. Effects of stomach acid on the larynx. *Proc Am Laryngol Assoc.* 1983;104:108–112.

8. Ohman L, Olofsson J, Tibbling L, Ericsson G. Esophageal dysfunction in patients with contact ulcer of the larynx. *Ann Otol Rhinol Laryngol.* 1983;92:228–230.

9. Bain WM, Harrington JW, Thomas LE, Schaefer SD. Head and neck manifestations of gastroesophageal reflux. *Laryngoscope.* 1983;93:175–179.

10. Orenstein SR, Orenstein DM, Whitington PF. Gastroesophageal reflux causing stridor. *Chest.* 1983;84: 301–302.

11. Ward PH, Berci G. Observations on the pathogenesis of chronic non-specific pharyngitis and laryngitis. *Laryngoscope.* 1982;92:1377–1382.

12. Ward PH, Zwitman D, Hanson D, Berci G. Contact ulcers and granulomas of the larynx: new insights into their etiology as a basis for more rational treatment. *Otolaryngol Head Neck Surg.* 1980;88:262–269.

13. Goldberg M, Noyek AM, Pritzker KP. Laryngeal granuloma secondary to gastro-esophageal reflux. *J Otolaryngol.* 1978;7:196–202.

14. Chodosh PL. Gastro-esophago-pharyngeal reflux. *Laryngoscope.* 1977;87;1418–1427.

15. Toohill RJ, Kuhn JC. Role of refluxed acid in pathogenesis of laryngeal disorders. *Am J Med.* 1997;103(5A): 100S–106S.

16. Wiener GJ, Koufman JA, Wu WC, et al. Chronic hoarseness secondary to gastroesophageal reflux disease: documentation with 24-hr ambulatory pH monitoring. *Am J Gastroenterol.* 1989;84:1503–1508.

17. Sataloff RT, Spiegel JR, Hawkshaw MJ. Strobovideolaryngoscopy: results and clinical value. *Ann Otol Rhinol Laryngol.* 1991;100(9):725–727.

18. Koufman JA, Wiener GJ, Wu WC, Castell DO. Reflux laryngitis and its sequelae: the diagnostic role of ambulatory 24-hour pH monitoring. *J Voice.* 1988; 2(1):78–89.

19. Toohill RJ, Ulualp SO, Shaker R. Evaluation of gastroesophageal reflux in patients with laryngotracheal stenosis. *Ann Otol Rhinol Laryngol.* 1998;107:1010–1014.

20. Ross JA, Noordzji JP, Woo P. Voice disorders in patients with suspected laryngo-pharyngeal reflux disease. *J Voice.* 1998;12:84–88.

21. Rothstein SG. Reflux and vocal disorders in singers with bulimia. *J Voice.* 1988;12:89–90.

22. Kuhn J, Toohill RJ, Ulualp SO, et al. Pharyngeal acid reflux events in patients with vocal cord nodules. *Laryngoscope.* 1998;108:1146–1149.

23. Gumpert L, Kalach N, Dupont C, Contencin P. Hoarseness and gastroesopahgeal reflux in children. *J Laryngol Otol.* 1998;112:49–54.

24. Halstead LA. Role of gastroesophageal reflux in pediatric upper airway disorders. *Otolaryngol Head and Neck Surg.* 1999;120:208–214.

25. Al Sabbagh G, Wo JM. Supraesophageal manifestations of gastroesophageal reflux disease. *Semin Gastrointest Dis.* 1999;10:113–119.

26. Hanson DG, Jiang JJ. Diagnosis and management of chronic laryngitis associated with reflux. *Am J Med.* 2000;108(suppl 4a):112S–119S.

27. Grontved AM, West F. pH monitoring in patients with benign voice disorders. *Acta Otolaryngol Suppl.* 2000; 543:229–231.

28. Koufman JA, Amin MR, Panetti M. Prevalence of reflux in 113 consecutive patients with laryngeal and voice disorders. *Otolaryngol Head Neck Surg.* 2000;123: 385–388.

29. Poelmans J, Tack J, Feenstra L. Chronic middle ear disease and gastroesophageal reflux disease: a causal relation? *Otol Neurotol.* 2001;22:447–450.

30. Tasker A, Dettmar PW, Panetti M, et al. Reflux of gastric juice and glue ear in children. *Lancet.* 2002;359–493.

31. Loehrl TA, Smith TL, Darling RJ, et al. Autonomic dysfunction, vasomotor rhinitis, and extraesophageal manifestations of gastroesophageal reflux. *Otolaryngol Head Neck Surg.* 2002;126:382–387.

32. Koufman JA. The otolaryngologic manifestations of gastroesophageal reflux disease (GERD): a clinical investigation of 225 patients using ambulatory 24-hour pH monitoring and an experimental investigation of the role of acid and pepsin in the development of laryngeal injury. *Laryngoscope.* 1991;101(4 Pt 2 suppl 53):1–78.

33. Sataloff RT. *Professional Voice: The Science and Art of Clinical Care.* 3rd ed. San Diego, CA: Singular Publishing Group; 2005.

34. Rosen DC, Sataloff RT. *The Psychology of Voice Disorders.* San Diego, CA: Singular Publishing Group; 1997:1–284.
35. Li Q, Castell JA, Castell DO. Manometric determination of esophageal length. *Am J Gastroenterol.* 1994;89: 722–725.
36. Gerhardt DC, Shuck TL, Bordeaux RA, Winship DH. Human upper esophageal sphincter. *Gastroenterology.* 1978;75:268–274.
37. Winans CS. Manometric asymmetry of the lower-esophageal high-pressure zone. *Am J Dig Dis.* 1977;22: 348–354.
38. Meyer GW, Austin RM, Brady CE, et al. Muscle anatomy of the human esophagus. *J Clin Gastroenterol.* 1986;8:131–134.
39. Weisbrodt NW. Neuromuscular organization of esophageal and pharyngeal motility. *Arch Intern Med.* 1976;136:524–531.
40. Meyer GW, Gerhardt DC, Castell DO. Human esophageal response to rapid swallowing: muscle refractory period of neural inhibition? *Am J Physiol.* 1981; 241:G129–G136.
41. Goyal RK, Rattan S. Genesis of basal sphincter pressure: effect of tetrodotoxin on the lower esophageal sphincter in opossum in vivo. *Gastroenterology.* 1976; 71:62–67.
42. Richter JE, Sinar DR, Cordova CM, Castell DO. Verapamil—a potent inhibitor of esophageal contractions in the baboon. *Gastroenterology.* 1982;82:882–886.
43. Richter JE, Spurling TJ, Cordova CM, Castell DO. Effects of oral calcium blocker, diltiazem, on esophageal contractions. *Dig Dis Sci.* 1984;29:649–656.
44. Dodds WJ, Dent J, Hogan WJ, Arndorfer RC. Effect of atropine on esophageal motor function in humans. *Am J Physiol.* 1981;240:G290–G296.
45. Pasricha PJ, Ravich WJ, Kalloo AN. Effects of intragastric botulinum toxin on the lower esophageal sphincter in piglets. *Gastroenterology.* 1993;105:1045–1049.
46. Goyal RK, Rattan S, Said SI. VIP as a possible neurotransmitter of non-cholinergic non-adrenergic inhibitory neurones. *Nature.* 1980;288:378–380.
47. Sanders KM, Ward SM. Nitric oxide as a mediator of nonadrenergic non-cholinergic neurotransmission. *Am J Physiol.* 1992;262(3 Pt1):C379–C392.
48. Castell DO. The lower esophageal sphincter. Physiologic and clinical aspects. *Ann Intern Med.* 1975;83: 390–401.
49. Christensen J, Lund GF. Esophageal responses to distention and electrical stimulation. *J Clin Invest.* 1969; 48:408–419.
50. *A Gallup Survey on Heartburn Across America.* New York, NY: The Gallup Organization Inc; 1968.
51. Locke GR III, Talley NJ, Fett SL, et al. Prevalence and clinical spectrum of gastroesophageal reflux: a population-based study in Olmstead County, Minnesota. *Gastroenterology.* 1997;112:448–456.
52. Nebel OT, Fornes MF, Castell DO. Symptomatic gastroesophageal reflux: incidence and precipitating factors. *Am J Dig Dis.* 1976;21:953–956.
53. Winters C Jr, Spurling TJ, Chobanian SJ, et al. Barrett's esophagus: a prevalent, occult complication of gastroesophageal reflux disease. *Gastroenterology.* 1987;92: 118–123.
54. Ollyo JB, Monnier P, Fontollier C, et al. The natural history, prevalence and incidence of reflux esophagitis. *Gullet.* 1993;3(suppl):3–10.
55. Pace F, Santalucia F, Bianchi Porro G. Natural history of gastro-oesophageal reflux disease without esophagitis. *Gut.* 1991;32:845–848.
56. Schnatz PF, Castell JA, Castell DO. Pulmonary symptoms associated with gastroesophageal reflux: use of ambulatory pH monitoring to diagnose and to direct therapy. *Am J Gastroenterol.* 1996;91:1715–1718.
57. Harding SM, Richter JE, Guzzo MR, et al. Asthma and gastroesophageal reflux: acid suppressive therapy improves asthma outcome. *Am J Med.* 1996;100: 395–405.
58. el-Serag HB, Sonnenberg A. Comorbid occurrence of laryngeal or pulmonary disease with esophagitis in United States military veterans. *Gastroenterology.* 1997; 113:755–760.
59. Harding SM, Guzzo MR, Richter JE. Prevalence of GERD in asthmatics without reflux symptoms. *Gastroenterology.* 1997;4:A141.
60. Sontag SJ, O'Connell S, Khandelwal S, et al. Most asthmatics have gastroesophageal reflux with or without bronchodilator therapy. *Gastroenterology.* 1990;99:613–618.
61. Irwin RS, French CL, Curley FJ, et al. Chronic cough due to gastroesophageal reflux. Clinical, diagnostic, and pathogenic aspects. *Chest.* 1993;194:1511–1517.
62. Katz PO, Castell DO. Approach to the patient with unexplained chest pain. *Am J Gastroenterol.* 2000;7:95 (8 suppl):S4–S8.
63. Hewson EG, Sinclair JW, Dalton CB, Ritcher JE. Twenty-four-hour esophageal pH monitoring: the most useful test for evaluating noncardiac chest pain. *Am J Med.* 1991;90:576–583.
64. Cherian P, Smith LF, Bardham KD, et al. Esophageal tests in the evaluation of non-cardiac chest pain. *Dis Esophagus.* 1995;8:129–133.
65. Larrain A, Carrasco E, Galleguillos F, et al. Medical and surgical treatment of non-allergic asthma associated with gastroesophageal reflux. *Chest.* 1991;99: 1330–1335.
66. Sontag SJ, Schnell TG, Miller TQ, et al. Prevalence of oesophagitis in asthmatics. *Gut.* 1992;33:872–876.
67. Achem SR, Kolts BE, MacMath T, et al. Effects of omeprazole versus placebo in treatment of noncardiac chest pain and gastroesophageal reflux. *Dig Dis Sci.* 1997;42(10):2138–2145.
68. Fass R, Fennerty B, Ofman JJ, et al. The clinical and economic value of a short course of omeprazole in patients with noncardiac chest pain. *Gastroenterology.* 1998;115:42–49.
69. Achem SR, DeVault KR. Unexplained chest pain at the turn of the century. *Am J Gastroenterol.* 1999;94(1):5–8.

70. Börjesson M, Albertsson P, Dellborg M, et al. Esophageal dysfunction syndrome X. *Am J Cardiol.* 1998;82:1187–1191.

71. O'Connor JF, Singer ME, Richter JE. The cost-effectiveness of strategies to assess gastroesophageal reflux as an exacerbating factor in asthma. *Am J Gastroenterol.* 1999;94(6):1472–1480.

72. Levin TR, Sperling RM, McQuaid KR. Omeprazole improves peak expiratory flow rate and quality of life in asthmatics with gastroesophageal reflux. *Am J Gastroenterol.* 1998;93(7):1060–1063.

73. Govil Y, Khoury R, Katz PO, et al. Anti-reflux therapy improves symptoms in patients with reflux laryngitis [Abstract]. *Gastroenterology.* 1998;114:562.

74. Spechler SJ. Complications of gastroesophageal reflux disease. In: Castell DO, ed. *The Esophagus.* Boston, MA: Little, Brown and Company; 1992:543–556.

75. Lieberman DA, Oehlke M, Helfand M. Risk factors for Barrett's esophagus in community based practice. *Am J Gastroenterol.* 1997;92:1293–1297.

76. Fouad YM, Koury R, Hattlebakk JG, Katz PO, Castell DO. Ineffective esophageal motility: the most common motility disorder in patients with GERD-associated respiratory symptoms. *Am J Gastroenterol.* 1999;94:1464–1467.

77. Johnson LF. New concepts and methods in the study and treatment of gastroesophageal reflux disease. *Med Clin North Am.* 1981;65:1195–1222.

78. Delahunty JE. Acid laryngitis. *J Laryngol Otol.* 1972;86(4):335–342.

79. Sataloff RT. The human voice. *Sci Am.* 1993;267:108–115.

80. Axford SE, Sharp N, Ross PE, et al. Cell biology of laryngeal epithelial defenses in health and disease: preliminary studies. *Ann Otol Rhinol Laryngol.* 2001;110(12):1099–1108.

81. Kamel PL, Hanson D, Kahrilas PJ. Omeprazole for the treatment of posterior laryngitis. *Am J Med.* 1994;96:321.

82. Sataloff RT. Professional singers: the science and art of clinical care. *Am J Otolaryngol.* 1981;8:251–266.

83. Spiegel JR, Sataloff RT, Cohn JR, et al. Respiratory function in singers: medical assessment, diagnoses and treatments. *J Voice.* 1988;2(1):40–50.

84. Hallewell JD, Cole TB. Isolated head and neck symptoms due to hiatus hernia. *Arch Otolaryngol.* 1970;92:499–501.

85. Ossakow SJ, Elta G, Colturi T, et al. Esophageal reflux and dysmotility as the basis for persistent cervical symptoms. *Ann Otol Rhinol Laryngol.* 1987;96:387–392.

86. Kuriloff DB, Chodosh P, Goldfarb R, Ongseng F. Detection of gastroesophageal reflux in the head and neck: the role of scintigraphy. *Ann Otol Rhinol Laryngol.* 1989;98:74–80.

87. Lumpkin SM, Bishop SG, Katz PO. Chronic dysphonia secondary to gastroesophageal reflux disease (GERD): diagnosis using simultaneous dual-probe prolonged pH monitoring. *J Voice.* 1989;3:351–355.

88. McNally PR, Maydonovitch CL, Prosek RA, et al. Evaluation of gastroesophageal reflux as a cause of idiopathic hoarseness. *Dig Dis Sci.* 1989;34:1900–1904.

89. Katz PO. Ambulatory esophageal and hypopharyngeal pH monitoring in patients with hoarseness. *Am J Gastroenterol.* 1990;85:38–40.

90. Freeland AP, Adran GM, Emrys-Roberts E. Globus hystericus and reflux oesophagitis. *J Laryngol Otol.* 1974;88:1025–1031.

91. Pesce G, Caligaris F. Le laringiti posteriori nella pathologia dell'apparato digerente. *Arch Ital Laringol.* 1966;74:77–92.

92. Vaughan CW, Strong MS. Medical management of organic laryngeal disorders. *Otolaryngol Clin North Am.* 1984;17:705–712.

93. Barkin RL, Stein ZL. GE reflux and vocal pitch. *Hosp Pract.* 1989;24(10A):20.

94. Jacob P, Kahrilas PJ, Herzon G. Proximal esophageal pH-metry in patients with "reflux laryngitis." *Gastroenterology.* 1991;100:305–310.

95. Wilson JA, White A, von Haacke NP, et al. Gastroesophageal reflux and posterior laryngitis. *Ann Otol Rhinol Laryngol.* 1989;98:405–410.

96. Cherry J, Margulies S. Contact ulcer of the larynx. *Laryngoscope.* 1968;78:1937–1940.

97. Delahunty JE, Cherry J. Experimentally produced vocal cord granulomas. *Laryngoscope.* 1968;78:1941–1947.

98. Gaynor EB. Gastroesophageal reflux as an etiologic factor in laryngeal complications of intubation. *Laryngoscope.* 1988;98:972–979.

99. Lillemoe KD, Johnson LF, Harmon JW. Role of the components of the gastrodudenal contents in experimental acid esophagitis. *Surgery.* 1982;92:276–284.

100. Johnson LF, Harmon JW. Experimental esophagitis in a rabbit model. Clinical relevance. *J Clin Gastroenterol.* 1986;(8 suppl 1):26–44.

101. Cherry J, Seigel CI, Margulies SI, Donner M. Pharyngeal localization of symptoms of gastroesophageal reflux. *Ann Otol Rhinol Laryngol.* 1970;79:912–914.

102. von Leden H, Moore P. Contact ulcer of the larynx. Experimental observations. *Arch Otolaryngol.* 1960;72:746–752.

103. Toohill RJ, Mushtag E, Lehman RH. Otolaryngologic manifestations of gastroesophageal reflux. In: Sacristan T, Alvarez-Vincent JJ, Bartual J, et al, eds. *Proceedings of XIV World Congress of Otolaryngology—Head and Neck Surgery.* Amsterdam, The Netherlands: Kugler & Ghedini Publications; 1990:3005–3009.

104. Koufman JA, Amin M. Laryngopharyngeal reflux and voice disorders. In: Rubin JS, Sataloff RT, Korovin GS. *Diagnosis and Treatment of Voice Disorders.* 2nd ed. Clifton Park, NY: Delmar Thomson Learning; 2003:381–392.

105. Ormseth EJ, Wong RK. Reflux laryngitis: pathophysiology, diagnosis and management. *Am J Gastroenterol.* 1999;94(10):2812–2817.

106. Richter JE, Hicks DM. Unresolved issues in gastroesophageal reflux-related ear, nose and throat problems. *Am J Gastroenterol.* 1997;92(12):2143–2144.

107. Sone M, Katayama N, Kato T, et al. Prevalence of laryngopharyngeal reflux symptoms: comparison between health checkup examinees and patients

with otitis media. *Otolaryngol–Head Neck Surg.* 2012; 146(4):562–566.

108. Habesoglu TE, Habesoglu M, Kalaycik C, et al. Gastroesophageal reflux disease and tympanoplasty surgical outcome: is there a relationship? *J Laryngol Otol.* 2012;126(6):580–585.

109. Brunworth JD, Mahboubi H, Garg R, et al. Nasopharyngeal acid reflux and Eustachian tube dysfunction in adults. *Ann Otol Rhinol Laryngol.* 2014;123(6):415–419.

110. Rodrigues MM, Dibbern RS, Santos VJ, Passeri LA. Influence of obesity on the correlation between laryngopharyngeal reflux and obstructive sleep apnea. *Braz J Otorhinolaryngol.* 2014;80(1):5–10.

111. Sung MW, Lee WH, Wee JH, et al. Factors associated with hypertrophy of the lingual tonsils in adults with sleep-disordered breathing. *JAMA Otolaryngol Head Neck Surg.* 2013;139(6):598–603.

112. Corvo MA, Eckley CA, Liquidato BM, Castilho GL, Arruda CN. pH salivary analysis of subjects suffering from Sjogren's syndrome and laryngopharyngeal reflux. *Braz J Otorhinolaryngol.* 2012;78(1):81.

113. Sole ML, Conrad J, Bennett M, et al. Pepsin and amylase in oral and tracheal secretions: a pilot study. *Am J Crit Care.* 2014;23(4):334–338.

114. Garland JS, Alex CP, Johnston N, Yan JC, Werlin SL. Association between tracheal pepsin, a reliable marker of gastric aspiration, and head of bed elevation among ventilated neonates. *J Neonatal Perinatal Med.* 2014;7(3):185–192.

115. Ali Mel-S, Bulmer DM, Dettmar PW, Pearson JP. Mucin gene expression in reflux laryngeal mucosa: histological and in situ hybridization observations. *Int J Otolaryngol.* 2014;2014:264075.

116. Eckley CA, Sardinha LR, Rizzo LV. Salivary concentration of epidermal growth factor in adults with reflux laryngitis before and after treatment. *Ann Otol Rhinol Laryngol.* 2013;122(7):440–444.

117. Falk GL, Beattie J, Ing A, et al. Scintigraphy in laryngopharyngeal and gastroesophageal reflux disease: a definitive diagnostic test? *World J Gastroenterol.* 2015; 21(12):3619–3627.

118. Falk M, Van der Wall H, Falk GL. Differences between scintigraphic reflux studies in gastrointestinal reflux disease and laryngopharyngeal reflux disease and correlation with symptoms. *Nucl Med Commun.* 2015; 36(6):625–630.

119. Günbey E, Gören I, Ünal R, Yilmaz M. An evaluation of olfactory function in adults with gastro-esophageal reflux disease [published online October 19, 2015]. *Acta Otolaryngol.* 2016;136(2):214–218.

120. Krawczyk M, Scierski W, Ryzkiel I, et al. Endoscopic evidence of reflux disease in the larynx. *Acta Otolaryngol.* 2014;134(8):831–837.

121. Ozmen S, Yücel OT, Sinici I, et al. Nasal pepsin assay and pH monitoring in chronic rhinosinusitis. *Laryngoscope.* 2008;118(5):890–894.

122. Bercin S, Kutluhan A, Yurttas V, et al. Evaluation of laryngopharyngeal reflux in patients with suspected laryngopharyngeal reflux, chronic otitis media and laryngeal disorders. *Eur Arch Otorhinolaryngol.* 2008; 265:1539–1543.

123. Kantas I, Balatsouras DG, Kamargianis N, et al. The influence of laryngopharyngeal reflux in the healing of laryngeal trauma. *Eur Arch Otorhinolaryngol.* 2009; 266:253–259.

124. Bock JM, Brawley MK, Johnston N, et al. Analysis of pepsin in tracheoesophageal puncture sites. *Ann Otol Rhinol Laryngol.* 2010;119:799–805.

125. Cengiz S, Cengiz MI, Sarac YS. Dental erosion caused by gastroesophageal reflux disease: a case report. *Cases J.* 2009;2:8018.

126. Roth DF, Ferguson BJ. Vocal allergy: recent advances in understanding the role of allergy in dysphonia. *Curr Opin Otolaryngol Head Neck Surg.* 2010;18:176–181.

127. Higo T, Mukaisho K, Ling ZG, et al. An animal model of intrinsic dental erosion caused by gastro-oesophageal reflux disease. *Oral Dis.* 2009;15:360–365.

128. Ranjitkar S, Kaidonis JA, Richards LC, Townsend GC. The effect of CPP-ACP on enamel wear under severe erosive conditions. *Arch Oral Biol.* 2009;54:527–532.

129. Becker S, Schmidt C, Berghaus A, Tschiesner U, Olzowy B, Reichel O. Does laryngopharyngeal reflux cause intraoral burning sensations? A preliminary study. *Eur Arch Otolaryngol.* 2011;268:1375–1381.

130. Chung JH, Tae K, Lee YS, et al. The significance of laryngopharyngeal reflux in benign vocal mucosal lesions. *Otolaryngol HNS.* 2009;141:369–373.

131. Saleh H. Rhinosinusitis, laryngopharyngeal reflux and cough: an ENT viewpoint. *Pulm Pharmacol Ther.* 2009;22:127–129.

132. Randhawa PS, Mansuri S, Rubin JS. Is dysphonia due to allergic laryngitis being misdiagnosed as laryngopharyngeal reflux? *Logoped Phoniatr Vocal.* 2010;35:1–5.

133. Eskiizmir G, Kezirian E. Is there a vicious cycle between obstructive sleep apnea and laryngopharyngeal reflux disease? *Med Hypotheses.* 2009;73:706–708.

134. Suzuki M, Saigusa H, Kurogi R, et al. Arousal in obstructive sleep apnea patients with laryngopharyngeal and gastroesophageal reflux. *Sleep Med.* 2010;11: 356–374.

135. Karkos PD, Leong SC, Benton J, Sastry A, Assimakopoulos DA, Issing WJ. Reflux and sleeping disorders: a systematic review. *J Laryngol Otol.* 2009;123:372–374.

136. Wang L, Liu X, Liu YL, et al. Correlation of pepsin-measured laryngopharyngeal reflux disease with symptoms and signs. *Otolaryngol HNS.* 2010;143: 765–771.

137. Eryuksel E, Dogan M, Olgun S, Kocak I, Celikel T. Incidence and treatment results of laryngopharyngeal reflux in chronic obstructive pulmonary disease. *Eur Arch Otorhinolaryngol.* 2009;266:1267–1271.

138. de la Hoz RE, Christie J, Teamer JA, et al. Reflux symptoms and disorders and pulmonary disease in former World Trade Center rescue and recovery workers and volunteers. *J Occup Environ Med.* 2008;50:1351–1354.

139. Ward PH, Berci G. Observations on the pathogenesis of chronic non-specific pharyngitis and laryngitis. *Laryngoscope.* 1982;92:1377–1382.

140. Von Leden H, Moore P. Contact ulcer of the larynx. Experimental observations. *Arch Otolaryngol.* 1960;72:746–752.

141. Kjellen G, Brudin L. Gastroesophageal reflux disease and laryngeal symptoms. Is there really a causal relationship? *ORL J Otorhinolaryngol Relat Spec.* 1994;56:287–290.

142. Groome M, Cotton JP, Borland M, et al. Prevalence of laryngopharyngeal reflux in a population with gastroesophageal reflux. *Laryngoscope.* 2007;117:1424–1428.

143. Lai YC, Wang PC, Lin JC. Laryngopharyngeal reflux in patients with reflux esophagitis. *World J Gastroenterol.* 2008;14:4523–4528.

144. Qua CS, Wong CH, Gopala K, Goh KL. Gastro-oesophageal reflux disease in chronic laryngitis: prevalence and response to acid-suppressive therapy. *Aliment Pharmacol Ther.* 2007;25:287–295.

145. Galli J, Calo L, Agostino S, et al. Bile reflux as possible risk factor in laryngopharyngeal inflammatory and neoplastic lesions. *Acta Otorhinolaryngol Ital.* 2003;23:377–382.

146. Koufman JA, Wiener GJ, Wu WC, Castell DO. Reflux laryngitis and its sequelae: the diagnostic role of ambulatory 24-hour pH monitoring. *J Voice.* 1988;2(1):78–89.

147. Belafsky PC, Postma GN, Koufman JA. The validity and reliability of the reflux finding score (RFS). *Laryngoscope.* 2001;111:1313–1317.

148. Belafsky PC, Postma GN, Koufman JA. The validity and reliability of the reflux symptom index (RSI). *J Voice.* 2002;16:274–277.

149. Carr MM, Nguyen A, Poje C, et al. Correlation of findings on direct laryngoscopy and bronchoscopy with presence of extraesophageal reflux disease. *Laryngoscope.* 2000;110:1560–1562.

150. McMurray JS, Gerber M, Stern Y, et al. Role of laryngoscopy, dual pH probe monitoring, and laryngeal mucosal biopsy in the diagnosis of pharyngoesophageal reflux. *Ann Otol Rhinol Laryngol.* 2001;110:299–304.

151. Hicks DM, Ours TM, Abelson T, et al. The prevalence of hypopharynx findings associated with gastroesophageal reflux in normal volunteers. *J Voice.* 2002;16:564–579.

152. Close LG. Laryngopharyngeal manifestations of reflux: diagnosis and therapy. *Eur J Gastroenterol Hepatol.* 2002;14(suppl 1):S23–S27.

153. Tauber S, Gross M, Issing WJ. Association of laryngopharyngeal symptoms with gastroesophageal reflux disease. *Laryngoscope.* 2002;112:879–886.

154. Vaezi MF. Ear, nose, and throat manifestations of gastroesophageal reflux disease. *Clin Perspect Gastroenterol.* 2002;5:324–328.

155. Book DT, Rhee JS, Toohill RJ, Smith TL. Perspectives in laryngopharyngeal reflux: an international survey. *Laryngoscope.* 2002;112(8 pt 1):1399–1406.

156. Branski RC, Bhattacharyya N, Shapiro J. The reliability of the assessment of endoscopic laryngeal findings associated with laryngopharyngeal reflux disease. *Laryngoscope.* 2002;112:1019–1024.

157. Noordzij JP, Khidr A, Desper E, et al. Correlation of pH probe-measured laryngopharyngeal reflux with symptoms and signs of reflux laryngitis. *Laryngoscope.* 2002;112:2192–2195.

158. Marambaia O, Andrade NA, Varela DG, et al. Laryngopharyngeal reflux: prospective study that compares early laryngoscopic findings and 2-channel 24-hour pH monitoring. *Rev Brasil Otorrinolaryngol.* 2002;68:527–531.

159. Siupsinskiene N, Adamonis K. Diagnostic test with omeprazole in patients with posterior laryngitis. *Medicina (Kaunas, Lithuania).* 2003;39:47–55.

160. Vaezi MF. Sensitivity and specificity of reflux-attributed laryngeal lesions: experimental and clinical evidence. *Am J Med.* 2003;115(suppl 3A):105S–108S.

161. Issing WJ. Gastroesophageal reflux—a common illness? [in German]. *Laryngorhinootologie.* 2003;82:118–122.

162. Maronian N, Haggitt R, Oelschlager BK, et al. Histologic features of reflux-attributed laryngeal lesions. *Am J Med.* 2003;115(suppl 3A):105S–108S.

163. Burati DO, Duprat ADC, Eckley CA, et al. Gastroesophageal reflux disease: analysis of 157 patients. *Rev Brasil Otorrinolaringol.* 2003;69:458–462.

164. Wang JH, Lou JY, Dong L, et al. Epidemiology of gastroesophageal reflux disease: a general population-based study in Xi-an of Northwest China. *World J Gastroenterol.* 2004;10:1647–1651.

165. Ahmad I, Batch AJ. Acid reflux management: ENT perspective. *J Laryngol Otol.* 2004;118:25–30.

166. Grillo C, Maiolino L, Caminiti D, et al. Gastroesophageal reflux and otolaryngologic diseases. *Acta Medica Mediterrancea.* 2004;20:155–158.

167. Lenderking WR, Hillson E, Crawley JA, et al. The clinical characteristics and impact of laryngopharyngeal reflux disease on health-related quality of life. *Value Health.* 2003;6:560–565.

168. Gaynor EB. Gastroesophageal reflux as an etiologic factor in laryngeal complications of intubation. *Laryngoscope.* 1988;98:972–979.

169. Lillemoe KD, Johnson LF, Harmon JW. Role of the components of the gastroduodenal contents in experimental acid esophagitis. *Surgery.* 1982;92:276–284.

170. Johnson LF, Harmon JW. Experimental esophagitis in a rabbit model. Clinical relevance. *J Clin Gastroenterol.* 1986;8(suppl 1):26–44.

171. Cherry J, Siegel CI, Margulies SI, Donner M. Pharyngeal localization of symptoms of gastroesophageal reflux. *Ann Otol Rhinol Laryngol.* 1970;79:912–914.

172. Chen MY, Ott DJ, Casolo BJ, et al. Correlation of laryngeal and pharyngeal carcinomas and 24-hr pH monitoring of the esophagus and pharynx. *Otolaryngol Head Neck Surg.* 1998;119:460–462.

173. Ludemann JP, Manoukian J, Shaw K, et al. Effects of simulated gastroesophageal reflux on the untraumatized rabbit larynx. *J Otolaryngol.* 1998;27:127–131.

174. Ward PH, Berci G. Observations on the pathogenesis of chronic non-specific pharyngitis and laryngitis. *Laryngoscope.* 1982;92:1377–1382.

175. Von Leden H, Moore P. Contact ulcer of the larynx. Experimental observations. *Arch Otolaryngol.* 1960;72:746–752.

176. Kjellen G, Brudin L. Gastroesophageal reflux disease and laryngeal symptoms. Is there really a causal relationship? *ORL J Otorhinolaryngol Relat Spec.* 1994;56:287–290.

177. Groome M, Cotton JP, Borland M, et al. Prevalence of laryngopharyngeal reflux in a population with gastroesophageal reflux. *Laryngoscope.* 2007;117:1424–1428.

178. Lai YC, Wang PC, Lin JC. Laryngopharyngeal reflux in patients with reflux esophagitis. *World J Gastroenterol.* 2008;14:4523–4528.

179. Qua CS, Wong CH, Gopala K, Goh KL. Gastrooesophageal reflux disease in chronic laryngitis: prevalence and response to acid-suppressive therapy. *Aliment Pharmacol Ther.* 2007;25:287–295.

180. Galli J, Calo L, Agostino S, et al. Bile reflux as possible risk factor in laryngopharyngeal inflammatory and neoplastic lesions. *Acta Otorhinolaryngol Ital.* 2003;23:377–382.

181. Adhami T, Goldblum JR, Richter JE, et al. The role of gastric and duodenal agents in laryngeal injury: an experimental canine model. *Ann J Gastroenterol.* 2004;99:2098–2106.

182. Eckley CA, Michelsohn N, Rizzo LV, et al. Salivary epidermal growth factor concentration in adults with reflux laryngitis. *Otolaryngol Head Neck Surg.* 2004;131:401–406.

183. Eckley CA, Costa HO. Salivary EGF concentration in adults with chronic laryngitis caused by laryngopharyngeal reflux. *Rev Brasil Otorrinolaringol.* 2003;69:590–597.

184. Altman KW, Haines GK III, Hammer ND, Radosevich JA. The H+/K+-ATPase (proton) pump is expressed in human laryngeal submucosal glands. *Laryngoscope.* 2003;113:1927–1930.

185. Johnston N, Dettmar PW, Lively MO, et al. Effect of pepsin on laryngeal stress protein (Sep70, Sep53, and Hsp70) response: role in laryngopharyngeal reflux disease. *Ann Otol Rhino Pharyngol.* 2006;115:47–58.

186. Johnson N, Knight J, Dettmar PW, et al. Pepsin and carbonic anhydrase isoenzyme III as diagnostic markers for laryngopharyngeal reflux disease. *Laryngoscope.* 2004;114:2129–2134.

187. Johnston N, Wells CW, Blumin JH, et al. Receptor-mediated uptake of pepsin by laryngeal epithelial cells. *Ann Otol Rhinol Laryngol.* 2007;116:934–938.

188. Johnston N, Bulmer D, Gill GA, et al. Cell biology of laryngeal epithelial defenses in health and disease: further studies. *Ann Otol Rhinol Laryngol.* 2003;112:481–491.

189. Johnston N, Dettmar PW, Bishworkarma B, et al. Activity/stability of human pepsin: implications for reflux attributed to laryngeal disease. *Laryngoscope.* 2007;117:1036–1039.

190. Ylitalo R, Thibeault SL. Relationship between time of exposure of laryngopharyngeal reflux and gene expression in laryngeal fibroblasts. *Ann Otol Rhinol Laryngol.* 2006;115:775–783.

191. Samuels TL, Handler E, Syring ML, et al. Mucin gene expression in human laryngeal epithelia: effect of laryngopharyngeal reflux. *Ann Otol Rhinol Laryngol.* 2008;117:688–695.

192. Habesoglu TE, Habesoglu M, Surmeli M, et al. Histological changes of rat soft palate with exposure to experimental laryngopharyngeal reflux. *Auris Nasus Larynx.* 2010;37:730–736.

193. Erickson E, Sivansakar M. Simulated reflux decreases vocal fold epithelial barrier resistance. *Laryngoscope.* 2010;120:1569–1575.

194. Johnston N, Wells CW, Samuels TL, Blumin JH. Pepsin in non-acidic refluxate can damage hypopharyngeal epithelial cells. *Ann Otol Rhinol Laryngol.* 2009;118:677–685.

195. Bulmer DM, Ali MS, Brownlee IA, Dettmar PW, Pearson JP. Laryngeal mucosa: its susceptibility to damage by acid and pepsin. *Laryngoscope.* 2010;120:777–782.

196. Samuels TL, Johnston N. Pepsin as a marker of extra-esophageal reflux. *Ann Otol Rhinol Laryngol.* 2010;119:203–208.

197. Richter JE. Role of gastric refluxate in gastroesophageal reflux disease: acid, weak acid and bile. *Am J Med Sci.* 2009;338:89–95.

198. Rees LEN, Pazmany L, Gutowska-Owsiad D, et al. The mucosal immune response to laryngopharyngeal reflux. *Am J Respir Crit Care Med.* 2008;177:1187–1193.

199. Wada T, Sasaki M, Kataoka H, et al. Gastroesophageal and laryngopharyngeal reflux symptoms correlate with histopathologic inflammation of the upper and lower esophagus. *J Clin Gastroenterol.* 2009;43:249–252.

200. Park S, Chun HJ, Keum B, et al. An electron microscope study—correlation of gastroesophageal reflux disease and laryngopharyngeal reflux. *Laryngoscope.* 2010;120:1303–1308.

201. Amin SM, Abdel Maged KH, Naser AY, Aly BH. Laryngopharyngeal reflux with sore throat: an ultrastructural study of oropharyngeal epithelium. *Ann Otol Rhinol Laryngol.* 2009;118:362–367.

202. Ossakow SJ, Elta G, Colturi T, et al. Esophageal reflux and dysmotility as the basis for persistent cervical symptoms. *Ann Otol Rhinol Laryngol.* 1987;96:387–392.

203. Fouad YM, Khoury RM, Hatlebakk JG, Katz PO, Castell DO. Ineffective esophageal motility (IEM) is more prevalent in reflux patients with respiratory symptoms. *Gastroenterology.* 1998;114(suppl 1):A123. Abstract 6506.

204. Postma GN, Tomek MS, Belafsky PC, Koufman JA. Esophageal acid clearance in otolaryngology patients with laryngopharyngeal reflux. *Ann Otol Rhinol Laryngol.* 2001;110:1114–1116.

205. Gerhardt DC, Shuck TJ, Bordeaux RA, Winship DH. Human upper esophageal sphincter. Response to volume, osmotic and acid stimuli. *Gastroenterology.* 1978;75:268–274.

206. Szczesniak MM, Williams RB, Brake HM, Maclean JC, Cole IE, Cook IJ. Upregulation of the esophago-UES relaxation response: a possible pathophysiological

mechanism in suspected reflux laryngitis. *Neurogastroenterol Motil.* 2010;22:381–386.

207. Vardouniotis AS, Karatzanis AD, Tzortzaki E, et al. Molecular pathways and genetic factors in the pathogenesis of laryngopharyngeal reflux. *Eur Arch Otorhinolaryngol.* 2009;266:795–801.

208. Cheng CM, Hsieh CC, Lin CS, et al. Macrophage activation by gastric fluid suggests MMP involvement in aspiration-induced lung disease. *Immunobiology.* 2010; 215:173–181.

209. Chong VH, Jalihal A. Heterotopic gastric mucosal patch of the esophagus is associated with higher prevalence of laryngopharyngeal reflux symptoms. *Eur Arch Otorhinolaryngol.* 2010;267:1793–1799.

210. Salminen P, Ovaska J. Heterotopic gastric mucosal patch in patients with reflux laryngitis: an entity of clinical interest? *Surg Laparosc Endosc Percutan Tech.* 2009;19:361–363.

211. Basseri B, Conklin JL, Mertens RB, Lo SK, Bellack GS, Shaye OA. Heterotopic gastric mucosa (inlet patch) in a patient with laryngopharyngeal reflux (LPR) and laryngeal carcinoma: a case report and review of literature. *Dis Esophagus.* 2009;22:E1–E5.

212. Clark CS, Kraus BB, Sinclair J, Castell DO. Gastroesophageal reflux induced by exercise in healthy volunteers. *JAMA.* 1989;261:3599–3601.

213. Castell DO, *The Esophagus.* 3rd ed. Philadelphia, PA: Lippincott; 1999:222–223.

214. Castell DO. *The Esophagus.* 3rd ed. Philadelphia, PA: Lippincott, 1999:582–583.

215. Castell DO. *The Esophagus.* 3rd ed. Philadelphia, PA: Lippincott; 1999:401.

216. Sataloff RT. The human voice. *Sci Am.* 1993;267:108–115.

217. Spiegel JR, Sataloff RT, Cohn JR, Hawkshaw M, Epstein J. Respiratory function in singers: medical assessment, diagnoses and treatments. *J Voice.* 1988;2: 40–50.

218. Koufmna JA, Wiener GJ, Wu WC, Castell DO. Reflux laryngitis and its sequelae: the diagnostic role of ambulatory 24-hour pH monitoring. *J Voice.* 1988;2(1): 78–89.

219. Gould WJ, Sataloff RT, Spiegel JR. *Voice Surgery.* St. Louis, MO: CV Mosby; 1993.

220. Teisanu E, Heciota D, Dimitriu T, et al. Tulburari Faringolaringiene la Bolnavii cu reflux gastroesofagian. *Rev Chir Oncol Radio ORL Oftalmol Stomatol Otorinolaringol.* 1978;23:279–286.

221. Miko TL. Peptic (contact ulcer) granuloma of the larynx. *J Clin Pathol.* 1989;42:800–804.

222. Bogdassarian RS, Olson NR. Posterior glottic laryngeal stenosis. *Otolaryngol Head Neck Surg.* 1980;88:765–772.

223. Fligny I, Francois M, Aigrain Y, et al. [Subglottic stenosis and gastroesophageal reflux]. *Ann Otolaryngol Chir Cervicofac.* 1989;106:193–196.

224. Havas TE, Priestley J, Lowinger DS. A management strategy for vocal process granulomas. *Laryngoscope.* 1999;109:301–306.

225. Koufman JA. Contact ulcer and granuloma of the larynx. In: Gates G, ed. *Current Therapy in*

*Otolaryngology–Head and Neck Surgery.* 5th ed. St. Louis, MO: Mosby; 1994:456–459.

226. Delahunty JE, Ardran GM. Globus hystericus: a manifestation of reflux oesophagitis? *J Laryngol Otol.* 1970; 84:1049–1054.

227. Wilson JA, Pryde A, Piris J, et al. Pharyngoesophageal dysmotility in globus sensation. *Arch Otolaryngol Head Neck Surg.* 1989;115:1086–1090.

228. Curran AJ, Barry MK, Callanan V, Gormley PK. A prospective study of acid reflux and globus pharyngeus using a modified symptom index. *Clin Otolaryngol Allied Sci.* 1995;20(6):552–554.

229. Shaker R, Milbrath M, Ren J, et al. Esophagopharyngeal distribution of refluxed gastric acid in patients with reflux laryngitis. *Gastroenterology.* 1995;109:1575–1582.

230. Hill J, Stuart RC, Fung HK, et al. Gastroesophageal reflux, motility disorders and psychological profiles in the etiology of globus pharyngis. *Laryngoscope.* 1997;107:1373–1377.

231. Smit CF, van Leeuwen AMJ, Mathus-Vliegen LMH, et al. Gastropharyngeal and gastroesophageal reflux in globus and hoarseness. *Arch Otolaryngol Head Neck Surg.* 2000;126:827–830.

232. Malcomson KG. Radiological findings in globus hystericus. *Br J Radiol.* 1966;39:583–586.

233. Koufman JA, Blalock PD. Functional voice disorders. *Otolaryngol Clin North Am.* 1991;24:1059–1073.

234. Loughlin CJ, Koufman JA. Paroxysmal laryngospasm secondary to gastroesophageal reflux. *Laryngoscope.* 1996;106:1502–1505.

235. Yelken K, Yilmaz A, Guven M, Eyibilen A, Aladag I. Paradoxical vocal fold motion dysfunction in asthma patients. *Respiratory.* 2009;14:729–733.

236. Murry T, Branski RC, Yu K, Cukier-Blaj S, Duflo S, Aviv JE. Laryngeal sensory deficits in patients with chronic cough and paradoxical vocal fold movement disorder. *Laryngoscope.* 2010;120:1576–1581.

237. Spechler SJ, Goyal RK. Barrett's esophagus. *N Engl J Med.* 1986;315:362–371.

238. MacDonald WC, MacDonald JB. Adenocarcinoma of the esophagus and/or gastric cardia. *Cancer.* 1987;60: 1094–1098.

239. Garewal HS, Sampliner R. Barrett's esophagus: a model premalignant lesion for adenocarcinoma. *Prev Med.* 1989;18:749–756.

240. Reid BJ. Barrett's esophagus and esophageal adenocarcinoma. *Gastroenterol Clin North Am.* 1991;20:817–834.

241. Chow WH, Finkle WD, McLaughlin JK, et al. The relation of gastroesophageal reflux disease and its treatment to adenocarcinomas of the esophagus and gastric cardia. *JAMA.* 1995;274(6):474–477.

242. Morrison M. Is chronic gastroesophageal reflux a causative factor in glottic carcinoma? *Otolaryngol Head Neck Surg.* 1988;99:370–373.

243. Olson NR. Aerodigestive malignancy and gastroesophageal reflux disease. *Am J Med.* 1997;103(5A):975–995.

244. Richtsmeier WJ, Eisele D. In vivo anergy reversal with cimetadine in patients with cancer. *Arch Otolaryngol Head Neck Surg.* 1986;112:1074–1077.

245. Richtsmeier WJ, Styczynski P, Johns ME. Selective, histamine-mediated, immunosuppression in laryngeal cancer. *Ann Otol Rhinol Laryngol.* 1987;96:569–572.

246. El-Serag HB, Hepworth EJ, Lee P, Sonnenberg A. Gastroesophageal reflux disease is a risk factor for laryngeal and pharyngeal cancer. *Am J Gastroenterol.* 2001;96:2013–2018.

247. Koufman JA, Burke AJ. The etiology and pathogenesis of laryngeal carcinoma. *Otolaryngol Clin North Am.* 1997;30:1–19.

248. Ward PH, Hanson DG. Reflux as an etiological factor of carcinoma of the laryngopharynx. *Laryngoscope.* 1988;98:1195–1199.

249. Freije JE, Beatty TW, Campbell BH, et al. Carcinoma of the larynx in patients with gastroesophageal reflux. *Am J Otolaryngol.* 1996;17(6):386–390.

250. Ling ZQ, Mukaisho K, Hidaka M, et al. Duodenal contents reflux-induced laryngitis in rats: possible mechanism of enhancement of the causative factors in laryngeal carcinogenesis. *Ann Otol Rhinol Laryngol.* 2007;116:471–478.

251. Del Negro A, Araujo MR, Tincani AJ, et al. Experimental carcinogenesis on the oropharyngeal mucosa of rats with hydrochloric acid, sodium nitrate, and pepsin. *Acta Cir Bras.* 2008;23:337–342.

252. Qadeer MA, Colabianchi N, Strome M, et al. Gastroesophageal reflux and laryngeal cancer: causation or association? *Am J Otolaryngol.* 2006;27:119–128.

253. Reavis KM, Morris CD, Gopal DV, et al. Laryngopharyngeal reflux symptoms better predict the presence of esophageal adenocarcinoma than typical gastroesophageal reflux symptoms. *Ann Surg.* 2004;239:849–858.

254. Reichel O, Issing WJ. Should patients with pH-documented laryngopharyngeal reflux routinely undergo oesophagogastroduodenoscopy? A retrospective analysis. *J Laryngol Otol.* 2007;121:1165–1169.

255. Perry KA, Enestvedt CK, Lorenzo CS, et al. The integrity of esophagogastric junction anatomy in patients with isolated laryngopharyngeal reflux symptoms. *J Gastrointest Surg.* 2008;12:1880–1887.

256. Kuipers EJ. *Helicobacter pylori* and the risk and management of associated diseases: gastritis, ulcer disease, atrophic gastritis and gastric cancer. *Aliment Pharmacol Ther.* 1997;11(S1):71–88.

257. Katsinelos P, Kountouras J, Chatzimavroudis G, et al. Should inspection of the laryngopharyngeal area be part of routine upper gastrointestinal endoscopy? A prospective study. *Dig Liver Dis.* 2009;41:283–288.

258. Sandner A, Illert J, Koitzsh S, Unverzagt S, Schon I. Reflux induces DNA strand breaks and expression changes of MMP1+9+14 in a human miniorgan culture model. *Exp Cell Res.* 2013;319(19):2905–2915.

259. Kelly EA, Samuels TL, Johnston N. Chronic pepsin exposure promotes anchorage-independent growth and migration of a hypopharyngeal squamous cell line. *Otolaryngol Head Neck Surg.* 2014;150(4):618–624.

260. LeBlanc B, Lewis E, Caldito G, Nathan CA. Increased pharyngeal reflux in patients treated for laryngeal cancer: a pilot study. *Otolaryngol Head Neck Surg.* 2015;153(5):791–794.

261. Samuels TL, Pearson AC, Wells CW, Stoner GD, Johnston N. Curcumin and anthocyanin inhibit pepsin-mediated cell damage and carcinogenic changes in airway epithelial cells. *Ann Otol Rhinol Laryngol.* 2013;122(10):632–641.

262. Little PJ, Matthews BL, Glock MS, et al. Extraesophageal pediatric reflux: 24-hour double-probe pH monitoring of 222 children. *Ann Otol Rhinol Laryngol Suppl.* 1997;169:1–16.

263. Wetmore RF. Effects of acid on the larynx of the maturing rabbit and their possible significance to the sudden infant death syndrome. *Laryngoscope.* 1993;103:1242–1254.

264. Landler U. Hollwarth ME, Uray E, et al. [Esophageal function of infants with sudden infant death—risk.] *Klin Padiatr.* 1990;202(1):37–42. German.

265. Kurza R, Schenkeli R, Hollwarth M, et al. [Sleep apnea in infants and the risk of SIDS.] *Monatsschr Kinderheilkd.* 1986; 134(10):17–20. German.

266. Benhamou PH, Dupont C. [Relationship between gastroesophageal reflux and severe malaise in infants.] *Presse Med.* 1992;21(35):1673–1676. French.

267. Spitzer AR, Boyle JT, Tuchman DN, et al. Awake apnea associated with gastroesophageal reflux: a specific clinical syndrome. *J Pediatr.* 1984;104:200–205.

268. McCulloch K, Vidyasagar D, Infantile apnea. *Am Fam Physician.* 1986;34(3):105–114.

269. Jeffery HE, Rahilly P, Read DJ. Multiple causes of asphyxia in infants at high risk for sudden infant death. *Arch Dis Child.* 1983;58(2):92–100.

270. Camfield P, Camfield C, Bagnell P, Rees E. Infant apnea syndrome. A prospective evaluation of etiologies. *Clin Pediatr.* 1982;21(11):684–687.

271. Mark JD, Brooks JG. Sleep-associated airway problems in children. *Pediatr Clin North Am.* 1984;31(4):907–918.

272. Rosen CL, Frost JD Jr, Harrison GM. Infant apnea: polygraphic studies and follow-up monitoring. *Pediatrics.* 1983;71(5):731–736.

273. Haney PJ. Infant apnea: findings on the barium esophagram. *Radiology.* 1983;148(2):425–427.

274. Kahn A, Rebuffat E, Sottiaux M, et al. Sleep apneas and acid esophageal reflux in control infants and in infants with an apparent life-threatening event. *Biol Neonate.* 1990;57(3–4):144–149.

275. Ramet J. Cardiac and respiratory reactivity to gastroesophageal reflux: experimental data in infants. *Biol Neonate.* 1994;6:240–246.

276. Paton JY, Macfadyen U, Williams A, Simpson H. Gastro-oesophageal reflux and apnoeic pauses during sleep in infancy—no direct relation. *Eur J Pediatr.* 1990;149(10):680–686.

277. Paton JY, Nanayakkara CS, Simpson H. Observations on gastro-oesophageal reflux, central apnoea and heart rate in infants. *Eur J Pediatr.* 1990;149(9):608–612.

278. Buts JP, Barudi C, Moulin D, et al. Prevalence and treatment of silent gastro-oesophageal reflux in children with recurrent respiratory disorders. *Eur J Pediatr.* 1986;145(5):396–400.

279. Rahilly PM. The pneumographic and medical investigation of infants suffering apparent life threatening episodes. *J Paediatr Child Health.* 1991;27(60):349–353.

280. Sacre L, Vandenplas Y. Gastroesophageal reflux associated with respiratory abnormalities during sleep. *J Pediatr Gastroenterol Nutr.* 1989;9(1):28–33.

281. Vandenplas Y, Deneyer M, Verlinden M, et al. Gastroesophageal reflux incidence and respiratory dysfunction during sleep in infants: treatment with cisapride. *J Pediatr Gastroenterol Nutr.* 1989;8(1):31–36.

282. Halpern LM, Jolley SG, Tunell WP, et al. The mean duration of gastroesophageal reflux during sleep as an indicator of respiratory symptoms from gastroesophageal reflux in children. *J Pediatr Surg.* 1991;26(6):686–690.

283. Graff MA, Kashlan F, Carter M, et al. Nap studies underestimate the incidence of gastroesophageal reflux. *Pediatr Pulmonol.* 1994;18(40):258–260.

284. Gomes H, Lallemand P. Infant apnea and gastroesophageal reflux. *Pediatr Radiol.* 1992;22(1):8–11.

285. Kurz R, Hollwarth M, Fasching M, et al. Combined disturbance of respiratory regulation and esophageal function in early infancy. *Prog Pediatr Surg.* 1985;18:52–61.

286. Singareddy R, Moole S, Calhoun S, Vocalan P, Tsaoussoglou M. Medical complaints are more common in young school-aged children with parent reported insomnia symptoms. *J Clin Sleep Med.* 2009;5:549–553.

287. Indrio F, Riezzo G, Raimondi F, Cavallo L, Francavilla R. Regurgitation in healthy and non-healthy infants. *Ital J Pediatr.* 2009;35:39.

288. Van Houtte E, Van Lierde K, Claeys S. Pathophysiology and treatment of muscle tension dysphonia: a review of the current knowledge. *J Voice.* 2011;25:202–207.

289. Ulualp SO, Rodriguez S, Cunningham S, et al. Pharyngeal pH monitoring in infants with laryngitis. *Otolaryngol Head Neck Surg.* 2007;137:776–779.

290. Block BB, Brodsky L. Hoarseness in children: the role of laryngopharyngeal reflux. *Int J Ped Otorhinolaryngol.* 2007;71:1361–1369.

291. Hoa M, Kingsley EL, Coticchia JM. Correlating the clinical course of recurrent croup with endoscopic findings: a retrospective observational study. *Ann Otol Rhinol Laryngol.* 2008;117:464–469.

292. Barreto VM, D'Avila JS, Sales NJ, et al. Laryngeal and vocal evaluation in untreated growth hormone deficient adults (IGHD). *Otolaryngol HNS.* 2009;140:37–42.

293. Dogru M, Kuran G, Haytoglu S, Dengiz R, Arikan OK. Role of laryngopharyngeal reflux in the pathogenesis of otitis media with effusion. *J Int Adv Otol.* 2015;11(1):66–71.

294. Abdel-Aziz MM, El-Fattah AM, Abdalla AF. Clinical evaluation of pepsin for laryngopharyngeal reflux in children with otitis media with effusion. *Int J Pediatr Otorhinolaryngol.* 2013;77(10):1765–1770.

295. Katra R, Kabelka Z, Jurovcik M, et al. Pilot study: association between *Helicobacter pylori* in adenoid hyperplasia and reflux episodes detected by multiple intraluminal impedance in children. *Int J Pediatr Otorhinolaryngol.* 2014;78(8):1243–1249.

296. Miura MS, Mascaro M, Rosenfeld RM. Association between otitis media and gastroesophageal reflux: a systematic review. *Otolaryngol Head Neck Surg.* 2012;146(3):345–352.

297. Martines F, Salvago P, Ferrara S, et al. Factors influencing the development of otitis media among Sicilian children affected by upper respiratory tract infections [published online July 21, 2015]. *Braz J Otorhinolaryngol.* 2016;82(2):215–222.

298. Nation J, Kaufman M, Allen M, Sheyn A, Coticchia J. Incidence of gastroesophageal reflux disease and positive maxillary antral cultures in children with symptoms of chronic rhinosinusitis. *Int J Pediatr Otorhinolaryngol.* 2014;78(2):218–222.

299. Luo HN, Yang QM, Sheng Y, et al. Role of pepsin and pepsinogen: linking laryngopharyngeal reflux with otitis media with effusion in children. *Laryngoscope.* 2014;124(7):E294–E300.

300. Iannella G, Di Nardo G, Plateroti R, et al. Investigation of pepsin in tears of children with laryngopharyngeal reflux disease [published online October 30, 2015]. *Int J Pediatr Otorhinolaryngol.* 2015;79(12):2312–2315.

301. Andrews TM, Orobello N. Histologic versus pH probe results in pediatric laryngopharyngeal reflux. *Int J Pediatr Otorhinolaryngol.* 2013;77(5):813–816.

302. Ott DJ. Gastroesophageal reflux: what is the role of barium studies? *Am J Roentgenol.* 1994;162:627–629.

303. Thompson JK, Koehler RE, Richter JE. Detection of gastroesophageal reflux: value of barium studies compared with 24-hour pH monitoring. *Am J Roentgenol.* 1994;162:621–626.

304. Ott DJ, Wu WC, Gelfand DW. Reflux esophagitis revisited: prospective analysis of radiologic accuracy. *Gastrointest Radiol.* 1981;6:1–7.

305. Richter JE, Castell DO. Gastroesophageal reflux. Pathogenesis, diagnosis, and therapy. *Ann Intern Med.* 1982;97:93–103.

306. Sellar RJ, DeCaestecker JS, Heading RC. Barium radiology: a sensitive test for gastro-oesophageal reflux. *Clin Radiol.* 1987;38:303–307.

307. Malmud LS, Fisher RS. Radionuclide studies of esophageal transit and gastroesophageal reflux. *Semin Nucl Med.* 1982;12(2):104–115.

308. Jenkins AF, Cowan RJ, Richter JE. Gastroesophageal scintigraphy: is it a sensitive test for gastroesophageal reflux disease? *J Clin Gastroenterol.* 1985;7:127.

309. Ismail-Beigi F, Horton PF, Pope CE Jr. Histological consequences of gastroesophageal reflux in man. *Gastroenterology.* 1970;58:163–174.

310. DeVault KR, Castell DO. Guidelines for the diagnosis and treatment of gastroesophageal reflux disease. *Arch Intern Med.* 1995;155:2165–2173.

311. Hetzel DJ, Dent J, Reed WD, et al. Healing and relapse of severe peptic esophagitis after treatment with omeprazole. *Gastroenterology.* 1988;95:903–912.

312. Koufman JA. Personal communication. June 2004.

313. Johnson LF. DeMeester TR. Twenty-four hour pH monitoring of the distal esophagus. *Am J Gastroenterol.* 1974;62:325–332.

314. Wiener GJ, Richter JE, Copper PA, et al. The symptom index: a clinically important parameter of ambulatory 24-hour esophageal pH monitoring. *Am J Gastroenterol.* 1988;83(4):358–361.

315. Dobhan R, Castell DO. Normal and abnormal proximal esophageal acid exposure: results of ambulatory dual probe pH monitoring. *Am J Gastroenterol.* 1993; 88:25–29.

316. Schnatz PE, Castell JA, Castell DO. Pulmonary symptoms associated with gastroesophageal reflux: use of ambulatory pH monitoring to diagnose and to direct therapy. *Am J Gastroenterol.* 1996;91:1715–1718.

317. Shi G, des Varannes SB, Scarpignato C, Le Rhun M Galmiche J-P. Reflux related symptoms in patients with normal oesophageal exposure to acid. *Gut.* 1995; 37:457–464.

318. Shaker R, Bardan E, Gu C, et al. Intrapharyngeal distribution of gastric acid refluxate. *Laryngoscope.* 2003; 113:1182–1191.

319. Bilgen C, Ogut F, Kesimli-Dinc H, et al. The comparison of an empiric proton pump inhibitor trial vs. 24-hour double-probe pH monitoring in laryngopharyngeal reflux. *J Laryngol Otol.* 2003;117:386–390.

320. Maldonado A, Diederich L, Castell D, et al. Laryngopharygeal reflux identified using a new catheter design: defining normal values and excluding artifacts. *Laryngoscope.* 2003;113:349–355.

321. Sato K, Umeno H, Chitose S, Nakashima T. Tetraprobe, 24-hour pH monitoring for laryngopharyngeal reflux: a technique for simultaneous study of hypopharynx, esophagus and stomach. *J Laryngol Otol.* 2009;123(suppl 31):117–122.

322. Sato K, Umeno H, Chitose S, Nakashima T. Patterns of laryngopharyngeal and gastroesophageal reflux. *J Laryngol Otol.* 2009;123(suppl 31):42–47.

323. Zelenik K, Matousek P, Urban O, Schwarz P, Starek I, Kominek P. Globus pharyngeus and extraesophageal reflux: simultaneous pH <4.0 and pH <5.0 analysis. *Laryngoscope.* 2010;120:2160–2164.

324. Vaezi MF, Richter J, Stasney CR, et al. A randomized double-blind placebo controlled study of acid suppression for the treatment of suspected laryngopharyngeal reflux. *Gastroenterology.* 2004;126:A40.

325. Ulualp SO, Toohill RJ, Shaker R, et al. Outcomes of acid suppressive therapy in patients with posterior laryngitis. *Otolaryngol Head Neck Surg.* 2001;124:16–22.

326. El-Sayed Ali M. Laryngopharyngal reflux: diagnosis and treatment of a controversial disease. *Curr Opin Allergy Clin Immunol.* 2008;8:28–33.

327. Reichel O, Issing WJ. Impact of different pH thresholds for 24-hour dual probe pH monitoring in patients with suspected laryngopharyngeal reflux. *J Laryngol Otol.* 2008;122(5):485–489.

328. Friedman M, Hamilton C, Samuelson CG, et al. The value of routine pH monitoring in the diagnosis and treatment of laryngopharyngeal reflux. *Otolaryngol Head Neck Surg.* 2012 Jun;146(6):952–958.

329. Carroll TL, Fedore LW, Aldahlawi MM. pH impedance and high-resolution manometry in laryngopharyngeal reflux disease high-dose proton pump inhibitor failures. *Laryngoscope.* 2012;122(11):2473–2481.

330. Komatsu Y, Hoppo T, Jobe BA. Proximal reflux as a cause of adult-onset asthma: the case for hypopharyngeal impedance testing to improve the sensitivity of diagnosis. *JAMA Surg.* 2013;148(1):50–58.

331. Vailati C, Mazzoleni G, Bondi S, et al. Oropharyngeal pH monitoring for laryngopharyngeal reflux: is it a reliable test before therapy? *J Voice.* 2013;27(1):84–89.

332. Jette ME, Gaumnitz EA, Birchall MA, Welham NV, Thibeault SL. Correlation between reflux and multichannel intraluminal impedance pH monitoring in untreated volunteers. *Laryngoscope.* 2014;124(10): 2345–2351.

333. Becker V, Graf S, Schlag C, et al. First agreement analysis and day-to-day comparison of pharyngeal pH monitoring with pH/impedance monitoring in patients with suspected laryngopharyngeal reflux. *J Gastrointest Surg.* 2012;16(6):1096–1101.

334. Gooi Z, Ishman SL, Bock JM, Blumin JH, Akst LM. Changing patterns in reflux care: 10-year comparison of ABEA members. *Ann Otol Rhinol Laryngol.* 2015; 124(12):940–946.

335. Pandolfino JE, Kahrilas PJ. Prolonged pH monitoring: Bravo capsule. *GI Clin North Am.* 2005;15:307–318.

336. Wu JCY. Combined multichannel intraluminal impedance and pH monitoring for patients with suspected laryngopharyngeal reflux: is it ready to use? *J Neurogastroenterol Motil.* 2010;16:108–109.

337. Lee BE, Kim GH, Ryu DY, et al. Combined dual channel impedance/pH-metry in patients with suspected laryngopharyngeal reflux. *J Neurogastroenterol Motil.* 2010;16:157–165.

338. Loots CM, Benninga MA, Davidson GP, Omari TI. Addition of pH-impedance monitoring (pH-MII) to standard pH monitoring increases the yield of symptom association analysis in infants and children with gastroesophageal reflux. *J Pediatr.* 2009;154:248–252.

339. Tutuian R, Castell DO. Reflux monitoring: role of combined multi-channel intraluminal impedance and pH. *GI Clin North Am.* 2005;15:361–371.

340. Musser J, Kelchner L, Nelis-Strunjas J, Montorse M. A comparision of rating scales used in the diagnosis of estraesophagel reflux. *J Voice.* 2011;25:293–300.

341. Park K, Choi S, Kwon S, Yon S, Kim S. Diagnosis of laryngopharyngeal reflux among globus patients. *Otolaryngol Head Neck Surg.* 2006;134:81–85.

342. Barry D, Vaezi M. Laryngoparyngeal reflux: more questions than answers. *Cleveland Clin J Med.* 2010; 77(5):327–334.

343. Qadeer MA, Phillips CO, Lopez AR, et al. Proton pump inhibitor therapy for suspected GERD-related chronic laryngitis: a meta-analysis of randomized controlled trials. *Am J Gastroenterol.* 2006;101(11):2646–2654.

344. Ford CN. Evaluation and management of laryngopharyngeal reflux. *JAMA*. 2005;294(12):1534–1540.
345. Belafsky PC, Postma GN, Koufman JA. Validity and reliability of the reflux symptom index (RSI). *J Voice*. 2002;16(2):274–277.
346. Wiener GJ, Tsukashima R, Kelly C, et al. Oropharyngeal pH monitoring for the detection of liquid and aerosolized supraesophagel gastric reflux. *J Voice*. 2009;23(4):498–504.
347. Koufman JA. The otolaryngologic manifestations of gastroesophageal reflux disease (GERD): a clinical investigation of 225 patients using ambulatory 24-hour pH monitoring and an experimental investigation of the role of acid and pepsin in the development of laryngeal injury. *Laryngoscope*. 1991;101(4 Pt 2, suppl 53):1–78.
348. Golub JS, Johns MM 3rd, Lim JH, DelGaudio JM, Klein AM. Comparison of an oropharyngeal pH probe and a standard duel pH probe for the diagnosis of laryngopharyngeal reflux. *Ann Otol Rhinol Laryngol*. 2009;118(1):1–5.
349. Friedman M, Hamiliton C, Samielson CG, et al. The value of routine pH monitoring in the diagnosis and treatment of laryngopharyngeal reflux. *Otolaryngol–Head Neck Surg*. 2012;146(6):952–958.
350. Vailati C, Mazzoleni G, Bondi S, Passaretti S, Bussi M, Testoni P. Oropharyngeal pH-monitoring with the Restech probe for laryngo-pharyngeal reflux: a new reliable test before PPI therapy? *Gastroenterology*. 2012;142(5 suppl 1):S-424.
351. Friedman M, Maley A, Kelley K, et al. Impact of pH monitoring on laryngopharyngeal reflux treatment: improved complicance and symptom resolution. *Otolaryngol Head Neck Surg*. 2011;144(4):558–562.
352. Barrett J, Peghini P, Katz P, et al. Ineffective esophageal motility (IEM): the most common manometric abnormality in GERD. (Abstract 66.) *Gastroenterology*. 1997;112.
353. Johnson PE, Koufman JA, Nowak LJ, et al. Ambulatory 24-hour double-probe pH monitoring: the importance of manometry. *Laryngoscope*. 2001;111:1970–1975.
354. Johnson LF, DeMeester TR. Twenty-four hour pH monitoring of the distal esophagus. *Am J Gastroenterol*. 1974;62:325–332.
355. Rosen SN, Pope CE Jr. Extended esophageal pH monitoring. An analysis of the literature and assessment of its role in the diagnosis and management of gastroesophageal reflux. *J Clin Gastroenterol*. 1989;11:260–270.
356. Mattox H III, Richter JE. Prolonged ambulatory esophageal pH monitoring in the evaluation of gastroesophageal reflux disease. *Am J Med*. 1990;89:345–356.
357. Richter JE, Bradley LA, DeMeester TR, Wu WC. Normal 24-hour ambulatory esophageal pH values: Influence of study center, pH electrode, age and gender. *Dig Dis Sci*. 1992;37:849–856.
358. Johansson KE, Tibbling L. Gastric secretion and reflux pattern in reflux oesophagitis before and during ranitidine treatment. *Scand J Gastroenterol*. 1986;21(4):487–492.
359. Haase GM, Ross MN, Gance-Cleveland B, Kolack KE. Extended four-channel esophageal pH monitoring: the importance of acid reflux patterns at the middle and proximal levels. *J Pediatr Surg*. 1988;23(1 Pt 2):32–37.
360. Lehamn G, Rogers D, Cravens E, Flueckiger J. Prolonged pH probe testing less than 5 cm above the lower esophageal sphincter (LES): establishing normal control values. *Gastroenterology*. 1990;98:77.
361. Weusten BL, Akkermans LM, vanBerge-Henegouwen GP, Smout AJ. Spatiotemporal characteristics of physiological gastroesophageal reflux. *Am J Physiol*. 1994;266(3 Pt 1):G357–G362.
362. Sloan S, Rademaker AW, Kahrilas PJ. Determinants of gastroesophageal junction incompetence: hiatal hernia, lower esophageal sphincter, or both? *Ann Intern Med*. 1992;117:977–982.
363. Palmer ED. The hiatus hernia-esophagitis-esophageal stricture complex. Twenty-year prospective study. *Am J Med*. 1968;44:566–579.
364. Sloan S. Kakrilas PJ. Impairment of esophageal emptying with hiatal hernia. *Gastroenterology*. 1991;100:596–605.
365. NIH. Consensus Conference. *Helicobacter pylori* in peptic ulcer disease. NIH Consensus Development Panel on Helicobacter pylori in peptic ulcer disease. *JAMA*. 1994;272:65–69.
366. World Health Organization. Schistosomes, liver flukes and *Helicobacter pylori*. *IARC Monograph on the Evaluation of Carcinogen Risks to Humans*. 1994;61:177–220.
367. Nilius M, Malfertheiner P. Diagnostische Verfahren bei *Helicobacter-pylori* Infektion. In: Malfertheiner P, Hrsg. *Helicobacter pylori: Von der Grundlage zur Therapie*. Stuttgart, Germany: George Thieme Verlag; 1996;139–147.
368. Yilmaz T, Bajin MD, Gunaydin RO, Ozer S, Sozen T. Laryngopharyngeal reflux and *Helicobacter pylori*. *World J Gastroenterol*. 2014;20(27):8964–8970.
369. Cekin E, Ozyurt M, Erkul E, et al. The association between *Helicobacter pylori* and laryngopharyngeal reflux in laryngeal pathologies. *Ear Nose Throat J*. 2012;91(3):E6–E9.
370. Siupsinskiene N, Jurgutaviciute V, Katutiene I, et al. *Helicobacter pylori* infection in laryngeal diseases. *Eur Arch Otorhinolaryngol*. 2013;270(8):2283–2288.
371. Islam A, Oguz H, Yucel M, et al. Does *Helicobacter pylori* exist in vocal fold pathologies and in the interarytenoid region? *Dysphagia*. 2013;28(3):382–387.
372. Wo JM, Grist WJ, Gussack G, et al. Empiric trial of high-dose omeprazole in patients with posterior laryngitis: a prospective study. *Am J Gastroenterol*. 1997;92:2160–2165.
373. Metz DC, Childs ML, Ruiz C, Weinstein GS. Pilot study of the oral omeprazole test for reflux laryngitis. *Otolaryngol Head Neck Surg*. 1997;16:41–46.
374. Kuo B, Castell DO. Optimal dosing of omeprazole 40 mg daily: effects on gastric and esophageal pH and serum gastrin in healthy controls. *Am J Gastroenterol*. 1996;91:1532–1538.

375. Jacobson BH, Johnson A, Grywalski C, et al. The Voice Handicap Index (VHI): development and validation. *J Speech-Lang Pathol.* 1997;6:66–70.

376. Belafsky PC, Postma GN, Koufman JA. The validity and reliability of the reflux finding score. *Laryngoscope.* 2001;111:1313–1317.

377. Rivicki DA, Wood M, Maton PN, et al. The impact of gastroesophageal reflux disease on health-related quality of life. *Am J Med.* 1998;104:252–258.

378. Lenderking WR, Hillson E, Rawler C, et al. The clinical characteristics and impact of laryngopharyngeal reflux disease on health-related quality of life. *Value Health.* 2003;6:560–565.

379. Andersson O, Rydén A, Ruth M, Moller RY, Finizia C. Development and validation of a laryngopharyngeal reflux questionnaire, the Pharyngeal Reflux Symptoms Questionnaire. *Scand J Gastroenterol.* 2010; 45:147–159.

380. Oyer SL, Anderson LC, Halum SL. Influence of anxiety and depression on the predictive value of the Reflux Symptom Index. *Ann Otol Rhinol Laryngol.* 2009;118:687–692.

381. Elam JC, Ishman SL, Dunbar KB, Clarke JO, Gourin CG. The relationship between depressive symptoms and Voice Handicap Index scores in laryngopharyngeal reflux. *Laryngoscope.* 2010;120:1900–1903.

382. Cheung TK, Lam PK, Wei WI, et al. Quality of life in patients with laryngopharyngeal reflux. *Digestion.* 2009;79:52–57.

383. Nishimura K, Fujita H, Tanaka Y, et al. Endoscopic classification for reflux pharyngolaryngitis. *Dis Esophagus.* 2010;23:20–26.

384. Bell NJ, Burget DL, Howden CW, et al. Appropriate acid suppression for the management of gastro-esophageal reflux disease. *Digestion.* 1992;51(suppl 1):59–67.

385. Johnson LF, DeMeester TR. Elevation of the head of the bed, bethanecol and antacid form tablets on gastroesophageal reflux. *Dig Dis Sci.* 1981;26:673.

386. Scott DR, Simon RA. Supraesophageal reflux: correlation of position and occurrence of acid reflux-effect of head-of-bed elevation on supine reflux. *J Allergy Clin Immunol Pract.* 2015;3(3):356–361.

387. Schallom M, Dykeman B, Metheny N, Kirby J, Pierce J. Head-of-bed elevation and early outcomes of gastrif reflux, aspiration and pressure ulcers: a feasibility study. *Am J Crit Care.* 2015;24(1):57–66.

388. Richter JE, Castell DO. Drugs, foods, and other substances in the cause and treatment of reflux esophagitis. *Med Clin North Am.* 1981;65:1223–1234.

389. Becker DJ, Sinclair J, Castell DO, Wu WC. A comparison of high and low fat meals on postprandial esophageal acid exposure. *Am J Gastroenterol.* 1989;84: 782–786.

390. Wright LE, Castell DO. The adverse effect of chocolate on lower esophageal sphincter pressure. *Am J Dig Dis.* 1975;20:703–707.

391. Dent J, Dodds WJ, Friedman RH, et al. Mechanism of gastroesophageal reflux in recumbent asymptomatic human subjects. *J Clin Invest.* 1980;65:256–267.

392. Koufman JA. Low-acid diet for recalcitrant laryngopharyngeal reflux: therapeutic benefits and their implications. *Ann Otol Rhinol Laryngol.* 2011;120:281–287.

393. Hamdan AL, Nassar J, Dowli A, Al Zaghal Z, Sabri A. Effect of fasting on laryngopharyngeal reflux disease in male subjects. *Eur Arch Otorhinolaryngol.* 2012; 269(11):2361–2366.

394. Jaworek A, Krane N, Lyons K, Sataloff RT. *Laryngopharyngeal Reflux and Gluten Sensitivity.* The Voice Foundation's 44th Annual Symposium on Care of the Professional Voice & International Association of Phonosurgery. Philadelphia, Pennsylvania, May 31, 2015.

395. Sapone A, Bai JC, Ciacci C, et al. Spectrum of gluten-related disorders: consensus on new nomenclature and classification. *BMC Med.* 2012;10:13.

396. Fasano A, Berti I, Gerarduzzi T, et al. Prevalence of celiac disease in at-risk and not-at-risk groups in the United States: a large multicenter study. *Arch Intern Med.* 2003;163(3):286–292.

397. Mansueto P, Seidita A, D'Alcamo A, Carrocio A. Non-celiac gluten sensitivity: literature review. *J Am Coll Nutr.* 2014;33(1):39–54.

398. Leonard M, Vasagar B. US perspective on gluten-related diseases. *Clin Exp Gastroenterol.* 2014;7:25–37.

399. Volta U, Tovoli F, Cicola R, et al. Serological tests in gluten sensitivity (nonceliac gluten intolerance). *J Clin Gastroenterol.* 2012;46:680–685.

400. Gujral N, Freeman H, Thomson ABR. Celiac disease: prevalence, diagnosis, pathogenensis, and treatment. *World J Gastroenterol.* 2012;46:680–685.

401. Fasano A, Berti I, Gerarduzzi T, et al. Prevalence of celiac disease in at-risk and not-at-risk groups in the United States, a large multicenter study. *Arch Intern Med.* 2003;163:286–292.

402. Iovino P, Ciacci C, Sabbatini F, et al. Esophageal impairment in adult celiac disease with steatorrhea. *Am J Gastroenterol.* 1998;93:1243–1249.

403. Lucendo AJ. Esophageal manifestations of celiac disease. *Dis Esophagus.* 2011;24:470–475.

404. Giorgetti GM, Tursi A, Brandimarte G, et al. Dysmotility-like dyspeptic symptoms in celiac patients: role of gluten and *Helicobacter pylori* infection. *Dig Liver Dis.* 2000;32:73–74.

405. Chiarioni G, Bassotti G, Germani U, et al. Gluten-free diet normalizes mouth-to-cecum transit of a caloric meal in adult patients with celiac disease. *Dig Dis Sci.* 1997;42:2100–2105.

406. Fraquelli M, Bardella MT, Peracchi M, et al. Gallbladder emptying and somatostatin and cholecystokinin plasma levels in celiac disease. *Am J Gastroenterol.* 1999;94:1866–1870.

407. Bai JC, Maurino E, Martinez C, et al. Abnormal colonic transit time in untreated celiacsprue. *Acta Gastroenterol Latinoam.* 1995;25:277–284.

408. Usai P, Manca R, Cuomo R, et al. Effect of gluten-free diet on preventing recurrence of gastroenterol reflux disease-related symptoms in adult celiac patients with nonerosive reflux disease. *J Gastroenterol Hepatol.* 2008;23:1368–1372.

409. Nachman F, Vazquez H, Gonzalez A, et al. Gastro-esophageal reflux symptoms in patients with celiac disease and the effect of a gluten-free diet. *Clin Gastroenterol Hepatol.* 2011;9:214–219.

410. Lamanda R, Panarese A, De Stefano S. Coeliac disease and gastroesophageal non-erosive reflux: prevalence and effect of gluten-free diet. *Dig Liver Dis.* 2009; 41(suppl 1):S90.

411. Revicki DA, Wood M, Wiklund I, Crawley J. Reliability and validity of the gastrointestinal symptom rating scale in patients with gastroesophagael reflux disease. *Qual Life Res.* 1998;7:75–83.

412. Tursi A. The treatment of gastro-esophagal reflux disease in adult celiac disease. *J Clin Gastroenterol.* 2004; 38(8):724–725.

413. Collin P, Mustalahti K, Kyronpalo S, et al. Should we screen reflux oesophagitis patients for celiac disease? *Eur J Gastroenterol Hepatol.* 2004;16:917–920.

414. Cuomo A, Romano M, Rocco A, et al. Reflux oesophagitis in adult celiac disease: beneficial effect of a gluten free diet. *Gut.* 2003;52:514–517.

415. Wex T, Monkemuller K, Kuester D. Zonulin is not increased in the cardiac and esophageal mucosa of patients with gastroesophageal reflux disease. *Peptides.* 2009;30:1082–1087.

416. Rubio-Tapia A, Hill ID, Kelly CP, et al. American College of Gastroenterology clinical guideline: diagnosis and management of celiac disease. *Am J Gastroenterol.* 2013;108(5):656–677.

417. Volta U, Tovoli F, Cicola R, et al. Serological tests in gluten sensitivity (nonceliac gluten intolerance). *J Clin Gastroenterol.* 2012;46:680–685.

418. Leffler DA, Schuppan D. Update on serologic testing in celiac disease. *Am J Gastroenterol.* 2010;105:2520–2524.

419. Kabbani TA, Vanga RR, Leffler DA, et al. Celiac disease or non-celiac gluten sensitivity? An approach to clinical differential diagnosis. *Am J Gastroenterol.* 2014; 109:741–746.

420. Castillo NE, Thimmaiah GT, Leffler DA. The present and future in the diagnosis and management of celiac disease. *Gastroenterol Rep.* 2015;3(1):3–11.

421. Lundin KEA, Alaedini A. Non-celiac gluten sensitivity. *Gastrointest Endoscopy Clin N Am.* 2012;22:723–734.

422. Kikendall JW, Friedman AC, Oyewole MA, et al. Pill-induced esophgeal injury: case reports and review of the medical literature. *Dig Dis Sci.* 1983;28:174–182.

423. de Groen PC, Lubbe DF, Hirsch LJ, et al. Esophagitis associated with the use of alendronate. *N Engl J Med.* 1996;335(14):1016–1021.

424. Curcic J, Schwizer A, Kaufman E, et al. Effects of baclofen on the functional anatomy of the oesophago-gastric junction and proximal stomach in healthy volunteers and patients with GERD assessed by magnetic resonance imaging and high-resolution manometry: a randomized controlled double-blind study. *Aliment Pharmacol Ther.* 2014;40(10):1230–1240.

425. Cossentino MJ, Mann K, Armbruster SP, Lake JM, Maydonovitch C, Wong RK. Randomised clinical trial: the effect of baclofen in patients with gastro-oesophageal

reflux—a randomized prospective study. *Ailment Pharmacol Ther.* 2012;35(9):1036–1044.

426. Abbasinazari M, Panahi Y, Mortazavi SA, et al. Effect of a combination of omeprazole plus sustained release baclofen versus omeprazole alone on symptoms of patients with gastroesophageal reflux disease (GERD). *Iran J Pharm Res.* 2014;13(4):1221–1226.

427. Scarpellini E, Boecxstaens V, Farre R, et al. Effect on baclofen on the acid pocket at the gastroesophageal junction. *Dis Esophagus.* 2015;28(5):488–495.

428. Li S, Shi S, Chen F, Lin J. The effects of baclofen for the treatment of gastroesophageal reflux disease: a meta-analysis of randomized controlled trials. *Gastroenterol Res Pract.* 2014;2014:307805.

429. Vadlamudi NB, Hitch MC, Dimmitt RA, Thame KA. Baclofen for the treatment of pediatric GERD. *J Pediatr Gastroenterol Nutr.* 2013;57(6):808–812.

430. Xu X, Chen Q, Luang S, Lu H, Qiu Z. Successful resolution of refactory chronic cough induced by gastroesophageal reflux with treatment of baclofen. *Cough.* 2012;8(1):8.

431. Xu XH, Yang ZM, Chen Q, et al. Therapeutic efficacy of baclofen in refractory gastroesophageal reflux-induced chronic cough. *World J Gastroenterol.* 2013; 19(27):4386–4392.

432. Blondeau K, Boecxstaens V, Rommel N, et al. Baclofen improves symptoms and reduces postprandial flow events in patients with rumination and supragastric bleching. *Clin Gastroenterol Hepatol.* 2012;10(4):379–384.

433. Orr WC, Goodrich S, Wright S, Shepherd K, Mellow M. The effect of baclofen on nocturnal gastroesophageal reflux and measures of sleep quality: a randomized, crossover trial. *Neurogastroenterol Motil.* 2012; 24(6):553–559.

434. Sontag S, Robinson M, McCallum RW, et al. Ranitidine therapy for gastroesophageal reflux disease. Results of a large double blind trial. *Arch Intern Med.* 1987;147:1485–1491.

435. Euler AR, Murdocck RH Jr, Wilson TH, et al. Ranitidine is effective therapy for erosive esophagitis. *Am J Gastroenterol.* 1993;88:520–524.

436. Vigneri S, Termini R, Leandro G, et al. A comparison of five maintenance therapies for reflux esophagitis. *N Engl J Med.* 1995;333:1106–1110.

437. Feldman M, Burton ME. Histamine 2-receptor antagonists: standard therapy for acid-peptic diseases. *N Engl J Med.* 1990;323:1672–1680.

438. Van Thiel DH, Gavaler JS, Smith WI Jr, Paul G. Hypothalamic-pituitary-gonadal dysfunction in men using cimetidine. *N Engl J Med.* 1979;300:1012–1015.

439. Enzmann GD, Leonard JM, Paulsen CA. Effects of cimetidine on reproductive function in men [Abstract]. *Clin Res.* 1981;29(1):26A.

440. Carlson HE, Ippoliti AF, Swerdloff RS. Endocrine effects of acute and chronic cimetidine administration. *Dig Dis Sci.* 1981;26(5):428–432.

441. Winters SJ, Lee J, Teoen P. Competition of the histamine $H_2$-antagonist cimetidine for androgen binding sites in man. *J Androl.* 1980;1(30):111–114.

442. Jensen RT, Collen MJ, Pandol SJ, et al. Cimetidine-induced impotence and breast changes with gastric hypersecretory states. *N Engl J Med.* 1989;308(15):383–387.

443. Malagelada JR, Edis AJ, Adson MA, et al. Medical and surgical options in the management of patients with gastrinoma. *Gastroenterology.* 1983;85:1524–1532.

444. DiPadova C, Roine R, Frezza M, et al. Effects of ranitidine on blood alcohol levels after ethanol ingestion. *JAMA.* 1992;267(1):83–86.

445. Sontag S, O'Connell SA, Greenlee HB, et al. Is gastroesophageal reflux a factor in some asthmatics? *Am J Gastroenterol.* 1987;82:119–126.

446. Harper PC, Bergner A, Kaye MD. Antireflux treatment for asthma: improvement in patients with associated gastroesophageal reflux. *Arch Intern Med.* 1987; 147:56–60.

447. Ekstrom T, Lindgren BR, Tibbling L. Effects of ranitidine treatment on patients with asthma and a history of gastro-oesophageal reflux: a double blind crossover study. *Thorax.* 1989;44:19–23.

448. Gustafsson PM, Kjellman NI, Tibbling L. A trial of ranitidine in asthmatic children and adolescents with or without pathologic gastroesophageal reflux. *Eur Respir J.* 1992;5:201–206.

449. Irwin RS, Curley FJ, French CL. Chronic cough. The spectrum and frequency of causes, key components of the diagnostic evaluation, and outcome of specific therapy. *Am Rev Respir Dis.* 1990;141:640–647.

450. Irwin RS, Zwacki JK, Curley FJ, et al. Chronic cough as the sole presenting manifestation of gastroesophageal reflux. *Am Rev Respir Dis.* 1989;140:1294–1300.

451. Fitzgerald JM, Allen CJ, Craven MA, Newhouse MT. Chronic cough and gastroesophageal reflux. *Can Med Assoc J.* 1989;140:520–524.

452. Waring JP, Lacayo L, Hunter J, et al. Chronic cough and hoarseness in patients with severe gastroesophageal reflux disease. Diagnosis and response to therapy. *Dig Dis Sci.* 1995;40:1093–1097.

453. Blum AL, Adami B, Bouzo MH, et al. Effect of cisapride on relapse of esophagitis. *Dig Dis Sci.* 1993;38:551–560.

454. Castell DO, Sigmund C, Patterson D, et al. Cisapride 20 mg bid provides symptomatic relief of heartburn and related symptoms in patients with symptoms of chronic mild to moderate gastroesophageal reflux disease. *Am J Gastroenterol.* 1998;93:547–552.

455. Wiseman LR, Faulds D. Cisapride. An updated review of its pharmacology and therapeutic efficacy as a prokinetic agent in gastrointestinal motility disorders. *Drugs.* 1994;47:116–152.

456. Dordal MT, Baltazar MA, Roca I, et al. Nocturnal spasmodic cough in the infant. Evolution after antireflux treatment. *Allerg Immunol* (Paris). 1994;26:53–58.

457. Dupont C, Molkhou P, Petrovic N, Freitag B. [Treatment using Motilium of gastroesophageal reflux associated with respiratory manifestations in children.] *Ann Pediatr* (Paris). 1989;36:148–150.

458. Ekstrom T, Tibbling T. Esophageal acid perfusion, airway function, and symptoms in asthmatic patients with marked bronchial hyperactivity. *Chest.* 1989;96:995–998.

459. Smyrnios NA, Irwin RS, Curley FJ. Chronic cough with a history of excessive sputum production. *Chest.* 1995;108:991–997.

460. Ing AJ, Ngu MC, Breslin AB. Chronic persistent cough and gastroesophageal reflux. *Thorax.* 1994;46:479–483.

461. Khoury R, Paoletti V, Cohn J, et al. Cisapride improves pulmonary function tests in patients with gastroesopahgeal (GE) reflux and chronic respiratory symptoms. *Gastroenterology.* 1998;114:712.

462. Glicksman JT, Mick PT, Fung K, Carroll TL. Prokinetic agents and laryngopharyngeal reflux disease: a systematic review. *Laryngoscope.* 2014;124(10):2375–2379.

463. Guo H, Ma H, Wang J. Proton pump inhibitor therapy for the treatment of laryngopharyngeal reflux: a meta-analysis of randomized controlled trials [published online April 16, 2015]. *J Clin Gastroenterol.* 2016; 50(4):295–300.

464. Luo H, Ma S, Gao Y, et al. The therapeutic effect of proton pump inhibitor on alleviation of hoarseness symptoms in patients with laryngopharyngeal reflux. *Lin Chung Er Bi Yan Hou Tou Jing Wai Ke Za Zhi.* 2015; 29(11):997–1001.

465. Sandmark S, Carlsson R, Fausa O, Lundell L. Omeprazole or ranitidine in the treatment of reflux esophagitis. *Scand J Gastroenterol.* 1988;23:625–632.

466. Castell DO, Richter JE, Robinson M, et al. Efficacy and safety of lansoprazole in the treatment of erosive esophagitis. *Am J Gastroenterol.* 1996;91:1749–1757.

467. Klinkenberg-Knol E, Festen HP, Jansen JB, et al. Long-term treatment with omeprazole for refractory esophagitis. *Ann Intern Med.* 1994;121:161–167.

468. Klinkenberg-Knol EC. Eleven years' experience of continuous maintenance treatment with omeprazole in GERD patients. [Abstract 180]. *Gastroenterology.* 1991;98:114.

469. Hatlebakk JG, Katz PO, Kuo B, Castell DO. Nocturnal gastric acidity and acid breakthrough on different regimes of omeprazole 40 mg daily. *Aliment Pharmacol Ther.* 1998;12:1235–1240.

470. Hatlebakk JG, Katz PO, Camacho-Lobato L, Castell DO. Proton pump inhibitors: better acid suppression when taken before a meal than without a meal. *Aliment Pharmacol Ther.* 2000;14:1267–1272.

471. Peghini PL, Katz PO, Bracy NA, Castell DO. Nocturnal recovery of gastric acid secretion with twice-daily dosing of proton pump inhibitors. *Am J Gastroenterol.* 1998;93:763–767.

472. Peghini PL, Katz PO, Castell DO. Ranitidine controls nocturnal gastric acid breakthrough on omeprazole: a controlled study in normal subjects. *Gastroenterology.* 1998;115:1335–1339.

473. Zimmerman A, Walters JK, Katona B, Souney P. Alternative methods of proton pump inhibitor administration. *Consultant Pharmacist.* 1886;19:990–998.

474. Kamel PL, Hanson D, Kahrilas PJ. Omeprazole for the treatment of posterior laryngitis. *Am J Med.* 1994; 96:321–325.

475. Belafsky PC, Postma GN, Koufman JA. Laryngopharyngeal reflux symptoms improve before changes in physical findings. *Laryngoscope.* 2001;111:979–981.

476. Kuipers EJ, Lundell L, Klinkenberg-Knol EC, et al. Atrophic gastritis and *Helicobacter pylori* infection in patients with reflux esophagitis treated with omeprazole or fundoplication. *N Engl J Med.* 1996;334:1018–1022.

477. Proton pump inhibitor relabeling for cancer risk not warranted. *FDA Report.* 1996;58(Nov 11):T&G-1–2.

478. Ford GA, Oliver PS, Prior JS, et al. Omeprazole in the treatment of asthmatics with nocturnal symptoms and gastro-oesopahgeal reflux: a placebo-controlled crossover study. *Postgrad Med J.* 1994;70:350–354.

479. Boeree MJ, Peters FT, Postma DS, Kleibbeuker JH. No effects of high dose omeprazole in patients with severe airway hyperresponsiveness and a symptomatic gastro-oesophageal reflux and pulmonary fucntion in patients with obstructive lung disease. *Eur Respir J.* 1998;11(5):1070–1074.

480. Meier JH, McNally PR, Punja M, et al. Does omeprazole (Prilosec) improve respiratory function in asthmatics with gastroesophageal reflux? *Dis Dis Sci.* 1994;39:2127–2133.

481. Hanson DG, Kamel PL, Kahrilas PJ. Outcomes of anti-reflux therapy for the treatment of chronic laryngitis. *Ann Otol Rhinol Laryngol.* 1995;104:550–555.

482. Wo JM, Grist WJ, Gussack G, et al. Empiric trial of high dose omeprazole in patients with posterior laryngitis: a prospective study. *Am J Gastroenterol.* 1997;92:2160–2165.

483. Metz DC, Child ML, Ruiz C, Weinstein GS. Pilot study of the oral omeprazole test for reflux laryngitis. *Otolaryngol Head Neck Surg.* 1997;116:41–46.

484. Jaspersen D, Draf W, Weber R, Hammar C-H. Effect of omeprazole on the course of treatment of reflux associated esophagitis and laryngitis. *Gastroenterology.* 1996;31:765–767.

485. El-Serag HB, Lee P, Buchner A, et al. Lansoprazole treatment of patients with chronic idiopathic laryngitis; a placebo-controlled trial. *Am J Gastroenterol.* 2001;96(4):979–983.

486. Amin MR, Postma GN, Johnson P, et al. Proton pump inhibitor resistance in the treatment of laryngopharyngeal reflux. *Otolaryngol Head Neck Surg.* 2001;125:374–378.

487. Chiverton SG, Howden CW, Burget DW, Hunt RH. Omeprazole (20 mg) daily given in the morning or evening: a comparison of effects on gastric acidity, and plasma gastrin and omeprazole concentration. *Aliment Pharmacol Ther.* 1992;6:103–111.

488. Portnoy JE, Gregory ND, Cerulli CE, et al. Efficacy of super high dose proton pump inhibitor administration in refractory laryngopharyngeal reflux: a pilot study. *J Voice.* 2014;28(3):369–377.

489. Lee YC, Lee JS, Kim SW, et al. Influence of age on treatment with proton pump inhibitors in patients with laryngopharyngeal reflux disease: a prospective multicenter study. *JAMA Otolaryngol Head Neck Surg.* 2013;139(12):1291–1295.

490. El-Serag HB, Sonnenberg A. Comorbid occurrence of laryngeal or pulmonary disease with esophagitis in United States military veterans. *Gastroenterology.* 1997;113:755–760.

491. Noordzij J, Khidir A, Evans BA, et al. Evaluation of omeprazole in the treatment of reflux laryngitis: a prospective, placebo-controlled, randomized, double-blind study. *Laryngoscope.* 2001;111:2147–2151.

492. Eherer AJ, Habermann W, Hammer HF, et al. Effect of pantoprazole on the course of reflux-associated laryngitis: a placebo-controlled double-blind crossover study. *Scand J Gastroenterol.* 2003;38:462–467.

493. Issing WJ, Tauber S, Folwaczny C, et al. Impact of 24-hour intraesophageal pH monitoring with 2 channels in the diagnosis of reflux-induced otolaryngologic disorders [in German]. *Laryngorhinootology.* 2003;82:347–352.

494. Bilgen C, Ogut F, Kesimli-Dinc H, et al. The comparison of an empiric proton pump inhibitor vs. 24-hour double-probe pH monitoring in laryngopharyngeal reflux. *J Laryngol Otol.* 2003;117:386–390.

495. Bruley des Varannes S, Coron E, Galmiche JP. Short and long-term PPI treatment for GERD. Do we need more-potent anti-secretory drugs? *Best Pract Res Clin Gastroenterol.* 2010;24:905–921.

496. Tighe MP, Afzal NA, Bevan A, Beattie RM. Current pharmacological management of gastro-esophageal reflux in children: an evidence-based systematic review. *Paediatr Drugs.* 2009;11:185–202.

497. Romano C, Chiaro A, Comito D, Loddo I, Ferrau V. Proton pump inhibitors in pediatrics: evaluation of efficacy in GERD therapy. *Curr Clin Pharmacol.* 2011;6:41–47.

498. Lam PK, Ng ML, Cheung TK, et al. Rabeprazole is effective in treating laryngopharyngeal reflux in a randomized placebo-controlled trial. *Clin Gastroenterol Hepatol.* 2010;8:770–776.

499. Masaany M, Marina MB, Ezat WP, Sani A. Empirical treatment with pantoprazole as a diagnostic tool for symptomatic adult laryngopharyngeal reflux. *J Laryngol Otol.* 2011;125:502–508.

500. Abou-Ismail A, Vaezi MF. Evaluation of patients with suspected laryngopharyngeal reflux: a practical approach. *Curr Gastroenterol Rep.* 2011;13:213–218.

501. Dadabhai A, Friedenberg FK. Raberprazole: a pharmacologic and clinical review for acid-related disorders. *Expert Opin Drug Saf.* 2009;8:119–126.

502. Fass R, Noelck N, Willis MR, et al. The effect of esomeprazole 20 mg twice daily on acoustic and perception parameters of the voice in laryngopharyngeal reflux. *Neurogastroenterol Motil.* 2010;22:134–141, e44–e45.

503. Johnston N, Bulmer D, Gill GA, et al. Cell biology of laryngeal epithelial defenses in health and disease: further studies. *Ann Otol Rhinol Laryngol.* 2003;112:481–491.

504. Reichel O, Dressel H, Wiederanders K, et al. Double-blind, placebo-controlled trial with esomeprazole for

symptoms and signs associated with laryngopharyngeal reflux. *Otolaryngol Head Neck Surg.* 2008;139: 414–420.

505. Belafsky PC, Rees CJ, Rodriguez K, et al. Esophagopharyngeal reflux. *Otolaryngol Head Neck Surg.* 2008; 138:57–61.

506. Belafsky PC, Postma GN, Koufman JA. Laryngopharyngeal reflux symptoms improve before changes in physical findings. *Laryngoscope.* 2001;111:979–981.

507. Reichel O, Keller J, Rasp G, et al. Efficacy of once-daily esomeprazole treatment in patients with laryngopharyngeal reflux evaluated by 24-hour pH monitoring. *Otolaryngol Head Neck Surg.* 2007;136:205–210.

508. Jin BJ, Lee YS, Jeong SW, et al. Change of acoustic parameters before and after treatment in laryngopharyngeal reflux patients. *Laryngoscope.* 2008;118:938–941.

509. Chapman DB, Rees CJ, Lippert D, Sataloff RT, Wright SC Jr. Adverse effects of long-term proton pump inhibitor use: a review for otolaryngologists. *J Voice.* 2011;25:236–240.

510. Sataloff RT. Proton pump inhibitor: adverse effects [Editorial]. *ENT J.* 2010;89(12):574–576.

511. Davies M, Wilton LV, Shakir SA. Safety profile of esomeprazole: results of a prescription-event monitoring study of 11,595 patients in England. *Drug Saf.* 2008;31:313–323.

512. Yang YX, Lewis JD, Epstein S, Metz DC. Long-term proton pump inhibitor therapy and risk of hip fracture. *JAMA.* 2006;296:2947–2953.

513. Solomon DH, Diem SJ, Ruppert K, et al. Bone mineral density changes among women initiating proton pump inhibitors or H2 receptor antagonists: a SWAN cohort study. *J Bone Miner Res.* 2015; 30(2):232–239.

514. Lam JR, Schneider JL, Zhao W, Corley DA. Proton pump inhibitor and histamine 2 receptor antagonist use and vitamin B12 deficiency. *JAMA.* 2013; 310(22):2435–2442.

515. Aseeri M, Schroeder T, Kramer J, Zackula R. Gastric acid suppression by proton pump inhibitors as a risk factor for *Clostridium difficile*–associated diarrhea in hospitalized patients. *Am J Gastroenterol.* 2008; 103(9):2308–2313.

516. Gilard M, Arnaud B, Cornily C, et al. Influence of omeprazole on the antiplatelet action of clopidogrel associated with aspirin: the randomized, double-blind OCLA (Omeprazole Clopidogrel Aspirin) study. *J Am Coll Cardiol.* 2008;51:256–260.

517. Pezalla E, Day D, Pulliadath I. Initial assessment of clinical impact of a drug interaction between clopidogrel and proton pump inhibitors. *J Am Coll Cardiol.* 2008;52:1038–1039.

518. Eslami L, Kalantarian S, Nasseri-Moghaddam S, Majdzadeh R. Long-term proton pump inhibitor (PPI) use and the incidence of gastric (pre)malignant lesions. *Cochrane Database Syst Rev.* 2008;CD007098.

519. Freston JW. Omeprazole, hypergastrinemia, and gastric carcinoid tumors. *Ann Intern Med.* 1994;121: 232–233.

520. Lazarus B, Yuan C, Wilson FP, et al. Proton pump inhibitor use and the risk of chronic kidney disease [published online January 11, 2016]. *JAMA Intern Med.* 2016;176(2):238–246.

521. Antoniou T, Macdonald EM, Hollands S, et al. Proton pump inhibitors and the risk of acute kidney injury in older patients: a population-based cohort study. *CMAJ Open.* 2015;3(2):E166–E171.

522. FDA Drug Safety Communication: Low magnesium levels can be associated with long-term use of Proton Pump Inhibitor drugs (PPIs) 2011. Rockville, MD: MedWatch.

523. Cheungpasitporn W, Thongprayoon C, Kittanamongkolchai W, et al. Proton pump inhibitors linked to hypomagnesemia: a systematic review and meta-analysis of observational studies. *Ren Fail.* 2015;37(7): 1237–1241.

524. Kwok CS, Arthur AK, Anibueze CI, et al. Risk of *Clostridium difficile* infection with acid suppressing drugs and antibiotics: meta-analysis. *Am J Gastroenterol.* 2012;107(7):1011–1019.

525. Bavishi C, Dupont HL. Systematic review: the use of proton pump inhibitors and increased susceptibility to enteric infection. *Aliment Pharmacol Ther.* 2011;34: 1269–1281.

526. Zhou B, Huang Y, Li H, Sun W, Liu J. Proton-pump inhibitors and risk of fractures: an update meta-analysis [published online October 13, 2015]. *Osteoporos Int.* 2016;27(1):339–347.

527. Eom CS, Jeon CY, Lim JW, et al. Use of acid-suppressive drugs and risk of pneumonia: a systematic review and meta-analysis. *CMAJ.* 2011;183(3):310–319.

528. Fillion KB, Chateau D, Targownik LE, et al. CNODES Investigators. Proton pump inhibitors and the risk of hospitalization for community-acquired pneumonia: replicated cohort studies with meta-analysis. *Gut.* 2014;63(4):552–558.

529. Focks JJ, Brouwer MA, von Oijen MG, et al. Concomitant use of clopidogrel and proton pump inhibitors: impact on platelet function and clinical outcome: a systematic review. *Heart.* 2013;99(8):520–527.

530. Melloni C, Washam JB, Jones WS, et al. Conflicting results between randomized trials and observational studies on the impact of proton pump inhibitors on cardiovascular events with coadministered with dual antiplatelet therapy: systematic review. *Circ Cardiovasc Qual Outcomes.* 2015;8(1):47–55.

531. Shin JM, Lee JY, Lee DY, et al. Proton pump inhibitors as a possible cause of vitiligo: an in vivo and in vitro study. *J Eur Acad Dermatol Venereol.* 2014;28(11): 1475–1479.

532. Shah NH, LePendu P, Bauer-Mehren A. Proton pump inhibitor usage and the risk of myocardial infarction in the general population. *Plos One.* 2015;10(6):e0124653.

533. Shih CJ, Chen YT, Ou SM, Li SY, Chen TJ, Wang SJ. Proton pump inhibitor use represents an independent risk factor for myocardial infarction. *Int J Cardiol.* 2014;177:292–297.

534. Targownik LE, Lix LM, Leung S, et al. Proton-pump inhibitor use is not associated with osteoporosis or accelerated bone mineral density loss. *Gastroenterology.* 2010;138:8896–8904.

535. Corley DA, Kubo A, Zhao W, et al. Proton pump inhibitors and histamine-2 receptor antagonists are associated with hip fractures among at-risk patients. *Gastroenterology.* 2010;139:93–101.

536. Ngamreungphong S, Leonatiadis GI, Radhi S, et al. Proton pump inhibitors and risk of fracture: a systematic review and meta-analysis of observational studies. *Am J Gastroenterol.* 2011;106:1209–1218; quiz 1219.

537. Targownik LE, Leslie WD, Davison KS, et al. The relationship between proton pump inhibitor use and longitudinal change in bone mineral density: a population-based study from the Canadian Multicentre Osteoporosis Study (CaMos). *Am J Gastroenterol.* 2012;107:1361–1369.

538. Kwok CS, Jeevanantham V, Dawn B, Loke YK. No consistent evidence of differential cardiovascular risk amongst proton-pump inhibitors when used with clopidogrel: meta-analysis. *Int J Cardiol.* 2013;167(3):965–974.

539. Ford GA, Oliver PS, Prior JS, et al. Omeprazole in the treatment of asthmatics with nocturnal symptoms and gastro-oesophageal reflux: a placebo-controlled cross-over study. *Postgrad Med J.* 1994;70:350–354.

540. Gomm W, von Holt K, Thome F, et al. Association of proton pump inhibitors with risk of dementia: a pharmacoepidemiological claims data analysis. *JAMA.* 2016;73(4):410–416.

541. Smoak BR, Koufman JA. Effects of gum chewing on pharyngeal and esophageal pH. *Ann Otol Rhinol Laryngol.* 2001;110:1117–1119.

542. Durkes A, Sivansakar MP. Bicarbonate availability for vocal fold epithelial defense to acidic challenge. *Ann Otol Rhinol Laryngol.* 2014;123(1):71–76.

543. Koufman JA, Johnston N. Potential benefits of pH 8.8 drinking water as an adjunct in the treatment of reflux disease. *Ann Otol Rhinol Laryngol.* 121(7):431–434.

544. Goddard A, Logan R. One-week low-dose triple therapy: new standards for *Helicobacter pylori* treatment. *Eur J Gastroenterol Hepatol.* 1995;7:1–3.

545. Katz PO, Anderson C, Khoury R, Castell DO. Gastrooesophageal reflux associated with nocturnal gastric acid breakthrough on proton pump inhibitor. *Aliment Pharmacol Ther.* 1998;12:1231–1234.

546. Katzka DA, Paoletti V, Leite L, Castell DO. Prolonged ambulatory pH monitoring in patients with persistent gastroesophageal symptoms reflux disease: testing while on therapy identifies need for more aggressive antireflux therapy. *Am J Gastroenterol.* 1996;91:2110–2113.

547. Peghini P, Katz P, Castell D. Bedtime ranitidine decreases gastric acid secretion and eliminates acid exposure overnight in a patient with Barrett's esophagus taking omeprazole, 20 mg BID. *Am J Gastroenterol.* 1997;92:1723.

548. Allison PR. Reflux esophagitis, sliding hiatal hernia, and the anatomy of repair. *Surg Gynecol Obstet.* 1951;92:419–431.

549. Hill LD. An effective operation for hiatal hernia: an eight-year appraisal. *Ann Surg.* 1967;166:681–692.

550. Nissen R. Eine einfache Operation zur Beeinflussung der Refluxoesophagitis. *Schweiz Med Wochenschr.* 1956;86:590.

551. Geagea T. Laparoscopic Nissen's fundoplication: preliminary report on ten cases. *Surg Endosc.* 1991;5:170–173.

552. Bittner HB, Meyers WC, Brazer SR, Pappas JN. Laparoscopic Nissen fundoplication: operative results and short-term follow-up. *Am J Surg.* 1994;167:193–200.

553. Collet D, Cadiere GB. Conversions and complications of laparoscopic treatment of gastroesophageal reflux disease. *Am J Surg.* 1995;169:622–626.

554. Cuschieri A, Hunter J, Wolfe B, et al. Multicenter prospective evaluation of laparoscopic antireflux surgery. *Surg Endosc.* 1993;7:505–510.

555. Fontaumard E, Espalieu P, Boulez J. Laparoscopic Nissen-Rossetti fundoplication. *Surg Endosc.* 1995;9:869–873.

556. Spechler SJ. Comparison of medical and surgical therapy for complicated gastroesophageal reflux disease in veterans. *New Engl J Med.* 1992;326:786–792.

557. Spechler SJ, Lee E, Ahnen D, et al. Long-term outcome of medical and surgical therapies for gastroesophageal reflux disease. *JAMA.* 2001;285(18):2331–2338.

558. So JB, Zeitels SM, Rattner DW. Outcomes of atypical symptoms attributed to gastroesophageal reflux treated by laparoscopic fundoplication. *Surgery.* 1998;124(1):28–32.

559. Geagea T. Laparoscopic Nissen-Rossetti fundoplication. *Surg Endosc.* 1994;8:1080–1084.

560. Hinder RA, Filipi CJ, Wetscher G, et al. Laparoscopic Nissen fundoplication is an effective treatment for gastroesophageal reflux disease. *Ann Surg.* 1994;220:472–483.

561. Jamieson GG, Watson DI, Britten-Jones R, et al. Laparoscopic Nissen fundoplication. *Ann Surg.* 1994;220:137–145.

562. McKernan JB, Laws HL. Laparoscopic Nissen fundoplication for the treatment of gastroesophageal reflux disease. *Am Surg.* 1994;60:87–93.

563. McKernan JB, Champion JK. Laparoscopic anti-reflux surgery. *Am Surg.* 1995;6:1530–1536.

564. Peters JH, Heimbucher J, Kauer WK, et al. Clinical and physiological comparison of laparoscopic and open Nissen fundoplication. *J Am Coll Surg.* 1995;180:385–393.

565. Rattner DW, Brooks DC. Patient satisfaction following laparoscopic and open antireflux surgery. *Arch Surg.* 1995;130:289–294.

566. Sataloff DM, Pursnani K, Hoyo S, et al. An objective assessment of laparoscopic antireflux surgery. *Am J Surg.* 1997;174:63–67.

567. Snow LL, Weinstein LS, Hannon JK. Laparoscopic reconstruction of gastroesophageal anatomy for

the treatment of reflux disease. *Surg Endosc.* 1995;9: 774–780.

568. Weerts JM, Dallemagne B, Hamoir E, et al. Laparoscopic Nissen fundoplication detailed analysis of 132 patients. *Surg Laparosc Endosc.* 1993;3:359–364.

569. Johnson WE, Hagen JA, DeMeester TR, et al. Outcome of respiratory symptoms after antireflux surgery on patients with gastroesophageal reflux disease. *Arch Surg.* 1996;131:489–492.

570. DeMeester TR, O'Sullivan GC, Bermudez G, Midell AI, Cimochowski GE, O'Drobinak J. Esophageal function in patients with angina-type chest pain and normal coronary angiograms. *Ann Surg.* 1982;196:488–498.

571. Perrin-Fayolle M, Gormand F, Braillon G, et al. Long-term results of surgical treatment for gastroesophageal reflux in asthmatic patients. *Chest.* 1989;96:40–45.

572. Deveney CW, Benner K, Cohen J. Gastroesophageal reflux and laryngeal disease. *Arch Surg.* 1993;128: 1021–1027.

573. Pitcher DE, Pitcher WD, Martin DT, Curet MJ. Antireflux surgery does not reliably correct reflux-related asthma. *Gastrointest Endosc.* 1996;43:433.

574. Hunter JG, Trus TL, Branum GD, et al. A physiological approach to laparoscopic fundoplication for gastroesophageal reflux disease. *Ann Surg.* 1996;223:673–687.

575. Weber B, Portnoy JE, Castellanos A, et al. Efficacy of anti-reflux surgery on refractory laryngopharyngeal reflux disease in professional voice users: a pilot study. *J Voice.* 2014;28(4):492–500.

576. Trad KS, Turgeon DG, Deljkich E. Long-term outcomes after transoral incisionless fundoplication in patients with GERD and LPR symptoms. *Surg Endosc.* 2012;26(3):650–660.

577. Fahin M, Vardar R, Ersin S, et al. The effect of antireflux surgery on laryngeal symptoms, findings and voice parameters. *Eur Arch Otorhinolaryngol.* 2015; 272(11):3375–3383.

578. Hoppo T, Sanz AF, Nason KS, et al. How much pharyngeal exposure is "normal"? Normative data for laryngopharyngeal reflux events using hypopharyngeal multichannel intraluminal impedance (HMII). *J Gastrointest Surg.* 2012;16(1):16–24.

579. Mazzoleni G, Vailati C, Lisma DG, Testoni PA, Passaretti S. Correlation between oropharyngeal pH-monitoring and esophageal pH-impedance monitoring in patients with suspected GERD-related extraesophageal symptoms. *Neurogastroenterol Motil.* 2014; 26(11):1557–1564.

580. Toomey P, Teta A, Patel K, et al. Transoral incisionless fundoplication: is it as safe and efficacious as a Nissen or Toupet fundoplication? *Am Surg.* 2014;80(9): 860–867.

581. Reimer C, Sendergaard B, Hilsted L, Bytzer P. Proton-pump inhibitor therapy induces acid-related symptoms in healthy volunteers after withdrawal of therapy. *Gastroenterology.* 2009;137:80–87.

582. Triadafilopoulos G, DiBaise JK, Nostrant TT, et al. The Stretta procedure for the treatment of GERD: 6 and 12 month follow-up of the US open label trial. *Gastrointest Endosc.* 2002;55:149–156.

583. Corley DA, Katz P, Wo JM, et al. Improvement of gastroesophageal reflux symptoms after radiofrequency energy: a randomized, sham-controlled trial. *Gastroenterology.* 2003;125:668–676.

584. Filipi CJ, Lehman GA, Rothstein RI, et al. Transoral, flexible endoscopic suturing for treatment of GERD: a multicenter trial. *Gastrointest Endosc.* 2001;53:416–422.

585. Rothstein RI, Pohl H, Grove M, et al. Endoscopic gastric plication for the treatment of GERD: two-year follow-up results. *Am J Gastroenterol.* 2001;96:S35. Abstract 107.

586. Chen YK, Raijman I, Ben-Menachem T, et al. Long-term outcomes of endoluminal gastroplication: a US multicenter trial. *Gastrointest Endosc.* 2005;61:659–667.

587. Mason RJ, Hughes M, Lehman GA, et al. Endoscopic augmentation of the cardia with a biocompatible injectable polymer (Enteryx) in a porcine model. *Surg Endosc.* 2002;16:386–391.

588. Cohen LB, Johnson DA, Ganz RA, et al. Enteryx implantation for GERD: expanded multicenter trial results and interim postapproval follow-up to 24 months. *Gastrointest Endosc.* 2005;61:650–658.

589. Deviere J, Costamagna G, Neuhaus H, et al. Nonresorbable copolymer implantation for gastroesophageal reflux disease: a randomized sham-controlled multicenter trial. *Gastroenterology.* 2005;128:532–540.

590. Pleskow D, Rothstein R, Lo S, et al. Endoscopic full-thickness plication for the treatment of GERD: 12-month follow-up for the North American open-label trial. *Gastrointest Endosc.* 2005;61:643–649.

591. Pleskow V. Endoscopic, endoluminal fundoplication for gastroesophageal reflux disease: initial experience and lessons learned. *Surgery.* 2010;148:646–651.

592. Velanovich V. Endoscopic, endoluminal fundoplication for gastroesophageal reflux disease: initial experience and lessons learned. *Surgery.* 2010;148;646–651.

593. Francis DO, Goutte M, Slaughter JC, et al. Traditional reflux parameters and not impedance monitoring predict outcome after fundoplication in extraesophageal reflux. *Laryngoscope.* 2011;121:1902–1909.

# 12

# Laryngeal Manifestations of Autoimmune Diseases

*Abdul-Latif Hamdan, Robert Thayer Sataloff, and Mary J. Hawkshaw*

## Laryngeal Manifestations of Rheumatoid Arthritis

Rheumatoid arthritis (RA) is a chronic inflammatory disease that affects the synovial membranes within diarthrodial joints. It is a destructive systemic entity characterized by the deposition of articular and extra-articular lesions in various organs of the body leading to functional and disability disorders.[1,2] Through remission and exacerbation, inflammatory changes of the synovial membranes often result in bony destruction and joint deformities. Although all joints can be targeted, there is a predilection for small joints and pressure joints. However, with progress of the disease, larger joints are affected as well. Women are more affected than men with a female to male ratio of 2:1 and an overall prevalence that increases with age to reach 1% of the general population.[3]

Given the musculoskeletal structure of the larynx and its joint framework, it is subject to involvement by rheumatoid arthritis. Both the cricoarytenoid Joints (CAJ) and the cricothyroid joints are encapsulated diarthrodial joints prone to be affected by this systemic disease. To that end, there has been a growing prevalence of laryngeal manifestations of RA since the early report by Lawry in 1960.[4] The disease can affect muscles, cartilages, and joints with a prevalence on histologic examination of 88%.[5-7]

The prevalence of vocal disorders in patients with laryngeal involvement is not always that obvious.[4,6,8-10] The manifestations can result in a plethora of symptoms often masked or shadowed by the systemic complaints and by confounding diseases such as laryngopharyngeal reflux disease and or allergic laryngitis. Nevertheless, despite the subtleness of these symptoms, the number of reports on the prevalence of laryngeal involvement in RA is on the rise. This has been attributed to the advances in the diagnostic methods, and to the increased physician's index of suspicion. The presence of vocal symptoms in patients with RA varies between 12% to 75%, with a mean of 35%.[11,12] The variation in prevalence depends on the outcome measures used whether objective or subjective, and on method of analysis.[6,13-18] Roy et al in his study of 100 patients with RA interviewed by phone, 35% had reported a voice disorder that impacted quality of life but none had pursued professional help. It is important to note that the prevalence rate was not affected by age, phonatory behavior, and intake of medications, or severity of the disease.[11] On the other hand, Hojna et al in their investigation of 72 patients with rheumatoid arthritis reported voice disorders in 44.44%, the frequency of which was higher with advanced activity of the disease.[15] Fisher et al has also confirmed the correlation between disease activity and severity of vocal disorders.[9] Similarly, Speyer et al in his investigation of risk and prevalence of dysphonia in a cohort study of 166 RA patients and 148 healthy controls, both the risk and the prevalence of dysphonia were higher in patients versus controls (12–27% vs 3–8%). Patients with RA were three times more likely to have vocal symptoms compared to healthy controls.[14] In this investigation, both Voice Handicap Index and three item outcome scale questionnaires were used as outcome measures. Likewise, Sanz et al in a transverse analytic study of 80 patients with RA, rheumatic patients had an odds ratio of 2.82 and 5.04 for dysphonia and three items outcome scales, respectively.[8] Despite these numerous reports corroborating the higher prevalence of vocal disorders in RA patients comparted to controls,[6,9,14,19,20] a recent study by Hah et al on 418 RA patients and 18,950 controls taking into account several confounding variables such as age, smoking, and stress level, revealed no association between RA and subjective voice discomfort or the odds ratio for subjective voice complaints. Moreover, the study failed to show a higher prevalence of organic laryngeal diseases in RA patients compared to controls.[21]

The type of symptoms varies with the stage of the disease and its chronicity. In the acute phase, symptoms related to sensation in the laryngopharyngeal mucosa are often reported, whereas in chronic cases airway symptoms secondary to cricoarytenoid fixation are more noticeable. Based on a study by Kara et al two-thirds of laryngeal symptoms are attributed to involvement of the CAJ.[22] To that end, reported laryngopharyngeal symptoms range from mild subtle throat discomfort to life-threatening conditions. These include foreign body sensation, throat soreness, tension in the neck, referred otalgia, change in voice quality, odynophonia, dysphagia, odynophagia, shortness of breath, and stridor.[4,23] An investigation by Castro et al showed that 19 out of 27 patients with RA had laryngeal symptoms described mainly as intermittent dysphonia and foreign body sensation.[24] The dysphonia in patients with RA is described as breathiness, roughness, asthenic, loss of range, and inability to project the voice. Based on Hojna et al a higher grade of dysphonia is observed in subjects with advanced disease.[15] In this study the most frequently reported vocal complaints were vocal fatigue (55.6%), hoarseness (52.76%), followed by cough, mucus retention, pain in the larynx, and foreign body sensation. In addition to the chronicity of the disease as an important variable in predicting the nature of vocal disorders in patients with RA, the degree of joint involvement that affects the position of the vocal fold also plays a role. If both vocal folds are fixed in the median position, patients are obviously more likely to develop respiratory symptoms often necessitating emergency tracheotomy.[25] On the other hand when one vocal fold is fixed in the lateral position patients report dysphonia and aspiration. This mandates a medialization procedure such as thyroplasty type I, injection laryngoplasty, or arytenoid adduction as reported by Kumai et al in an RA patient with aphonia.[26] Few studies have examined the acoustic changes in patients with RA to substantiate the aforementioned vocal changes.[4,15] In 2007 Amernick et al reported increased perturbation parameters, namely, jitter and shimmer, and decreased fundamental frequency in their analysis of 77 patients with RA compared to controls.[5] Similar findings were reported by Castro et al and later by Hojna et al. The increase in the perturbation parameters invariably correlated with the severity of the disease.[15,24]

In the presence of laryngopharyngeal symptoms, patients with RA need to undergo laryngeal examination using both telescopic and fiberoptic endoscopy. The telescopic examination is crucial for delicate assessment of the anatomical structures of the larynx and in particular for visualization of any signs of erythema and edema of the cricoarytenoid joints. The flexible fiberoptic examination on the other hand allows proper assessment of the laryngeal biomechanics which may be altered in the presence of vocal fold pathology or impaired mobility of the vocal folds. Indeed, one out of two patients with RA and vocal symptoms may exhibit laryngeal changes on endoscopy. The most common laryngeal findings are: Edema and erythema of the vocal folds and/or the cricoarytenoid joints, dryness of the vocal folds, impaired mobility and or fixation of one or both vocal folds, presence of rheumatoid nodules, or bamboo nodes.[4,5,15,24]

Impaired mobility or fixation of one or both vocal folds is reported often in patients with RA and is mostly attributed to cricoarytenoid joint arthritis. See Figure 12–1. Based on numerous histologic studies there is inflammation of the synovial lining with spread to the articulating surfaces of the diarthrodial joint leading to destruction of the articular surfaces with subsequent fibrosis and ankyloses.[1,2,27] In view of its critical role in respiration, phonation, and swallowing, cricoarytenoid joint (CAJ) involvement by RA has received much attention in the 1950s and 1960s with a growing number of reports describing the arthritic changes in this joint. Most of these reports focused on obstructive respiratory symptoms and less on phonation.[28–32] In 1957 Baker and Bywaters described a case of laryngeal stridor in a 42-year-old female patient with classical RA. The patient had fixed left vocal fold and limited abduction of the right fold.[30] In 1958, Bates reported a 63-year-old woman who had rheumatoid arthritis for 14 years and continuous increase of stridor since its onset. Direct laryngoscopy revealed bilateral fixed vocal folds with a 2-mm chink in between. Due to difficulty in breathing, a permanent tracheotomy with a speaking valve was performed.[33] In 1963, Bienenstock et al has emphasized the frequent involvement of the cricoarytenoid joint in patients with RA. In their study on 64 randomly selected patients with RA, 17 had symptoms that were attributed to CAJ involvement.

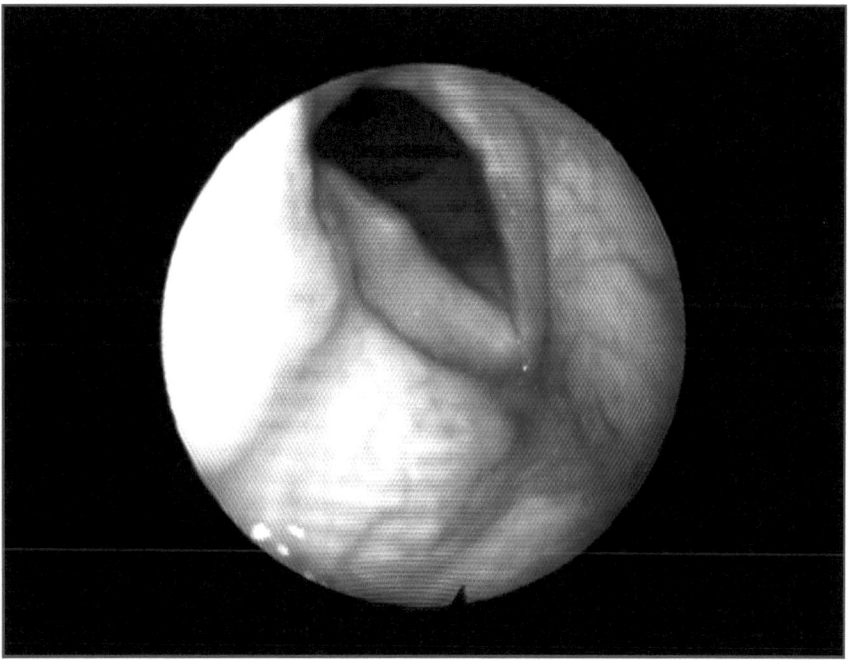

**Figure 12–1.** Fixation of the right vocal fold secondary to cricoarytenoid joint fixation in a 53-year-old patient diagnosed with rheumatoid arthritis and receiving methotrexate.

Seven out of eight patients had post-mortem histopathologic evidence of arthritis.[2] In 1996, Bossingham and Simpson reported a case of a 55-year-old woman with advanced RA who was admitted with acute stridor necessitating steroid administration and tracheotomy for relief of her symptom.[31] In 2002 Kolman and Morris reported a patient with rheumatoid arthritis who developed inspiratory stridor twice that led to an awake tracheotomy. Laryngoscopic examination showed inflammation of the cricoarytenoid joint with subsequent narrowing of the airway.[34] In 2016 Pradan et al reported another 52-year-old female who presented with respiratory distress and hoarseness that necessitated tracheotomy. On exam there was total fixation of both vocal folds in the paramedian position in addition to the presence of edema and a nodule over the left arytenoid.[35]

Based on the aforementioned, most of the reports describe bilateral cricoarytenoid joint involvement in both acute and chronic RA. In the acute phase of inflammation, patients complain of neck pain, difficulty in swallowing and talking, referred pain to the ears, and hoarseness, whereas in the chronic phase patients present more with shortness of breath and obstructive airway symptoms. The report by Copeman exemplifies the various degrees of cricoarytenoid involvement in three RA patients.[28] In the first case,

RA was moderate in intensity and patient reported hoarseness and difficulty in speaking loud, at times associated with shortness of breath. These symptoms were secondary to impaired mobility of the left vocal fold with evidence of peri-arthritic inflammation around the arytenoid cartilage that resolved with medical treatment. In the second case there was total fixation of the vocal fold with edema of the periarytenoid area that resulted in frequent attacks of hoarseness and shortness of breath. In the third case there was complete fixation of both vocal folds resulting in dysphonia and stridor. It is worth noting that despite the high rate of cricoarytenoid joint involvement in patients with RA, which ranges between 15 to 75%,[36-38] patients may not have vocal fold fixation and may not suffer from vocal symptoms. This can be attributed to the insidious onset of the disease that allows ample of time for patients to adapt. It is also important to note that impaired mobility of the vocal folds is not always secondary to CAJ involvement but may also be secondary to involvement of the recurrent laryngeal nerve or to cervicomedullary compression due to cervical spine involvement.[39-40] Demyelination of the recurrent laryngeal nerve with subsequent paralysis leading to stridor has been reported by Darke et al.[39]

Other laryngeal findings in patients with RA include rheumatoid nodules. Laryngeal rheumatoid nodules were first described by Raven et al in 1948.[41] Since then rheumatoid nodules have been reported in the larynx at various sites.[42–44] These are more likely to appear at pressure sites or areas subject to repeated trauma. To that end there have been reports of rheumatoid nodules in the cricoarytenoid joint, periarytenoid area, and vocal folds with the mid-membranous portion being the most common site.[45] Other authors have reported the presence of these nodules in the posterior third of the vocal folds. Woo et al in 1994 reported two cases of RA who presented with hoarseness secondary to involvement of the vocal folds. In the first case, there was evidence of decreased amplitude of the mucosal waves secondary to bilateral submucosal nodules that were resected through a cordotomy approach. The second case had bilateral subcordal masses that were also treated surgically.[44] Given the ubiquity of reports on laryngeal rheumatoid nodules, the American Rheumatism Association has included the presence of submucosal nodules in the criteria for classification of rheumatoid arthritis.[46] These lesions consist of focal areas of fibrinoid necrosis surrounded by palisading histiocytes with outer rims of fibrosis. See Figure 12–2. The treatment of these lesions is primarily aimed at restoring the function of the vocal folds while preserving its anatomical structure. When there is reduction in the mucosal waves resulting in dysphonia, surgical removal thru a cordotomy approach is often recommended.

Bamboo nodes of the vocal folds are also rare laryngeal manifestations of RA in addition to other autoimmune diseases. These have been described initially by Hosako et al in 1993 as transverse yellowish or whitish submucosal lesions of the vocal folds.[47] See Figure 12–3. These lesions occur mainly in patients with autoimmune diseases, primarily systemic lupus erythematosus, Sjogren's syndrome, and rheumatoid arthritis. Unlike rheumatoid nodules which are well-rounded submucosal lesions, bamboo nodes are frequently fusiform in shape and have ill-defined margins that are hard to delineate.[48–51] These lesions consist of central necrosis surrounded by macrophages and inflammatory cells. In 2007 Immerman and Sulica reported a 24-year-old female who presented with hoarseness and effortful voice production that were secondary to bilateral vocal fold bamboo nodes. The patient was managed with systemic steroids with no recurrence at 4 months follow-up.[52] A year later Hilgert et al reported another case of RA who had hoarseness with multiple submucosal cysts that were treated by logopedic speech therapy.[50] The management of these lesions varies according to the authors' preference and availability of resources. One option is conservative and focuses on controlling the confounding variables and risk factors for dysphonia such as laryngopharyngeal reflux disease and allergy, in addition to vocal therapy for rehabilitation of the phonatory behavior.[50] The second option

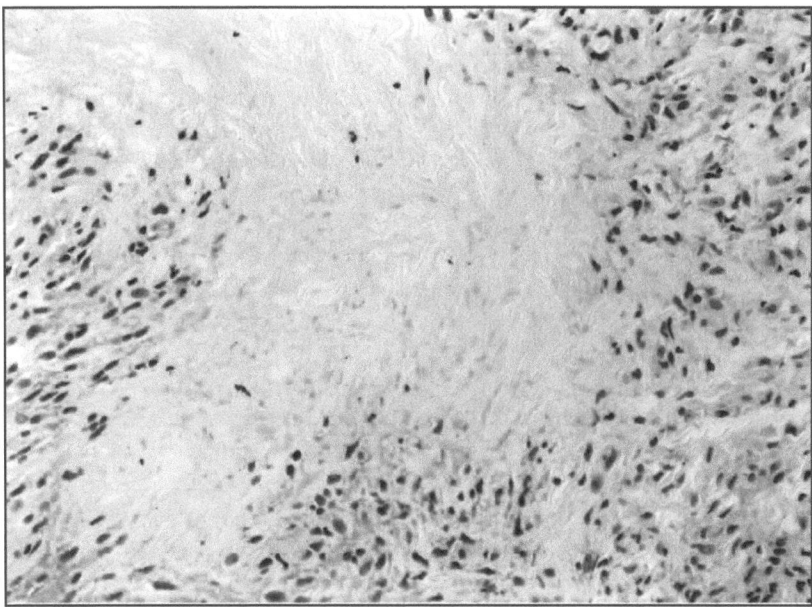

**Figure 12–2.** Hematoxylin and Eosin staining (power 10x): Rheumatoid nodule. Irregular areas of necrosis surrounded by palisade of elongated and epithelioid histiocytes with occasional lymphocytes.

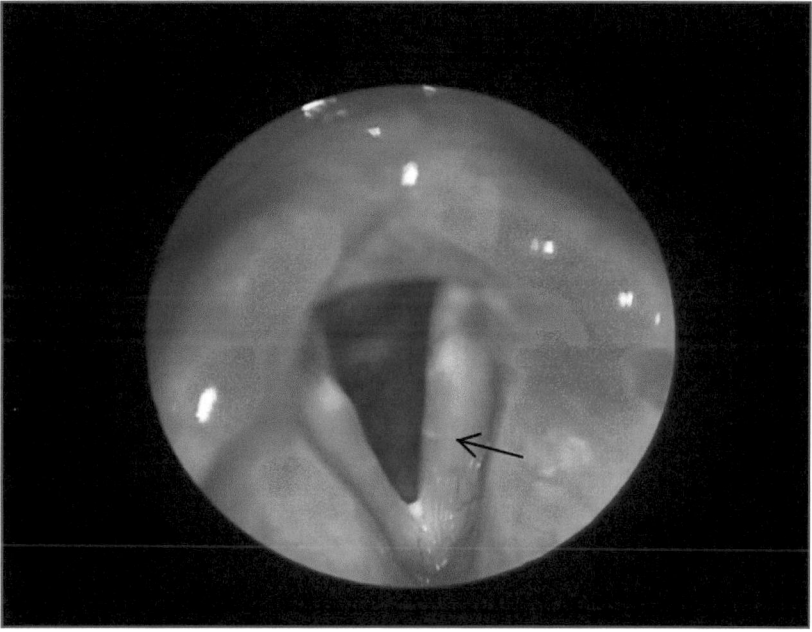

**Figure 12–3.** Bilateral bamboo nodes in the midmembranous portion of the vocal folds in a 24-year-old female who presented with dysphonia, vocal fatigue, and inability to project the voice.

is surgical removal of these lesions under suspension microlaryngoscopy.

It is important to note that all the aforementioned laryngeal pathologies, namely, rheumatoid nodules and bamboo nodes seen on telescopic examination can be supplemented with stroboscopic imaging which provides further information on the malleability and behavior of the vocal fold cover. It can also assist in diagnosing mild mucosal changes and subtle submucosal lesions. Wojnowski et al described decrease in vibration amplitude and mucosal irregularities in two out of the three RA subjects.[6] Hojna et al reported features of hypofunctional dysphonia confirmed by high-speed digital imaging and videokymography in RA patients with moderate activity of the disease.[15] Similarly in a recent investigation by Puerta et al using videolaryngostrobosopy in patients with RA, abnormal findings were reported in almost two-thirds of the 36 patients examined. The most common findings were signs and symptoms of laryngopharyngeal reflux (64%), followed by muscle tension dysphonia (31%), and presence of bamboo node in one patient.[20]

Other important diagnostic tests include computerized tomographic evaluation of the larynx and in particular of the cricoarytenoid joint and cricothyroid joint. The most common radiologic findings include narrowing of the joint, prominence, ankylosis,

erosion, and increased soft tissue densities. The rate of CAJ abnormalities varies with the sensitivity of the imaging technique and resolution used. The figure can reach up to 72% with the presence of osseous destruction in close to 50% of the cases.[53] Other reported findings include sublaxation of the joint, joint irregularities, space narrowing, and joint irregularities.[22] Interestingly, the presence of radiologic changes in the CAJ does not always correlate with the presence of symptoms. In a study by Grossman et al close to half of patients with radiologic findings were asymptomatic.[16] On the other hand the study by Amernick in 2007 and the one by Hojna et al in 2015 showed a correlation between vocal disorders and radiologic changes.[5,15] It is also worth mentioning that not only the CAJ is amenable to involvement by RA but also the cricothyroid joint (CTJ). In a study by Berjawi et al on 11 patients with advanced RA receiving methotrexate, the CTJ abnormalities were investigated using high-resolution computerized tomography. The results indicated CTJ abnormalities in 10 out of the 11 patients. The involvement was mainly unilateral, with narrowing of the joint space (defined as decrease in volume) present in more than 2/3 of the cases. Other radiologic findings included changes in density (45.5% of the cases) and thickening of the vocal folds (27.3% of cases). See Figures 12–4, 12–5, 12–6, and 12–7. It is worth noting that these radiologic changes in the CTJ were commensurate with a decrease in vocal range in almost half the subjects.[54]

The management of laryngeal manifestations of RA requires a multidisciplinary approach. The internist, the otolaryngologist, as well as the speech-language pathologist play a role. The internist needs to control the systemic disease using steroids in order to mitigate the development of permanent changes within the affected joints. Corticosteroids may also be delivered via intra or periarticular injections.[55,56] Dockery et al has reported five cases of RA with laryngeal manifestations who were treated successfully by systemic and intra-articular steroids. The symptoms of hoarseness, dysphagia, and shortness of breath improved following speech therapy. The authors highlighted the importance of early diagno-

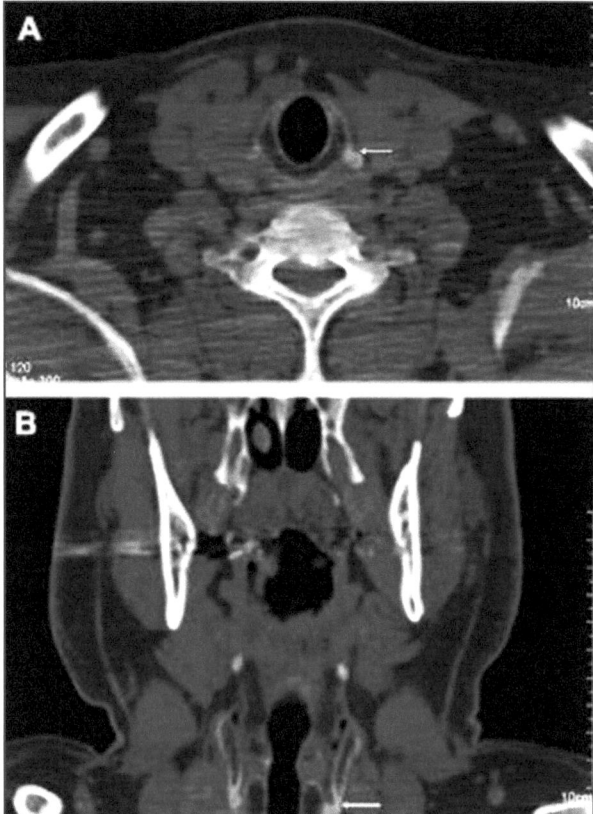

Figure 12–6. **A.** Axial cut of a CT scan showing left CTJ ankyloses. **B.** Coronal cut of a CT scan showing left CTJ ankyloses.

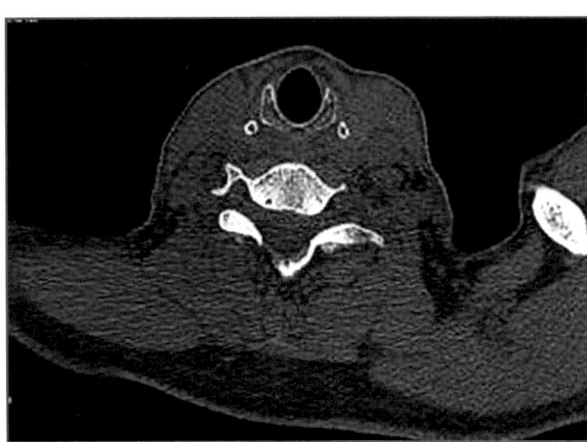

Figure 12–4. Axial cut of a CT scan showing normal CTJ space.

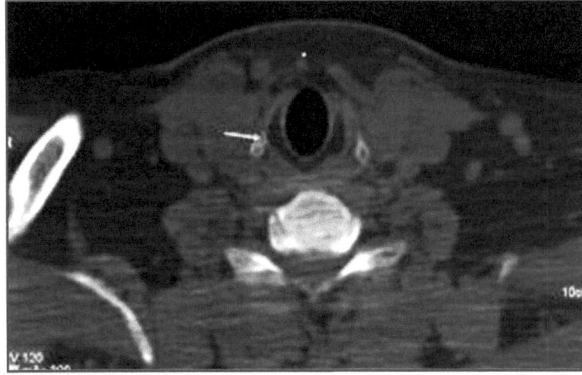

Figure 12–5. Axial cut of a CT scan showing narrowing of right CTJ space.

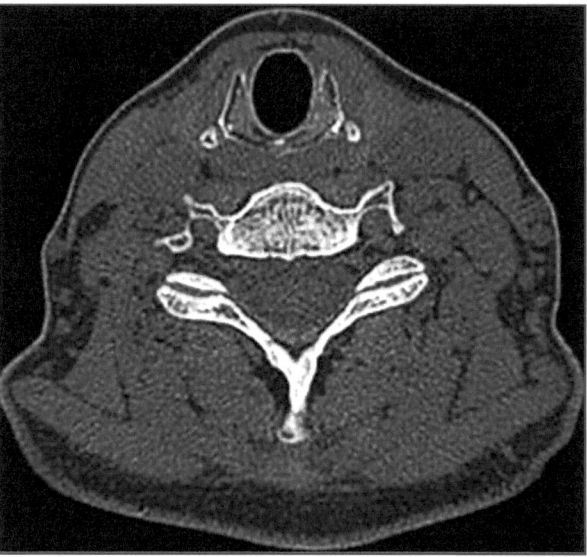

Figure 12–7. Axial cut of HRCT scan showing an increase in the density of right CTJ.

sis and intervention in these cases.[13] Simpson et al has reported 6 cases of RA who were treated successfully with periarticular injections and had adequate improvement. The authors highlighted the many added values of this mode of therapy, namely, the ease of performance, short duration of the procedure, and minimal training needed to perform such an injection.[55]

In advanced cases that do not respond to steroid therapy, the use of methotrexate or Leflunomide might be indicated.[19,57] In these refractory cases securing the airway obstruction by performing a tracheotomy is often required. This is followed by a lateralization procedure to widen the glottis inlet permanently. Endoscopic laser arytenoidectomy is the most commonly used procedure with very promising results. Variations on its theme have been described over the last two decades, such as laser posterior partial cordectomy by Dennis and Kashima in 1989, endoscopic laser medial cordectomy by Crumley in 1993, or subtotal arytenoidectomy by Remacle et al in 1996.[58-60]

## Laryngeal Manifestations of Systemic Lupus Erythematosus

Systemic lupus erythematosus (SLE) is an autoimmune disease characterized by the deposition of autoantibodies in different sites in the body, namely, joints, pleura, kidneys, central nervous system, and less commonly in the larynx.[61] Since the first description of laryngeal involvement in patients with SLE by Sacarpelli et al in 1959 there has been a growing number of cases in the literature.[62-64] Today laryngeal pathology is estimated to be present in one out of three patients with SLE with a reported incidence that ranges between 0.3 to 30% based on numerous studies.[63,64] The symptoms are many and can range from foreign body sensation, mild change in voice quality and throat discomfort, to life-threatening difficulty in breathing. In a review by Teitel et al of 97 patients with SLE, the most common reported symptoms were hoarseness, throat discomfort, dysphagia, and dyspnea.[65] Other rare manifestations include acute airway obstruction and respiratory distress often necessitating tracheotomy. Three possible mechanisms for laryngeal involvement have been suggested: One is the deposition of the immune complexes in the laryngeal structures such as muscles and mucosa,[65,66] second, is involvement of the recurrent laryngeal nerve either by reduction in its vascularity or by compression, last, is infection and diffuse chondritis of the thyroid cartilage and cricoid.[65,67-74] It is important to note that symptoms related to the laryngopharyngeal complex may not always prevail during the active stage of the disease. Korbet et al in 1984 reported a case of hoarseness and dyspnea in a patient with inactive SLE. The early detection of laryngeal involvement allowed adjustment of steroid dosage and thus spared the patient undue complications.[75]

When phonatory symptoms are present, laryngeal findings are neither rare nor isolated.[65] These may range from mucosal changes such as edema, inflammation, and ulceration at the level of the arytenoids and or aryepiglottic folds, to vocal fold paralysis and life-threatening necrotizing vasculitis. These findings may be evident on radiologic imaging as shown in the two cases reported by Ozcan et al, where CT scan of the larynx showed thickening of the laryngeal mucosa at the aryepiglottic fold with evidence of arytenoid asymmetry.[76] Mucosal inflammation is usually the most common clinical finding in patients with SLE and may be present in almost one-third of the cases. In 1992 Martin et al in their review of 158 cases of SLE reported 4 cases of upper airway obstruction.[77] In rare cases patients may present with epiglottitis, diffuse mucosal edema, irregular shaped epiglottic mass, and/or superficial mucosal ulcerations as reported by Toomey et al.[78] Acute epiglottitis can be the sole presentation of the disease as reported by Charuvanij and Houghton in a 5-year-old girl who developed sepsis.[79] The most common pathogens in epiglottitis in patients with SLE are pneumococcal and *Haemophilus influenzae*.[79-81] When nonspecific laryngeal findings are present in patients with SLE, other causes such as infection laryngitis, smoke-induced injury, allergic angioedema, irradiation, and phonotrauma should be ruled out.[82,83] Less frequently encountered etiology presenting with laryngeal edema is relapsing polychondritis which results in laryngeal perichondritis often occurring with other connective tissue disorders and complicated by tracheomalacia.[78] Other laryngeal manifestations of SLE include the presence of vasculitis resulting in a polypoid or nodular lesion.[84,85] In cases of vasculitis, biopsy shows evidence of fibrinoid necrosis and inflammatory infiltrates with disruption of the submucosal arterial walls. Other reported findings include perivascular lymphocytic infiltrates, thickening of the vessel walls, and hyalinization.[62,86]

Phonatory symptoms in patients with SLE can also be secondary to the presence of rheumatoid nodules or bamboo nodes in addition to the aforementioned laryngeal inflammatory changes. In 1993, Hosako et al was the first to describe the presence of a transverse yellowish submucosal lesion of the vocal folds

**Table 12–1.** Reported Cases of Bamboo Nodes in Patients with SLE and Connective Tissue Disease

| Study | Subjects | Sex | Age (years) | Disease | Disease duration (years) | Presentation |
|---|---|---|---|---|---|---|
| Hosako et al 1993[87] | 4 | F | 28 | SLE | 2 | Dysphonia and diplophonia |
| Tsunoda and Soda 1996[88] | 1 | F | 51 | Autoimmune hepatitis and SLE | N/A | Hoarseness as the initial manifestation of systemic lupus erythematosus |
| Murano et al 2001[89] | 2 | F | 28 | SLE | 0 | Sudden onset of hoarseness |
| Todic et al 2014 [French][90] | 1 | F | 18 | TTP, hemolytic anemia, SLE | N/A | Hoarseness |
| Hilgert et al* 2008[91] | 3 | F | 29 | Mixed connective tissue disease | 8 | Hoarseness |
| | | F | 31 | Mixed connective tissue disease | 9 | Hoarseness |
| Schwemmle et al 2013[94] | 1 | F | 43 | Mixed connective tissue disease | 6 | Sudden onset of hoarseness |

F: Female; M: Male; UCTS: Undifferentiated connective tissue syndrome; N/A: Not available; TTP: Thrombotic thrombocy-topenic purpura; SLE: Systemic lupus erythematosus.

*: Study reporting bamboo nodes in a patient with rheumatoid arthritis

in a patient with SLE in reference to its similarity to the bamboo and its nodes. The lesion was described as a "bamboo joint-like lesion."[87] In 1996 Tsunoda and Soda reported a 51-year-old case who developed "bamboo joint-like nodules" as a result of lupus laryngitis, and improved on systemic therapy.[88] Five similar cases have been reported in the literature and the term was later modified to "vocal fold bamboo nodes" by Murano et al in 2001.[89] Another report on bamboo nodes was reported by Todic et al in 2014.[90] See Table 12–1. Although these lesions occur primarily in patients with SLE, other underlying autoimmune diseases such as Sjogren's disease and progressive systemic sclerosis must be ruled out.[87,88,92,93] The management strategy for these lesions mandates steroid injection as a first line of treatment and surgery as the second line for those who fail to achieve the desired voice outcome. Schwemmle in 2007 was the first to

report local steroid injection as a first line of therapy in a 43-year-old female patient with Sharp syndrome and bilateral bamboo nodes.[94] The injection was made locally in the vocal folds 4 times before taking the patient to the operating room for suspension microlaryngoscopy and excision. Intraoperatively there was fixation of the mucosal cover to the submucosal structures.[94]

Vocal fold paralysis is also another less frequently encountered laryngeal manifestation of SLE that can result in dysphonia, aspiration, and dyspnea. There are many reports of unilateral and bilateral vocal fold paralysis that can be temporary or permanent with a prevalence rate of 11% according to Teitel et al.[65-75,82,95,96] In 2001 Nanke et al was the first to report a case of overlap syndrome who had respiratory distress secondary to bilateral cricoarytenoid joint arthritis which mandated a tracheotomy.[97] In 2008 Lee et al

| Type of Laryngeal examination | Laryngeal findings | Management | Recurrence of symptoms |
|---|---|---|---|
| Laryngoscopy, stroboscopy | Transverse cream-yellow band lesions protruding from the surface of the vocal folds in the middle portions | Surgery | No |
| Laryngoscopy, stroboscopy | Transverse lesion encircling the vocal fold | Surgery and systemic steroids | N/A |
| Rigid laryngeal endoscopy, stroboscopy | White transverse band lesion in the submucosal space slightly protruded from surface | Systemic steroids | Yes |
| Laryngoscopy, stroboscopy | Submucosal oval lesions in middle third of both vocal folds | Systemic steroids then local steroids (twice) | No, at 6 months follow-up after second injection |
| Laryngoscopy, stroboscopy | Multiple cystic shaped yellowish lesions protruding from the surface of both vocal folds | Logopedic therapy | No |
| Laryngoscopy, stroboscopy | Small cream yellow transparent transverse cystic lesions of the vocal folds | Logopedic therapy | No, at 6 months follow-up |
| Rigid laryngeal endoscopy, stroboscopy | Bilateral whitish transverse band stripes in the submucosa which lent a slightly protruded aspect to the vocal folds | Intralesional steroid injection 4 times followed by surgery | No (short intervals of speech therapy) |

has reported a 41-year-old female diagnosed with SLE who presented with hoarseness and dyspnea. Fiberoptic examination showed fixed left vocal fold in the paramedian position. The paralysis was confirmed using electromyography of the left thyroarytenoid muscle that revealed positive sharp waves and fibrillation at rest. Hypothesized etiologies included vasculitis of the vasa nervosa of the recurrent laryngeal nerve, thrombolytic events, pulmonary hypertension, and cricoarytenoid arthritis.[98] Karim et al has reported a 52-year-old female who presented with acute airway obstruction secondary to cricoarytenoid arthritis as the only presentation of SLE following several years of quiescence.[99] In 2009, Hughes and Hill reported a case of isolated left vocal fold palsy in the absence of cranial nerve deficit in a patient with SLE who developed hoarseness. The patient was treated with immunosuppression to partial avail.[100] A year

later Jayachandran et al reported a 17-year-old girl with active SLE who presented with hoarseness and shortness of breath. On laryngeal exam she had bilateral vocal fold paralysis with oral ulcerations. The patient was treated with intravenous hydrocortisone with significant improvement in her condition.[101] In 2013 Leszczynski and Pawlak-Bus also reported a case of a 38-year-old female patient diagnosed with SLE who presented with bilateral vocal fold paralysis. Her condition was complicated by the morbidities of other diseases, namely, myasthenia gravis and Hashimoto thyroiditis. She was managed with pulsed steroid intake and immunosuppressive therapy.[102] It is important to note that vocal fold paralysis may also be drug induced as reported by Hari et al following the intake of Hydralazine.[103] Other airway manifestations of SLE include subglottic stenosis that again can be life threatening. Smith and Ferguson have reported a 63-year-old female with active SLE who presented with shortness of breath and dyspnea on exertion. Endoscopy revealed subglottic stenosis that failed medical therapy and dilatation and required tracheotomy.[104]

With respect to treatment, unlike patients with rheumatoid arthritis, SLE patients with cricoarytenoid joint involvement respond to steroid therapy[63] and few may require a tracheotomy to secure the airway. The lack of mucosal changes such as inflammation or necrosis on laryngeal examination and the lack of response to steroid treatment make the etiology of arthritis and muscle inflammation unlikely. The presence of dilated pulmonary vessel on chest X-ray or echocardiography in the absence of any laryngeal lesions favors recurrent laryngeal nerve compression as the cause of the paralysis.

## Laryngeal Manifestations of Sjögren's Syndrome

Sjögren's syndrome (SS) is an autoimmune disease characterized by the presence of lymphocytic infiltrates within the exocrine glands resulting in systemic dryness that affects several systems in the body.[105,106] These include the central nervous system, the respiratory and digestive systems, in addition to many organs such as the lacrimal and salivary glands. The clinical picture may vary from non-specific symptoms of ocular and oral dryness, to marked exacerbation of sicca-related symptoms.[107,108] When Sjögren's syndrome coexists with other autoimmune diseases such as systemic lupus erythematosus, rheumatoid arthritis, and scleroderma, it is referred to as secondary, otherwise it is considered primary. Secondary SS accounts for 60% of the cases whereas the overall prevalence of primary SS is 1% of the adult population, an underestimated figure given the large number of underdiagnosed cases.[108] Sjögren's syndrome affects mainly women in their 4th and 5th decades and seems to be exacerbated by occupational factors and lifestyle. Pierce et al has reported in a large survey of 101 patients with SS that had vocally demanding jobs and exposure to inhalant irritants and dust, which are considered as significant risk factors that worsen the laryngeal symptoms in affected patients.[109] Other risk factors reported in this study are excessive jaw tension, neck tension, and history of lower airway disease such as pneumonia and bronchitis.

The etiology of SS remains unknown and many factors have been implicated such as viral infections and hormonal disturbances in addition to genetic predisposition.[110,111] A large array of antibodies has been incriminated in the pathophysiology of this disease among which is the antinuclear antibody (ANA) and rheumatoid factor (RA). The autoantibodies to the minor and major salivary glands and in particular to the glandular tissues in the laryngopharyngeal mucosa can cause severe reduction in the amount of saliva produced resulting in significant complaints. Irrespective of the culprit, the laryngeal symptoms in patients with SS are similar. These are usually gradual in onset with progression toward chronicity in 83% of the cases. The overall current prevalence of voice disorders can range between 41.9% up to 59.4% compared to a figure of 6.6% seen in the normal population.[109,112,113] In a study by Ruiz et al of 31 patients with SS, the disease was secondary in 87% of the cases. Associated symptoms of dysphagia and dysglossia were present in 70.9% and 35.4% of the cases, respectively.[113] The prevalence of these symptoms correlated with the severity of the disease but not with age, gender, duration of the disease, and its associated co-morbidities.[109] When present, the laryngeal symptoms of Sjögren's syndrome affect the quality of life to variable degrees. In a study by Heller et al of 11 patients with SS, the Voice Handicap Index scores were mild to moderate with a mean of 43 and a SD of 23.[114] Similarly Salturk et al has reported a higher Voice Handicap Index score in 10 women with SS patients compared to controls.[115] In a large study by Tanner et al on 101 patients with SS who completed interviews using Voice-Related Quality of Life (V-RQOL) and the general health-related quality of life short Form 36 (SF-36) questionnaire, the results indicated that patients with vocal symptoms had a higher burden on quality of life, and those with specific symptoms such as throat clearing, soreness, and vocal discomfort had significantly reduced SF-36 scores.[116] The results of this large cohort study not only supports the strong association between autoimmune diseases and voice but also substantiates the mild to moderate reduction in quality of life of patients with SS irrespective whether patients had voice disorders or not. Nevertheless, despite the aforementioned, only a few affected individuals seek medical attention (15.8%). This has been attributed either to the fact that the overall disease severity may mask or shadow the vocal symptoms, or to the shortage in education and level of awareness regarding the management modalities readily available for the treatment of these symptoms.

The symptoms in patients with SS are mainly related to physical sensations in the laryngopharyngeal complex. These include throat clearing, throat dryness, hoarseness, increased effort to talk, vocal fatigue, and dysphagia.[113,114,117,118] The phonatory symptoms are not always substantiated by disturbances in the acoustic parameters as shown on spectral and speech analysis. Heller et al has reported a significant difference in the fundamental frequency and perturbation parameters in her study of 11 patients with SS compared to normative values.[114] Similarly Ruiz et al has reported abnormalities in one or more of the acoustic parameters in 28 patients with SS.[113] These findings were further corroborated by Ogut et al who has reported a significant difference in all the voice quality parameters except for the noise to harmonic ration (NHR) in patients with SS compared to controls.[118] According to the authors, these findings were attributed to the aperiodic vibration of the vocal folds and to inadequate adduction. On the other hand, Salturk et al failed to show any significant difference in any of the acoustic or aerodynamic measures in his study on 10 patients with SS.[115]

In parallel with the aforementioned phonatory and swallowing symptoms, patients with Sjogren's syndrome exhibit diverse laryngeal pathology. These include impaired mobility of the vocal folds secondary to fixation of the cricoarytenoid joint or recurrent laryngeal nerve palsy,[119] presence of granulomatous and non-granulomatous nodules,[120–124] vocal nodules,[125] lymphocytic infiltrates,[126] lesions such as bamboo nodes,[127] dryness and crusting, and erythema and edema. In 2005 Seve et al reported a rare case of a 50-year-old female with SS who presented with dysphonia and oral dryness. On videostroboscopy she had cricoarytenoid joint (CAJ) arthritis with joint fixation that was managed successfully with prednisolone.[128] Arthritis of the CAJ has also been previously reported by Montgomery in 1963 and by Gresham and Kellaway in 1958.[129,130] Prytz reported the case of a 31-year-old female teacher who had persistent dysphonia following removal of bilateral vocal fold nodules. The patient was later diagnosed with SS and the recurrence of her vocal symptoms was attributed to edema and hyperemia of the vocal folds that resolved with medical treatment.[125] Ito et al reported a case who had recurrent swelling of the false vocal folds that necessitated repeated excisions of the false cords to alleviate obstructive airway symptoms. The pathology revealed atrophic glandular changes and cystic dilation suggestive of SS.[131] Korst has also reported another laryngotracheal manifestation of SS in a 61-year-old women who complained of dyspnea and stridor that was attributed to a circumferential narrowing of the subglottic region 3 cm below the true vocal folds. The patient was managed by subglottic resection and reconstruction of the mucosal membrane after excision of the stenotic segment. The pathology was consistent with mucosal associated lymphoid tissue lymphoma.[126]

The edema and erythema of the laryngeal mucosa most commonly seen in patients with SS can be secondary either to the effect of the disease itself on the seromucinous glands of the laryngeal mucosa or to precipitation and worsening of pre-existent or silent laryngopharyngeal reflux disease.[113,125,127,128,132–135] Patients with SS are more predisposed to reflux symptoms because of deficiencies in their anti-reflux barriers in addition to the inherent susceptibility of the laryngeal and pharyngeal mucosa to the refluxate material. The limited buffering of the saliva in patients with SS makes the esophagus more vulnerable to acid. Confounded with further reduction in acid clearance, there is exacerbation and worsening of the reflux symptoms as reported by Belafsky and Postma in 2003.[132] In a study by Ogut et al on 77 patients with SS, both the Reflux Symptoms Index and Reflux Finding Scores were statistically significantly higher compared to the control group.[118]

Despite the description of an array of laryngeal pathologies in patients with SS, in many instances patients present with vocal symptoms in the absence of frank or gross laryngeal pathology on endoscopy. Instead patients present with subtle abnormalities hardly perceived on routine examination. Using the Stroboscopy Evaluation Rating Form (SERF), Salturk et al has reported that the smoothness, straightness, regularity, and closure of the vocal folds in patients with SS differed significantly from normal subjects.[115] Similarly in a study by Ruiz et al on 31 subjects with SS, 41.9% of whom had dysphonia, vocal fold mucosal changes and reduced amplitude have been reported in 90% of the cases and altered nasopharyngeal and laryngeal mucosa in 77.41% of the cases. The most common mucosal changes were hyperemia and thick secretions. In parallel with the phonatory symptoms there was dysphagia in 70.9% and abnormalities in swallowing mechanism in 90.3%.[113] A study by Heller et al revealed mild reduction in the laryngeal function with normal vibratory behavior and mobility of the vocal folds.[114]

Treatment of SS is frustrating both to the patient and to the physician. There is no cure for this disease and the treatment consists of controlling the symptoms. Most commonly used regimens include topical lubricants, use of nebulizers, and cholinergic medications. The use of nebulizers has gained popularity because of the known effect of local hydration on the voice in addition to systemic hydration. Hydration correlates with the phonatory threshold pressure (PTP) which is the pressure needed to set the vocal folds into vibration, and subsequently with the phonatory effort. Subjects who are well hydrated have lower PTP and need less effort to phonate compared to subjects who are poorly hydrated. Similarly, osmotically induced dehydration as reported by Chan and Tayama and by Finkelhor et al increases vocal fold stiffness and viscosity.[136,137] This correlation has also been demonstrated in regard to systemic dehydration.[138–141] As the vocal fold surface consists of water and mucus, humidifiers, nasal breathing, and use of nebulizers assist in replenishing surface tissue hydration which secures epithelial cell homeostasis and helps protect the existing mucus of the vocal folds from external irritants.[142–144] Various concentrations of nebulized saline have been prescribed for the treatment of autoimmune related symptoms of the upper and lower airway.[145–149] Tanner et al has recently reported the effects of nebulized saline in a longitudinal study on eight patients with SS. Cepstral Spectral Index of Dysphonia improved by 20% during treatment and worsened with withdrawal. Patients on treatment had less vocal effort, less laryngeal dryness, and better voice production. Thus, nebulized saline has been recommended by the authors as a topical hydration treatment for the vocal folds that can be used temporary and intermittently.[150]

## Laryngeal Manifestations of Relapsing Polychondritis

Relapsing polychondritis (RP) is an inflammatory disease that affects cartilaginous structures and connective tissues in the body leading to functional disorders and disabilities.[151] It has multiple systemic manifestations among which are arthritic, vascular, and ocular, often leading to degenerative changes and deformities. It was first described as polychondropathy by Jaksch-Wartenhorst in 1923 and later coined as relapsing polychondritis in view of the relapsing and episodic nature of the disease.[152] All ethnic groups are affected and the prevalence is around 3.5 cases per million, affecting almost equally men and women between their fourth to sixth decades of life. Its association with cancer has been reported in two cases by Quinsat et al in 1989.[153] The etiology is believed to be autoimmune based on the high prevalence of other autoimmune diseases present in almost one out of three patients and on the high titers of circulating antibodies to type II collagen in two out of three affected individuals.[154] In a study by Buckner et al, T cells against CII were identified in patients with RP and the cloning of which was specific for CII peptide 261–273.[155] To that end, Navarro et al has reported the successful use of oral CII in the treatment of a child with relapsing polychondritis.[156] More so, studies by Lang et al and later by Zeuner et al have docu-

mented the presence of HLA-DR4 antigen in patients with RP.[157,158]

In view of its overlap with many autoimmune diseases, the diagnosis of the otolaryngologic manifestations of RP can be masked by non-specific symptoms. The otolaryngologic manifestations are many with chondritis being the hallmark feature of the disease and a key diagnostic feature. It may present in one out of two patients, and is usually limited to the ear, nose, and laryngotracheal structures. The ears are affected first in 40% to 90% of the cases. Patients usually complain of ear pain, redness, and severe tenderness upon slight touching which often is mistaken for an acute infection.[159,160] The recurrent bouts of inflammation often lead to collapse, calcification, and cauliflower deformity in 10% of the cases.[161] Audiovestibular manifestations can also be present in up to 40% of the cases with a sudden onset of sensorineural hearing loss. Nasal chondritis is the second most common presentation of this disease. It affects primarily the dorsum or bridge of the nose with subsequent, atrophy of the cartilage, and nasal septal collapse. Nasal crusting, pain, and epistaxis are the primary symptoms of nasal chondritis which is present in one out of four patients with RP. Repeated episodes of nasal inflammation may result in destruction of the nasal cartilage with subsequent saddle nose deformity. Systemic vasculitis has been reported to be a poor prognostic indicator of nasal involvement

Laryngotracheal manifestations of RP can occur in one out of two patients along the course of the disease often leading to fatal complications.[162] The associated symptoms are usually present in 25% of the cases as reported by Isaak et al in 1986 in his cohort study of 112 patients. When the larynx is affected patients often report a change in voice quality, cough, difficulty in breathing, wheezing, neck pain at the site of the laryngotracheal complex, and choking.[160] What is alarming is that the airway symptoms may be the initial symptoms in affected patients. Childs et al reported three cases of laryngeal manifestation of relapsing polychondritis, all of whom presented with airway symptoms that necessitated aggressive medical therapy and or surgical intervention.[162] Similarly the summary article by Kent et al on the clinical manifestations of RP indicated that almost half the subjects had respiratory tract symptoms, namely, wheezing, stridor, and dyspnea in addition to change in voice quality.[163] These results were further corroborated by numerous studies indicating the high prevalence of airway and phonatory symptoms in patients with relapsing polychondritis.[164–166] Hong and Kim have reported that in patients with airway involvement, the larynx is affected in 25% of the cases.[165] In Michet et al's review of 112 cases, airway involvement was the cause of death in 10% of the cases.[166] The laryngotracheal symptoms have been attributed to inflammatory changes, cicatricial formation with subsequent subglottic stenosis, infection of the proximal and distal airway, and last to collapse of the airway, all of which lead to obstruction of the endolaryngeal or tracheal lumen. The rheumatologic manifestations of the disease in patients with airway involvement have been reported by Hong and Kim in 2013 in their review of 12 patients with RP and airway involvement. In addition to the tracheal and laryngeal involvement in 100% and 25%, respectively, other rheumatologic manifestations included the nose, ears, and eyes.[165]

The diagnosis of RP is based on meeting 3 out of the 6 criteria set by McAdam's criteria which represent a compilation of signs and symptoms of chondritic and inflammatory changes in various organs of the body.[154] Additional histologic features and extent of response to therapy were later added to these diagnostic criteria by Damiani and Levine.[167] Based on the aforementioned, for a patient to be diagnosed with RP he or she has to have not only 3 out of the 6 diagnostic criteria set by McAdam but also histologic confirmation of one or more of McAdam's signs, and response to therapy, namely, steroids and or Dapsone. Laryngotracheal manifestations of relapsing polychondritis mandate proper assessment not only of the static extent of involvement in terms of site and severity but also of the dynamic impairment of affected patients given the pliability of the airway during inspiration and expiration. Numerous diagnostic methods have been used, including flow-volume loop studies to assess extra-thoracic airway obstruction and resistance, plain radiography such as laryngotracheograms, or more advanced radiologic imaging such as computerized tomography which allows three-dimensional reconstruction of the airway while breathing. Krell et al in 1986 reported on the utility of pulmonary function testing (PFT) in 5 patients with RP. In three out of the five patients the PFT showed evidence of both inspiratory and expiratory obstruction, findings that were not reflected or evident on bronchoscopy during quiet breathing.[168] Mohsenifar et al has also advocated the usefulness of maximal expiratory and inspiratory flow-volume in the assessment of the dynamic nature of the tracheobronchial tree in patients with RP and airway symptoms.[169]

The treatment of relapsing polychondritis is individually based on the patient's condition, and extent and severity of the disease. It is invariably tailored given the disparities in the clinical presentation and the response to therapy. The mainstay medication given chronically or as bolus is glucocorticoid steroids. The dosage in patients with laryngotracheal manifestations is 1mg/kg/day that is tapered over time.[151,170–172] In the study by McAdam on 23 patients, three-fourths were on corticosteroid therapy, the effect of which was promising except in cases of severe respiratory tract involvement.[173] Less commonly used medications include colchicine and Dapsone, the intake of which mandates close observation in view of their adverse effects. In severe cases, immunosuppressive agents such a methotrexate are advocated with caution regarding hematologic complications.[171] In the investigation of the clinical characteristics of patients with RP and airway involvement, Hong and Kim recommended the use of both steroid and methotrexate as a therapeutic option.[165] Childs et al also reported the usage of steroids with methotrexate in two patients with hoarseness and dyspnea, one of whom needed laser treatment for the control of the laryngeal mass.[154] Biologic agents such as infliximab have been used experimentally but several patients experienced fatal infections.[174] Infliximab is a monoclonal antibody that has been used successfully for the treatment of disease mediated by tumor necrosis factors. Mpofu et al has described the usage of infliximab in the treatment of a 51-year-old female with RP who had relapse following cessation of methyl prednisolone therapy and had developed methemoglobinemia following administration of Dapsone.[175]

## Laryngeal Manifestations of Sarcoidosis

Sarcoidosis is a slowly progressive disease characterized by the occurrence of non-caseating granuloma in various sites of the body. It rarely occurs below the age of 15 years and is most common in the third to fifth decade of life affecting women more than men, and African Americans more than Caucasians.[176,177] Based on the ACCESS study (A Case Control Etiologic Study of Sarcoidosis) designed to characterize sarcoidosis in the United States, women are likely to suffer from neurologic and ocular involvement whereas men are more likely to develop hypercalcemia. The study has also shown that Blacks were more likely to have skin, liver, eye, and bone marrow involvement.[178] The etiology of sarcoidosis is still unknown. Many theories have been suggested, none of which are confirmative. These include infectious, toxic, and abnormal immune regulation.[176,179] For a subject to develop sarcoidosis, three elements must coincide: a stimulus or an allergen be it environmental or infectious, a genetic predisposition, and a host reaction that is most likely immunologic. Today there is limited understanding of the gene-environment interactions in sarcoidosis as in many other disease entities. An external stimulus can modulate gene expression and similarly a genetic variant is context-dependent, meaning it is only expressed upon exposure to the right stimulus.[180] The notion that sarcoidosis is familial has been supported by the increased odds ratio among siblings by five and by the presence of familial clustering.[181] HLA-related genes have also been suggested in the genetic predisposition in some of the affected patients, namely, the HLA-DQB1 in African-American families, alluding to racial differences.[180–182] To that end, sarcoidosis has an inherited susceptibility and future genotyping may further elucidate the true genetic makeup of affected patients.[182]

The starting point in the histology of sarcoidosis is a granuloma that forms as a reaction to an antigenic agent that leads to the clustering of different inflammatory cells as an immune mediated response. Several antigens such as mycobacteria or Propionibacteria have been incriminated as stimuli and "Interferon-gamma" and cytokines such as TNF-alpha, IL-12 and IL-18[183,184] have been suggested to play a role in the formation of the granuloma. A recent study by Moller supported the notion that *Mycobacterium tuberculosis* catalase-peroxidase protein (mKatG) is an antigenic stimulus in a subset of sarcoidosis patients.[184] His results were in accordance with a recent review that further substantiates that infectious agents, namely, mycobacteria and proprionibacteria are considered to be etiologic antigens in some cases of sarcoidosis.[185] Once exposed to these antigens, there is an immune-mediated response. These include "reduced lymphocyte blastogenesis, circulating immune complexes or delayed hypersensitivity reactions."[185] However, it is important to note that whether the autoimmune response is primary or secondary remains a controversial issue.

The course of the disease is characterized by remissions and relapses often leading to functional impairment. At times it can be self-attenuating within one to three years leaving behind residual end organ damage.[179] The disease has a predilection for lungs and chest lymph nodes. Other organs less likely to be involved are spleen, liver, skin, bones, and nervous system.[178,186–189] The otolaryngologic manifestations of this disease may be present in 10 to 15% of patients with sarcoidosis with involvement of the nasopharynx, nose, paranasal sinuses, tongue, tonsils, and larynx.[176,179,183,189] Laryngeal sarcoidosis is a rare entity with the first case being reported by Poe in 1940.[190]

Since then the estimated prevalence of laryngeal sarcoidosis is 0.5 to 1.4% within the context of otolaryngologic manifestations of this disease which is within the range of 9 to 15%.[189,191] Laryngeal sarcoidosis is invariably accompanied by systemic manifestations such as relapsing fever, polyarthritis that is migratory, fatigue, and weight loss. When accompanied by head and neck manifestations, symptoms such as nasal crusting, bleeding, and multiple cranial neuropathies related to central nervous system involvement may prevail. A limited number of isolated laryngeal sarcoidosis have been reported in the literature.[192,193] In the review of the Mayo Clinic by Neel and McDonald in 1982, almost half the patients with laryngeal sarcoidosis had systemic manifestations and similarly in the review of Benjamin et al of five cases of laryngeal sarcoid, only one had disease not confined to the larynx.[193,194] Nevertheless, before stating that sarcoidosis is isolated to the larynx, a systematic inquiry must be made and a long-term follow-up is needed to ensure that no other organ is involved.[195]

The clinical presentation of sarcoidosis is mosaic as demonstrated in the report of 4 cases by Mayerhoff et al.[196] Although the symptoms of laryngeal sarcoidosis are invariably confined to the laryngopharyngeal complex, these can vary in nature and severity. The most common symptoms reported are cough, change in voice quality, difficulty in swallowing, and airway obstruction.[194,197] Based on a report of 13 cases of laryngeal sarcoidosis by Neel and McDonald, the most common symptoms by order of frequency were hoarseness followed by dysphagia and dyspnea.[194] This order of frequency of symptoms was confirmed by numerous studies with an estimated presence of hoarseness in 70 to 85% of the cases followed by dysphagia in up to 85%, dyspnea in 47% to 60%, and non-specific symptoms such as globus and cough in one out of 10 patients. Note that up to 18% of patients with laryngeal sarcoidosis may be asymptomatic.[191,194,197,198] Indeed in the report by Neel and McDonald one patient out of the 13 had incidental findings of laryngeal sarcoidosis in the absence of any symptoms.

All the aforementioned reports alluded further to the heterogeneity of the laryngeal findings in patients with sarcoidosis. The most common site of laryngeal involvement is the supraglottis in 80% of cases, followed by subglottis in 15 to 20% of the cases, and the true vocal folds in 1%.[192,194,197,198] In the review by Neel and McDonald the supraglottis was the site most commonly involved in 9 out of 13 patients, followed by the subglottis in two patients and the vocal folds in one.[194] The sites most commonly involved in the supraglottis are the epiglottis, aryepiglottic folds, and false vocal folds.[191] The rarity of involvement of the true vocal folds is due to the scarcity of lymphatics and lymphoid tissue within these structures. Nevertheless, the report by Bower et al revealed abnormalities in the vocal folds in 24% of the cases.[197] When affected, non-specific findings of inflammatory changes in the anteroinferior segments are present.

Despite the presence of edema, inflammation, and diffuse mucosal thickening in any area of the larynx,[199] the classic appearance of an epiglottic rim that is fully rounded with a turban-like thickening is pathognomonic of laryngeal sarcoidosis.[195] Note that laryngeal involvement may not be limited to one laryngeal segment but instead multiple laryngeal sites can be involved as reported by Sims and Thakkar in 2007, where two-thirds of patients with laryngeal sarcoidosis had extensive disease necessitating surgical management.[200] When these lesions are sporadic and non-specific the otolaryngologist must also rule out allergic reactions and infectious diseases such as tuberculosis, blastomycosis, histoplasmosis, or syphilis. It is also important to keep in mind that similar mucosal changes may be found following irradiation or in patients with connective tissue disorders such as amyloidosis.[201] A less frequently encountered finding is an exophytic lesion well localized, mimicking laryngeal neoplasms.[192,202,203] Sakamato et al has reported a rare case of laryngeal sarcoidosis presenting as a polypoid mass pedunculated arising from the right arytenoid and aryepiglottic fold in a 45 year women who presented with stridor.[203] In similar cases, the otolaryngologist must rule out other neoplastic lesions and laryngeal malignant tumors such as lymphoma or cartilaginous neoplasms.

Sarcoidosis may also cause unilateral or bilateral vocal fold paralysis as reported by many authors.[204–209] The paralysis can be isolated or in combination with multiple cranial neuropathies involving the facial and optic nerves in addition to the hypoglossal, trigeminal, spinal accessory, auditory, and vagal nerves. When present in the absence of polyneuritis, the etiology is usually compression of the recurrent laryngeal nerve along its course in the chest. Significant hilar or peritracheal lymphadenopathy is usually present on computerized tomography of the chest. Based on a literature review only eight cases of vocal fold paralysis have been reported with the majority being unilateral and on the left side given the long course of the recurrent laryngeal nerve on the left.[204–209] Only two cases of bilateral vocal fold paralysis have been reported, one by Witt attributed to both polyneuritis and compression of the recurrent laryngeal nerve and one by Coffey et al that was attributed to

intrathoracic lymphadenopathy, a common finding in patients with sarcoidosis present in up to 90% of the cases.[206–209] The majority of these patients improve on corticosteroid therapy within few days after the initiation of therapy.

In the absence of systemic complaints and when the disease is confined to the larynx the diagnosis of laryngeal sarcoidosis may be challenging to the Otolaryngologist. It is more so when the laryngeal findings are non-specific, which mandates a good index of suspicion in order to make the proper diagnosis. It should be based on clinical findings, exclusion of other infectious and inflammatory diseases that have similar presentations, and on histopathologic confirmation. To that end a complete workup to assess the extent of the disease systemically and to assess the response to treatment is crucial. This includes laboratory studies to check for abnormal protein electrophoresis, the presence of hyperglobulinenia, hypercalcemia, hypercalciuria in case of abnormal vitamin D3 metabolism, decreased albumin, and abnormal electrophoresis, in addition to electrocardiogram and chest x-ray to rule out the presence of hilar, paratracheal or mediastinal lymphadenopathy, and/or the presence of pulmonary infiltrates.[179,210] Other required tests include PPD skin testing to exclude tuberculosis, and last pulmonary function testing which may show signs of upper airway obstruction in cases of laryngeal involvement.[191,195,197] Gallium-67 citrate may be used to detect granulomatous inflammation in other sites of the body such as the salivary glands that may not be clinically apparent at the time of presentation.[194,211] The Kveim test to elicit an allergic reaction at the site of injection is not commonly used in view of its low accuracy and the difficulty in procuring the antigen of right consistency.[194,195,212]

The diagnosis is confirmed on histologic examination with the presence of noncaseating nonnecrotic granuloma formation that consists of inflammatory cells such as epithelioid cells, Langerhans' giant cells, macrophages, and lymphocytes. With time, there is hyalinization, fibrosis, and scarring. That is why a biopsy taken late in the course of the disease may be non-diagnostic and reveals only non-specific inflammatory infiltrates. It is preferable to have more than one laryngeal biopsy in order to demonstrate the presence of noncaseating granulomatous lesion. Cultures for acid-fast bacilli and fungus in addition to Ziehl-Neelsen staining must be taken to exclude other infections and disease entities. However, if the clinical picture is typical and the laryngeal findings are highly suggestive, biopsies taken from other sites of the body showing noncaseating granulomatous disease may be used to make the diagnosis as reported by Neel and McDonald.[194] The physician must also exclude other disease entities as discussed earlier in this chapter.

The management of laryngeal sarcoidosis aims at restoring the airway while preserving good voice quality. To that end, it is empirical to remain conservative as much as possible. The mainstays of medical treatment are corticosteroids and cytotoxic agents such as methotrexate and cyclophosphamide.[191,202,213,214] Fortune and Courey have reported the successful management of a 28-year-old woman diagnosed with sarcoidosis with systemic steroids. The patient had severe supraglottic swelling that resulted in dysphagia, shortness of breath, and dysphonia. All the symptoms improved on systemic steroids that was tapered over the course of three weeks.[192] In another report, Hensderson et al discussed the treatment of a 50-year-old man who had failed steroid therapy with methotrexate 10 mg/ week. The methotrexate resulted in marked improvement of both cutaneous and nasolaryngeal lesions.[202]

Given the natural course of the disease, namely, remission and relapse with spontaneous regression, sometimes it is very hard to assess the effect of medical treatment in particular the use of glucocorticoids. Nevertheless, steroids still are recommended as the first line of treatment for systemic manifestations such as pulmonary disease, ocular myasthenia gravis (MG), central nervous system or skin involvement. Steroids may also be used as intralesional injections in patients with localized laryngeal lesions.[191,198] A report by Gallivan and Landis of two teachers who presented with a "honking" voice secondary to laryngeal sarcoidosis with the typical pathognomonic appearance were successfully treated with intralesional steroid injection. This mode of therapy in addition to early diagnosis of laryngeal involvement of this disease may spare the patient unnecessary morbidity such as tracheotomy.[191] Similarly Dean et al has reported successful treatment of a 64-year-old female case of sarcoidosis with laryngeal intralesional steroid injections in addition to steroid inhalers. Three months after initiation of therapy, the patient had marked improvement in both voice quality and breathing.[198]

Surgical resection is also an alternative that is mainly performed endoscopically. James and Simpson have reported a 60-year-old woman who failed intralesional steroid and dilation and presented with symptoms of airway obstruction. The stenotic area was treated successfully with $CO_2$ laser followed by the application of mytomycin C (0.4 mg/mL saline).[215] More aggressive and extensive lesions that fail conservative transoral or microlaryngeal resection may require surgery through open approaches such as laryngofissure for excision of subglottic lesions or supraglottic laryngectomy. Low-dose irradiation confined to the site of the lesion is also a viable alternative. Additionally, tracheotomy may be considered as a last resort in order to secure the airway.

## Laryngeal Manifestations of Wegener's Granulomatosis

Wegener's granulomatosis, initially named after Friedreich Wegener in 1939, is a necrotizing granulomatous inflammatory disease characterized by vasculitis that involves small and medium-sized blood vessels. Recently, the preferred name has been changed to granulomatosis with polyangiitis. Also described as granulomatosis with polyangiitis (GPA), Wegener's granulomatosis affects 3 out 100,000 individuals in the United States with a predilection for whites compared to blacks.[216,217] Information on geographic variation is conflicting despite the numerous reports indicating a higher prevalence in Europe compared to the United States.[216,218-220] Patients are usually in their 5th, 6th, and 7th decades of life.[216,217] Unlike adults, when children are affected, the course of the disease may be undulant with life-threatening dyspnea and respiratory distress.[221]

Wegener's granulomatosis can present either as a syndrome with the classic involvement of the respiratory tract, kidneys, and lungs, or as a local disease affecting mainly the upper and lower airway. When the disease is systemic, patients present with systemic complaints such as malaise, arthritic pain, generalized weakness, myalgia, and night sweats, in addition to the presence of cutaneous lesions mainly on the lower extremities. When the lungs are involved, which occurs in 50 to 90% of cases, hemoptysis and cough are the most common symptoms. Evidence of pulmonary cavitated parenchymal lesions are often mistaken for fibrosis or pulmonary vascular diseases on radiologic imaging.[222,223] When the kidneys are affected the prognosis is worse and patients present with hematuria and protenuria secondary to necrotizing glomerulonephritis.[217] Criteria for distinguishing GPA from other systemic vasculitis have been defined by the American College of Rheumatology. Two of the following 4 criteria must be present in order to make the diagnosis: (1) "sinus involvement, (2)"lung radiograph demonstrating nodules, fixed infiltrates, or cavities," (3) abnormal urine cytology, and (4)" histologic evidence of granulomas in or around an artery or

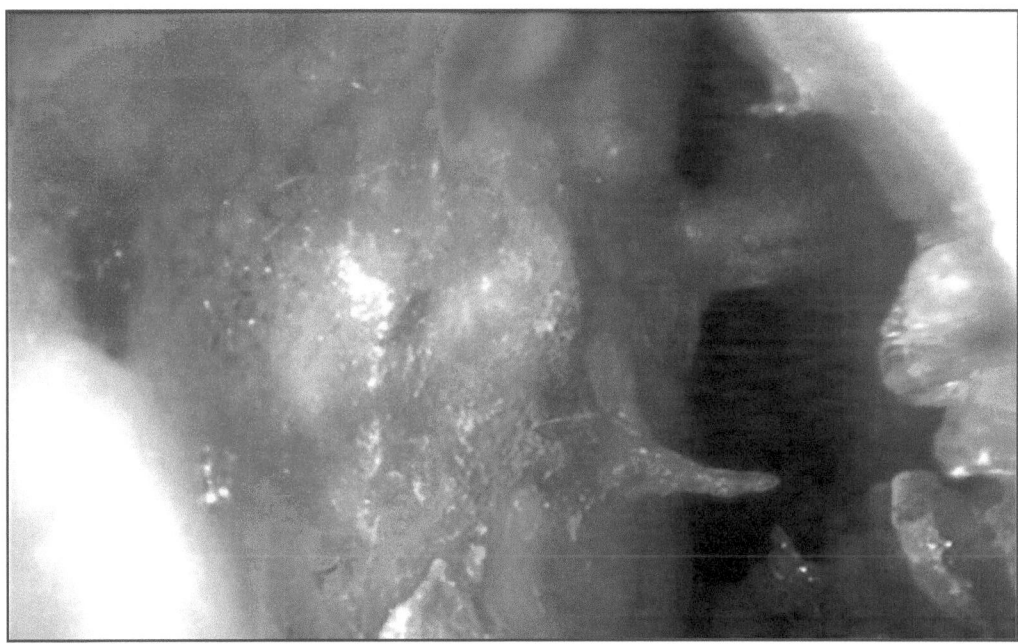

**Figure 12–8.** Crusting and ulcerations of the nasal septum in a 40-year-old woman diagnosed with Wegener's granulomatosis.

arteriole."[224] Depending on the severity of the disease, the Birmingham Vasculitis Activity Score can be used to grade the extent of the disease.[225]

It is important to note that the otolaryngologic manifestations may be the first presenting symptoms occurring in up to 92% of patients affected with Wegener's granulomatosis. The most common prevalent site in the head and neck region is the sinonasal tract, mainly the septum in up to 85% of the cases, followed by the ears in around 44% with a predilection to the middle ear, and the laryngotracheal complex in up to 23%.[226–228] When the sinonasal tract is affected, patients present with history of excessive nasal crusting, epistaxis, and nasal obstruction in addition to facial heaviness and pain over the nasal dorsum. On physical examination there is irregular granular thickening of the mucosa with ulceration and necrosis often leading to septal perforation.[229,230] See Figure 12–8. The septal perforations have been attributed to vasculitis affecting the Kiesselbach triangle leading to cartilage necrosis. In rare cases there is nasal saddle deformity secondary to loss of support to the nasal dorsum.[231–233] Based on a report by Cannady et al of 120 patients with nasal manifestations, the most common findings were nasal crusting and chronic sinusitis in 69% and 61%, respectively. Nasal obstruction was present in more than 50% and nasal saddle deformity in almost one out of 5.[231]

Involvement of the ear which occurs in 20 to 70% of the cases may be the first sign of Wegener's disease. When affected, the external ear is rarely involved, instead patients present with recurrent or persistent serous otitis media resistant to treatment.[232–234] The etiology is thought to be eustachian tube dysfunction. Suppurative otitis media is often complicated by mastoiditis and associated facial nerve palsy in up to 10% of the cases.[235,236]

Involvement of the airway and in particular the larynx is not rare.[237–240] In children, the prevalence can be as high as 86% as reported by Fowler et al.[237] The sites most commonly affected are the subglottic region and the trachea. This stands to reason given the high affinity of this disease to the respiratory ciliated epithelium. The presence of subglottic stenosis (SGS) in the absence of history of laryngeal or tracheal manipulation should greatly increase suspicion of Wegener's granulomatosis. It is important to note that SGS more often than not represents the limited or localized form of the disease rather than its systemic form.[236] At times the stenosis may extend to the glottic region and cricoarytenoid joint resulting in fixation of these joints. The incidence of having CAJ involvement in patients with subglottic stenosis is not well reported; however, the rate of subglottic stenosis (SGS) is estimated to be 16%.[220,237] See Figure 12–9. It is important to note that the progress of SGS in affected patients does not

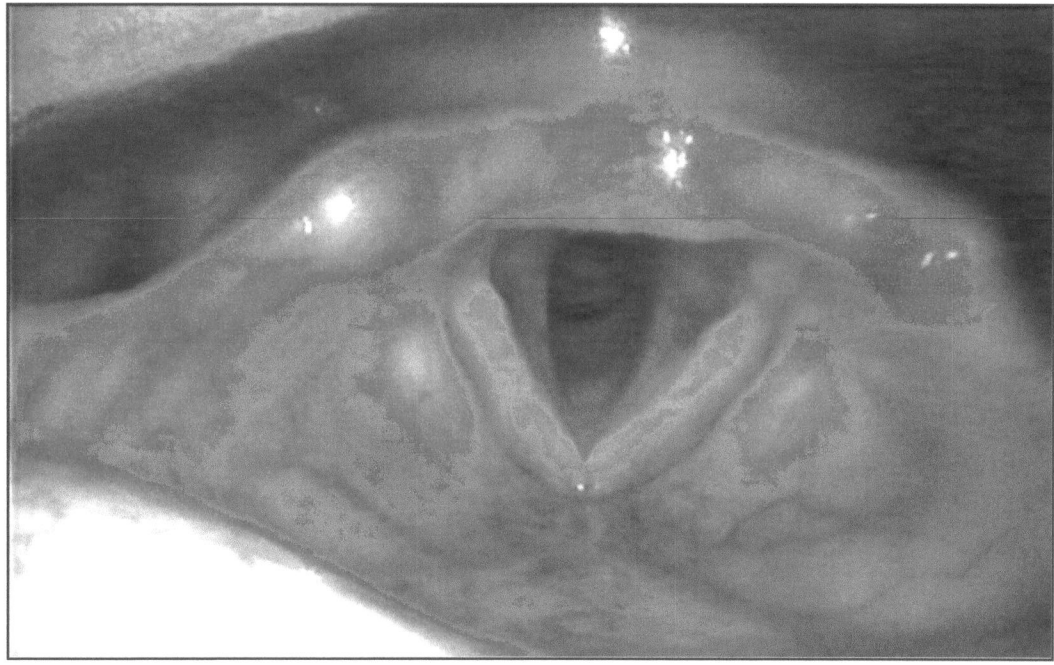

**Figure 12–9.** Subglottic stenosis in a 40-year-old woman diagnosed case of Wegener's granulomatosis presenting with history of shortness of breath and dyspnea.

always correlate with the extent and stage of the disease. Subsequently, the pathologic findings on tissue examination of biopsies taken from the subglottis may vary from scar tissue and nonproliferative fibroblasts to the presence of necrotizing granuloma diagnostic of granulomatosis with polyangiitis.[240] Nevertheless, the differential diagnosis should include infectious diseases such as tuberculosis, syphilis, lupus, leprosy, candidosis, mucormycosis, and aspergillosis in addition to non-specific inflammatory or autoimmune disorders such as sarcoidosis.[241]

The diagnosis of Wegener's is both clinical and pathologic. It is based on positive serologic studies for ANCA and on histologic evidence of necrotizing granulomatous inflammation with evidence of vasculitis affecting mainly small and medium-sized vessels. Anti-proteinase 3 antibody, known as c-ANCA is commonly used as a serologic marker for the disease activity. Although Wegener's granulomatosis is believed to be an immunologically mediated disease, the etiology behind the release of pro-inflammatory cytokines and ANCA has not been elucidated in the literature.[242,243] To that end, several hypotheses have been suggested and these include infection, drug-induced, genetic background, and environmental factors.[244] Nevertheless, it is important to note that the yield of both ANCA serologies and laryngeal tissue biopsy findings are more often than not negative and unreliable for pathologic diagnosis especially in

the presence of extensive scarring.[236,245] Paraclinical diagnosis may also include a complete blood count, urine analysis, chemistry studies, C-reactive proteins, and other serologic tests such as anticytoplasmic autoantibodies and rheumatoid factors, as patients with Wegener's granulomatosis may also present with anemia, high sedimentation rate, and high ACPA. The high ACPA is based on the IgG against the cytoplasms of neutrophils presenting with a diffuse cytoplasmic granular staining in cytopsin preparations of neutrophils of affected patients.[241]

The treatment of Wegener's granulomatosis with laryngotracheal involvement is both medical and surgical. The medical management consists of immunosuppressive agents such as steroids, cyclophosphamide, and methotrexate or the usage of trimethroprim-sulfamethoxazol.[223,245–247] The treatment may be given either in stages or in pulse doses and its duration is crucial in relation to the extent of relapse as 50% of the relapses occur when the patient is not on treatment.[248] Medical therapy has been shown to attenuate the severity of the disease and at times reduce the need for surgical intervention. However, when medical therapy fails to improve patients' airway symptoms, which is more likely to occur when the disease is localized to the upper airway, surgical therapy is indicated. The latter is more reserved for the treatment of subglottic stenosis and tracheal lesions, and is usually advised when the disease is in its inactive phase. When indicated, surgical intervention should be conservative with the least amount of intervention. The surgical intervention may vary from simple repeated dilatation, to dilatation with steroid injections, dilatation with stent placement, laryngofissure with or without skin grafting, laryngotracheal reconstruction, and or segmental tracheal resection with end-to-end anastomosis.[249-251]

The laser plays a major role as a cutting and coblation tool for the resection and or ablation of the stenotic segment. To that end there are numerous reports on the usage of both the $CO_2$ laser and other photocoagulating lasers such as the Nd:YAG. The main added values lie in: (1) The use of an endoscopic approach versus the open approach commonly adopted in laryngotracheal reconstruction or segmental tracheal resection, (2) the short operative time and hospital stay of the patient compared to other surgical procedures, (3) the low rate of complications during and following the procedure pertaining to bleeding and injury to the recurrent laryngeal nerve, and (4) the lack of need for a tracheotomy because of minimal edema.[252] The added value of using the laser is mostly pronounced in patients with high subglottic stenosis in close proximity to the vocal folds. Strong et al was among the first to use laser for the treatment of glottic and subglottic stenosis.[253] Since then the successful outcome and usefulness of laser therapy has been reported further by many authors. Dedo et al and Ossoff in their report on the microtrapdoor technique for the treatment and resection of glottis and subglottic stenosis showed marked improvement in both phonation and breathing in patients.[254] On the other hand there were reports on the recurrence and even worsening of subglottic scarring following laser therapy.[226] In a study by Lebovics et al on 25 cases who underwent treatment for their subglottic scarring, multimodality and frequent interventions using dilatation, $CO_2$ laser and laryngotracheoplasty were often needed. The authors indicated that the course of treatment of subglottic stenosis is more often than not complex. This has led many to recommend minimal manipulation especially during the active phase of the disease.[226] Gluth et al in his study of 27 patients with Wegener's granulomatosis and subglottic stenosis strongly advise the least amount of surgical intervention when the disease is active. A tracheotomy is often done in order to secure the airway in times of respiratory distress.[245]

## Laryngeal Manifestations of Systemic Sclerosis

Systemic sclerosis (SS) is an autoimmune disease that affects various tissues in the body. Since its initial description by Carlo Curzio in 1753 as hardening of the skin, numerous terms have been used alternatively to describe the same disease entity.[255] It is characterized initially by chronic inflammation that is followed by interstitial fibrosis and vasculopathy that often leads to dysfunction of many organs.[256] See Figure 12–10. Based on an autopsy study of 58 cases of systemic sclerosis, the organs most commonly affected are the skin and gastrointestinal tract followed by the lungs, kidneys, and skeletal muscles.[257] It is also associated with an increased incidence of cancer, namely, bladder, breast, and cervical cancer.[258] The incidence in the United States is estimated to be 10 cases in a million adults with a prevalence of 276 cases per million. Based on a random sample of 6,998 subjects from South Carolina, the prevalence ranged from 67 to 265 per 100,000 with the ratio of non-definite cases, that is, not meeting the American Rheumatism Association criteria, to definite cases being 2:5. This leads us to believe that SS is underdiagnosed and a high index of suspicion is needed in order to have a proper estimate of its prevalence which seems to be on the rise.[259] Women are usually three to four times more affected than men with preponderance in the fourth to sixth decade of life.[260,261] More so, blacks are twice as likely to be affected as whites.[262] In addition to race, age is also considered as a factor that negatively affects survival. Subjects below the age of 25 are rarely involved whereas the onset at an older age carries a worse prognosis in view of multisystem involvement.

Afflicted patients present with an array of clinic-pathologic manifestations. In its mild form, systemic sclerosis affects only the skin with subsequent thickening, induration, and disfigurement often referred to as scleroderma. Initially, there is lymphocytic infiltration ($CD^4$+T cells) which is followed by deposition of collagen type 1, fibronectin, elastin, and other proteoglycans leading to marked disturbance in the extracellular matrix architecture. The cutaneous form may also include "calcinosis, Raynaud's, esophageal dysmotility, sclerdactily and telangiectasias" known as CREST syndrome.[263] In its more extensive form, systemic sclerosis occurs in conjunction with other autoimmune diseases such as rheumatoid arthritis, often referred to as part of "Overlap syndrome." Associated autoantibodies include "antinuclear autoantibodies (ANA), anticentromere, anti-topoisomerase 1, anti-RNA polymerase I/III, antifibrillarin" with the majority, that is, over 95%, having a positive serum for ANA.[256,264]

The otolaryngologic manifestations of SS are few with the primary focus being on muscles of mastication, tongue, and the laryngopharyngeal complex. Patients often present with trismus secondary to

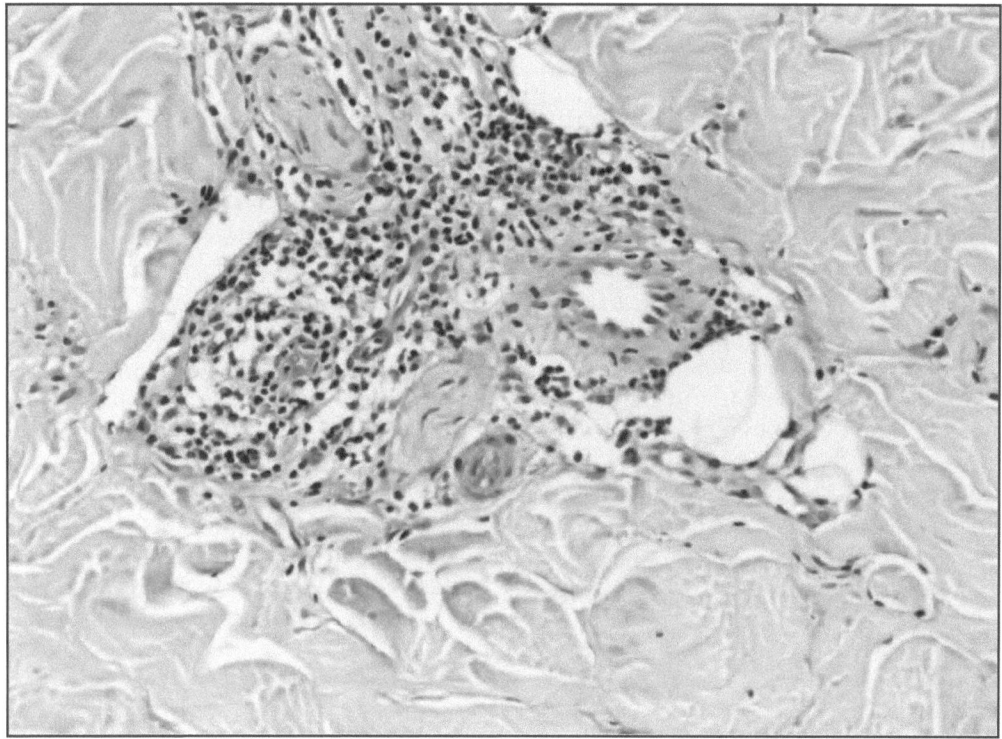

**Figure 12–10.** Hematoxylin and Eosin staining (power 10x): Deposition of swollen collagen bundles with lymphoplasmacytic infiltrates.

fibrosis of the muscles of mastication, ankyloglossia, and difficulties in swallowing and phonation. The laryngeal symptoms are the result of either primary laryngeal involvement or secondary to the gastroesophageal manifestation of this disease. Aside from skin involvement and Raynaud's phenomenon, the gastroesophageal system is third in the manifestation of progressive systemic sclerosis.[260] The high prevalence of gastrointestinal involvement (90%) and reflux in affected patients is secondary to reduced esophageal peristalsis, decreased lower esophageal sphincter pressure, autonomic dysfunction, and associated hiatal hernia.[257] Subsequent to these pathophysiologic alterations, namely, absent peristalsis in the distal two-thirds of the esophagus and to incompetent lower esophageal sphincter,[265] patients often complain of gastroesophageal and laryngopharyngeal reflux symptoms such as heartburn and regurgitation in addition to throat discomfort and globus sensation.

There are only a few reports in the literature describing vocal disorders in patients affected by this disease which leads us to believe that laryngeal involvement in systemic sclerosis is rather rare and variable in its course. When the larynx is affected, the most common phonatory complaints are dys-

phonia, vocal fatigue, increased pitch perturbations, reduced vocal intensity, and decrease in vocal range. These phonatory changes are associated with a large array of reflux-related symptoms as previously discussed such as heartburn, dysphagia, globus, and symptoms of regurgitation. The associated laryngeal findings include diffuse thickening of the vocal folds, increased perivascularity, yellowish submucosal lesions in the upper surface or free edge of the vocal folds, impaired mobility of the vocal folds or paralysis, and cricoarytenoid joint involvement.[264,266–272] Pepper et al has reported a 47-year-old woman with SS who presented with slowly progressive onset of hoarseness along with a reduced maximum phonation time. Laryngeal examination revealed multiple vocal fold submucosal yellowish lesions located centrally and associated with reduction in the mucosal waves' amplitude. These were removed surgically through a cordotomy approach with microdissection using both cold steel instrument and the carbon dioxide laser followed by local injection of long-acting steroids. Histopathologic examination revealed fibrinoid degeneration of ill-defined margins.[264] Sataloff et al also reported a 46-year-old singer who had dysphonia during the exacerbation of her scleroderma that affected both the larynx and esophagus at the time. The patient had a decrease in vocal range and ability to control her singing voice which markedly affected her vocal performance. These vocal symptoms were attributed to thickening of the vocal folds with hypervascularity and dilated varices, findings commonly seen in patients with collagen vascular disease.[266] Ramos et al reported 11 cases of SS who presented with various laryngeal signs suggestive of reflux. Diffuse mucosal thickening of the vocal folds was present in all subjects, vocal fold nodularity in two patients, and signs of laryngeal hypertrophy in one. It is worth noting that all patients with scleroderma had laryngeal involvement and almost half had clinical complaints.[267] Aside from nodularity and hypervascularity, more subtle laryngeal findings such as vocal fold atrophy may be responsible for the phonatory changes often described by these patients. Belenotti et al has reported dysphonia in a 45-year-old patient with diffuse cutaneous systemic sclerosis. The vocal symptoms and associated acoustic and aerodynamic changes, namely, the increase in Jitter, and reduced vocal range and maximum phonation time were attributed to an atrophic vocal fold. The suggested mechanism behind the atrophy is chronic inflammation, followed by fibrosis and atrophic changes. The patient was successfully treated with voice rehabilitation.[268]

All the aforementioned phonatory symptoms can be accompanied by upper respiratory obstructive symptoms such as dyspnea, shortness of breath, and respiratory discomfort. Kanter and Barash presented a case of undiagnosed scleroderma that necessitated retrograde wire intubation for an elective cardiac bypass surgery. The patient was found to have a difficult airway with redundant oropharyngeal soft tissues that impeded proper visualization of the larynx. Skin biopsies taken after the surgery were consistent with progressive systemic sclerosis.[269] Other causes of airway obstruction in patients with SS are unilateral or bilateral vocal fold paralysis. Ingegnoli et al described a rare case of an overlap syndrome, namely, rheumatoid arthritis and systemic sclerosis who presented with dyspnea and dysphonia that were progressive in nature over the course of 5 months. These symptoms were secondary to bilateral vocal fold paralysis nearly in the median position in the absence of postcricoid edema.[270] Similarly Viner et al reported a 40-year-old man diagnosed with scleroderma who presented with mild respiratory distress and inspiratory stridor in addition to change in voice quality.[271] On examination the patient had bilateral fixed vocal folds in the median position with edematous changes in the postcricoid region secondary to non-specific inflammatory changes as shown on biopsy of the arytenoid mucosa. Although arthritis is a rare manifestation of scleroderma, when present there is evidence of lymphocytic and plasma cell infiltration with subsequent development of a fibrin layer and fibrosis of the affected joint.[272] In a nutshell, laryngeal involvement in patients with progressive SS is rare and the treating physician should always be on the alert for any change in voice quality or airway symptoms in afflicted patients.

To that end, immediate medical attention is warranted in order to prevent undue complications. The management of SS depends on the clinical presentation of the patient and extent of functional impairment. The decision is often individualized and based on a mosaic variety of medications. The two pillars of therapy are systemic steroid administration and administration of immunosuppressive agents. These may be coupled with adjunctive procedures for the control of symptoms and signs of laryngeal and esophageal involvement. These are often managed conservatively with voice therapy and or steroid injection. Surgical intervention should be contemplated only in cases refractory to medical therapy.

## Laryngeal Manifestations of Amyloidosis

Amyloidosis is rare with an overall incidence of around 5 to 10 per million. It affects men more than women (M:F ratio 3:1) in their fifth and sixth decades of life.[273] Children are rarely affected with only few cases being reported in the literature.[274–280] Amyloidosis is characterized by the extracellular deposition of insoluble fibrillary proteins in various organs and tissues of the body, with a predilection to the heart, kidney, and liver.[281–285] Although this proteinaceous material may have a uniform appearance microscopically, there are different types of fibril proteins according to which the type of amyloid disease is designated. Currently, there are more than 36 biochemical forms in the human species with the amyloid light (AL) type accounting for close to 90% of the cases. The major ones are the AL referred to as immunoglobulin light chain and the amyloid associated (AA). The former is usually associated with myeloma and primary systemic amyloidosis whereas the latter is associated with secondary amyloidosis. The disease can be either localized where the plasma cells secrete light chain in a localized fashion at a given site, or systemic where the deposition is more widespread reaching various tissues and organs.[281,282] The head and neck region is affected in 20% of the cases with the most common sites of occurrence being the nasopharynx, oral cavity, orbit, and tracheobronchial

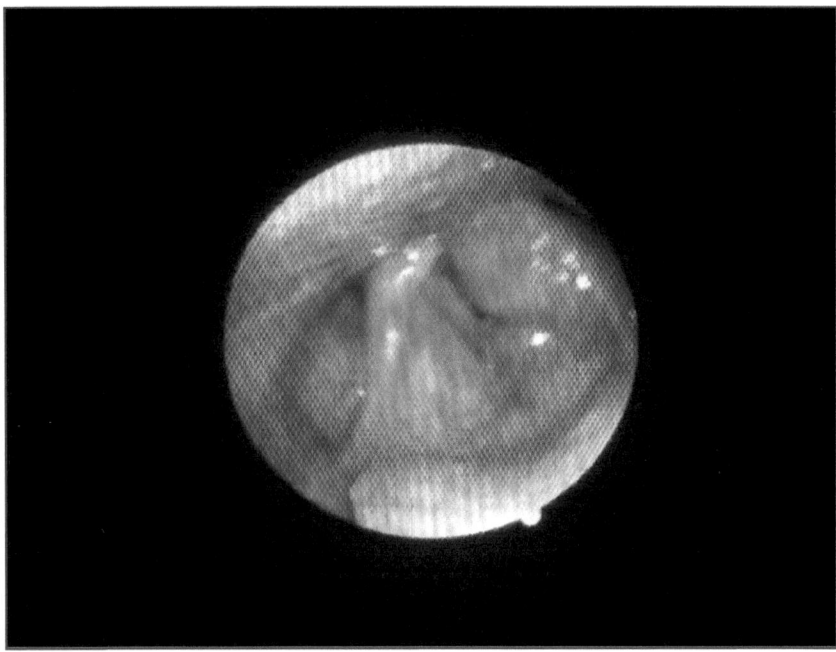

**Figure 12–11.** A 59-year-old woman, known case of amyloidosis, presented with history of shortness of breath and change in voice quality of a few months duration. On fiberoptic laryngeal exam there is a large supraglottic mass, mostly submucosal, involving the left aryepiglottic fold, false vocal fold, and reaching the apex of the arytenoid.

tree.[286] The larynx is most commonly affected and laryngeal amyloidosis accounts for 0.2 to 1.5% of all benign laryngeal lesions.[287–290] In a large review of 89 patients by Xu et al, localized amyloidosis affecting the larynx and trachea was present in only 2 cases.[291] Amyloidosis localized to the larynx is rarely associated with systemic diseases or plasma cell dyscrasia, and thus the characteristic signs and symptoms of AL amyloidosis are rarely reported in these cases.[290] In a retrospective review of 16 patients with amyloidosis treated at the Department of Otolaryngology at a university setting, 15 had isolated laryngeal amyloidosis and the majority were not suspected initially.[292]

The laryngeal findings in patients with isolated laryngeal amyloidosis may vary markedly depending on the extent of the disease and site of involvement. The lesion may appear either as nodular, cystic, or as diffuse swelling with thickening of the overlying tissues.[293] More often than not the lesion is reported as submucosal, smooth, whitish, sometimes described as a degenerative polyp, and often mistaken as a tumor. In rare cases, amyloidosis may be diffuse with ill-defined or demarcated margins.[294] Any part of the larynx may be involved with variations in the reports on the most commonly affected site. In the review by Wierzbicka et al, the most com-

mon site was the glottis (8 out of 16) followed by the epiglottis (7 cases).[292] In the report by Thompson et al, six out of 11 cases had transglottic lesions. The second-most common site in this study was the glottis (4 cases).[289] In brief, we can fairly assume that the ventricular folds, aryepiglottic folds, and vocal folds are the sites most commonly affected.

The clinical picture varies with the site involved as well as the duration of the disease. When the lesion is underneath the mucosa of the vocal fold, patients complain of change in voice quality that is often described as raspy, whereas when the lesion is in the supraglottis, the course of the disease may be insidious and patients may remain asymptomatic until there is significant narrowing of the airway. See Figure 12–11. In such cases, patients will present with progressive dyspnea and shortness of breath that is worsening with time.[295] In cases of thickening of the laryngeal and pharyngeal mucosa or with the presence of a large mass, patients may report dysphagia and difficulty swallowing. In brief the most common symptoms are related to phonation and breathing. Patients often complain of a change in voice quality with or without dyspnea, cough, and shortness of breath. Other reported symptoms include difficulty in swallowing and hemoptysis. The time lapse between the laryngeal involvement of the disease and emergence of the aforementioned symptoms or complaints varies markedly between a few months, 4 or 5, up to 20 years.[291,292,296] Note that the laryngeal lesion may be found incidentally on routine laryngeal examination or during microlaryngoscopy. In the report by Wierzbicka et al, laryngeal involvement was found in 0.52% of cases who underwent microlaryngoscopy over the course of 9 years. In the majority of cases there was no suspicion of a lesion preoperatively.[292]

For proper diagnosis, a tissue biopsy is invariably needed in order to perform proper histopathologic examination. See Figure 12–12. Congo red staining is used and the pathognomonic finding is the apple-green birefringence appearance using polarized light.[273,274] Once the diagnosis of amyloidosis is made, a comprehensive evaluation is needed given the systemic nature of the disease and its possible complications. The workup of patients diagnosed with amyloidosis includes hematologic assessment, in addition to radiologic imaging. Radiologic imaging may assist the otolaryngologist in assessing the extent of the disease and the different sites of involvement given that it is multifocal in many instances. Both computerized tomography as well as magnetic resonance imaging can be used with a preference for the latter in view of its specificity for soft tissue changes. On computerized tomography there is evidence of tissue thickening whereas on magnetic res-

onance imaging there is "Intermediate T1-weighted signal intensity and low T2-weighted signal intensity" as reported by Philips et al in 2017.[297]

The treatment of laryngeal amyloidosis mandates a thorough understanding of the course and nature of this disease. The treating physician has to keep in mind that laryngeal amyloidosis is benign and unless there is airway obstruction, a conservative management strategy following a comprehensive evaluation is advocated. Given the high rate of recurrence and the importance of preserving good voice quality, the least amount of intervention, just necessary enough to secure the airway without jeopardizing the malleability of the vocal folds is recommended. To that end, treatment varies between observation in cases of slowly progressive lesions to surgical intervention. When surgery is indicated, the two main goals should be improvement of airway and voice preservation. With these concepts in mind, a large array of treatment options ought to be considered ranging from serial local excision in cases of localized lesions to hemilaryngectomy.[291] The surgical approaches are most commonly the endoscopic and external approaches. With the advances in technology and the increased accessibility to different lasers, repeated endoscopic laser resection has been commonly adopted. This multi-stage endoscopic laser resection approach is advocated by many authors with promising results.[291,298–300] The main advantages of the laser are precision, better

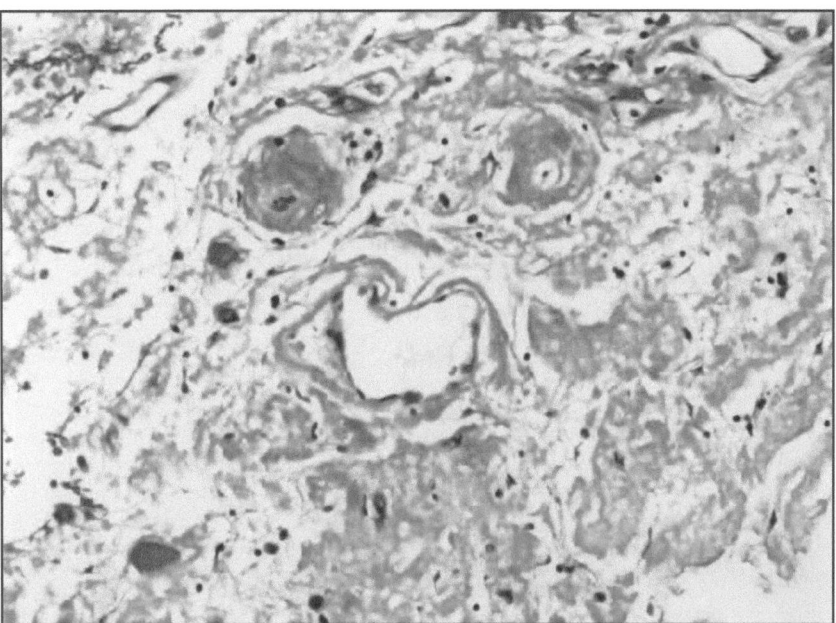

**Figure 12–12.** Hematoxylin and Eosin staining (power 20x): Deposition of amorphous eosinophilic material situated around the vessels.

hemostasis, faster recovery, and better healing. Deviprasad et al has reported the successful usage of KTP laser in the treatment of three cases of localized laryngeal amyloidosis. There was no need for further surgical intervention in any of the three cases throughout a follow-up period of 4 years on the average.[301] However, in severe cases an open approach such as laryngofissure may be advocated. Supraglottic laryngectomy remains a controversial option and should be reserved only for severe cases of diffuse involvement.[289]

This mosaic approach in treatment is best exemplified in the report of Xu et al of 16 cases of laryngeal amyloidosis where the spectrum of conservative endoscopic resection to stenting and use of tracheotomy has been described.[291] The report by Celenk et al on the management of three cases of laryngeal amyloidosis, two of whom were treated with combination of surgery and radiotherapy, highlights the importance of radiation therapy as an adjuvant or primary modality of treatment in affected patients.[302] The main added value occurs when the lesion is primarily submucosal and in cases of recurrence after surgery.

## References

1. Geterud Å. Rheumatoid arthritis in the larynx. *Scand J Rheumatol.* 1991; 20(3):215.
2. Bienenstock H, Ehrlich GE, Freyberg RH. Rheumatoid arthritis of the cricoarytenoid joint: a clinicopathologic study. *Arth Rheum.* 1963;6(1):48–63.
3. Linos A, Worthington JW, O'Fallon MI, Kurland LT. The epidemiology of rheumatoid arthritis in Rochester Minnesota: a study of incidence, prevalence, and mortality. *Am J Epidemiol.* 1980;111(1):87–98.
4. Lawry GV, Finerman ML, Hanafee WN, Mancuso AA, Fan PT, Bluestone R. Laryngeal involvement in rheumatoid arthritis. *Arth Rheum.* 1984;27 (8):873–882.
5. Amernik K. Glottis morphology and perceptive—acoustic characteristics of voice and speech in patients with rheumatoid arthritis [in Polish]. *Ann Acad Med Stetin.* 2007;53 (3):55–65.
6. Wojnowski W, Karlik M, Wiskirska-Woz´nica B, Walczak M. Voice disorders in rheumatoid arthritis [in Polish]. *Otolaryngol Pol.* 2005;59(4):603–606.
7. Voulgari PV, Papazisi D, Bai M, Zagorianakou P, Assimakopoulos D, Drosos AA. Laryngeal involvement in rheumatoid arthritis. *Rheumatol Int.* 2005; 25(5):321–325.
8. Sanz L, Sistiaga JA, Lara AJ, Cuende E, García-Alcántara F, Rivera T. The prevalence of dysphonia, its association with immunomediated diseases and correlation with biochemical markers. *J Voice.* 2012;26(2):148–153.
9. Fisher BA, Dolan K, Hastings L, McClinton C, Taylor PC. Prevalence of subjective voice impairment in rheumatoid arthritis. *Clin Rheumatol.* 2008;27(11):1441–1443.
10. Hamdan AL, El-Khatib M, Dagher W, Othman I. Laryngeal involvement in rheumatoid arthritis. *Middle East J Anesthesiol.* 2007;19:335–344.
11. Roy N, Tanner K, Merrill RM, Wright C, Miller KL, Kendall KA. Descriptive epidemiology of voice disorders in rheumatoid arthritis: prevalence, risk factors, and quality of life burden. *J Voice.* 2016;30(1):74–87.
12. Roy N, Merrill RM, Gray SD, Smith EM. Voice disorders in the general population: prevalence, risk factors, and occupational impact. *Laryngoscope.* 2005;115(11):1988–1995.
13. Dockery KM, Sismanis A, Abedi E. Rheumatoid arthritis of the larynx: the importance of early diagnosis and corticosteroid therapy. *South Med J.* 1991;84(1):95.
14. Speyer R, Speyer I, Heijnen MAM. Prevalence and relative risk of dysphonia in rheumatoid arthritis. *J Voice.* 2008;22:232–237.
15. Kosztyła-Hojna B, Moskal D, Kuryliszyn-Moskal A. Parameters of the assessment of voice quality and clinical manifestation of rheumatoid arthritis. *Adv Med Sci.* 2015;60(2):321–328.
16. Grossman A, Martin JR, Root HS. Rheumatoid arthritis of the crico-arytenoid joint. *Laryngoscope.* 1961; 71(5):530–544.
17. Guerra LG, Lau KY, Marwah RA. Upper airway obstruction as the sole manifestation of rheumatoid arthritis. *J Rheumatol.* 1992;19(6):974–976.
18. Benjamin B. Laryngeal manifestations of systemic diseases. In: *Endolaryngeal Surgery.* London, UK; Martin Dunitz:1998.
19. Hamdan AL, Sarieddine D. Laryngeal manifestations of rheumatoid arthritis. *Autoimm Dis.* 2013.
20. Gómez-Puerta JA, Cisternas A, Hernández MV, Ruiz-Esquide V, Vilaseca I, Sanmartí R. Laryngeal assessment by videolaryngostroboscopy in patients with rheumatoid arthritis. *Reumatolog Clín* (English ed.). 2014;10(1):32–36.
21. Hah JH, An SY, Sim S, et al. A population-based study on the association between rheumatoid arthritis and voice problems. *Clin Rheumatol.* 2016:1–6.
22. Kara SA, Altinok D, Orknn S, Bayar N, Keleç I, Koç C. Cricoarytenoiditis in rheumatoid arthritis: radiologic and clinical study. *J Otolaryngol.* 2003;32(6).
23. Masilamani K, Gandhi A. Cricoarytenoid arthritis presenting as croup. *J Royal Soc Med.* 2009;102(11): 491–492.
24. Castro MA, Dedivitis RA, Pfuetzenreiter EG, Barros AP, dos Santos Queija D. Videolaryngostroboscopy and voice evaluation in patients with rheumatoid arthritis. *Brazil Otorhinolaryngol.* 2012;78(5):121–127.
25. Tarnowska C, Amernik K, Matyja G, Brzosko I, Grzelec H, Burak M. [Fixation of the crico-arythenoid joints in rheumatoid arthritis—preliminary report]. *Otolaryngol Polska. Polish Otolaryngology.* 2003; 58(4):843–849.
26. Kumai Y, Murakami D, Masuda M, Yumoto E. Arytenoid adduction to treat impaired adduction of the vocal fold due to rheumatoid arthritis. *Auris Nasus Larynx.* 2007;34(4):545–548.

27. Bastian RW. Chronic non-specific disease of the larynx. In: Ballenger, JJ. ed., *Diseases of the Nose, Throat, Ear, Head and Neck.* Lea & Febiger; 1991: 616–630.

28. Copeman WS. Rheumatoid arthritis of the crico-arytenoid joints. *Brit Med J.* 1957;1(5032):1398–1399.

29. Montgomery WW. Cricoarytenoid arthritis. *Laryngoscope.* 1963;73(7):801–836.

30. Baker OA, Bywaters EG. Laryngeal stridor in rheumatoid arthritis due to crico-arytenoid joint involvement. *Brit Med J.* 1957;1(5032):1400.

31. Bossingham DH, Simpson FG. Acute laryngeal obstruction in rheumatoid arthritis. *Brit Med J.* 1996; 312(7026):295.

32. Lofgren RH, Montgomery WW. Incidence of laryngeal involvement in rheumatoid arthritis. *New Engl J Med.* 1962;267(4):193–195.

33. Bates CP. *Proc Roy Soc Med.* 1958; 57: 333.

34. Kolman J, Morris I. Cricoarytenoid arthritis: a cause of acute upper airway obstruction in rheumatoid arthritis. *Canad J Anaesthe.* 2002;49(7):729–793.

35. Pradhan P, Bhardwaj A, Venkatachalam VP. Bilateral cricoarytenoid arthritis: a cause of recurrent upper airway obstruction in rheumatoid arthritis. *Malaysian J Med Sci.* 2016;23(3):89.

36. Beirith SC, Ikino CM, Pereira IA. Laryngeal involvement in rheumatoid arthritis. *Brazil J Otorhinolaryngol.* 2013;79(2):233–238.

37. Geterud Å, Bake B, Berthelsen B, Bjelle A, Ejnell H. Laryngeal involvement in rheumatoid arthritis. *Acta Oto-laryngol.* 1991;111(5):990–998.

38. Gresham GA, Kellaway TD. Rheumatoid disease in the larynx and lung. *Ann Rheum Dis.* 1958;17(3): 286.

39. Darke CS, Wolman L, Young A. Laryngeal stridor in rheumatoid arthritis. *Brit Med J.* 1958;1(5082):1279.

40. Link DT, McCaffrey TV, Link MJ, Krauss WE, Ferguson MT. Cervicomedullary compression: an unrecognized cause of vocal cord paralysis in rheumatoid arthritis. *Ann Otol Rhinol Laryngol.* 1998;107(6):462–471.

41. Raven RW, Weber FP, Price LW. The necrobiotic nodules of rheumatoid arthritis. *Ann Rheum Dis.* 1948; 7: 63–75.

42. Webb JO, Payne WH. Rheumatoid nodules of the vocal folds. *Ann Rheum Dis.* 1972; 31(2):122.

43. Abadir WF, Forster PM. Rheumatoid vocal cord nodules. *J Laryngol Otol.* 1974; 88:473–478.

44. Woo P, Mendelsohn J, Humphrey D. Rheumatoid nodules of the larynx. *Otolaryngol Head Neck Surg.* 1994;113(1):147–150.

45. Titze IR. Mechanical stress in phonation. *J Voice.* 1994; 8(2):99–105.

46. Arnett FC, Edworthy SM, Bloch DA, et al. The American Rheumatism Association 1987 revised criteria for the classification of rheumatoid arthritis. *Arthr Rheum.* 1988;31(3):315–324.

47. Hosako Y, Nakamura M, Tayama N, et al. Laryngeal involvements in systemic lupus erythematosus: a case report. *Larynx Jpn.* 1993;5:171–175.

48. Murano E, Hosako-Naito Y, Tayama N, et al. Bamboo node: primary vocal fold lesion as evidence of autoimmune disease. *J Voice.* 2001;15(3):441–450.

49. Brooker DS. Rheumatoid arthritis: otorhinolaryngological manifestations. *Clin Otolaryngol Alli Sci.* 1988; 13(3):239–246.

50. Hilgert E, Toleti B, Kruger K, Nejedlo I. Hoarseness due to bamboo nodes in patients with autoimmune diseases: a review of literature. *J Voice.* 2008; 22(3): 343–350.

51. Ylitalo R, Heimbürger M, Lindestad PÅ. Vocal fold deposits in autoimmune disease—an unusual cause of hoarseness. *Clin Otolaryngol All Sci.* 2003; 28(5): 446–450.

52. Immerman S, Sulica L. Bamboo nodes. *Otolaryngol Head Neck Surg.* 2007;137(1):162–163.

53. Jurik AG, Pedersen U. Rheumatoid arthritis of the crico-arytenoid and crico-thyroid joints: a radiological and clinical study. *Clin Radiol.* 1984;35(3):233–236.

54. Berjawi G, Uthman I, Mahfoud L, et al. Cricothyroid joint abnormalities in patients with rheumatoid arthritis. *J Voice.* 2010;24(6):732–737.

55. Simpson GT, Javaheri A, Janfaza P. Acute cricoarytenoid arthritis: local periarticular steroid injection. *Ann Otol Rhinol Laryngol.* 1980;89(6):558–562.

56. Habib MA. Intra-articular steroid injection in acute rheumatoid arthritis of the larynx. *J Laryngol Otol.* 1977;91(10):909–910.

57. Greco A, Fusconi M, Macri GF, et al. Cricoarytenoid joint involvement in rheumatoid arthritis: radiologic evaluation. *American J Otolaryngol.* 2012;33(6):753–755.

58. Dennis DP, Kashima H. Carbon dioxide laser posterior cordectomy for treatment of bilateral vocal cord paralysis. *Ann Otol Rhinol Laryngol.* 1989;98(12):930–934.

59. Crumley RL. Endoscopic laser medial arytenoidectomy for airway management in bilateral laryngeal paralysis. *Ann Otol Rhinol Laryngol.* 1993 Feb;102(2):81–84.

60. Remacle M, Mayné A, Lawson G, Jamart J. Subtotal carbon dioxide laser arytenoidectomy by endoscopic approach for treatment of bilateral cord immobility in adduction. *Ann Otol Rhinol Laryngol.* 1996;105(6):438–445.

61. Curley JW, Byron MA, Bates GJ. Crico-arytenoid joint involvement in acute systemic lupus erythematosus. *J Laryngol Otol.* 1986;100 (6):727–732.

62. Scarpelli DG, McCoy FW, Scott JK. Acute lupus erythematosus with laryngeal involvement. *New Engl J Med.* 1959; 261(14):691–694.

63. Langford CA, Van Waes C. Upper airway obstruction in the rheumatic diseases. *Rheum Dis Clin North Am.* 1997; 23(2):345–363.

64. Smith GA, Ward PH, Berci G. Laryngeal lupus erythematosus. *J Laryngol Otol.* 1978; 92(01):67–73.

65. Teitel AD, MacKenzie CR, Stern R, Paget SA. Laryngeal involvement in systemic lupus erythematosus. *Semi Arth Rheumat.* 1992; 22: 203–214.

66. Gilliam JN, Cheatum DE. Immunoglobulins in the larynx in systemic lupus erythematosus. *Arch Dermatol.* 1973; 108(5):696–697.

67. Asherson RA, Hughes GR. Vocal cord paralysis in systemic lupus erythematosus complicated by pulmonary hypertension. *J Rheumatol.* 1985;12(5):1029–1030.

68. Aszkenasy OM, Clarke TJ, Hickling P, Marshall AJ. Systemic lupus erythematosus, pulmonary hypertension, and left recurrent laryngeal nerve palsy. *Ann Rheum Dis.* 1987; 46(3):246–247.

69. Espana A, Gutierrez JM, Soria C, Gila L, Ledo A. Recurrent laryngeal palsy in systemic lupus erythematosus. *Neurology.* 1990; 40(7):1143.

70. Imauchi Y, Urata Y, Abe K. Left vocal cord paralysis in cases of systemic lupus erythematosus. *ORL.* 2001; 63(1):53–55.

71. Kraus A, Guerra-Bautista G. Laryngeal involvement as a presenting symptom of systemic lupus erythematosus. *Ann Rheum Dis.* 1990; 49(6):421.

72. Saluja S, Singh RR, Misra A, et al. Bilateral recurrent laryngeal nerve palsy in systemic lupus erythematosus. *Clin Exp Rheumatol.* 1989; 7(1):81.

73. Sharma A, Singh RR, Malaviya AN. Vocal cord palsy in a patient of systemic lupus erythematosus. *J Assn Phys India.* 1988; 36(11):674–675.

74. Toubi E, Naschitz JE, Kessel A, Fradis M. Vocal cord paralysis in a patient with active systemic lupus erythematosus. *Israel Med Assn J.* 2000;2(3):243–244.

75. Korbet SM, Block LJ, Lewis EJ. Laryngeal complications in a patient with inactive systemic lupus erythematosus. *Arch Int Med.* 1984; 144(9):1867–1868.

76. Ozcan KM, Bahar S, Ozcan I, et al. Laryngeal involvement in systemic lupus erythematosus: report of two cases. *J Clin Rheumatol.* 2007; 13(5):278–279.

77. Martin L, Edworthy SM, Ryan JP, Fritzler MJ. Upper airway disease in systemic lupus erythematosus: a report of 4 cases and a review of the literature. *J Rheumatol.* 1992; 19(8):1186–1190.

78. Toomey JM, Snyder GG, Maenza RM, Rothfield NP. Acute epiglottitis due to systemic lupus erythematosus. *Laryngoscope.* 1974; 84(4):522–527.

79. Charuvanij S, Houghton KM. Acute epiglottitis as the initial presentation of pediatric. 2009.

80. Isenberg DA, Lipkin DP, Mowbray JF, Fisher C, Davies R. Fatal pneumococcal epiglottitis in lupus overlap syndrome. *Clin Rheumatol.* 1984; 3(4):529–532.

81. Shalit ME, Gross DJ, Levo YO. Pneumococcal epiglottitis in systemic lupus erythematosus on high-dose corticosteroids. *Ann Rheum Dis.* 1982; 41(6):615–616.

82. Van den Broek P. Acute and chronic laryngitis; leukoplakia. *Scott-Brown's Otolaryngol.* 1987; 5:103,105.

83. Shumrick KA. Benign diseases of the hypopharynx and larynx. In: *Textbook of Otolaryngology and Head and Neck Surgery.* New York, NY: Elsevier; 1989:619.

84. Weiser GA, Forouhar FA, White WB. Hydralazine hoarseness: A new appearance of drug-induced systemic lupus erythematosus. *Arch Int Med.* 1984; 144(11): 2271–2272.

85. Chatelanat F, Rauch S. Angeite necrosante du larynx chez un homme atteint par ailleurs d'un lupus discoide. *Rev Laryngol Otol Rhinol.* 1959; 80:233–240.

86. Minchina RA, Fastovskiĭ I, Antonova NA. [Changes in the larynx in systemic lupus erythematosus and systemic scleroderma]. *J Otol Rhinol Laryngol.* 1969; 30(4):67–73.

87. Hosako Y, Nakamura M, Tayama N, et al. Laryngeal involvements in systemic lupus erythematosus: a case report. *Larynx Jpn.* 1993;5:171–175.

88. Tsunoda K, Soda Y. Hoarseness as the initial manifestation of systemic lupus erythematosus. *J Laryngol Otol.* 1996;110(05):478–479.

89. Murano E, Hosako-Naito Y, Tayama N, et al. Bamboo node: primary vocal fold lesion as evidence of autoimmune disease. *J Voice.* 2001;15(3):441–450.

90. Todic J, Schweizer V, Leuchter I. [Bamboo nodes of vocal folds: case report and review of literature]. *Rev Med Suisse.* 2014;10(444):1811–1812.

91. Hilgert E, Toleti B, Kruger K, Nejedlo I. Hoarseness due to bamboo nodes in patients with autoimmune diseases: a review of literature. *J Voice.* 2008; 22(3): 343–350.

92. Hosako-Naito Y, Tayama N, Niimi S, et al. Diagnosis and physiopathology of laryngeal deposits in autoimmune disease. *ORL.* 1999; 61(3):151–157.

93. Nishinarita M, Ohta S, Uesato M, Oka Y, Kamoshida T, Takahashi A. [Undifferentiated connective tissue syndromes (UCTS) accompanied by laryngeal involvement and autoimmune hepatitis]. *Jap J Clin Immunol.* 1995; 18(5):559–565.

94. Schwemmle C. Bamboo nodes als Ursache von Dysphonien bei Autoimmunkrankheiten. *HNO.* 2007; 55(7):564–568.

95. Burgess ED, Render KC. Hypopharyngeal obstruction in lupus erythematosus. *Ann Int Med.* 1984; 100(2):319.

96. Maxwell D, Silver R. Laryngeal manifestations of drug induced lupus. *J Rheumatol.* 1987; 14(2):375–577.

97. Nanke YU, Kotake SH, Yonemoto KO, Hara M, Hasegawa M, Kamatani NA. Cricoarytenoid arthritis with rheumatoid arthritis and systemic lupus erythematosus. The *J Rheumatol.* 2001; 28(3):624–626.

98. Lee JH, Sung IY, Park JH, Roh JL. Recurrent laryngeal neuropathy in a systemic lupus erythematosus (SLE) patient. *Amer J Phys Med Rehab.* 2008; 87(1):68–70.

99. Karim A, Ahmed S, Siddiqui R, Marder GS, Mattana J. Severe upper airway obstruction from cricoarytenoiditis as the sole presenting manifestation of a systemic lupus erythematosus flare. *CHEST J.* 2002; 121(3):990–993.

100. Hughes M, Hill J. Left vocal cord paralysis in systemic lupus erythematosus. *Mod Rheumatol.* 2009; 19(4):441–442.

101. Jayachandran NV, Agrawal S, Rajasekhar L, Narsimulu G. Bilateral vocal cord palsy as a manifestation of systemic lupus erythematosus. *Lupus.* 2009; 19(1).

102. Leszczynski P, Pawlak-Bus K. Vocal cords palsy in systemic lupus erythematosus patient: diagnostic

and therapeutic difficulties. *Rheumatol Int*. 2013;33(6): 1577–1580.

103. Hari CK, Raza SA, Clayton MI. Hydralazine-induced lupus and vocal fold paralysis. *J Laryngol Otol*. 1998; 112(9):875–877.

104. Smith RR, Ferguson GB. Systemic lupus erythematosus causing subglottic stenosis. *Laryngoscope*. 1974; 86(5):734–738.

105. Ito I, Nagai S, Kitaichi M, et al. Pulmonary manifestations of primary Sjögren's syndrome: a clinical, radiologic, and pathologic study. *Am J Resp Crit Care Med*. 2005; 171(6):632–638.

106. Patel R, Shahane A. The epidemiology of Sjögren's syndrome. *Clin Epidemiol*. 2014; 6:247.

107. Chambers MS. Sjogren's syndrome. *ORL Head Neck Nurs: Offic J Soc Otorhinolaryngol Head Neck Nurses*. 2004; 22(4):22–30.

108. Kassan SS, Moutsopoulos HM. Clinical manifestations and early diagnosis of Sjögren syndrome. *Arch Int Med*. 2004; 164(12):1275–1284.

109. Pierce JL, Tanner K, Merrill RM, et al. Voice disorders in Sjögren's syndrome: Prevalence and related risk factors. *Laryngoscope*. 2014;125(6):1385–1392.

110. Mathews SA, Kurien BT, Scofield RH. Oral manifestations of Sjögren's syndrome. *J Den Res*. 2008; 87(4): 308–318.

111. Skálová S, Minxová L Slezák R. Hypokalemic paralysis revealing Sjögren's syndrome in a 16-year-old girl. *Ghana Med J*. 2008; 42:124–128.

112. Roy N, Merrill RM, Gray SD, Smith EM. Voice disorders in the general population: prevalence, risk factors, and occupational impact. *Laryngoscope*. 2005; 115(11):1988–1995.

113. Ruiz AL, Hernández LX, Arreguín PJ, Velasco RR, Pacheco DV, Pérez GA. Alterations in voice, speech and swallowing in patients with Sjögren's syndrome. *Acta Otorrinolaringol Espan*. 2011; 62(4):255–264.

114. Heller A, Tanner K, Roy N, et al. Voice, speech, and laryngeal features of primary Sjögren's syndrome. *Ann of Otol Rhinol Laryngol*. 2014; 123(11):778–785.

115. Saltürk Z, Özdemir E, Kumral TL, et al. Subjective and objective voice evaluation in Sjögren's syndrome. *Logoped Phoniatri Vocol*. 2015:1–3.

116. Tanner K, Pierce JL, Merrill RM, Miller KL, Kendall KA, Roy N. The quality of life burden associated with voice disorders in Sjögren's syndrome. *Ann of Otol Rhinol Laryngol*. 2015; 124(9):721–727.

117. Doig JA, Whaley K, Dick WC, Nuki G, Williamson J, Buchanan WW. Otolaryngological aspects of Sjögren's syndrome. *Br Med J*. 1971; 4(5785):460–463.

118. Ogut F, Midilli R, Oder G, Engin EZ, Karci B, Kabasakal Y. Laryngeal findings and voice quality in Sjögren's syndrome. *Auris Nasus Larynx*. 2005;32(4):375–380.

119. Wolman L, Drake CS, Young A. The larynx in rheumatoid arthritis. *J Laryngol Otol*. 1965; 79 (5):403–434.

120. Chatelanat F, Rauch S. Angeite necrosante du larynx chez un homme atteint par ailleurs d'un lupus discoide. *Rev Laryngol Otol Rhinol*. 1959; 80:233–240.

121. Sinclair DS, Rosen PS, Noyek AM. Systemic lupus erythematosus with a vocal cord granulomatous nodule. *J Otolaryngol*. 1976; 5(4):337–342.

122. Webb JO, Payne WH. Rheumatoid nodules of the vocal folds. *Ann Rheum Dis*. 1972; 31(2):122.

123. Friedman BA, Rice DH. Rheumatoid nodules of the larynx. *Acta Otolaryngol*. 1975; 101(6):361–363.

124. Luchsinger R, and Arnold GE. In: *Voice, Speech and Language. Clinical Communicology: Its Physiology and Pathology*. Vocal nodules and polyps. 1965; 176–187.

125. Prytz S. Vocal nodules in Sjögren's syndrome. *J Laryngol Otol*. 1980; 94(02):197–203.

126. Korst RJ. Primary lymphoma of the subglottic airway in a patient with Sjögren's syndrome mimicking high laryngotracheal stenosis. *Ann Thorac Surg*. 2007; 84(5):1756–1758.

127. Murano E, Hosako-Naito Y, Tayama N, et al. Bamboo node: primary vocal fold lesion as evidence of autoimmune disease. *J Voice*. 2001; 15(3):441–450.

128. Sève P, Poupart M, Bui-Xuan C, Charhon A, Broussolle C. Cricoarytenoid arthritis in Sjögren's syndrome. *Rheumatol Int*. 2005; 25(4):301–302.

129. Montgomery WW. Cricoarytenoid arthritis. *Laryngoscope*. 1963;73(7):801–836.

130. Gresham GA, Kellaway TD. Rheumatoid disease in the larynx and lung. *Ann Rheum Dis*. 1958;17 (3):286.

131. Ito K, Yuyama S, Yamashita K, Hiiragi K, Tsukuda M, Ohishi K. A case report of Sjögren's syndrome with repeated false cord swelling. *ORL*. 1994; 56(3):173–176.

132. Belafsky PC, Postma GN. The laryngeal and esophageal manifestations of Sjögren's syndrome. *Curr Rheumatol Rep*. 2003; 5(4):297–303.

133. Hilgert E, Toleti B, Kruger K, Nejedlo I. Hoarseness due to bamboo nodes in patients with autoimmune diseases: a review of literature. *J Voice*. 2006; 22:343–350.

134. Bitter T, Volk GF, Lehamnn P, Wittekindt C, Guntinas-Lichius O. [Progressive hoarseness] [in German]. *HNO*. 2011;59:283–285. doi: 10.1007/s00106-010-2207-6

135. Cheung S-M, Chen C-J, Hsin Y-J, Tsai Y-T, Leong C-P. Effect of neuromuscular electrical stimulation in a patient with Sjogren's syndrome with dysphagia: a real time videofluoroscopic swallowing study. *Chang Gung Med J*. 2010; 33:338–345.

136. Chan RW, Tayama N. Biomechanical effects of hydration in vocal fold tissues. *Otolaryngol Head Neck Surg*. 2002; 126(5):528–537.

137. Finkelhor BK, Titze IR, Durham PL. The effect of viscosity changes in the vocal folds on the range of oscillation. *J Voice*. 1988;1(4):320–325.

138. Jiang J, Ng J, Hanson D. The effects of rehydration on phonation in excised canine larynges. *J Voice*. 1999; 13(1):51–59.

139. Jiang J, Verdolini K, Jennie NG, Aquino B, Hanson D. Effects of dehydration on phonation in excised canine larynges. *Ann Otol Rhinol Laryngol*. 2000; 109(6): 568–575.

140. Verdolini K, Titze IR, Fennell A. Dependence of phonatory effort on hydration level. *J Speech Lang Hear Res*. 1994; 37(5):1001–1007.

141. Verdolini-Martson K, Titze IR, Druker DG. Changes in phonation threshold pressure with induced conditions of hydration. *J Voice*. 1990; 4 (2): 142–151.

142. Sivasankar MP, Carroll T, Kosinski AM, Rosen CA. Quantifying the effects of altering ambient humidity on ionic composition of vocal fold surface fluid. *Laryngoscope*. 2013; 123:1275–1278.

143. Widdicombe, J. Airway surface fluid: concepts and measurements. In: Rogers DF, Lethem MI, eds. *Airway Mucus: Basic Mechanisms and Clinical Perspectives*. Basel, Switzerland: Birkhauser Verlag; 1997:1–17.

144. Suk JS, Boylan J, Trehan K, et al. N-acetylcysteine enhances cystic fibrosis sputum penetration and airway gene transfer by highly compacted DNA nanoparticles. *Mol Ther*. 2011; 19:1981–1989.

145. Badami KG, McKellar M. Allogeneic serum eye drops: time these became the norm? *Br J Ophthalmol*. 2012; 96:1151–1152.

146. Reeves EP, Molloy K, Pohl K, McElvaney NG. Hypertonic saline in treatment of pulmonary disease in cystic fibrosis. *Sci World J*. 2012; 2012:465230. doi: 10.1100/2012/465230

147. Tanner K, Roy N, Merrill RM, Elstad M. The effects of three nebulized osmotic agents in the dry larynx. *J Speech Lang Hear Res*. 2007; 50:635–646.

148. Tanner K, Roy N, Merrill RM, et al. Comparing nebulized water versus saline after laryngeal desiccation challenge in Sjögren's syndrome. *Laryngoscope*. 2013; 123:2787–2792.

149. Tanner K, Roy N, Merrill RM, et al. Nebulized isotonic saline versus water following a laryngeal desiccation challenge in classically trained sopranos. *J Speech Lang Hear Res*. 2010; 53:1555–1566.

150. Tanner K, Nissen SL, Merrill RM, et al. Nebulized isotonic saline improves voice production in Sjögren's syndrome. *Laryngoscope*. 2015; 125(10):2333–2340.

151. Lahmer T, Treiber M, von Werder A, et al. Relapsing polychondritis: an autoimmune disease with many faces. *Autoimm rev*. 2010; 9(8):540–546.

152. Pearson CM, Kline HM, Newcomer VD. Relapsing polychondritis. *New Engl J Med*. 1960; 263(2):51–58.

153. Quinsat D, Harle JR, Durand JM, Weiller PJ, Mongin M. Relapsing polychondritis and cancer. Two cases. *Ann Med Interne* 1989; 140:422–423.

154. Childs LF, Rickert S, Wengerman OC, Lebovics R, Blitzer A. Laryngeal manifestations of relapsing polychondritis and a novel treatment option. *J Voice*. 2012; 26(5):587–589.

155. Buckner JH, Van Landeghen M, Kwok WW, Tsarknaridis L. Identification of type II collagen peptide 261–273-specific T cell clones in a patient with relapsing polychondritis. *Arth Rheumat*. 2002; 46(1):238–244.

156. Navarro MJ, Higgins GC, Lohr KM, Myers LK. Amelioration of relapsing polychondritis in a child treated with oral collagen. *Am J Med Sci*. 2002; 324(2): 101–103.

157. Lang B, Rothenfusser A, Lanchbury JS, et al. Susceptibility to relapsing polychondritis is associated with HLA-DR4. *Arth Rheum*. 1993; 36:660–664.

158. Zeuner M, Straub RH, Rauh G, et al. Relapsing polychondritis: clinical and immunogenetic analysis of 62 patients. *J Rheumatol*. 1997; 24:96–101.

159. Loehrl TA, Smith TL. Inflammatory and granulomatous lesions of the larynx and pharynx. *Am J Med*. 2001; 111:113S–117S.

160. Isaak BL, Liesegang TJ, Michet CJ. Ocular and systemic findings in relapsing polychondritis. *Ophthalmology*. 1986; 93:681–689.

161. Puéchal X, Terrier B, Mouthon L, Costedoat-Chalumeau N, Guillevin L, Le Jeune C. Relapsing polychondritis. *Joint Bone Spine*. 2014;81(2):118–124.

162. Childs LF, Rickert S, Wengerman OC, Lebovics R, Blitzer A. Laryngeal manifestations of relapsing polychondritis and a novel treatment option. *J Voice*. 2012;26(5):587–589.

163. Kent PD, Michet CJ, Luthra HS. Relapsing polychondritis. *Cur Opin Rheumatol*. 2004; 16(1):56–61.

164. 15 Kong KO, Vasoo S, Tay NS, Chng HH. Relapsing polychondritis—an Oriental case series. *Sing Med J*. 2003; 44(4):197–200.

165. Hong G, Kim H. Clinical characteristics and treatment outcomes of patients with relapsing polychondritis with airway involvement. *Clin Rheumatol*. 2013; 32(9):1329–1335.

166. Michet CJ, McKenna CH, Luthra HS, O'Fallon WM. Relapsing polychondritis. *Ann Intern Med*. 1986; 104:74–78.

167. Damiani JM, Levine HL. Relapsing polychondritis—report of ten cases. *Laryngoscope*. 1979; 89(6):929–946.

168. Krell WS, Staats BA, Hyatt RE. Pulmonary function in relapsing polychondritis 1–3. *American Review of Respiratory Disease*. 1986; 133(6):1120–1123.

169. Mohsenifar Z, Tashkin DP, Carson SA, Bellamy PE. Pulmonary function in patients with relapsing polychondritis. *Chest*. 1982; 81(6):711–717.

170. Luthra HS. Relapsing polychondritis. In: KlippelJH, Dieppe PA, eds. *Rheumatology*. St Louis: Mosby; 1998; 27: 1–4.

171. Trentham DE, Le CH. Relapsing polychondritis. *Ann Intern Med*. 1998; 129:114–122.

172. Mathew SD, Battafarano DF, Morris MJ. Relapsing polychondritis in the Department of Defense population and review of the literature. *Sem Arth Rheum*. 2012; 42:70–83.

173. McAdam LP, O'hanlan MA, Bluestone R, Pearson CM. Relapsing polychondritis: prospective study of 23 patients and a review of the literature. *Medicine*. 1976; 55(3):193–215.

174. Kemta Lekpa F, Kraus VB, Chevalier X. Biologics in relapsing polychondritis: a literature review. *Sem Arth Rheum*. 2012; 41:712–719.

175. Mpofu S, Estrach C, Curtis J, Moots RJ. Treatment of respiratory complications in recalcitrant relapsing polychondritis with infliximab. *Rheumatology*. 2003; 42(9):1117–1118.

176. Aladesanmi OA. Sarcoidosis: an update for the primary care physician. *Med Gen Med*. 2004; 6(1):7–14.

177. Rybicki BA, Maliarik MJ, Major M, Popovich Jr J, Iannuzzi MC. Epidemiology, demographics, and genetics of sarcoidosis. *Sem Resp Infect.* 1998; 13(3): 166–173.
178. Baughman RP, Teirstein AS, Judson MA, et al. Clinical characteristics of patients in a case control study of sarcoidosis. *Am J Respir Crit Care Med.* 2001;164(10): 1885–1889.
179. Baughman RP, Lower EE, du Bois R. Sarcoidosis. *Lancet.* 2003; 361:1111–1118.
180. Culver DA, Newman LS, Kavuru MS. Gene-environment interactions in sarcoidosis: challenge and opportunity. *Clin Dermatol.* 2007;25(3):267–275.
181. Iannuzzi MC. Advances in the genetics of sarcoidosis. *Proc Am Thorac Soc.* 2007;4(5):457–460.
182. Iannuzzi MC, Rybicki BA (2007) Genetics of sarcoidosis. *Proc Am Thorac Soc.* 4(1):108–116.
183. Nunes H, Bouvry D, Soler P, Valeyre D. Sarcoidosis. *Orphan J Rare Dis.* 2006; 2:46–57.
184. Moller DR. State of the art. Potential etiologic agents in sarcoidosis. *Proc Am Thorac Soc.* 2007;4(5):465–468.
185. Drake WP, Newman LS. Mycobacterial antigens may be important in sarcoidosis pathogenesis. *Curr Opin Pulmon Med.* 2006;12(5):359–363.
186. Aytemur ZA, Erdinc M, Erdinc E, Ateş H, Akyürekli O. Clinical features and diagnostic approach to sarcoidosis according to stages. *Tuberkuloz Toraks.* 2003;51(1): 11–16.
187. Handa R, Aggarwal P, Wali JP, Wig N, Dinda AK, Biswas A. Sarcoidosis presenting with peripheral lymphadenopathy. *Sarcoid Vascul Diff Lung Dis: Official J WASOG/World Assn Sarcoidosis Other Granulomat Dis.* 1998;15(2):192.
188. Saleh S, Saw C, Marzauk K, Sharma O. Sarcoidosis of the spinal cord: literature review and report of eight cases. *J Natl Med Assoc.* 2006; 98(6):965–976.
189. Kolokotronis AE, Belazi MA, Haidemanos G, Zaraboukas TK, Antoniades DZ. Sarcoidosis: oral and perioral manifestations. *Hippokratia.* 2009; 13(2):119–121.
190. Poe DL. Sarcoidosis of the larynx. *Arch Otolaryngol.* 1940; 32:315–320.
191. Gallivan GJ, Landis JN. Sarcoidosis of the larynx: preserving and restoring airway and professional voice. *J Voice.* 1993 Mar 1;7(1):81–94.
192. Fortune S, Courey MS. Isolated laryngeal sarcoidosis. *Otolaryngol Head and Neck Surg.* 1998;118(6):868–870.
193. Benjamin B, Dalton C, Croxson G. Laryngoscopic diagnosis of laryngeal sarcoid. *Ann Otol Rhinol Laryngol.* 1995;104(7):529–531.
194. Neel III HB, McDonald TJ. Laryngeal sarcoidosis: report of 13 patients. *Ann Otol Rhinol Laryngol.* 1982;91(4):359–362.
195. Devine KD. Sarcoidosis and sarcoidosis of the larynx. *Laryngoscope.* 1965;75(4):533–569.
196. Mayerhoff RM, Pitman MJ. Atypical and disparate presentations of laryngeal sarcoidosis. *Ann Otol Rhinol Laryngol.* 2010;119(10):667–671.
197. Bower JS, Belen JE, Weg JG, Dantzker DR. Manifestations and treatment of laryngeal sarcoidosis. *Am Rev Respir Dis.* 1980;122:325–332.
198. Dean CM, Sataloff RT, Hawkshaw MJ, Pribitkin E. Laryngeal sarcoidosis. *J Voice.* 2002;16(2):283–288.
199. Pillsbury HC, Sasaki CT. Granulomatous diseases of the larynx. *Otolaryngol Clin North Am.* 1982;15(3): 539–551.
200. Sims HS, Thakkar KH. Airway involvement and obstruction from granulomas in African-American patients with sarcoidosis. *Resp Med.* 2007;101(11):2279–2283.
201. Djalilian M, McDonald TJ, Devine KD, Weiland LH. Nontraumatic, nonneoplastic subglottic stenosis. *Ann Otol Rhinol Laryngol.* 1975;84(6):757–763.
202. Henderson CA, Ilchyshyn A, Curry AR. Laryngeal and cutaneous sarcoidosis treated with methotrexate-case report. *J R Soc Med.* 1994; 87:632–633.
203. Sakamoto M, Ishizawa M, Kitahara N. Polypoid type of laryngeal sarcoidosis—case report and review of the literature. *Eur Arch Otorhinolaryngol.* 2000;257(8):436–438.
204. Jaffe R, Bogomolski-Yahalom V, Kramer MR. Vocal cord paralysis as the presenting symptom of sarcoidosis. *Respir Med.* 1994;88:633–636.
205. Tobias JK, Santiago SM, Williams AJ. Sarcoidosis as a cause of left recurrent laryngeal nerve palsy. *Arch Otolaryngol Head Neck Surg.* 1990;116: 971–972.
206. Coffey CS, Vallejo SL, Farrar EK, Judson MA, Halstead LA. Sarcoidosis presenting as bilateral vocal cord paralysis from bilateral compression of the recurrent laryngeal nerves from thoracic adenopathy. *J Voice.* 2009;23(5):631–634.
207. Swinburn CR, Pozniak AL, Davies DG, Treasure T, Johnson NM. Left recurrent laryngeal nerve palsy as the presenting feature of sarcoidosis. *Sarcoidosis.* 1986;3:67–68.
208. Chijimatsu Y, Tajima J, Washizaki M, Homma H. Hoarseness as an initial manifestation of sarcoidosis. *Chest.* 1980;78:779–781.
209. Witt RL. Sarcoidosis presenting as bilateral vocal fold paralysis. *J Voice.* 2003;17:265–268.
210. Chesnutt AN. Enigmas in sarcoidosis. *West J Med.* 1995; 162:519–526.
211. Lauver JW, Gooneratne NS. Lacrimal, parotid and mediastinal uptake of gallium-67 in sarcoidosis. *Brit J Radiol.* 1979;52(619):582–584.
212. Krespi YP, Husain S, Mitrani M, Meltzer CJ. Treatment of laryngeal sarcoidosis with intralesional steroid injection. *Ann Otol Rhinol Laryngol.* 1987;96(6):713–715.
213. Grutters JC, Van den Bosch JM. Corticosteroid treatment in sarcoidosis. *Eur Resp J.* 2006;28(3):627–636.
214. Roberts SD, Wilkes DS, Burgett RA, Knox KS. Refractory sarcoidosis responding to infliximab. *CHEST J.* 2003;124(5):2028–2031.
215. James JC, Simpson CB. Treatment of laryngeal sarcoidosis with CO2 laser and mitomycin-C. *Otolaryngol Head Neck Surg.* 2004;130(2):262–264.
216. Cotch MF, Hoffman GS, Yerg DE, Kaufman GI, Targonski P, Kaslow RA. The epidemiology of Wegener's granulomatosis. Estimates of the five-year period prevalence, annual mortality, and geographic disease

distribution from population-based data sources. *Arth Rheum.* 1996; 39(1):87–92.

217. Comarmond C, Cacoub P. Granulomatosis with polyangiitis (Wegener): clinical aspects and treatment. *Autoimmun Rev.* 2014;13(11):1121–1125.

218. Watts RA, Lane SE, Bentham G, Scott DG. Epidemiology of systemic vasculitis (sv)—a 10-year study. *Arth Rheum.* 1998;41(9):S122.

219. Haugeberg G, Bie R, Bendvold A, Larsen AS, Johnsen V. Primary vasculitis in a Norwegian community hospital: a retrospective study. *Clin Rheumatol.* 1998; 17(5):364–368.

220. Reinhold-Keller E, Zeidler A, Mock C, Raspe H, Gutfleisch J, Peter H. Epidemiology of primary systemic vasculitis in North and South Germany. *Sarcoidosis.* 1996;13(suppl 3):272.

221. Lee PY, Adil EA, Irace AL, et al. The presentation and management of granulomatosis with polyangiitis (Wegener's granulomatosis) in the pediatric airway. *Laryngoscope.* 2017;127(1):233–240.

222. Bhanji A, Karim M. Pulmonary fibrosis—an uncommon manifestation of anti-myeloperoxidase-positive systemic vasculitis? *NDT Plus.* 2010;3(4):351–353.

223. Hamada K, Nagai S, Kitaichi M, et al. Cyclophosphamide-induced late-onset lung disease. *Internal Med.* 2003;42(1):82–87.

224. Leavitt RY, Fauci AS, Bloch DA, et al. The American College of Rheumatology 1990 criteria for the classification of Wegener's granulomatosis. *Arth Rheum.* 1990;33(8):1101–1107.

225. Mahr AD, Neogi T, Lavalley MP, et al. Assessment of the item selection and weighting in the Birmingham vasculitis activity score for Wegener's granulomatosis. *Arth Care Res.* 2008;59(6):884–891.

226. Lebovics RS, Hoffman GS, Leavitt RY, et al. The management of subglottic stenosis in patients with Wegener's granulomatosis. *Laryngoscope.* 1992;102(12):1341–1345.

227. Del Pero MM, Rasmussen N, Chaudhry A, Jani P, Jayne D. Structured clinical assessment of the ear, nose and throat in patients with granulomatosis with polyangiitis (Wegener's). *Eur Arch Oto-Rhino-Laryngol.* 2013;270(1):345–354.

228. Waxman J, Bose WJ. Laryngeal manifestations of Wegener's granulomatosis: case reports and review of the literature. *J Rheumatol.* 1986;13(2):408–411.

229. Gottschlich S, Ambrosch P, Kramkowski D, et al. Head and neck manifestations of Wegener's granulomatosis. *Rhinology.* 2006;44(4):227–233.

230. Haris M, Koulaouzidis A, Yasir M, Clark S, Kaleem M, Mallya R. Clinical vistas briefs: Wegener's granulomatosis. *Canad Med Ass J.* 2008;178(1):25.

231. Cannady SB, Batra PS, Koening C, et al. Sinonasal Wegener granulomatosis: a single-institution experience with 120 cases. *Laryngoscope.* 2009;119(4):757–761.

232. McDonald TJ, DeRemee RA. Wegener's gramulomatosis. *Laryngoscope*, 1983, 93 (2):220–231.

233. Mcdonald TJ, Deremee RA, Kern EB, Harrison EG. Nasal manifestations of Wegener's granulomatosis. *Laryngoscope.* 1974;84(12):2101–2112.

234. Jennings CR, Jones NS, Dugar J, Powell RJ, Lowe J. Wegener's granulomatosis—a review of diagnosis and treatment in 53 subjects. *Rhinology.* 1998;36(4):188–191.

235. Mokoka MC, Ullah K, Curran DR, O'Connor TM. Rare causes of persistent wheeze that mimic poorly controlled asthma. *BMJ Case Reports.* 2013;2013: bcr2013201100.

236. Stone JH. Limited versus severe Wegener's granulomatosis: baseline data on patients in the Wegener's granulomatosis etanercept trial. *Arth Rheum.* 2003;48(8):2299–2309.

237. Fowler NM, Beach JM, Krakovitz P, Spalding SJ. Airway manifestations in childhood granulomatosis with polyangiitis (Wegener's). *Arth Care Res.* 2012;64(3):434–440.

238. Murty GE. Wegener's granulomatosis: otorhinolaryngological manifestations. *Clin Otolaryngol All Sci.* 1990;15(4):385–393.

239. Bevelaqua F, Schicchi JS, Haas F, Axen K, Levin N. Aortic arch anomaly presenting as exercise-induced asthma. *Am Rev Resp Dis.* 1989;140:805–808.

240. Case records of the Massachusetts General Hospital. Weekly clinicopathological exercises. Case 31-1986. A 39-year-old woman with stenosis of the subglottic area and pulmonary artery. *N Engl J Med.* 1986;7:378–387.

241. Sarău CA, Lighezan DF, Doroş IC, et al. The involvement of upper airway in Wegener's granulomatosis—about four cases. *Roman J Morphol Embryol.* 2014; 56(2):613–618.

242. Hoare TJ, Jayne D, Evans PR, Croft CB, Howard DJ. Wegener's granulomatosis, subglottic stenosis and antineutrophil cytoplasm antibodies. *J Laryngol Otol.* 1989;103(12):1187–1191.

243. Rasmussen N, Petersen J. Cellular immune responses and pathogenesis in c-ANCA positive vasculitides. *J Autoimmunity.* 1993;6(2):227–236.

244. Scott DG, Watts RA. Systemic vasculitis: epidemiology, classification and environmental factors. *Ann Rheum Dis.* 2000;59(3):161–163.

245. Gluth MB, Shinners PA, Kasperbauer JL. Subglottic stenosis associated with Wegener's granulomatosis. *Laryngoscope.* 2003;113(8):1304–1307.

246. Utzig MJ, Warzelhan J, Wertzel H, Berwanger I, Hasse J. Role of thoracic surgery and interventional bronchoscopy in Wegener's granulomatosis. *Ann Thorac Surg.* 2002;74(6):1948–1952.

247. Stegeman CA, Tervaert JW, de Jong PE, Kallenberg CG. Trimethoprim-sulfamethoxazole (co-trimoxazole) for the prevention of relapses of Wegener's granulomatosis. Dutch Co-Trimoxazole Wegener Study Group. *N Engl J Med.* 1996;335:16–20.

248. Springer J, Nutter B, Langford CA, Hoffman GS, Villa-Forte A. Granulomatosis with polyangiitis (Wegener's): impact of maintenance therapy duration. *Medicine* (Baltimore). 2014; 93(2):82–90.

249. McDonald TJ, Neel HB, DeRemee RA. Wegener's granulomatosis of the subglottis and the upper portion of the trachea. *Ann Otol Rhinol Laryngol.* 1982; 91(6):588–592.

250. Eliachar I, Chan J, Akst L. New approaches to the management of subglottic stenosis in Wegener's granulomatosis. *Cleveland Clin J Med*. 2002;69: SII149–51.

251. Herridge MS, Pearson FG, Downey GP. Subglottic stenosis complicating Wegener's granulomatosis: surgical repair as a viable treatment option. *J Thorac Cardiovasc Surg*. 1996;111(5):961–966.

252. Shvero J, Shitrit D, Koren R, Shalomi D, Kramer MR. Endoscopic laser surgery for subglottic stenosis in Wegener's granulomatosis. *Yonsei Med J*. 2007;48(5): 748–753.

253. Strong MS, Healy GB, Vaughan CW, Fried MP, Shapshay S. Endoscopic management of laryngeal stenosis. *Otolaryngol Clin North Am*. 1979;12(4):797–805.

254. Dedo HH, Sooy CD. Endoscopic laser repair of posterior glottic, subglottic and tracheal stenosis by division or micro-trapdoor flap. *Laryngoscope*. 1984;94(4): 445–450.

255. LeRoy EC. Scleroderma (systemic sclerosis). *Textbook of Rheumatology*. 1981:2.

256. Varga J, Denton CP. Systemic sclerosis and the scleroderma-spectrum disorders. In: Firestein GS, ed. *Kelley's Textbook of Rheumatology*. 8th ed. Philadelphia, PA: WB Saunders Co-Elsevier; 2008.

257. D'Angelo WA, Fries JF, Masi AT, et al. Pathologic observations in systemic sclerosis (scleroderma), a study of 58 autopsy cases and 58 matched controls. *Am J Med*. 1969;46:428–440.

258. Kaşifoğlu T, Bilge ŞY, Yıldız F, et al. Risk factors for malignancy in systemic sclerosis patients. *Clin Rheumatol*. 2016;35(6):1529–1533.

259. Maricq HR, Weinrich MC, Keil JE, et al. Prevalence of scleroderma spectrum disorders in the general population of South Carolina. *Arth Rheum*. 1989;32(8): 998–1006.

260. Le Roy EC, Black C, Fleischemajer R, et al. Scleroderma (systemic sclerosis): classification, subsets, and pathogenesis. *J Rheumatol*. 1988;15:202–205.

261. Steen VD, Oddis CV, Conte CG, Janoski J, Casterline GZ, Medsger TA. Incidence of systemic sclerosis in Allegheny county, Pennsylvania. A twenty-year study of hospital-diagnosed cases, 1963–1982. *Arth Rheumatol*. 1997;40(3):441–445.

262. Mayes MD, Lacey JV, Beebe-Dimmer J, et al. Prevalence, incidence, survival, and disease characteristics of systemic sclerosis in a large US population. *Arth Rheumatol*. 2003;48(8):2246–2255.

263. Wipff J, Allanore Y, Soussi F, et al. Prevalence of Barrett's esophagus in systemic sclerosis. *Arth Rheum*. 2005; 52:2882–2888. [PubMed: 16142744].

264. Pepper JP, Kupfer RA, McHugh JB, Hogikyan ND. Histopathologic findings and clinical manifestations in a patient with dysphonia and vocal fold involvement by systemic sclerosis. *Arch Otolaryngol Head Neck Surg*. 2011;137(8):816–819.

265. Ebert EC. Esophageal disease in scleroderma. *J Clin Gastroenterol*. 2006;40(9):769–775.

266. Sataloff RT, Spiegel JR, Rosen DC. Vocal fold consequences of scleroderma. *Ear Nose Throat J*. 1996;75(1): 12–13.

267. Ramos HV, Pillon J, Kosugi EM, Fujita R, Pontes P. Laryngeal assessment in rheumatic disease patients. *Braz J Otorhinolaryngol*. 2005;71(4): 499–503.

268. Belenotti P, Lagier A, Granel B, Serratrice J, Giovanni A, Weiller PJ. Atrophy of the vocal fold: an usual cause of hoarseness in scleroderma. *Joint Bone Spine*. 2015:206–.

269. Kanter GJ, Barash PG. Undiagnosed scleroderma in a patient with a difficult airway. *Yale J Biol Med*. 1998;71(1):31.

270. Ingegnoli F, Galbiati V, Bacciu A, Zeni S, Fantini F. Bilateral vocal fold immobility in a patient with overlap syndrome rheumatoid arthritis/systemic sclerosis. *Clin Rheumatol*. 2007;26(10):1765–1767.

271. Viner DD, Sabri A, Tucker HM. Bilateral cricoarytenoid joint ankylosis in scleroderma. *Otolaryngol Head Neck Surg*. 2001;124(6):696–697.

272. Blocka KLN, Bassett LW. Furst DE, et al. The arthropathy of advanced progressive systemic sclerosis. *Arth Rheum*. 1981; 24:874–884.

273. Pribitkin E, Friedman O, O'Hara B, et al. Amyloidosis of the upper aerodigestive tract. *Laryngoscope*. 2003;113: 2095–2101.

274. Balbani AP, Formigoni GG, Sennes LU, Jacob F, Miniti A, de Carvalho TS. Primary laryngeal amyloidosis in a child. *J Otolaryngol*. 1999;28:171–172.

275. Godbersen GS, Leh JF, Hansmann ML, Rudert H, Linke RP. Organ-limited laryngeal amyloid deposits: clinical, morphological, and immunohistochemical results of five cases. *Ann Otol Rhinol Laryngol*. 1992;101:770–775.

276. Nagasaka T, Lai R, Kuno K, Nakashima T, Nakashima N. Localized amyloidosis and extramedullary plasmacytoma involving the larynx of a child. *Hum Pathol*. 2001;32:132–134.

277 Hurbis CG, Holinger LD. Laryngeal amyloidosis in a child. *Ann Otol Rhinol Laryngol*. 1990;99:105–107.

278. Mitrani M, Biller HF. Laryngeal amyloidosis. *Laryngoscope*. 1985;95:1346–1347.

279. O'Halloran LR, Lusk RP. Amyloidosis of the larynx in a child. *Ann Otol Rhinol Laryngol*. 1994;103:590–594.

280. Clevens RA, Wiatrak BJ, Myers MW. Multifocal amyloidosis of the pediatric airway. *Arch Otolaryngol Head Neck Surg*. 1995; 121:229–232.

281. Sipe JD, Benson MD, Buxbaum JN, et al. Nomenclature 2014: amyloid fibril proteins and clinical classification of the amyloidosis. *Amyloid*. 2014; 21:221–224.

282. Gertz MA. Immunoglobulin light chain amyloidosis: 2013 update on diagnosis, prognosis, and treatment. *Am J Hematol*. 2013;88:416–425.

283. Merlini G, Westermark P. The systemic amyloidoses: clearer understanding of the molecular mechanisms offers hope for more effective therapies. *J Intern Med*. 2004;255:159–178.

284. Rokitansky KF. *Handbuch der Pathologischen Anatomie*. Vienna, Austria: Braumuller und Seidel; 1842: 209–249.

285. Virchaw R. Bav and Zussmmersetzying der Corporci Amalacca des Menschen. *Vehr Phys Med Geswurzlurg.* 1851; 2: 51–53.

286. Simpson GT 2nd, Skinner M, Strong MS, Cohen AS. Localized amyloidosis of the head and neck and upper aerodigestive and lower respiratory tracts. *Ann Otol Rhinol Laryngol.* 1984;93: 374–379.

287. Szmeja Z, Wierzbicka M, Kruk-Zagajewska A, Turczuk-Bierla I. [Amyloidosis of the larynx]. *Otolaryngol Pol.* 1999; 53:617–621.

288. Morawska A, Wiatr M, Skladzien J. Ways of treatment of non-malignant laryngeal tumors in older patients—laryngeal amyloidosis. *Otolaryngol Pol.* 2008; 62:141–144.

289. Thompson LD, Derringer GA, Wenig BM. Amyloidosis of the larynx: a clinicopathologic study of 11 cases. *Mod Path.* 2000; 13:528–535.

290. Lebowitz RA, Morris L. Plasma cell dyscrasias and amyloidosis. *Otolaryngol Clin North Am.* 2003; 36:747–764.

291. Xu L, Cai BQ, Zhong X, Zhu YJ. Respiratory manifestations in amyloidosis. *Chin Med J.* 2005; 118:2027–2033.

292. Wierzbicka M, Budzyński D, Piwowarczyk K, Bartochowska A, Marszałek A, Szyfter W. How to deal with laryngeal amyloidosis? Experience based on 16 cases. *Amyloid.* 2012; 19(4):177–181.

293. Barnes EL, Zafar T. Laryngeal amyloidosis: clinicopathologic study of seven cases. *Ann Otol Rhinol Laryngol.* 1977; 86: 856–863.

294. Gallivan GJ, Gallivan HK. Laryngeal amyloidosis causing hoarseness and airway obstruction. *J Voice.* 2010; 24(2):235–239.

295. Dedo HH, Izdebski K. Laryngeal amyloidosis in 10 patients. *Laryngoscope.* 2004; 114: 1742–1746.

296. Penner CR, Muller S. Head and neck amyloidosis: a clinicopathologic study of 15 cases. *Oral Oncol.* 2006; 42:421–429.

297. Phillips NM, Matthews E, Altmann C, Agnew J, Burns H. Laryngeal amyloidosis: diagnosis, pathophysiology and management. *J Laryngol Otol.* 2017; 131(S2):S41–47.

298. Pino Rivero V, González Palomino A, Trinidad Ruíz G, et al. Amyloidosis of the larynx. A clinical case and literature review. *Ann Otorrinolaringol Ibero Am.* 2004; 31:1–7.

299. Motta G, Salzano FA, Motta S, Staibano S. CO2-laser treatment of laryngeal amyloidosis. *J Laryngol Otol.* 2003; 117:647–650.

300. Bartels H, Dikkers FG, van der Wal JE, Lokhorst HM, Hazenberg BP. Laryngeal amyloidosis: localized versus systemic disease and update on diagnosis and therapy. *Ann Otol Rhinol Laryngol.* 2004; 113:741–748.

301. Deviprasad D, Pujary K, Balakrishnan R, Nayak DR. KTP laser in laryngeal amyloidosis: five cases with review of literature. *Ind J Otolaryngol Head Neck Surg.* 2013; 65(1):36–41.

302. Celenk F, Durucu C, Baysal E, et al. Management of upper aerodigestive tract amyloidosis. *Ann Otol Rhinol Laryngol.* 2013; 122(8):535–540.

# Laryngeal Manifestations of Endocrine Disorders

*Abdul-Latif Hamdan, Robert Thayer Sataloff, and Mary J. Hawkshaw*

## Sex Hormones

The larynx is a hormonal target. It is markedly influenced by the hormonal profile that shapes our vocal identity. Sex hormones in particular play a major role in the development of the vocal characteristics that identify a speaker as a man or woman. The effect is thought to be mediated via hormonal receptors in the various laryngeal structures. Estrogen, progesterone, as well as androgenic receptors in the vocal folds have been described by some authors and refuted by others.[1-5] In 1987 Večerina-Volić et al demonstrated the presence of androgen cytoplasmic and nuclear receptors in normal and cancerous tissues of the larynx in 16 subjects. The authors highlighted the etiologic role of androgen and the possible benefits of hormonal therapy.[4] In 2000, Newman et al reported the presence of hormonal receptors in both cytoplasm and nuclei within the vocal folds of 42 subjects.[1] The study was performed using immune-histochemical staining on fresh cadavers. The authors demonstrated an association between gender and androgen receptor staining in glandular cytoplasm. These results were later corroborated by Voelter et al in their study using monoclonal antibodies on 104 patients with different laryngeal pathologies. Their results confirmed the presence of sex hormones receptors in the vocal folds with predominance of androgen receptors followed by estrogen receptors. Their investigation did not demonstrate any evidence of progesterone receptors.[2] A report by Schneider et al in 2007 failed to show evidence of estrogen alpha, progesterone, and androgen receptors in the muscles, glands, lamina propria, and mucosa of the vocal folds in 15 autopsied patients. Their findings contradicted those of previ-

ous reports that found the presence of sex hormone expression in the larynx.[5] Nacci et al corroborated the report of Schneider and suggested the possible role of growth factors in the development of laryngeal tissues.[6]

Despite these contradictory reports, the phonatory conversion that occurs in parallel with the change in the hormonal climate at puberty is irrefutable. The sex hormones induce growth and differentiation of the laryngeal structures in both genders.[7,8] In females, estrogen and progesterone induce feminization of the voice, whereas in males androgen induces vocal masculinization. As a result of this hormonal influence, the vocal pitch drops by one-third-octave in females and by one octave in males. The "breaking" of voice is generally thought to be caused by the increase in muscle mass that negatively correlates with vocal pitch. As the vocal folds develop more bulk, their rate of vibration becomes slower resulting in a decrease in the fundamental frequency. During puberty, the development and prominence of the thyroid cartilage with widening of the cricothyroid membrane occurs also. This results in the descent of the larynx which is more pronounced in males compared to females. This accentuated drop of the laryngeal structures results in further lengthening of the vocal tract with subsequent decrease in all formants.

The following sections on the female voice and male voice illustrate the vital role of sex hormones in voice maturation, during and after puberty. For the female voice, we discuss voice and menstruation, the premenstrual vocal syndrome, and the postmenopausal vocal syndrome. This will be followed by a section on hormonal therapy and role of adipose tissue, pregnancy and voice, oral contraceptives, and

313

a section on androgen excess and voice. Last there is a section on the male voice.

# I. The Menstrual Cycle and Voice

The prevalence of phonatory symptoms in relation to the menstrual cycle has been established. The fluctuation of various sex hormones, mainly estrogen and progesterone, leads to a constellation of systemic changes that can affect the voice either directly or indirectly. The discussion below is focused on the premenstrual syndrome and postmenopausal vocal syndrome. Additional literature review on the impact of sex hormones fluctuation during the menstrual cycle is covered in the section on oral contraceptives and voice.

## Pre-Menstrual Vocal Syndrome

It is well established that through the activity of the follicular stimulating hormone and the luteinizing hormone controlled by the hypothalamo-hypophysical axis, the menstrual cycle is regulated. During the follicular phase, estrogen induces endometrial mucosal thickening of the endometrial mucosa and progesterone results in thickening of the endo-cervical mucus.[9] Androgen on the other hand causes thickening of the cervical mucosa with reduction in its malleability. With this hormonal climate and cyclic changes in estrogen, progesterone, and androgen, an entity called "premenstrual syndrome" was described in 1953 by Dalton and Green in reference to a constellation of symptoms that recur cyclically in parallel with these hormonal fluctuations.[10] The symptoms include depression, decreased concentration, bloating, nausea, water retention, palpitations, and other systemic manifestations. To confirm the diagnosis of "premenstrual syndrome," these symptoms must be more problematic or pronounced in the "paramenstrum" period and must resolve between the end of menstrual period and ovulation.[11–16] It is important to note that although this syndrome is based on patient's complaints primarily, there is some scientific evidence that supports the symptoms reported. The symptoms of the "premenstrual syndrome" can be induced by the administration of ovarian hormones and suppressed following the cessation of ovulation and menstruation.[17] Several theories have been suggested in attempt to explain this syndrome of unknown etiology. These include the increase and decrease in estrogen and progesterone levels, deficiencies in vitamin B6, disturbances in glucose metabolism, and other biomechanical abnormalities.[18,19]

The premenstrual syndrome has several components to it that include psychological, auditory, metabolic, neurologic, respiratory, as well as phonatory symptoms. The phonatory symptoms associated with premenstruation have been investigated by several authors. In 1978 Silverman and Zimmer evaluated the degree of premenstrual hoarseness in a group of 20 women with no vocal training. The vocal samples recorded at ovulation and few days before menses consisted of sustained vowels /a/, /i/, and /u/ for three seconds. The results suggested rare prevalence of hoarseness at premenstruation in vocally non-trained subjects.[20] On the other hand, 15 years later a survey conducted by Clarissa Behr Davis and Michael Lee Davis evaluating vocal changes associated with premenstrual syndrome revealed that singers on average had three vocal symptoms. The study was conducted on 104 female singers and included 67 general symptoms among which 20 were related to voice. Difficulties in singing the high notes was the most frequent symptom reported by the singers.[21] The aforementioned two studies confirm the differential effect of the menstrual cycle on subjects who are vocally trained versus those who are not.

These reports substantiate the well-known relationship between voice and the reproductive system that was initially described in the 4th century BC and further reported by many authors.[8, 22–26] It has often been referred to as laryngopathia premenstrualis, in reference to the phonatory symptoms experienced mostly by singers, and which often entailed a grace period that exempted these singers from performing.[27,28] It has been established that the effects of sex hormones are not limited to the genitourinary tract alone, but involve the vocal apparatus as well. The vocal symptoms that were once attributed to psychological factors are now explained on the basis of factual changes in the vocal folds, namely, rheological, vascular, and secretory.[25] Estrogen has been shown to have a proliferative and hypertrophic effect on vocal fold mucosa with a marked increase in glandular secretions above and below the true vocal folds. In addition it reduces the extent of desquamation and increases capillary permeability. At its peak on the 21st day of the menstrual cycle, estrogen enhances polymerization of mucopolysaccharides within the vocal fold. Following that peak, there is a decrease in the concentration of these polymers that further break down into smaller molecules. This change in the submucosal ground substance of the vocal folds, together with the increase in tissue permeability of the small vessels, increases the bulk of the vocal folds resulting in deepening of the voice.[8, 26] On the other hand progesterone has an antiproliferative effect and enhances desquamation with reduction in the amount of secretions. As a result there is dryness of the vocal folds with increased viscosity and acidity of the secretions. Progesterone also induces congestion by reducing capillary permeability with subsequent entrapment of extracellular fluids. Similarly androgens cause dehydration with a decrease in glandular secretions. These findings have been supported by the report of Jean Abitbol et al on the cytological similarities between vocal folds smears and smears taken from the cervix.[8]

As a result of these changes in the vocal fold mucosa prior to menstruation, namely, edema, dilated microvarices, and thickened secretions, patients experience a compilation of vocal symptoms today referred to as premenstrual vocal syndrome. These include vocal fatigue, loss of power, and decrease in vocal range more so for the high notes. These symptoms may also occur during ovulation and may more present in professional voice user as previously reported by the survey of Davis and Davis.[21] A study by Abitbol conducted on 97 professional voice users suffering from premenstrual vocal symptoms revealed mucosal, vascular, as well as muscular inflammatory signs in the majority of the participants. Vascular signs such as dilatation of microvarices, edema, and/ or submucosal hematoma were present in 71 patients. Muscular changes such as hypotonicity and diminished power of contraction were observed in 59 patients.[7] It is important to note that the phonatory symptoms experienced by women in their premenstrual period may also be accentuated by the presence of laryngopharyngeal reflux, gastric dismotility, and abdominal bloating experienced by these patients.

## Postmenopausal Vocal Syndrome

At menopause, following the decreased resistance of the remaining oocytes to the follicular stimulating hormone and luteinizing hormone, and subsequent to the cessation of ovulation, there is depletion of the major source of estrogen and progesterone. The drop in estrogen and progesterone levels at menopause results in a plethora of symptoms related to many systems in the body including the phonatory system. The prevalence of vocal symptoms has been reported as high as 77% depending on the methodology and outcome measures used. Symptoms reported most commonly were dryness of the oropharyngeal mucosa, frequent throat clearing, vocal fatigue, and decrease in vocal pitch. These symptoms are often

coupled with acoustic changes, including a decrease in the fundamental frequency, loss of high frequencies, and an increase in the perturbation parameters.[7]

The vocal complaints and acoustic changes experienced by menopausal women are based on the known effect of sex hormones on the vocal folds. With the decrease in estrogen and progesterone at menopause, there is evidence of atrophic changes, both at the mucosal and muscular levels. There is evidence of "sub atrophic mucosa with basophils and reduction in glandular cells in the mucosa of the ventricular band" on vocal fold cytology as reported by Jean Abitbol et al.[7] Similar findings were reported by Caruso et al in their cytology study of 36 menopausal women. There was evidence of atrophy-dystrophy in vocal fold smears similar to what was observed in vaginal smears.[29] As a result of the reduction of glandular cells in in the subglottic and supraglottic mucosa, and the decrease in glandular activity, the concentration of laryngeal mucus increases. This is coupled with mucosal edema secondary to the decrease in the permeability of blood vessels.[30] In his study of 100 menopausal women, Abitbol et al reported that 17% had the clinical presentation of postmenopausal vocal syndrome, namely, a decrease in vocal intensity and range, vocal fatigue, and loss of timber described as "flat and colorless." These symptoms were coupled with endoscopic findings of muscular atrophy, mucosal atrophy, and thinning of the vocal folds.[7] Similarly, in a survey used by Schneider et al, 49 menopausal women out of 107 reported vocal changes that were associated with subjective discomfort in 70% of the cases. In view of this high prevalence of vocal complaints the authors suggested "—additional systematic registration of voice impairment in future menopause rating scales."[30] Boulet and Oddnes also reported that more than half of all women in their fifth decade experience vocal changes related to menopause. The most common problem in female singers was attaining the high register. The authors alluded to the vulnerability of the female voice around the time of menopause.[31] Raj et al in their acoustic analysis of 20 menopausal women reported a lower fundamental frequency, a decrease in vocal intensity, and an increase in the perturbation parameters compared to 35 women in their reproductive years. These acoustic changes were attributed theoretically to the variations in vocal fold thickness secondary to the drop in of estrogen and increase in testosterone.[32] On the other hand, Laureano et al failed to show any statistically significant difference in jitter and shimmer between menopausal women, those during menarche, and those on hormonal replacement therapy (HRT). Their study evaluated 15 women with regular menstrual cycles, 15 menopausal not on HRT, and 15 menopausal on HRT. The acoustic analysis was performed while subjects were asked to sustain the vowel /i/.[33] The controversies in the aforementioned reports can be attributed to two main factors as reported by Friedman: One is the aging effect. The age difference between menopause and menarche is an imperative confounding factor to consider in the analysis of results. The aging process results in an accumulation of phonotrauma that may skew the true effect of hormonal changes. The second important factor is the limitation in the outcome measures used. Laryngeal videostroboscopy has its limitations in detecting very subtle changes in the lamina propria and acoustic analysis has little value in severely dysphonic subjects.[34]

## II. Hormonal Therapy and Role of Adipose Tissue

The benefits of hormonal replacement therapy in menopausal women has been reported extensively. The intake of estrogen/progesterone has proven to reverse the phonatory changes described by menopausal women. Most of the investigations involved professional voice users, with strong emphasis on the role of estrogen therapy in mitigating the acoustic changes, namely, the drop in fundamental frequency and elevated perturbation parameters. The studies of D'haeseleer et al clearly indicate that menopausal women on hormonal therapy have higher fundamental frequency and habitual pitch compared to those not on therapy, namely, 187.7 Hz versus 178.9 Hz, respectively. These findings were further corroborated by the same authors in another cross-sectional study looking at the effect of menopause on voice and nasal resonance.[35,36] Another investigation of 53 menopausal women, of whom 19 were on hormonal therapy and 34 not on therapy, revealed that those on hormonal therapy had significantly higher habitual pitch compared to those not on hormonal therapy ($p$-value 0.022). This acoustic finding did not change when body mass index (BMI) was taken into consideration. On the other hand, it is important to note that the study failed to show any significant difference in the prevalence of phonatory symptoms among the two groups.[37]

Along those lines it is empirical to highlight the important role of adipose tissue as a source of estrogen that is shadowed in the premenopause period because of the cyclic high peaks of estrogen during menstruation. The report by Abitbol J et al "Sex Hormones and the Female Voice" classified women into two types, the "Modigliani type" with little fat and "Rubenesque" with more fat and rounded figure.[7] Given that the ovaries remain a source of androgens, androstenedione, and testosterone after menopause, the biosynthesis of estrones from androgens derivatives in lipocytes thru cytochrome P450 becomes a crucial substitute for the loss of estrogen and progesterone. To that end, the Rubenesque type of women encumbered with the large adipose tissue reserve, tend to mitigate the loss of estrogen.

Few studies have demonstrated the positive correlation between Body Mass Index and the speaking fundamental frequency in menopausal women.[35,36,38] In the study by D'Haeseller et al, on 26 women, menopausal women with high Body Mass Index tended to have higher fundamental frequency than those with low Body Mass Index.[35] This association was not present in those on hormonal therapy or those with low body mass index. In a recent report, Hamdan et al compared the prevalence of phonatory symptoms in 34 menopausal and 35 premenopausal women taking into consideration the impact of Body Mass Index as a confounding variable. Outcome measures included phonatory and laryngopharyngeal symptoms in addition to acoustic analysis and Voice Handicap Index-10. The results indicated no statistically significant difference in any of the phonatory symptoms or acoustic parameters between high Body Mass Index in menopausal women and in premenopausal women. The results substantiated the important role of adipose tissue and the conventional vocal symptoms attributed to menopause.[39]

## III. Pregnancy and Voice

The dramatic increase in hormonal levels in women during pregnancy imposes major physiologic adaptations. Many systems are affected among which is the phonatory apparatus. Changes in posture, level of hydration, as well as impaired breathing secondary to reduced lung capacity, all impact voice and result in phonatory changes that are often experienced by professional voice users. In a study by Cassiraga et al on 44 third-trimester women, the authors reported a higher prevalence of breathiness and shortness of breath in pregnant women compared to controls.[40] They reported an increase in the intensity of speech and a decrease in the maximum phonation time. The decrease in the maximum phonation time was based on the reported overall changes in the respiratory system during pregnancy. There are alterations in pulmonary function, namely, a decrease in the "functional residual capacity, expiratory reserve volume, residual volume, and total lung volume."[41] In another study conducted on 25 pregnant women, the authors reported an increase in the maximum phonation time right after delivery. There was also an increase in the fundamental frequency and a decrease in the voice turbulence index.[42] The increase in the fundamental frequency was attributed to the drastic decrease in the body water content that follows delivery. It is important to note that toward the end of pregnancy the increase in water content is estimated to be 6.5 to 8.5 L.[43]

The surge in sex hormones with its potential effect on voice is also observed in patients undergoing in vitro fertilization (IVF). The severity and frequency of vocal symptoms during three visits along the course of in vitro fertilization were investigated in a group of 31 women. The most common symptom reported throughout the visits was throat clearing. Other symptoms such as vocal fatigue and globus sensation occurred in 9.68% of the women. There was no significant change in either the severity or the frequency of these phonatory symptoms between the visits, probably due to the short time window in between and to the wide intersubject variation in the level of estradiol during induction. Noteworthy was that the severity and frequency of throat clearing correlated with the level of estradiol levels in this study population.[44] These symptoms were attributed to the proliferative lubrication effect of the high estradiol level in the second and third visit (424,16 pg/mL and 1433.48 pg/mL, respectively). Two years later, a prospective study looking at acoustic measures in relation to estradiol level in a group of 10 women undergoing IVF was reported. The results indicated a decrease in F0 and F0 range with the increase in the estradiol level. This was expected given the associated edematous changes observed and with the documented increase in estrogen level. With edema of the vocal folds there is an increase in mass and subsequently a drop in the mean fundamental frequency.[45]

## IV. Oral Contraceptives

The impact of sex hormones on the voice is well known. The interaction is thought to be complex and involves direct effects on laryngeal structures through hormonal receptors.[1] During the menstrual cycle, the interplay between sex hormones and voice becomes more accentuated. The fluctuation in estrogen and progesterone levels carries a significant physiologic effect on the vocal folds similar to that seen on the cervix.[7] During the first phase of the menstrual cycle, estrogen level surges gradually inducing a hypertro-

phic effect on the vocal folds with an increase in the amount of mucus secretion. After its peak at day 14, it starts declining until day 21 when it peaks again before declining further toward the end of the cycle. The level of progesterone on the other hand starts rising after ovulation and reaches its peak on day 21 causing a decrease in glandular cell secretions, and an increase in mucous viscosity and acidity, with subsequent dehydration of the vocal folds.[46,47] Oral contraceptive pills (OCP) abort the aforementioned fluctuation in sex hormones that occurs during the menstrual cycle. The steady intake of progesterone and estrogen suppresses the luteinizing hormone secretion and follicular stimulating hormone during the luteal and follicular phases. The effect is thought to be compounded resulting in inhibition of ovulation.[48,49]

Despite the well-known interplay between sex hormones and phonation, the impact of OCP on voice is still not very clear. Following the introduction of the first generation of OCP that contained nortestosterone derivative, androgenic side effects in particular voice virilization, became an issue of major concern particularly in professional voice users.[48] Ismail in 1966 reported 87 cases of vocal virilization that were attributed to hypertrophy of the vocal folds' muscles.[50] This adverse effect was further substantiated by other investigations reported in 1969. Significant acoustic changes, namely, lowering of the fundamental frequency and increased vocal intensity, have been reported following the usage of oral contraceptives that contained a mixture of chlormadinone acetate and mestranol.[51,52] These reports have led to the development of pills with lesser amount of hormones. The second generation of pills introduced in the 1970s, made of a combination of progesterone derivative (levonorgestrel) and an estrogen derivative (ethinylestradiol), became very popular in view of is scarce side effects. The third generation made of "progestins, gestodene and desogestrel"[53] and the fourth generation containing Drospirenone as its progestine component, were also launched in the 1980s but were not as widely used as the second generation.[53]

Today these modern generations of OCP have led to 30% of women using OCP in their reproductive years.[54] Despite this high figure, there is still no clear consensus on the impact of OCP on voice.

### Where Does the Literature Stand on Usage of Oral Contraceptives Today?

With the increased importance of voice as a means of communication and the rising usage of OCP, a better understanding of the effect of these pills on voice has become paramount. To that end, numerous investigations on vocal changes associated with OCP usage have emerged. Most of these investigations are based on auditory perceptual evaluation, subjective ratings, laryngeal videostroboscopic examination, as well as objective measures such as acoustic, electro-laryngographic, and aerodynamic analysis. Below is a brief review of the literature on the impact of OCP on voice, stratified according to different outcome measures.

## Perceptual, Acoustic and Phono-articulatory Changes

In 1995, Wendler et al et reported a thorough perceptual and acoustic analysis of sustained vowels /a/, /e/, /i/, and /u/, while comparing two types of OCPs, one containing "2 mg cyproterone acetate and 0.035 mg ethinylestradiol "(Diane-35) and another containing "0.15 mg levonorgestrel and 0.03 mg ethinylestradiol "(Microgynon).[55] The study was conducted on 91 patients throughout a one-year period during which patients had stroboscopic examination in addition to subjective assessment and phoniatric investigation. Subjective information included complaints such as vocal fatigue and throat symptoms, whereas perceptual assessment comprised vocal characteristics such as onset of voice, mean speaking frequency, as well as the overall sound quality. The mean speaking fundamental frequency, voice range profile, and dynamic range were also measured. The results of this study indicated the lack of any vocal/throat symptoms, or audio-acoustic changes as side effects to the usage of OCP. These findings were commensurate with normal laryngeal stroboscopic examination. More so, there were no significant differences in any of the measured parameters between the two preparations used. The authors concluded that OCPs used in this investigation were rather safe compared to the first generation introduced in the 1960s.[55] This conclusion was corroborated by other investigators who furthermore alluded to the beneficial effect of these medications. In a study in 2002 by Amir et al, the authors reported a favorable effect of OCP on voice in terms of stability. The analysis of two sustained vowels /i/ and /a/ recorded during six intervals of the menstrual cycle in 10 patients (five on OCP and five not on OCP) revealed lower perturbation parameters for intensity and frequency in subjects on pills versus those not on pills (five on pills and five not on pills). The authors attributed vocal stabilization to the reduced fluctuation in the hormonal profile naturally witnessed during a menstrual cycle.[56] More so, there was no significant difference in the fundamental frequency between the two

groups unlike the results of previous studies on the first generation of OCP. However, there were changes in F0 toward the middle of the menstrual cycle in the pill group that were not present in the group not on pills, and to which the authors had no clear explanation. It is worth noting that the recordings were made over the course of 40 days and all 10 participants were non-professional voice users with no formal singing training. In conclusion the authors advocated the safety and beneficial effect of the new generation of OCP. Similarly in 2003, the same authors evaluated the effect of low dose monophasic OCP on voice in six women compared to six controls. All participants were non-professional voice users and the recordings were made during six intervals of one to two menstrual cycles. The same findings were reported, namely, lower values for variations in frequency and amplitude in subjects on pills versus those not on pills (0.86% vs 1.27% for jitter and 0.24 db vs 0.37 db for shimmer). The authors alluded to the stabilizing effect of the monophasic low dose OCP on these acoustic parameters,[57] although the study was limited because of the small number of subjects.

In 2004, Amir and Kishon-Rabin expanded their acoustic analysis to include additional perturbation parameters such as "relative average perturbation, pitch period perturbation quotient and amplitude average perturbation quotient."[58] The authors reported lower values for all acoustic variables except F0 in a group of seven women using low-dose monophasic OCP in comparison to controls. The recordings and analysis were conducted on sustained vowels /a/ and /i/ over the course of 36 to 45 days.[58] These results were in alignment with the results of previous reports substantiating the favorable effect of OCP on voice. Based on the study by Higgins and Saxman, the fluctuation in sex hormones around the time of ovulation may result in an increase in cycle-to-cycle variations in pitch and intensity. This increase is secondary to alterations in the speed of neural transmission and or to changes in the laryngeal mechanoreceptor sensitivity.[59] With the intake of OCP this hormonal fluctuation is obviously attenuated with subsequent reduction in the aforementioned perturbation parameters. During the same year, Gorham-Rowan corroborated the aforementioned stabilizing effect of OCP on voice by reporting "—greater stability during phonation" in subjects on OCP. The authors have investigated 28 women, 18 on OCP and 10 not on any OCP. The acoustic recordings were made prior to menses and included two phonatory tasks, a sustained vowel /a/ and reading of the "Rainbow Passage." There was a significant effect of OCP on shimmer and amplitude perturbation quotient APQ, with higher values being reported in the non OCP group. These findings were again attributed to the steadiness of the hormonal profile induced by the intake of oral contraceptives. On the other hand, the authors disagreed with Amir et al with respect to the effect of OCP on the fundamental frequency. During sustained vowel analysis, the group on OCP had higher fundamental frequency values F0 compared to the non OCP group (230.51 Hz vs 205.11 Hz). Similarly, during connected speech the speaking fundamental frequency in the OCP was also higher (213.62 Hz vs 199.14 Hz). The difference in the results between the two studies could be attributed to the difference in time of voice recording, which were primarily done prior to menses in the study by Gorham-Rowan. However, it is worth noting that there was no significant difference in the standard deviation of the speaking fundamental frequency between those on pills and those not on pills, which probably means that the stabilizing effect of OCP is more pronounced or effective in sustained vowel production rather than in connected speech.[60]

In 2005, Amir et al compared the effect of different formulations of OCP on voice in 29 women. These were divided into 3 groups, Drospirenones, Desogestrol, and Gestodone. An acoustic evaluation performed twice during the cycle revealed similar results between the three groups except for slight difference between the Drospirenone group and the remaining two groups.[61] One year later they increased the sample size to 30 women using different OCP with different progestin levels in comparison to 10 who were not on pills. The results revealed no significant difference in all acoustic measures between the two groups. More so, a meta-analysis combining the previous studies showed lower perturbation parameters in subjects on OCP compared to controls.[62] In that same year, Van Lierde et al investigated vocal changes in 24 women using monophasic pills. Assessment of two vocal recordings were made using various subjective and objective measures, one a few days before or after ovulation (day 10–17) and one during the first three days of menses. The results indicated no significant differences between the two assessments in terms of voice quality, dysphonia severity index, maximum phonation time, voice range, and acoustic parameters. To that end the authors concurred the stabilizing effect of OCP on sex hormones during the menstrual cycle. Nevertheless, it is worth noting the limitations of this study, namely, the lack of vocal samplings during the luteal phase and the lack of a control group.[63]

La et al in 2007 conducted the first randomized placebo controlled trial investigating variations in pitch and amplitude in a group of nine classical singers (one mezzo-soprano and 7 sopranos) taking a combined monophasic OCP (containing drospirenone) and a matched placebo over the course of three menstrual cycles. Using electrolaryngography, the authors analyzed period-to-period variations in frequency peaks (CFx) and period-to-period variations in amplitude peaks (CAx), as quantitative measures of variations in pitch and amplitude. The results indicated less irregularities in these measures when OCP were used. The period-to period amplitude peaks was higher in the menstrual and follicular phases while using placebo.[64] During the luteal phase, there were no differences in pitch and amplitude variations between women on OCP and placebo, which means that the variations seen in the follicular and menstrual phases are not necessarily secondary to hormonal fluctuations as suggested by Amir et al. Two years later, a similar study by the same authors was conducted on 20 professional voice users, 10 using OCP and 10 controls. Unlike the previous investigation, not all participants were classical singers and other professional voice users such as teachers were included. More so, both reading and singing samples were recorded for analysis ("Rainbow Passage" and "Yesterday" sung by the Beatles). In contrary to the previous investigation, the results of this study showed no effect of OCP on the two aforementioned electrographic parameters, namely, CFx and CAx.[65] The authors attributed this controversy to the study design, short duration of OCP intake and to the less demanding singing task of the song chosen in comparison to the German Classical song. In 2012, La et al reported different findings in a study investigating vibrato rate and pitch control in nine singers. Using audio-electrolaryngograph recordings during all phases of the menstrual cycle, the authors reported significant differences for pitch control at F5.[66] The results of this investigation highlight the importance of the phonatory task used in recording and analysis, which plays a crucial role in the interpretation of the results.

Voice onset time (VOT) and the vocal folds vibratory pattern have also been investigated in women receiving OCP. Morris et al examined the effect of OCP on VOT during two phases of two menstrual cycles, with the hypothesis that VOT variations are less evident in women on OCP compared to those not on OCP.[67] This hypothesis stemmed from the fact that fluctuation in sex hormones do affect VOT as reported by Whiteside et al.[68] The findings of their investigation on 20 women divided equally into two groups, one on OCP and another not on pills, contradicted those of Whiteside et al. There was no significant difference in the mean VOT between the two phases of the menstrual cycle in either groups. More so, the differences in the means of VOT between those on OCP and those not on pills did not reach any statistical significance either. Nevertheless, it is worth noting that the non OCP group had longer mean VOT for the /b/ phoneme whereas the OCP had longer VOT for the /p/ phoneme.[67] Two years later in 2011, Morris et al conducted a longitudinal study in order to better evaluate the effect of shifting to OCP use in a women with a natural menstrual cycle. The voice recordings of a 23-year-old women were collected during 2 cycles when she was naturally menstruating and in six cycles when she was on OCP. The recordings consisted of 3 sustained /ae/ vowels at comfortable pitch and loudness. Acoustic measures that correlated with closed quotient duration, glottal width, and vocal fold speed of closure were obtained. Unlike the previous study that showed no effect of OCP on VOT, the results of this investigation indicated changes in H1-H2 differences and in H1-A1 differences, which correlated with closed quotient duration and glottal width, respectively. In the follicular phase, there was a reduction in the H1-H2 difference and H1-A1 difference, whereas in the luteal phase, there was an increase in the difference of H1-H2 and H1-A1. On the other hand there were no changes in the difference H1-A3 before and after intake of OCP. The results also showed an increase in jitter level in both follicular and leuteal phases after intake of OCP but with no difference in shimmer and noise-to-harmonic ratio.[69]

The more recent literature on acoustic changes associated with OCP usage is in partial agreement with the previous reports but still not conclusive. In 2015, Meurer et al conducted a cross-sectional study investigating phonoarticulatory changes in four groups of women, two using low dosage OCP and two not on pills. Using both sustained vowels and connected speech, the authors reported better voice acuity for the sustained vowels in the groups not on pills, but slower speech in both midfollicular and midluteal phases. On the other hand, patients on OCP had higher frequency modulation for the connected speech.[70] In 2017, the effect of OCP on vocal folds vibration have been investigated by Kunduk et al in a group of 13 women divided in two subgroups, six on OCP and 7 not on pills. Voice recordings of sustained vowel /i/ coupled with high-speed video-endoscopic imaging were collected at three phases of the menstrual cycle; premenstruation, ovulation, and postmenstruation. Using several acoustic measures such as fundamental frequency, harmonic-to-noise ratio, harmonic richness factor, in addition to

subjective ratings such as perceptual evaluation, the authors reported no significant effect of OCP on vocal fold vibration. Their results, in particular the lack of significant difference on fundamental frequency deviation and harmonic-to-noise ratio in women on OCP were not in total agreement with the results of Amir et al who have reported lower perturbation parameters, jitter and shimmer, and lower noise-to-harmonic ratio in women using OCP compared to those not on pills.[62] Based on the author's interpretation, the discrepancy might be attributed to the high sensitivity of videoendoscopy to frequency perturbation and to possible differences in the background noise characteristics between the two studies.[71] On the other hand, the higher value of the harmonic richness factor and lower mean value of H1-H2, speak for a voice rich in harmonics, which is in keeping with the "better voice quality" as reported by Amir et al.[62] In the same year, Meurer et al 2017 investigated the impact of monophasic low dose OCP on vocal range in a group of 72 women (48 on pills and 24 controls). Subjects were asked to read a sentence in six variations. The authors reported that the "highest vocal tones for the same sentence uttered using an exclamatory fashion"[72] were lower in the OCP group compared to those not on pills. Similarly, the lowest vocal tones in the sentence uttered in a joyful intonation were higher in the OCP group. In conclusion the authors demonstrated that OCP have an effect on vocal range in women during their reproductive years.[72]

## Aerodynamic Measures and OCP

The aerodynamic measures in patients on OCP have also been investigated with the purpose of providing more information on the vibratory behavior of the vocal folds during a stable hormonal environment. In 2008 Mary Gorham-Rowan and Linda Fowler measured peak flow, minimum and alternating flows, in addition to the sound pressure level and fundamental frequency in a group of 16 women, eight of whom were receiving OCP. The subjects were asked to repeat the vowel /a/ three times at two phases of the menstrual period, directly after menstruation and around time of ovulation. The authors reported significant difference in some of the airflow measures between those on pills versus controls, with higher peaks and alternating flow rates reported in those on pills. However, after having eliminated the outliers, the results revealed no significant difference in the glottal airflow measurements between the two groups At this point, the authors emphasized that the aforementioned airflow measures may not be very useful in depicting vocal changes in patients using OCP.[73] A year later, the same authors reported different findings in another study where subjects were asked to repeat the syllable /pa/ instead of a vowel. The study which was conducted on 16 women (eight on OCP and eight not on OCP) and voice recordings were obtained at two phases in the menstrual cycle. The authors concluded that OCP have no effect on laryngeal airflow,[74] which is in keeping with the findings of La et al, namely, the lack of significant differences in the vocal vibrational pattern between subjects on OCP pills versus those not on pills.

**Vocal Resonance and OCP**

Resonance is defined as amplification of sound by mechanism of reflection. In phonation, the vocal signal is amplified in the vocal tract, nose, and paranasal sinuses. As such the nose plays an important role in vocal resonance, diseases of which may markedly impact voice quality. During pregnancy, the etiologic role of sex hormones in nasal congestion and hypersecretion has been well investigated in the literature. Several hypothesis have been suggested to explain the compilation of nasal symptoms in the last trimester of pregnancy. These include interstitial edema, reduction in apha-adrenergic supply resulting in venous sinusoidal congestion within the nasal mucosa, and last an upsurge in estrogen level.[75] The pathogenic role of the latter has been substantiated by the therapeutic usage of topical estrogen in cases of atrophic rhinitis and the presence of estrogen receptor in the nasal mucosa.[76,77] Nevertheless, conflicting studies on the pathogenic role of estrogen in patients with nasal symptoms have been reported. Ellegard and Karlsson investigated the extent of nasal obstruction during a menstrual cycle. The study was conducted on 27 women using nasal peak expiratory flow and subjective grading of nasal stuffiness from 0 to 4. Unexpectedly, the degree of nasal obstruction correlated negatively with the estrogen level. In the menstrual phase during which estrogen level is low, the nasal resistance was high.[75] These findings were further corroborated by a report by Paulson et al, which included three studies on the relationship between sex hormones and nasal congestion. All three studies failed to demonstrate an association between estrogen, progesterone, and nasal congestion. The outcome measures used in the first two studies included both subjective rating of nasal stuffiness and objective measures such as acoustic rhinometry and nasal expiratory peak-flow. These findings were in keeping with the absence of estrogen and progesterone receptors in biopsies taken from the nasal

mucosa in the third study of this same report.[78] On the other hand, two other reports, one by Haeggstrom et al and another by Philpott et al confirmed the interplay between estrogen surge and nasal congestion. The study by Haeggstrom et al did show that with an increase in estrogen level, at the pre-ovulatory stage of the menstrual cycle, there is hyperactivity of the nasal mucosa to histamine. The investigation was carried out on 10 women whose nasal mucosa was examined at baseline and after being challenged with histamine. The examination was performed three times during the menstrual cycle using acoustic rhinometry and rhinostereometry.[79] Similarly, the study by Philpott et al did show that nasal congestion occurs with an increase in estrogen level. The study included several diagnostic measures, self reported questionnaire on rhinitis, nasal airflow measures, examination of the nasal cavity, and acoustic rhinometry.[80]

With all the aforementioned data on the speculative association between estrogen level and nasal congestion, it was intuitive to investigate the clinicpathologic effects of OCP on the nasal mucosa and hence on vocal resonance. Indeed, the first histologic study on nasal mucosal changes in patients on OCP was reported by Toppozada et al in 1984. The authors took a punch biopsy from the inferior turbinates of 15 women who were on OCP, five of whom had nasal symptoms and the others were symptom free. Using histochemical and ultramicroscopic analysis of the human respiratory nasal mucosa, the authors demonstrated the presence of high acid mucoplysaccharide content and increased glandular and phagocytic activity in the symptom-free subjects. In those with nasal symptoms, there was evidence of "squamous metaplasia, intra-epithelial edema, glandular hyperplasia and histiocytic proliferation."[81] More than 2 decades later, the effect of OCP on resonance and other vocal parameters were investigated by Van Lierde et al in 2006. The study was conducted on 24 professional voice users during two phases of the menstrual cycle, around the time of ovulation and within three days after menses. The comparative analysis indicated no significant difference in nasality, nasalance, or any of the various subjective and objective measures used in this investigation. The authors concluded that OCP do provide a stable hormonal profile that works in favor of professional voice users who desire no phonatory disturbance during performance. However, the results of this study may not be as conclusive to non-professional voice users who lack the adaptive skills of professional voice users.[63] A similar study that includes singers, non-singers, and a control group may ascertain or refute the impact of OCP on resonance.

## Conclusion

In conclusion, thorough review of the literature reveals no clear consensus on the effect of OCP on voice. The lack of uniformity in the results can be attributed to several factors thoroughly discussed in Chapter 39 "The Effects of Oral Contraceptives and Voice" in the 4th edition of "*Professional Voice: The Science and Art of Clinical Care.*"[48] In brief these include: (1) the type of OCP used, taking into consideration the large variety of pills available in the market, (2) the voice sample analyzed, whether sustained vowels or connected speech, (3) lack of standardization of the time or phase of the menstrual cycle during which voice recordings were made, (4) variations in the voice outcome measures, and (5) the disparity in subject selection, whether professional voice users or non-professional voice user. This issue is of paramount importance knowing that singers have more adaptive skills to hormonal variations in comparison to subjects with no history of vocal training.[48] More evidence-based studies are needed to clearly elucidate the interplay between OCP and voice.

## V. Androgen Excess and Voice

### Endogenous Excess of Androgen

The pre-pubertal surge of testosterone is responsible for the growth and development of laryngeal structures in both genders. In concert with estrogen and progesterone, testosterone and its derivatives define our sexual identity. Despite the ubiquity of reports on the pre-and pubertal effect of sex hormones on voice, less has been reported on the pathogenic role of androgenic hormones in vocal virilization in the post-pubertal phase. To that end, various hormones have been implicated among which are testosterone, dihydrotestosterone (DHT), or dehydroepiandrosterone (DHEAS), complemented with metabolic hormonal disorders.[82] When androgen levels are high enough to induce symptoms and signs of virilization, a thorough investigation looking for the source of androgen excess should be undertaken. In parallel, medical treatment of hypernadrogenism should be initiated. This may include androgen receptor blockers such as cyproterone acetate, adrenal androgen production blockers such as glucocorticoid, and ovarian androgen production blockers.[83] Early initiation of therapy is crucial in reversing many of the androgenic signs except for voice deepening which invariably is irreversible.

The workup of androgen associated endocrinopathy is a challenging task that requires a high index of suspicion and a diligent stepwise approach. Both clinical perspective as well as hematologic/radiologic investigation are crucial in making the right diagnosis. A detailed history and physical examination looking for symptoms and signs of androgen excess in addition to voice deepening are of paramount importance. Important clues include the presence of hirsutism, pattern of hair loss, insulin resistance, increased libido, and cliteromegaly. Other important symptoms suggestive of an enlarged ovarian producing tumors are abdominal distention, amenorrhea, or irregular menses. Blood tests for free testosterone, DHEAS, and ratio of luteinizing hormone to follicular stimulating hormones are very important.[83,84] Based on a study by Waggoner et al looking at the predictive value of these tests in 478 hyperandrogenic cases, the authors reported the positive predictive value of testosterone level (above 8.67 nmol/L) for a neoplasm to be 9%. More so, none of 10 patients with elevated DHEAS (above 16.3 micomol/L) had adrenocortical tumor. The results of this investigation clearly questions the validity and usefulness of these tests and emphasizes the importance of the clinical picture instead.[85] Nevertheless, although the association between high blood level of testosterone and androgen-producing tumors has its controversies, baseline levels are still being adopted in the workup of patients with excess androgens. For instance, a blood level of total testosterone above 12 nmol/L is indicative of a virilizing tumor and a basal level of DHEAS above 18,5 micomol/L is more suggestive of an adrenal tumor.[84] Along the same line of investigation, an elevated ratio of LH to FSH is suggestive of PCOS despite the fact that almost half of patients with PCOS may have a normal ratio. The dexamethasone test has also been used to differentiate androgen excess of adrenal versus ovarian origin. After being administered for 4 days, a complete suppression is suggestive of adrenal origin whereas an incomplete suppression is suggestive of an ovarian origin. More so, morning levels of 17-hydroxyprogesterone level less than 6 nmol/L have also been used to exclude nonclassic congenital adrenal hyperplasia invariably due to 21-hydroxylase deficiency.[84] In addition to the hormonal evaluation, a radiologic workup is also valuable. It includes transabdominal or transvaginal ultrasonography, computerized tomographic imaging, and magnetic resonance imaging. Transvaginal ultrasonography in particular has been the standard diagnostic test of PCOS documenting the presence of increased stroma and distended ovaries.

As the origin of androgenic excess is sought with diligence using the aforementioned blood tests and radiologic imaging, physicians should keep in mind the cross-cutting between the various causes of virilization such as androgen associated endocrinopathy and androgen producing neoplasms. In a review of 950 cases of clinical hyperandrogenism, the most common causes were PCOS (72.1%), and idiopathic hyperandrogenism and idiopathic hirsutims in 15.8% and 7.6%, respectively. Twenty-one hydroxylase-deficient non-classic adrenal hyperplasia and androgen-secreting tumors accounted for only 4.3% and 0.2% of the total cases.[86] To that end, it is important to note the rarity of androgen-producing tumors as a cause of hyeprandrogenism and vocal virilization.

## Androgen-Associated Ovarian Disorders

### Polycystic Ovary Syndrome

Polycystic ovary syndrome (PCOS) is described as a common endocrine disorder with metabolic manifestations affecting close to 6 to 15% of women during their reproductive years.[87] The criteria used for diagnosis include oligo or anovulation, the presence of polycystic ovaries, and biochemical hyperandrogenism. This latter is key in the diagnosis of PCOS and may be present in 50% to 90% of affected women although the androgen level rarely exceeds 200 ng/dL, the level that results in severe virilization and deepening of the voice.[88] In a recent investigation on the prevalence of vocal symptoms and associated acoustic changes in 17 patients with PCOS, there was a statistically significant difference in the prevalence of "throat clearing, deepening of the voice, sensation of lump in the throat and difficulty being heard" in affected patients compared to controls.[89] There was also a statistically significant difference in the relative average perturbation and maximum phonation time between the two groups. These significant differences were attributed hypothetically to excessive laryngeal secretions and to possible congestion of the vocal folds that occurs with elevated estrogen levels in patients with PCOS. It is important to note that in the population studied, only three subjects had testosterone levels above 90 ng/dL. The treatment of PCOS consists of either behavioral modification, particularly dietary changes, given the fact that 80% of affected patients are obese, or the use of oral contraceptives. In a meta-analysis that included 13 randomized trials comparing metformin with placebo, the results indicated that metformin can increase ovulation by almost four times.[90] This concurred with previous studies that reported an ovulation rate of up to 89% using metformin especially when combined with Clomiphene, an anti-estrogenic medication that stimulates ovulation.[91]

### Androgen-Producing Ovarian Tumors

There are many reports in the literature on androgen-secreting ovarian tumors presenting with deepening of voice as one of many virilizing symptoms. Among these are the Sertoli-Leydig cell tumors (SLCT) referred to as androblastomas or arrhenoblastomas,[92] the virilizing ovarian steroid cell tumors, sclerosing-stromal tumors, thecoma tumors, virilizing teratomas, and transitional cell carcinoma.[93-110] Below is a brief review of the common androgen-secreting ovarian tumors.

*Sertoli-Leydig cell tumors* are rare ovarian tumors that originate from the pluripotential cells within the stroma and account for less than 0.5% of neoplasms of the ovaries.[95] They occur predominantly in women in their third decade of life with one out of three having excess androgen. As such these are considered as the most common virilizing ovarian tumors. In a review of 64 cases by Zaloudek and Norris, the authors reported virilization in 38% of the cases. Most of the lesions were unilateral, at an early stage of the disease, and had a favorable prognosis.[97] In another review of a large series of 207 cases, Young and Scully reported that most of these tumors are non-malignant (usually stage I) and more than half (58%) have a mixed nature (solid and cystic).[96] Based on a report by Jung et al on 15 cases of SLCT, the CT imaging of these lesions often reveals an enhancing mass with a cystic component. Magnetic resonance imaging usually shows hypointense lesions with various signal intensity of T2-weighted images.[98]

*Sclerosing stromal tumor of ovary (SST)*: SST is an uncommon neoplasm of the ovaries that affects women in their third decade of life and is more often than not considered as non-functioning tumor. Nevertheless, steroidogenesis does occur causing estrogenic symptoms such as irregular menses and infertility. Only a few cases of virilizing SST have been reported in the literature alluding to the rare possibility of these tumors to present with androgenic symptoms and signs such as deepening of the voice.[99-102] The main presentation is irregular menses with pelvic pain and evidence of a large heterogeneous mass with cystic component and high signal intensity on T2-weighed images.[98] Based on a literature review there are only four cases of SST presenting with virilization.[99-102] In 1990 Ismail and Walker presented an ovarian sclerosing stromal tumor with virilizing symptoms in a patient diagnosed with Gorlin's syndrome.[102] A year later Cashell and Cohen reported another case of sclerosing stromal tumor in a 27-year-old women during her pregnancy. The 3-cm ovarian mass was resected and the patient's hormonal profile reverted back to normal.[101] More than a decade later Park et al in 2011 reported an 11-year-old girl whose main presentation was deepening of her voice with hirsutism and hypertrophy of the clitoris. Radiologic imaging showed a pelvic mass that was resected with oopherctomy following which the patient had normalization of her testosterone level.[100] Boussaid et al in 2013 reported a 24-year-old woman with McCune Albright syndrome who was diagnosed with a virilizing sclerosing stromal tumor. The patient presented also with deepening of her voice in addition to other virilizing symptoms such as hirsutism, acne, and amenorrhea. Blood test showed a very high level of testosterone and abdominal CT revealed a 45-mm solid ovarian tumor on the left side.[99]

*Steroid cell tumors*: are rare tumors of the ovaries that affect women in their fifth and sixth decade of life. They are considered as a subtype of Leydig tumor with typical findings of "crystalloids of Reinke" on periodic acid-Shiff staining. These tumors are invariably virilizing tumors that present with excessive testosterone secretion leading to a constellation of noticeable androgenic symptoms including deepening of voice.[103,104] Radiologic imaging may be misleading because virilizing steroid cell tumors are usually small, almost of equal size to the ovaries with hypoechoic or hyperechoic structure on ultrasound.[105,106] On MRI there is evidence of intense enhancement on T1-weighted images.[98] Early diagnosis is important given the prevalence of malignant transformation in one-third of the cases. Salim et al described a 40-year-old woman with steroid cell ovarian tumor who presented with symptoms and signs of virilization.[107] Her symptoms included frontal balding, hirsutism, increased muscle mass, and deepening of her voice. Her high level of free and total testosterone and radiologic findings of a mass lesion in the uterine fundus with two oval lesions in the pelvis led to the diagnosis. The patient underwent staging laparotomy and abdominal hysterectomy. Microscopic examination of the ovaries revealed stromal hyperplasia with a well-differentiated steroid cell tumor of the left ovary.

*Thecoma tumors*: are rare benign tumors of the ovaries that are usually nonfunctional. When they contain luteinized theca cells they are referred to as luteinized thecoma. The latter may demonstrate signs of hyperestrogenism in 50% of the cases and virilization in one out of 10 patients.[108] These tumors may occur in young and postmenopausal females resulting in deepening of the voice in addition to other virilizing symptoms that may not improve following surgical resection of the tumor. A rare case of ovarian thecoma occurring concurrently with steroid cell tumor was reported in a 49-year-old postmenopausal woman. The patient had deepening of her voice also, that was commensurate with an elevated serum testosterone level.[109]

*Granulosa cell tumors*: are rare androgenic tumors of the ovaries that may present with a constellation of androgenic symptoms including deepening of the voice. In a review by Nakashima et al of 17 cases that included prepubertal, postpubertal, and pregnant women, the authors reported masculinized features with acne, clitorimegaly, and lowered pitch in more than two-thirds of the patients.[110]

### Androgen-Associated Adrenal Disorders

Androgen excess originating from the adrenal glands is secondary either to adrenocortical tumors or to adrenal hyperplasia. Below is a discussion of the clinical presentation of these entities in the context of vocal virilization.

*Adrenocortical carcinoma* is a rare entity with an incidence rate of 2.0 cases per million.[111] The age at diagnosis varies between 20 to 54 years with a bimodal distribution occurring in the first decade and fourth decade of life.[112] Affected children have better prognosis than adults and adults below the age of 40 years seem to do better than those above the age of 40 years.[113] Both sexes are equally affected, with a predominance in whites compared to blacks and Asians.[114,115] The majority of these tumors are functional tumors (59%) secreting either excessive active hormones or their precursors.[112] According to a Wooten and King epidemiologic study, there is an inverse relationship between age and functionality of these tumors with predominance of functional tumors in subjects below the age of 30 years.[112] Based on a clinical and diagnostic review by Muller, the clinical picture of these tumors can be stratified according to the nature of their hormonal secretions. Hence these tumors can be estrogenic, androgenic, or hypercortisolism. Clinically we may encounter adrenocortical carcinoma with Cushing syndrome, virilization syndrome, feminization syndrome, or a mixed picture.[116]

Of interest to Otolaryngologists, speech-language pathologists, and vocal teachers, is the pathogenic role of these tumors in a female patient with vocal virilization. Although as previously discussed, androgen-secreting tumors account only for 0.25% of all cases of androgen excess in women,[86] voice care professionals should be on the alert for the rare occurrence of these tumors given that early diagnosis may improve prognosis.[117,118] In adults the clinical presentation is that of a mixed secreting tumor, hypercortisolism, and virilization, whereas in children the predominant presentation is that of virilization. Indeed there are a few case reports in the literature that concur with the prevalence of virilizing symptoms and signs in pre-pubertal boys and girls, commensurate with elevated serum androgen levels.[119–121] That being said, physicians should be attentive to the presence of virilizing symptoms and signs in patients with deepening of the voice. Systemic clinical manifestations aside from those related to virilizations must also be looked for. These include symptoms of generalized weakness, myalgia, abdominal or pelvic pain, nausea, weight loss, hypertension, edema of the lower extremities, and urinary symptoms.[122] The diagnosis is further suggested based on the presence of abnormal hormonal findings, such as elevated levels of testosterone (ranging from 30 ng/dL to 2300 ng/dL), androstenedione (A), and dehydroepiandrosterone (DHEA), and DHEAS.[122] Various imaging studies are also used to confirm the diagnosis. These include ultrasonography, computerized tomography, and magnetic resonance imaging. Most of these tumors have a well-rounded and smooth appearance in comparison to the crescentic-shaped normal configuration of the adrenal gland.[123] Computerized tomography is the most commonly ordered radiologic test. Radiologic signs of attenuation, change in adrenal gland tissue consistency, and lack of homogeneity in enhancement, are often used to discriminate between various tumors. Treatment is usually surgical excision for early stages of the disease with some controversies on the outcome in advanced cases. The 5-year survival rate after surgical resection does not exceed 30% and poor prognosis in cases of metastasis has been reported.[124,125] Medical therapy in the form of adrenal cortex inhibitors such as mitotane, or chemotherapy using cisplatin, cyclophosphamide, and 5-flurouracil have been advocated in cases of resistance or poorly differentiated tumors.[122]

*Congenital adrenal hyperplasia* (CAH) is a well-known endogenous source of androgen excess. It is an autosomal recessive disorder mostly due to 21-hydroxylase deficiency, characterized by "cortisol and often aldosterone deficiency and excess production of precursor steroids with androgen effect."[126] It is categorized in three forms, the classic form that includes salt wasting and simple virilizing, and the non-classic NC, which occurs at a later onset of age.[127] Despite the rarity of this disease, there are few reports in the literature on deepening of the voice in women with CAH who had late diagnosis or were not treated appropriately.[128–130] Two major studies investigating vocal characteristics and phonatory changes have been reported in the literature.[130,131] In 2009 Nygren et al investigated the vocal symptoms in a group of 38 women with CAH in comparison to 24 healthy controls. The subjects were asked to rate their voice according to four statements that describe vocal function, namely, "my voice is hoarse, my voice is dark,

my voice is a problem in my daily life, and I get tired in my throat when speaking."[130] In addition to the self-rating, acoustic and perceptual analysis were performed on voice recording while reading a standard text. The results indicated a significant difference in the rating of the statement "my voice is a problem in my daily life" among the two groups. More so, affected patients had significantly lower mean fundamental frequency (F0) in comparison to controls. The low F0 was attributed to hypertrophic changes in the vocal folds given that almost half of the patients with low pitch and dark voice timbre had either late start of treatment or were not treated adequately. This hypothesis was further substantiated by the higher lean body mass index found in patients with deep voice compared to those with normal voice.[130] Four years later, the same authors reported vocal changes in 42 women diagnosed with CAH. The study was based on a questionnaire that included the Swedish version of the Voice Handicap Index, and questions pertaining to vocal virilization. The results were comparable to the previous study with the majority of women reporting a dark voice and being perceived as a man on the phone. These vocal changes were attributed again to hypertrophic changes in the vocal folds given the inappropriate treatment or delay in the start of the treatment in a good percentage of these patients.[131] In a recent imaging study using MRI, the same authors confirmed the anatomic basis for the low F0 in women with CAH. Affected patients had a larger thyroarytenoid cross-sectional area compared to controls.[132]

## VI. Exogenous Causes of Voice Virilization

### Exogenous Androgen

The indications for using testosterone in women are many. These include: (1) replacement therapy in cases of hormonal deficiency, (2) treatment of medical conditions and diseases such as endometriosis, and (3) increase in physical performance. A brief review of the literature on the current usage of testosterone replacement, anabolic androgenic steroids, and androgen derivatives is presented.

### *Testosterone Replacement and Voice*

The change in hormonal climate with menopause and aging has prompted many women to start testosterone (T) therapy as a remedy to many physiologic alterations. The main concern, however, has been the adverse effect on voice with the myth that testosterone replacement causes an irreversible drop in vocal pitch. To that end, numerous investigations were conducted in order to confirm or refute the vocal virilization in women on testosterone replacement. Huang et al investigated the dose dependent effect of T administration on voice in 71 women who were treated with various doses of transdermal T in a randomized trial over the course of 24 weeks. Sustained vowel "Ah" and reading of the first sentence of the Rainbow Passage were used as voice samples for assessment. Both the self-reported questionnaire (VHI) and acoustic analysis were used as outcome measures. The results indicated a significant decrease in the average pitch associated with an increase in free testosterone in the subgroups treated with a 12.5 and 25-mg dose of testosterone. Similarly, there was a significant decrease in average pitch while reading the sentence test in the subgroup treated with 25 mg of testosterone. However, there was no significant difference in the VHI score between any of the treated subgroups and placebo.[133] These results, to an extent, were commensurate with the adverse effects reported by the same authors a year before in their investigation on the effect of testosterone therapy on sexual function. In that previous study, only two patients treated with 25 mg T had a change in voice quality that was attributed to reflux and not to hormonal changes.[134] Both of the aforementioned studies were in alignment with the study by Nordenskjold et al who reported no androgenic effect on voice after the intake of 600 mg of Danazol for 6 months.[135]

Along the same line of investigation, Glaser et al in 2016 reported the effect of testosterone on the female voice in a prospective study conducted on 10 women, four post-menopause and six pre or perimenopausal.[136] Testosterone was delivered by subcutaneous implants and serum testosterone levels were computed before treatment, at 3 months, 6 months, and one year after treatment. Using various voice samples (sentences, Rainbow Passage, and conversation), the authors reported no significant differences in the average fundamental frequency before and after treatment (3 and 12 months). The authors concluded that testosterone therapy delivered through transdermal implants have no adverse effect on voice. It is worth noting that the amount of testosterone released using the dermal implants in this study did not exceed 1.4 mg/day although the therapeutic dosages of testosterone was above the normal endogenous range (471.6 + 148.1 ng/dL). This is an important variable to consider given that supraphysiologic dosage of anabolic steroids used in other studies resulted in irreversible vocal changes.[137–139]

Although there are conflicting reports on the effect of T replacement on the fundamental frequency, no vocal changes have been reported. This is in keeping with a more recent meta-analysis and systemic review of the literature on the safety of transdermal testosterone usage in postmenopausal women.[140] Seven randomized controlled trials were included with 3,035 participants. In addition to the beneficial effect of transdermal T on sexual performance and overall distress score, there were some adverse effects such as acne and hirsutism, but deepening of voice was not one of them.[140] To that end, the authors advocated the safety of T replacement with respect to voice.

### Anabolic-Androgenic Steroid (AAS) Usage and Voice

A practice that has increased over the last decade or so is the usage of anabolic-androgenic steroid (AAS) among athletes and non-athletes. Based on a recent report by Pope et al in 2014, 3 to 4 million of overall Americans between the age of 13 and 50 years use AAS in the United States.[141] Its usage in women has also increased markedly over the last few years with an estimated lifetime prevalence of 1.6%.[142] The rationale behind this surge in usage is enhancing the physical image in terms of muscle mass and contour, and improving physical performance in terms of muscle strength and endurance. In 2017 the ergogenic effect of anabolic-androgenic steroids on performance in women was reviewed by Huang and Basari.[143] Even though there was relatively substantial evidence to support improvement in physical performance among users, the authors emphasized the virilizing effect of these supplements, most common of which were alopecia, clitoromegaly, aggression, hirsutism, and deepening of voice.[144] The deepening of voice has been attributed hypothetically to hypertrophic changes in the vocal folds. Indeed, based on a histologic study conducted on mice, hypertrophic changes mostly on the inner aspect of the thyroarytenoid muscle in addition to hyperplasia and parakeratosis of the epithelium have been reported.[139] Given the irreversibility of vocal changes as a result of AAS intake, both physicians and patients should exert due diligence while using these medications. Any signs of androgen excess should be alarming.

### Androgen Derivatives in the Treatment of Endometriosis and in Gender Re-assignment

Another indication for the usage of androgen derivatives are medical conditions such as endometriosis irregularities in the menstrual cycle and fibrocystic breast disease.[145] Hormonal treatments such as Danazol, Gestrinone, and testosterone derivatives have been associated with adverse voice reactions. The reported deepening of voice and huskiness seem to be related to the duration of treatment, with more permanent changes occurring after prolonged therapy.[146–148] These irreversible vocal changes have been attributed to mucosal and muscular changes in the vocal folds.[139]

### Endometriosis

Endometriosis is one of the most common gynecologic diseases that affects up to 5% of women during their reproductive years. Patients may present with a history of infertility or recurrent pelvic pain. A large adnexal mass often referred to as endometria may be found on radiologic imaging or laparoscopy.[149] What is of relevance to otolaryngologists is the side effects of the treatment in the management of this disease as previously mentioned. Danazol, which is one out of four hormonal medications often prescribed for the treatment of endometriosis, is commonly associated with androgenic side effects that can affect voice. In a prospective study by Barbeiri on 100 patients with endometriosis who were successfully treated with Danazol 800 mg/day, 85% developed side effects including deepening of the voice.[150] In 1990 Boothroyd and Lepre reported permanent vocal masculinization in a 20-year-old woman after 3 to 4 months of therapy with Danazol 800 mg per day. Changes in the vocal folds included inflammation and edema, probably secondary to the increased water binding in the ground substance of the lamina propria.[148,151,152] Along the same line, Gerritsma et al reported loss of the high notes and more vocal instability in women following the intake of Deca-Durabolin.[153] Similarly, Janet Baker reported four women with vocal changes following the intake of medications with androgenic effect, namely, Danazol, nandrolene decanoate, and testosterone. Perceptual evaluation and acoustic analysis revealed voices that were in keeping with men's voice and fundamental frequencies commensurate with those of men even after treatment (112 Hz–120 Hz). The vocal range was also affected with a residual loss of four semitones to on octave mainly in the upper range. The authors attributed the vocal changes hypothetically to an increase in vocal fold muscle mass, and dysfunction in muscle coordination and proprioception.[154]

### Female to Male Gender Re-assignment

Other rare indications for androgen therapy are female to male gender reassignment. Lowering the patient's fundamental frequency in the direction of the male sex has become common practice given the known virilizing effect of androgens and androgen derivatives. The impact on the mean fundamental frequency is thought to be profound after three months of therapy, commensurate with a decrease in pitch range.[155] In a study by Damrose on a 33-year-old woman undergoing gender reassignment, the author reported a decrease in mean fundamental frequency from 228.45 Hz to 116.52 Hz following intramuscular androgen therapy.[155] Nevertheless, the change in voice in female-male transsexuals is not that straightforward as many other considerations such as prosodic features of speech and articulation should be considered and addressed using voice therapy.[156]

## VII. The Male Voice

As previously discussed, voice is an acoustic expression of our sexual identity. Sexual dimorphism is recognized by the difference in the mean fundamental frequencies between male and female voices. Examples commonly used to illustrate the disparities between vocal characteristics and gender identity are the castrato singers who were promoted in the 16th century, and athletic females who receive anabolic steroids or androgenic supplements. The "castrati voice" is the end result of lack of exposure of the laryngeal structures to testosterone. The effect of delayed laryngeal development is surmounted by the powerful breathing capacity given the tall stature of castrato singers.[157] Similarly, the intake of anabolic steroids or exogenous androgens has a major impact on voice quality with often irreversible deepening of the voice.[158] Other examples that illustrate the strong impact of sex hormones on voice in the pre-pubertal years include patients with isolated hypogonadotropic hypogonadism, characterized by failure of sexual maturation, and patients with chromosome abnormalities such as Werner's syndrome, Prader-Willi syndrome, and Kallmann syndrome.[159]

The acoustic stratification among men and women is primarily attributed to morphological changes in the phonatory apparatus, namely, in the configuration of the vocal tract and laryngeal framework. The exposure of the larynx to sex hormones at puberty results in growth of the laryngeal muscles and cartilages with subsequent alteration in their shape and dimensions. The anatomical study utilizing a sheep model by Beckford et al in 1985, demonstrated the impact of androgen stimulation on laryngeal structures. There was a differential growth of the thyroid cartilage in comparison to the cricoid and arytenoid cartilages with further sharpening of the angle between the two thyroid lamina. These changes were coupled with an increase in various dimensions within structures of the arytenoid cartilages.[160] In another study by Kahane on the growth of the prepubertal and pubertal larynges, he reported enlargement of the male vocal fold to be twice as much as the female vocal fold with further enlargement and prominence of the thyroid cartilage.[161] The study was performed on cadaveric human larynges, prepubertal and pubertal, in comparison to other adult cadaveric larynges. These morphologic changes can be attributed to the direct effect of sex hormones on the laryngeal structures as discussed earlier in this chapter, via estrogen, progesterone, and androgen receptors.[1] In parallel with these hypertrophic changes of the musculoskeletal laryngeal structures, there is further voice maturation secondary to the downward descent of the larynx and its differentiation of the vocal ligament in the pubertal years as reported by Hirano et al.[162]

Among the different acoustic parameters, mean fundamental frequency and habitual pitch are commonly used as indicators of our sexual identity. Several studies have supported the role of these acoustic measures in reflecting our hormonal profile. Evans et al reported the inverse relationship between salivary testosterone level and fundamental frequency.[163] Likewise, Dabbs et al reported the predictive value of testosterone level in assessing vocal pitch in men. In their investigation on 61 males, the authors reported a negative correlation between vocal pitch and salivary testosterone level. These findings were based on the increase in vocal fold mass and acquired vocal characteristics associated with the male hormones.[164] Similarly Brucket et al demonstrated narrower formants' dispersion in male subjects with higher testosterone levels compared to those with lower levels.[165] A study by Meuser and Nieschlag correlated voice classification with testosterone levels. In their investigation of 102 singers, bass and baritones had higher concentrations of testosterone compared to tenors.[166]

Despite the ubiquity of reports on the interplay between sex hormones and voice at pre-puberty and puberty, little has been written on the impact of male hormones on the post-pubertal voice. With the increase in the intake of testosterone by middle-aged men recently, a better understanding of the impact of androgen on the overall health and voice in particular becomes of paramount importance. The study by Griggs et al has shown that testosterone can lead to an increase in muscle mass secondary to an increase in muscle protein synthesis rather than an increase in muscle fiber diameter. The investigation was conducted on only four subjects in whom the muscle mass was estimated by measuring the creatinine level.[167] An animal study conducted on South African clawed frogs revealed that testosterone exposure can stimulate cell division in laryngeal muscles and cartilages. This hormonal induced myogenesis and chondrogenesis was not observed following estrogen exposure.[168] Another animal study by Beckford et al on 48 lambs stimulated with various degrees of testosterone found a dose dependent growth of both thyroid and arytenoid cartilages. Animals with hypoandrogenic levels of exposure had an inhibitory growth effect in comparison to controls.[160]

Conversely, androgen ablation may also affect voice. Akcam et al reported that male patients with isolated hypogonadotropic hypogonadism (IGHD) have a higher mean fundamental frequency compared to controls (229.33Hz vs 150.40 Hz). More so, there was a decrease in the mean fundamental frequency in these patients following the intake of androgen therapy. The drop in the mean F0 from 229 Hz to 173 Hz was attributed to the possible hypertrophic effect of androgen on laryngeal muscles despite the lack of a significant correlation between the MF0 and serum hormonal levels in this study.[169] In an investigation on the impact of androgen ablation on voice in a group of patients[18] with prostatic cancer, the results indicated a significant difference in the habitual pitch in comparison with controls. The higher habitual pitch in patients (131.76 Hz vs 114.11 Hz) was attributed to the loss of the deepening effect of testosterone on voice.[170] On the other hand, in the study by Gugatschka et al on the association between sex hormones and voice, the authors failed to demonstrate any significant difference in the voice parameters between eugonade and hypogonade patients. It is worth noting in this study that those with low levels of estrogen had higher fundamental frequencies.[171]

## The Thyroid Gland and Voice

The thyroid gland regulates body metabolism through the secretion of hormones that govern the rate of metabolism within our body. It is markedly affected by the amount of productivity we ensue, by tissue needs such as protein synthesis, and by the extent of environmental stresses. Despite the infinite neural control on the thyroid gland function, neuroendocrine imbalance may occur secondary to autoimmune diseases, viral infections, surgical intervention, and/or trauma. As a result of this imbalance, defective or excessive release of thyroid hormone takes place leading to a plethora of symptoms affecting various systems in the body.[172,173]

Given the delicate neuromuscular structure of the larynx and the intricate control needed for phonation, it stands to reason that voice is vulnerable to thyroid hormonal imbalance. This assumption firmly depends on the presence of thyroid hormonal receptors within various laryngeal structures. Altman et al reported positive immunostaining for thyroid receptors in two human cadaveric larynges. Thyroid hormonal receptor type alpha (TR-alpha) was found in the lamina propria, glandular structures, fibrous connective tissues, and thyroid cartilage, whereas thyroid hormonal receptor type beta (TR-beta) was found only in the lamina propria, in particular within its fibrous connective tissue component.[172] The authors emphasized the role of the thyroid gland in regulating laryngeal tissue metabolism, growth, and synthesis. That being stated, thyroid hormonal imbalance, be it hypo or hyperthyroidism, can lead to phonatory changes.

## Hypothryoidism and Voice

Hypothyroidism is an underdiagnosed entity that may affect up to 10% of the elderly.[173,174] Its clinical manifestations affect many systems in the body including the phonatory system. Patients with hypothyroidism usually present with systemic complaints such as generalized weakness, lethargy, bradychardia, and cold intolerance. Symptoms in relation to the laryngopharyngeal complex are often subtle and less prevailing.[175] These include globus sensation, dysphagia, dryness, change in voice quality, and a reduced vocal range.[176–178] Based on a report by Bicknell in a group of 27 patients with mild hypothyroidism, the prevalence of vocal symptoms varied in relation to the severity of the disease. Other complaints may include excessive vocal strain, lowering of the pitch, weakness of the voice, and inability to sing.[179]

Gupta et al reported phonatory symptoms in 77% of patients with idiopathic hypothyroidism with hoarseness and vocal fatigue being most common (40.9% and 25.8%, respectively).[180] In Mohammadzadeh et al's study of 120 patients with hypothyroidism, the prevalence of dryness, dyspnea, and globus sensation were significantly higher in affected subjects compared to controls. These phonatory and throat symptoms were substantiated by an abnormal soft phonation index, elevated amplitude variation, and noise-to-harmonic ratio.[181] On the other hand, a more recent investigation on phonatory changes in patients with non-myxedematous hypothyroidism versus controls revealed no significant changes in any of the perceptual parameters. More so, there was no significant difference in any of the acoustic

parameters between the two groups as well.[182] One possible explanation for these findings is that all subjects enrolled in that study had non-myxedematous hypothyroidism. Moreover, as these subjects didn't undergo a laryngeal examination, the lack of myxedematous changes as reported by their referring endocrinologist implies that it was unlikely that they had laryngeal involvement. Another less frequently reported symptom in hypothyroidism is dysarthria. Stollberger et al described a 43-year-old man who presented with dysarthria as the primary symptom of hypothyroidism. Other associated symptoms included cramps in the extremities, dizziness, and severe snoring. The patient improved markedly following initiation of hormonal replacement.[183]

Although dysphonia in patients with hypothyroidism has been described by many authors, the reason behind it is not very clear. Three suggested mechanisms have been proposed in the literature:

First is myxedematous involvement of the vocal folds. With a drop in thyroid hormonal secretion, a decrease in the overall rate of body metabolism including that of the phonatory apparatus occurs. As a result, excessive deposition of acidic mucopolysaccharides within various organs occurs, leading to alterations in tissue viscosity. The term myxedema has often been used to describe these histologic changes, in parallel with the clinical picture of non-pitting edema. When confined to the larynx, "myxedematous hoarseness" denotes the change in voice quality secondary of the aforementioned histologic changes. It is important to note that laryngeal manifestations of hypothyroidism usually precede the systemic picture of myxedema and may present as early as three days after diagnosis of hypothyroidism.[184] The excessive deposition of muco-polysaccharides within the superficial layer of the lamina propria results in distortion in its histologic architecture leading to alteration in its rheologic properties.

The hypothesis of myxedematous involvement of the vocal folds has been substantiated by numerous animal and human studies.[175,185,186] Ritter in his study on rats that were made hypothyroid, demonstrated submucosal myxedematous infiltrations of the submucosal surface of the vocal folds.[175] Similar findings were reported in the histologic study by Altman et al using colloidal iron stain.[172] The authors have confirmed the presence of hyaluronic acid within mucoprotein in hypothyroid larynges. In another study by Bicknell on 27 patients with mild hypothyroidism, the vocal folds were described as edematous, thickened, floppy, or polypoidal, a clinical appearance comparable to Reinke's edema often reported in middle-aged women with a history of smoking.[179] More so, vocal fold biopsies stained with Alcian blue revealed distinctive blue staining of the subepithelial space that was commensurate with the abundance of mucin in the vocal folds. Subsequent to the increase in mass associated with the excessive deposition of mucoploysaccharide, there is a drop in vocal pitch with an increase in cycle-to-cycle variation in intensity and frequency.

The second suggested mechanism is vocal fold paralysis or paresis secondary to enlargement of the thyroid gland often seen in patients with hypothyroidism. In a study on the prevalence of phonatory symptoms in 40 patients with goiter, the authors reported a significantly higher prevalence of vocal straining in affected patients compared to controls.[187] Hyperplasia of the thyroid gland, which is commonly encountered in patients with goiter, may impair vocal fold mobility in many ways. These include stretching or compression of the recurrent laryngeal nerve, vascular compromise via thrombosis of the vasa nervosa, mechanical fixation with erosion or direct involvement of the cricoarytenoid joint, and last inflammation of the recurrent laryngeal nerve with impairment in neural conduction.[188–191]

The third suggested mechanism is edema of the nucleus ambiguus.[184] Ficcara suggested that as brain tissue can easily become edematous and as edema is the early sign of myxedema, edema of the nucleus ambiguus may be one of the early manifestations of hypothyroidism.

Ficcara suggested also the mechanism of edema of the cricothyroid muscle which in parallel with edema of the nucleus ambiguus, edematous changes within the cricothyroid muscle may occur. When present, the contractile strength of this tensor muscle is markedly reduced resulting in lowering of the vocal pitch with subsequent change in voice quality.[184]

Another possible mechanism that may also contribute to the development of vocal symptoms in patients with hypothyroidism, is the high prevalence of laryngopharyngeal reflux disease (LPRD) in this group of patients. Fiorentino et al[192] reported laryngopharyngitis and alterations in swallowing in 67% and 90% of patients with goiter commonly associated with hypothyroidism. The authors emphasized the

relationship between symptoms of reflux and those of goiter, such as globus pharyngeus, throat discomfort, and dysphagia. The pathogenic role of LPRD in patients with goiter is further substantiated by the persistence of many of these symptoms following thyroidectomy. Close to 75% of patients with goiter who underwent surgery in their study still had the same complaints that were initially attributed to thyroid glandular enlargement. In another study conducted on a group of 52 patients with goiter, the authors failed to demonstrate a significant difference in the prevalence of LPRD in affected patients compared to controls.[193] Nevertheless, the study had its limitations, most importantly was the lack of an objective diagnostic measure of LPRD, such as double-probe pH monitoring or esophageal manometry.

## Hyperthyroidism, Thyroiditis, and Voice

Hyperthyroidism results from excess secretions of thyroid hormones, namely, triiodothyronine or thyroxine. As a result of this hormonal excess, patients may present with a variety of symptoms such as tremor, anorexia, palpitations, weight loss, and excessive nervousness. Fatigability has been attributed to the neuromuscular manifestation of the disease[194] whereas nervousness has been linked to the overproduction of cateholamines.[195] More focal symptoms include visual disturbances secondary to the associated ophthalmopathy, and symptoms of neck compression secondary to enlargement of the thyroid gland.

The literature is scarce on the interplay between hyperthyroidism and voice. Most of the studies on hyperthyroidism and the laryngopharyngeal complex focus on swallowing and pressure symptoms in the neck.[26] Many authors have reported the presence of these symptoms in patients with hyperthyroidism and their subsequent alleviation following thyroidectomy.[196,197] Only a few studies have reported the phonatory changes in patients with hyperthyroidism or thyroiditis. In 1987 Warren Tripp et al reported the prevalence of vocal symptoms in 2 out of five cases of hyperthyroidism.[198] The authors alluded to the heterogeneity in the clinical picture of hyperthyroidism and to the wide spectrum of symptoms and signs seen in this group of patients. In another study by Heman-Ackah et al, looking at the prevalence of thyroid disease in patients with vocal fold paralysis, the authors reported a figure of 47.4% in comparison to 16.5% in a control group of patients with sensorineural hearing loss and no vocal fold paresis selected from the authors' practice. Among those with thyroid disease, hyperthyroidism was the culprit in 4.5% of the cases.[199] In another study on the prevalence of vocal symptoms in a group of 22 patients with subacute thyroiditis, the most commonly reported symptoms were vocal fatigue, lump sensation, and aphonia (40.9%, 40.9%, and 31.8%, respectively). Aphonia was significantly more prevalent in affected patients compared to controls. More so, in 13.6% of the cases, the impact of dysphonia on quality of life was significant.[200] On the other hand, in another study conducted on 17 patients with thyroiditis, there was no significant difference in either the perceptual evaluation or the acoustic analysis in comparison to controls. The results of this investigation were attributed to the small sample size, the short duration of disease in patients enrolled in that study, and last to the fact that only two subjects had Hashimoto's thyroiditis, the subtype of thyroiditis that is most commonly associated with vocal fold paralysis.[201]

There are several few case reports of vocal fold paralysis as a complication of an acute thyroid infection or thyroidectomy.[202–204] Lucarotti et al described a case of recurrent laryngeal nerve paralysis in a patient with thyroiditis.[202] Likewise Dedivitis and Coelho et al reported a similar case of vocal fold paralysis in a patient with subacute thyroiditis who recovered following the intake of steroids. Dedivitis and Coelho have also reported the case of a 43-year-old woman who presented with a painful cervical node in the anterior neck and an elevated free thyroxin level, and an acute onset of dysphonia that was secondary to right vocal fold paralysis. The patient's symptoms improved markedly three days following the intake of steroids.[204]

## Growth Hormone and Voice

Growth hormone (GH) has a major role at several fronts in the development and composition of our body. It is a key player in bone apposition, cardiovascular stability, metabolism regulation, and somatic growth. Its otolaryngologic manifestations are also diverse and complex, highlighting the strong interplay of body stature, craniofacial morphology and voice. In a study Kuan et al reported the otolaryngologic manifestations in 25 patients with acromegaly who underwent resection of the pituitary adenoma thru the transnasal transphenoidal approach. The information was retrieved by reviewing their medical charts and completing a validated questionnaire, namely, the Sinonasal Outcome Test SNOT-22. The results showed that 52% of the patients had sleep disordered breathing, probably secondary to the

high prevalence of macroglossia in 60%. In addition, sinonasal symptoms and hearing loss/tinnitus were present in 16% and 20% of the cases, respectively.[205]

The effect of growth hormone on voice has been a subject of investigation for decades with only few studies being reported. The scarcity in information is partially due to the rarity of the disease and the early initiation of replacement therapy soon after the diagnosis is made. Most of the studies investigated phonatory changes in patients with growth hormone deficiency (GHD) as in cases of isolated growth hormone deficiency (IGHD), and in patients with hypersecretory state of growth hormones, as in cases of acromegaly.

Barreto et al reported on perceptual and acoustic features of adults with growth hormone deficiency. The study was conducted on a group of 23 patients with isolated growth hormone deficiency (IGHD), caused by a " homozygous mutation in the splice donor site of intron 1(IVSI+1G-A) of the GH-releasing hormone receptor (GHRHR) gene" in comparison to 22 controls. The voices of patients with IGHD were perceived as more rough, breathy, and strained compared to controls. According to the authors, this can be attributed to a higher level of laryngeal constriction associated with the increased level of "vocal-self assurance." In parallel with these perceptual findings, there was a significant difference in the fundamental frequency between the two groups. The higher fundamental frequency in patients with IGHD was attributed to the association between voice, craniofacial, and laryngeal dimensions.[206] Another study by Valenca et al on 33 patients with IGHD revealed lower Voice-Related Quality of Life scores compared to controls and to subjects with short stature.[207] Moore et al also reported the vocal characteristics in two groups of patients, those with congenital growth hormone deficiency and adult acquired GHD. The authors used spectral analysis and approximate Entropy (ApEn) in order to assess the acoustic characteristics and spectral complexity of voice. The results showed that those with congenital and untreated GHD had a higher fundamental frequency F0 in addition to abnormalities in the harmonic spectrum compared to controls. These findings were attributed to the known relationship between vocal pitch and laryngeal dimensions, in particular the length and mass of the vocal folds. In the group with adult acquired GHD, F0 was normal but patients had abnormal vocal fold function as shown by the low ApEn. The authors speculated that short stature and craniofacial abnormalities in patients with GHD contribute to the abnormal voice recordings in affected subjects.[208] Indeed the study by Valenca et al comparing voice quality in patients with IGHD, short stature (SS), and controls substantiates the association between craniofacial dimensions and voice. In their cross-sectional study on 73 adults, the fundamental frequency was higher in males with IGHD compared to the male group with short stature. Given that patients with IGHD have lower values for the cephalic perimeter than those with SS, the authors strongly suggested that craniofacial growth is linked to the fundamental frequency.[207] Another interesting finding in this study is that IGHD abolished the affect of aging on voice. The same authors have also reported the voice formants F1, F2, F3, F4 for seven oral vowels in 33 subjects with IGHD. They concluded that affected patients had higher formant values compared to controls. Again these findings were interpreted in the context of the natural variations in the vocal tract dimensions, namely, the oropharyngeal cavity, in patients with IGHD.[209]

Similar to growth hormone deficiency, growth hormone excess also impacts voice quality. Given that acromegaly patients are three times more likely to die by respiratory disease compared to the general population, the main focus in the literature has been on the airway with only few reports on the vocal characteristics in patients with acromegaly. Williams et al in their investigation of eight patients with acromegaly undergoing hypophysectomy, reported a lower mean fundamental frequency compared to controls.[210] Similarly, Bogazzi et al reported lower mean fundamental frequency in a group of 13 patients with acromegaly compared to controls. The perturbation parameters were also elevated more so in men.[211] Aydin et al have investigated the vocal characteristics of 37 patients with acromegaly in comparison with 30 controls using the Multi-Dimensional voice program. The authors reported significant differences in the perturbation parameters between the two groups. Both shimmer and jitter correlated with insulin like growth factor 1 but not significantly.[212] In all these studies, the acoustic characteristics were attributed to the known alterations in vocal fold mass and elasticity secondary to the excess exposure to growth hormone. Another potential cause for change in voice quality, although rare, is impaired mobility of the vocal folds. Cooper et al reported a case of a 56-year-old patient with acromegaly who presented with stridor and difficulty in breathing. The patient was diagnosed with bilateral vocal fold immobility that returned to normal following endoscopic resection of the pituitary adenoma. Several hypotheses were suggested by the author to explain the impaired mobility. These included arthritic changes within the

cricoarytenoid joint, overgrowth of the contiguous cartilaginous structures, and last compression of the recurrent laryngeal nerve resulting in axon demyelination and subsequent myopathy.[213]

## Diabetes and Voice

Type 2 diabetes mellitus is a common endocrine disorder that affects millions of people above the age of 65 years.[214] The main pathophysiology lies in insulin resistance at various tissue sites with subsequent decrease in glucose transfer and the breakdown of fat. The etiology is based on a genetic component, namely, genes related to pancreatic beta-cells, surmounted by a diabetogenic style of living.[214-216] Several morbidities have been associated with diabetes mellitus type 2. These include neuropathy affecting the sensory, motor, and autonomic system, vasculopathy leading to repeated thrombosis and ischemia, cardiac diseases, renal diseases, and many others. It is a major cause of renal failure in close to 50% of the cases and the leading cause of blindness according to the National Eye Institute and National Institute of Diabetes and Digestive and Kidney Diseases.[217,218]

Given the neural and musculoskeletal structures of the larynx, it is highly plausible that diabetic patients develop phonatory disturbances. A study looking at the presence of phonatory symptoms in a group of 105 patients with type 2 diabetes mellitus revealed a significantly higher prevalence of hoarseness and vocal straining compared to a control group. The most relevant finding in this study was the significant correlation between dysphonia and neuropathy, and between dysphonia and the degree of glycemic control based on HbA1c levels. Patients with average to poor control of glycemia and patients with neuropathy were more likely to have phonatory symptoms compared to controls. This correlation was attributed mainly to the impaired breathing capacity and the associated muscle weakness reported in patients with diabetic neuropathy.[219] A review by Krishnan et al on the association between diabetes and lung function indicated that patients with type 2 diabetes mellitus (DM) have decreased vital capacity, forced vital capacity, and diffusion capacity among other pulmonary function parameters. Similarly, there is a decrease in muscle strength associated with neuropathy that prevails in almost one out of two patients with type 2 diabetes mellitus.[220] Given the importance of breathing and the delicate muscle strength needed for phonation, it is not surprising that diabetic subjects have more vocal complaints compared to controls. These findings were partially corroborated by another study by Hamdan et al on 82 patients who underwent audio-perceptual evaluation. Although there was no statistically significant difference in any of the perceptual parameters in patients versus controls, further analysis revealed that those with neuropathy and poor glycemic control had a higher mean score for the overall grade of dysphonia.[221] Again these findings were attributed to the high prevalence of diabetic myopathy, atrophy, and neuropathy in up to 38% and 50% of the cases.[222,223] It is important to note that the study by Hamdan et al looking at the vocal characteristics in patients with type 2 diabetes mellitus failed to show any statistically significant difference in any of the acoustic variables between the diabetic group and controls. The authors had anticipated the opposite in view of possible alterations in thyroarytenoid muscle mass secondary to inflammation or atrophy.

Another feared complication of diabetes mellitus is diabetic neuropathy. In the head and neck region, single or multiple cranial neuropathies have been reported in the literature. Trigeminal neuralgia, ophthalmoplegia, and involvement of other cranial nerves have been described.[224] In the larynx, laryngeal sensory neuropathy has also been reported as a potential complication in patients with diabetes mellitus type 2. Laryngeal sensory neuropathy is a neurologic entity characterized by decreased sensory threshold of the laryngeal mucosa. Alteration in the afferent feedback has been suggested as a possible pathogenic mechanism. The abnormal laryngeal sensation precipitates abnormal laryngeal behavior and reflexes. As a result, patients may complain of throat clearing, globus pharyngeus, cough, foreign body sensation, and at times laryngeal spasm. The diagnosis can be made using fiberoptic endoscopic evaluation with sensory testing, laryngeal electromyography, and using surface evoked laryngeal sensory action potential waveform analysis.[225–227] Alternatively, the diagnosis can be made by exclusion after having rule out laryngopharyngeal reflux, allergy, drug-induced cough, and psychiatric disorders. In a study conducted on 50 patients with DM and 36 controls, the authors reported a significant difference in the prevalence of LSN between the two groups (42% vs 19%). This high prevalence of laryngeal sensory neuropathy (LSN) in the diabetic group was attributed to vagal neuropathy which is commonly seen in patients with DM. Affected patients invariably may report gastroparesis and laryngopharyngeal reflux secondary to gastroesophageal dismotilty. The prevalence of GI symptoms has been linked to the glycemic control and duration of the disease.[228]

# References

1. Newman SR, Butler J, Hammond EH, et al: Preliminary report on hormone receptors in the human vocal fold. *J Voice*. 2000;14: 72–81.
2. Ch Voelter, N. Kleinsasser, P. Joa, I. Nowack, R. Martinez, R. Hagen, and H. U. Voelker, Detection of hormone receptors in the human vocal fold. *Eur Arch Otorhinolaryngol*, 265 (2008), 1239–1244.
3. Cohen C, Lawson D, DeRose PB. Sex and androgenic steroid receptor expression in hepatic adenomas. *Hum Pathol*. 1998;29(12):1428–1432.
4. Večerina-Volić S, Romić-Stojković R, Krajina Z, Gamulin S. Androgen receptors in normal and neoplastic laryngeal tissue. *Arch Otolaryngol Head Neck Surg*. 1987;113(4):411–413.
5. Schneider B, Cohen E, Stani J, et al. Towards the expression of sex hormone receptors in the human vocal fold. *J Voice*. 2007;21(4):502–507.
6. Nacci A, Fattori B, Basolo F, et al. Sex hormone receptors in vocal fold tissue: a theory about the influence of sex hormones in the larynx. *Folia Phoniatr Logop*. 2010;63:77–82.
7. Abitbol J, Abitbol P, Abitbol B. Sex hormones and the female voice. *J Voice*. 1999;13:424–446.
8. Abitbol J, de Brux J, Millot G, et al. Does a hormonal vocal cord cycle exist in women? Study of vocal premenstrual syndrome in voice performers by videostroboscopy-glottography and cytology on 38 women. *J Voice*. 1989;2:157–162.
9. Macdonald PC, Dombroski RA, Caset ML. Recurrent secretion of progesterone in large amounts: an endocrine/metabolic disorder unique to young women? *Endocri Rev*. 1991;12(4):372–401.
10. Dalton K. *The Premenstrual Syndrome and Progesterone Therapy*. Chicago, IL: Year Book Medical Publishers; 1977:20–55.
11. Speroff L. Historical and social perspectives. In: Keye WR Jr, ed. *The Premenstrual Syndrome*. Philadelphia, PA: WB Saunders; 1988:3–4.
12. Sataloff RT. Endocrine Function. In: Sataloff RT. *Professional Voice: The Science and Art of Clinical Care*. 4th ed. San Diego, CA: Plural Publishing: 2017: 655–669.
13. Bender SD. PMS: questions and answers. Los Angeles, CA: The Body Press; 1989:18–19.
14. Norris R, Sullivan C. PMS: *Premenstrual Syndrome*. New York, NY: Rawson Associates; 1983:12.
15. Maxson WS, Hargrove IT. A practical approach to evaluation and treatment. In: Keye WR Jr, ed. *The Premenstrual Syndrome*. Philadelphia, PA: WB Saunders Company; 1988:172.
16. Speroff L. The clinical approach. In: Keye WR Jr, ed. *The Premenstrual Syndrome*. Philadelphia, PA: WB Saunders; 1988:169–170.
17. Keye WR Jr, Trunnell EP. A biopsychosocial model. In: Keye WR Jr, ed. *The Premenstrual Syndrome*. Philadelphia, PA: WB Saunders; 1988:207–208.

18. Reid R. Etiology: medical theories. In: Keye WR Jr, ed. *The Premenstrual Syndrome*. Philadelphia, PA: WB Saunders; 1988:66–93.

19. Chihal HI. *Premenstrual Syndrome: A Clinic Manual*. 2nd ed. Dallas, TX: Essential Medical Information Systems Inc; 1990: t8–47.

20. Silverman EM, Zimmer CH. Effect of the menstrual cycle on voice quality. *Arch Otolaryngol*. 1978;104(1): 7–10.

21. Davis CB, Davis ML. The effects of premenstrual syndrome (PMS) on the female singer. *J Voice*. 1993;7(4):337–353.

22. Luchsinger R, Arnold GE. *Voice-Speech-Language*. Belmont, CA: Wadsworth Publishing; 1965:189.

23. Flach M, Schwickardi H, Simon R. Welchen Einfluss haben Menstruation und Schwangerschaft aus die ausgebildete Gesangsstimme? *Folia Phoniatr (Basel)*. 1968;21: 199–210.

24. Smith-Frable MA. Hoarseness, a symptom of premenstrual tension. *Arch Otolaryngol*. 1961;75:66–68.

25. Punt NA. Laryngology applied to singers and actors. *J Laryngol Otol (suppl)*. 1983;6:1–24.

26. Valenta LJ. Cyclic laryngeal edema with aphonia. *Ann Intern Med*. 1975;82:62–63.

27. Van Gelder L. Psychosomatic aspects of endocrine disorders of the voice. *J Comm Dis*. 1974;7(3):257–262.

28. Schiff M. The influence of estrogens on connective tissue. In: *Hormones and Connective Tissue*. Copenhagen, Denmark: Munksgaard Press; 1967:282–341.

29. Caruso S, Roccasalva L, Sapienza G, Zappalá M, Nuciforo G, Biondi S. Laryngeal cytological aspects in women with surgically induced menopause who were treated with transdermal estrogen replacement therapy. *Fertil Steril*. 2000;74(6):1073–1079.

30. Schneider B, van Trotsenburg M, Hanke G, et al: Voice impairment in the menopause. *Menopause*. 2004; 11:151–158.

31. Boulet MJ, Oddens BJ: Female voice changes around and after the menopause: an initial investigation. *Maturitas*. 1996;23:15–21.

32. Raj A, Gupta B, Chowdhury A, Chadha S. A study of voice changes in various phases of menstrual cycle and in postmenopausal women. *J Voice*. 2010; 24(3):363–368.

33. Laureano JM, Sá MF, Ferriani RA, Romao GS. Variations of jitter and shimmer among women in menacme and postmenopausal women. *J Voice*. 2009;23(6):687–689.

34. Friedman AD. The impact of menopause on voice: past, present, and future. *Menopause*. 2011;18(3):248–250.

35. D'haeseleer E, Depypere H, Claeys S, et al. The relation between body mass index and speaking fundamental frequency in premenopausal and postmenopausal women. *Menopause*. 2011;18:754–758.

36. D'haeseleer E, Van Lierde K, Claeys S, et al. The impact of menopause and hormone therapy on voice and nasal resonance. *Facts Views Vis Obgyn*. 2012;4: 38.

37. Hamdan AL, Tabet G, Fakhri G, Sarieddine D, Btaiche R, Seoud M. Effect of hormonal replacement therapy on voice. *J Voice*. In press.

38. D'haeseleer E, Depypere H, Van Lierde K. Comparison of speaking fundamental frequency between premenopausal women and postmenopausal women with and without hormone therapy. *Folia Phoniatr Logopaed*. 2013;65(2):78–83.

39. Hamdan AL, Ziade G, Tabet G, et al. Vocal symptoms and acoustic findings in menopausal women in comparison to pre-menopause women with body mass index as a confounding variable. *J Menopaus Med*. 2017;23(2):117–123.

40. Cassiraga VL, Castellano AV, Abasolo J, Abin EN, Izbizky GH. Pregnancy and voice: changes during the third trimester. *J Voice*. 2012;26(5):584–586.

41. Weinberger S, Weiss S, Cohen W, et al. Pregnancy and the lung. *Am Rev Respir Dis*. 1980;121:L559.

42. Hamdan AL, Mahfoud L, Sibai A, Seoud M. Effect of pregnancy on the speaking voice. *J Voice*. 2009;23(4):490–493.

43. Theunissen I, Parer J. Fluid and electrolytes in pregnancy. *Clin Obstet Gynecol*. 1994;37:3.

44. Hamdan AL, Al Barazi R, Kanaan A, Sinno S, Soubra A. Vocal symptoms in women undergoing in vitro fertilization. *Am J Otolaryngol*. 2012;33(2):239–243.

45. Amir O, Lebi-Jacob N, Harari O. The effect of in vitro fertilization treatment on women's voice. *J Voice*. 2014; 28(4):518–522.

46. Speroff L, Glass RH, Kase NG. *Clinical Gynecologic Endocrinology and Infertility*. 6th ed. Baltimore, MD: Lippincott Williams & Wilkins; 1999;201–246.

47. Walker AE. *The Menstrual Cycle*. New York, NY: Routledge; 1997.

48. Sataloff RT. The effects of hormonal contraception on the voice. In: Sataloff RT. *Professional Voice: The Science and Art of Clinical Care*. 4th ed. San Diego, CA: Plural Publishing: 2017.

49. Speroff L, Darney P. *Clinical Guide for Contraception*. 5th ed. Philadelphia, PA: Lippincott Williams & Wilkins; 2011.

50. Ismail HK. The oto-rhino-laryngological manifestations of oral contraceptives. *Poc Nase, Hals und Ohr. 8th Int Congr ORL*. 1966:764–766.

51. Wendler J. Die physiologische Variabilitat der Frauenstimme-experimentell-phoniatrische Untersuchungen. *Med Habil-Schr Halle (Saale)*. 1969.

52. Wendler J. Zyklusabhangige Leistungsschwankungen der Stimme und ihre Beeinfhrssung durch Ovnlationshemmer. *Folia Phoniatr*. 1972;24:259–277.

53. Dhont M. History of oral contraception. *Eur J Contracep Reprod Health Care*. 2010;15(suppl 2):S12–18.

54. Well-Connected (webpage). What is Female Contraception? Lycos Health with WebMD 2000; Retrieved January 22, 2001, from: http://webmd.lycos.com/content/dmk/dmk_article_4461594.

55. Wendler J, Siegert C, Schelhorn P, et al. The influence of Microgynon® and Diane-35®, two sub-fifty ovula-

tion inhibitors, on voice function in women. *Contraception*. 1995;52(6):343–348.

56. Amir O, Kishon-Rabin L, Muchnik C. The effect of oral contraceptives on voice: preliminary observations. *J Voice*. 2002;16(2):267–273.

57. Amir O, Biron-Shental T, Muchnik C, Kishon-Rabin L. Do oral contraceptives improve vocal quality? Limited trial on low-dose formulations. *Obstetr Gynecol*. 2003;101(4):773–777.

58. Amir O, Kishon-Rabin L. Association between birth control pills and voice quality. *Laryngoscope*. 2004; 114(6):1021–1026.

59. Higgins MB, Saxman JH. Variations in vocal frequency perturbation across the menstrual cycle. *J Voice*. 1989; 3: 233–243.

60. Gorham-Rowan MM. Acoustic measures of vocal stability during different speech tasks in young women using oral contraceptives: a retrospective study. *Eur J Contracept Reprod Health Care*. 2004;9(3):166–172.

61. Amir O, Biron-Shental T, Tzenker O, Barer T. Different oral contraceptives and voice quality—an observational study. *Contraception*. 2005;71(5):348–352.

62. Amir O, Biron-Shental T, Shabtai E. Birth control pills and nonprofessional voice: acoustic analyses. *J Speech Lang Hear Res*. 2006;49(5):1114–1126.

63. Van Lierde KM, Claeys S, De Bodt M, Van Cauwenberge P. Response of the female vocal quality and resonance in professional voice users taking oral contraceptive pills: a multiparameter approach. *Laryngoscope*. 2006;116(10):1894–1898.

64. Lã FM, Ledger WL, Davidson JW, Howard DM, Jones GL. The effects of a third generation combined oral contraceptive pill on the classical singing voice. *J Voice*. 2007;21(6):754–761.

65. Lã FM, Howard DM, Ledger W, Davidson JW, Jones G. Oral contraceptive pill containing drospirenone and the professional voice: an electrolaryngographic analysis. *Logoped Phoniatr Vocal*. 2009;34(1):11–19.

66. Lã FM, Sundberg J, Howard DM, Sa-Couto P, Freitas A. Effects of the menstrual cycle and oral contraception on singers' pitch control. *J Speech Lang Hear Res*. 2012;55(1):247–261.

67. Morris RJ, Gorham-Rowan MM, Herring KD. Voice onset time in women as a function of oral contraceptive use. *J Voice*. 2009;23(1):114–118.

68. Whiteside S, Cowell P, Hanson A. Hormones and temporal components of speech: sex differences and effects of menstrual cyclicity on speech. *Neurosci Lett*. 2004;367:44–47.

69. Morris RJ, Gorham-Rowan MM, Harmon AB. The effect of initiating oral contraceptive use on voice: a case study. *J Voice*. 2011;25(2):223–229.

70. Meurer EM, Fontoura GV, von Eye Corleta H, Capp E. Speech articulation of low-dose oral contraceptive users. *J Voice*. 2015;29(6):743–750.

71. Kunduk M, Vansant MB, Ikuma T, McWhorter A. The effects of the menstrual cycle on vibratory characteristics of the vocal folds investigated with high-speed digital imaging. *J Voice*. 2017;31(2):182–187.

72. Meurer EM, Moura AD, Rechenberg L, von Eye Corleta H, Capp E. Vocal range in the speech of users of low-dose oral contraceptives. *J Voice*. 2017;31(3):390-e17.

73. Gorham-Rowan M, Fowler L. Aerodynamic assessment of young women's voices as a function of oral contraceptive use. *Folia Phoniatr Logopaed*. 2008; 60(1):20–24.

74. Gorham-Rowan M, Fowler L. Laryngeal aerodynamics associated with oral contraceptive use: preliminary findings. *J Comm Dis*. 2009;42(6):408–413.

75. Ellegård E, Karlsson G. Nasal congestion during the menstrual cycle. *Clinical Otolaryngol*. 1994; 19(5):400–403.

76. Ruskin SL. Rationale of estrogen therapy of primary atrophic rhinitis (ozena). *Arch Otolaryngol*. 1941; 36: 632–649.

77. Molteni A., Warphea RL, Brizio-Molteni, Fdrs EM. Estradiol receptor-binding protein in head and neck neoplastic and normal tissue. *Arch Surg*. 1981; 116: 207–210.

78. Paulsson B, Gredmark T, Burian P, Bende M. Nasal mucosal congestion during the menstrual cycle. *J Laryngol Otol*. 1997;111(4):337–339.

79. Haeggström A, Östberg B, Stjerna P, Graf P, Hallen H. Nasal mucosal swelling and reactivity during a menstrual cycle. *ORL*. 2000;62(1):39–42.

80. Philpott CM, El-Alami M, Murty GE. The effect of the steroid sex hormones on the nasal airway during the normal menstrual cycle. *Clin Otolaryngol*. 2004; 29(2):138–142.

81. Toppozada H, Toppozada M, El-Ghazzawi I, Elwany S. The human respiratory nasal mucosa in females using contraceptive pills. An ultramicroscopic and histochemical study. *J Laryngol Otol*. 1984;98(1):43–51.

82. Thiboutot D. Acne: hormonal concepts and therapy. *Clin Derm*. 2004;22: 419–428.

83. Thiboutot DM. Endocrinological evaluation and hormonal therapy for women with difficult acne. *J Eur Acad Dermatol Venereol*. 2001;15(suppl 3):S57–S61.

84. Harrisons. *Principles of Internal Medicine*. 19th ed. 2015; 331–335.

85. Waggoner W, Boots LR, Azziz R. Total testosterone and DHEAS levels as predictors of androgen-secreting neoplasms: a populational study. *Gynecologi Endocrinol*. 1999;13(6):394–400.

86. Carmina E, Rosato F, Janni A, Rizzo M, Longo RA. Relative prevalence of different androgen excess disorders in 950 women referred because of clinical hyperandrogenism. *J Clin Endocrinol Metab*. 2006; 91(1):2–6.

87. Dokras A, Witchel SF. Are young adult women with polycystic ovary syndrome slipping through the healthcare cracks? *J Clin Endocrinol Metab*. 2014; 99(5):1583–1585. doi:10.1210/jc.2013-4190.

88. Ehrmann DA. Polycystic ovary syndrome. *N Engl J Med*. 2005;352:1223–1236.

89. Hannoun A, Zreik T, Husseini ST, Mahfoud L, Sibai A, Hamdan AL. Vocal changes in patients with polycystic ovary syndrome. *J Voice*. 2011;25(4):501–504.

90. Lord JM, Flight IHK, Norman RJ. Metformin in polycystic ovary syndrome: systematic review and meta-analysis. *Br Med J*. 2003; 327:951–953.

91. Nestler JE, Jakubowicz DJ, Evans WS, Pasquali R. Effects of metformin on spontaneous and clomiphene-induced ovulation in the polycystic ovary syndrome. *N Engl J Med*. 1998;338:1876–1880.

92. Dickerson RD, Putman MJ, Black ME, et al. Selective ovarian vein sampling to localize a Leydig cell tumor. *Fertil Steril*. 2005;84(1):218-e19.

93. Baldwin LJ, Singh N, Tiltman A. Virilisation in a case of transitional cell carcinoma of the ovary. *J Clinic Pathol*. 2004;57(12):1331–1332.

94. López-Beltrán A, Calañas AS, Jimena P, et al. Virilizing mature ovarian cystic teratomas. *Virchows Archiv*. 1997;431(2):149–151.

95. Schorge JO. Ovarian germ cell and sex cord stromal tumors. In: *Williams Gynecology*. McGraw-Hill; 2008:749.

96. Young RH, Scully RE. Ovarian sertoli-leydig cell tumors. A clinicopathological analysis of 207 cases. *Am J Surg Pathol*. 1985;9:543–569.

97. Zaloudek C, Norris HJ. Sertoli-Leydig tumors of the ovary. A clinicopathologic study of 64 intermediate and poorly differentiated neoplasms. *Amer J Surg Pathol*. 1984;8(6):405–418.

98. Jung SE, Rha SE, Lee JM, et al. CT and MRI findings of sex cordstromal tumor of the ovary. *AJR Am J Roentgenol*. 2005;185:207–215.

99. Boussaïd K, Meduri G, Maiza JC, et al. Virilizing sclerosing-stromal tumor of the ovary in a young woman with McCune Albright syndrome: clinical, pathological, and immunohistochemical studies. *J Clinic Endocrinol Metab*. 2013;98(2):E314–320.

100. Park SM, Kim YN, Woo YJ, et al. A sclerosing stromal tumor of the ovary with masculinization in a premenarchal girl. *Kor J Pediatr*. 2011;54(5):224–227.

101. Cashell AW, Cohen ML. Masculinizing sclerosing stromal tumor of the ovary during pregnancy. *Gynecol Oncol*. 1991;43:281–285.

102. Ismail SM, Walker SM. Bilateral virilizing sclerosing stromal tumours of the ovary in a pregnant woman with Gorlin's syndrome: implications for pathogenesis of ovarian stromal neoplasms. *Histopathology*. 1990;17:15963.

103. Scully RE. Ovarian tumors. A review. *Am J Pathol*. 1977: 87 (3): 686–720.

104. Young RH, Scully RE: Sex-cord stromal steroid cell and other ovarian tumors with endocrine, paraendocrine, and paraneoplastic manifestations. In: Kurman RJ, ed. *Blaustein's Pathology of the Female Genital Tract*. 4th ed. New York, NY: SpringerVerlag; 1994:783–847.

105. Monteagudo A, Heller D, Husami N, Levine RU, McCaffrey R, TimorTritsch IE: Ovarian steroid cell tumors: sonographic characteristics. *Ultrasound Obstetr Gynecol*. 1997;10:282–288.

106. Wang PH, Chao HT, Lee RC, et al. Steroid cell tumors of the ovary: clinical, ultrasonic, and MRI diagnosis—a case report. *Eur J Radiol*. 1998, 26:269–273.

107. Salim S, Shantha GP, Patel AD, et al. Virilizing ovarian steroid cell tumor in a 40-year-old South Indian female: a case report. *Cases J*. 2009;2(1):7521.

108. Zhang J, Young RH, Arseneau J, et al: Ovarian stromal tumors containing lutein or Leydig cells (luteinized thecomas and stromal Leydig cell tumors): a clinico-pathological analysis of fifty cases. *Int J Gynecol Pathol*. 1982; 1:270.

109. Cserepes E, Szücs N, Patkos P, et al. Ovarian steroid cell tumor and a contralateral ovarian thecoma in a postmenopausal woman with severe hyperandrogenism. *Gynecologic Endocrinol*. 2002;16(3):213–216.

110. Nakashima N, Young RH, Scully RE. Androgenic granulosa cell tumors of the ovary. A clinicopathologic analysis of 17 cases and review of the literature. *Arch Pathol Labor Med*. 1984;108(10):786–791.

111. Public Health Service, National Cancer Institute. *Third National Cancer Survey: Incidence data* [NCI monograph]. Bethesda, MD: U.S. Department of Health, Education, and Welfare; Public Health Service, National Institutes of Health, 1975.

112. Wooten MD, King DK. Adrenal cortical carcinoma. Epidemiology and treatment with mitotane and a review of the literature. *Cancer*. 1993;72:3145–3155.

113. Luton J-P, Cerdas S, Billaud L, et al. Clinical features of adrenocortical carcinoma, prognostic factors, and the effect of mitotane therapy. *N Engl J Med*. 1990;322: 1195–1201.

114. Nader S, Hickey RC, Sellin RV, et al. Adrenal cortical carcinoma. A study of 77 cases. *Cancer*. 1983;52:707–711.

115. King DR, Lack EE. Adrenal cortical carcinoma. A clinical and pathologic study of 49 cases. *Cancer*. 1979;44:239–244.

116. Müller J. Adrenocortical tumors: clinical and diagnostic findings. *Results Cancer Res*. 1990;118:106–112.

117. Bodie B, Novick AC, Pontes JE, et al. The Cleveland Clinic experience with adrenal cortical carcinoma. *J Urol*. 1989;141:257–260.

118. Henley DJ, van Heerden JA, Grant CS, et al. Adrenal cortical carcinoma. A continuing challenge. *Surgery*. 1983;94:926–931.

119. Eliakim A, Cale-Benzoor M, Klinger-Cantor B, et al. A case study of virilizing adrenal tumor in an adolescent female elite tennis player—insight into the use of anabolic steroids in young athletes. *J Strength Condi Res*. 2011;25(1):46–50.

120. Ko JH, Lee HS, Hong J, Hwang JS. Virilizing adrenocortical carcinoma in a child with Turner syndrome and somatic TP53 gene mutation. *Euro J Pediatr*. 2010; 169(4):501–504.

121. Miyoshi Y, Oue T, Oowari M, et al. A case of pediatric virilizing adrenocortical tumor resulting in hypothalamic-pituitary activation and central precocious puberty following surgical removal. *Endocri J*. 2009;56(8):975–982.

122. Wajchenberg BL, Albergaria Pereira MA, Medonca BB, et al. Adrenocortical carcinoma. *Cancer.* 2000; 88(4):711–736.

123. Ferruci JT Jr. Body ultrasonography (medical progress). *N Engl J Med.* 1979;300:590–602.

124. Zografos GC, Driscoll DL, Karakousis CP, et al. Adrenal carcinoma: a review of 53 cases. *J Surg Oncol.* 1994;55:160–164.

125. Hogan TF, Gilchrist KW, Westring DW, et al. A clinical and pathological study of adrenocortical carcinoma. Therapeutic implications. *Cancer.* 1980;45:2880–2883.

126. White PC, Speiser PW. Congenital adrenal hyperplasia due to 21-hydroxylase deficiency. *Endocri Rev.* 2000; 21: 245–291.

127. Pinto G, Tardy V, Trivin C, et al. Follow-up of 68 children with congenital adrenal hyperplasia due to 21-hydroxylase deficiency: relevance of genotype for management. *J Clin Endocrinol Metab.* 2003; 88: 2624–2633.

128. Fürst-Recktenwald S, Dörr HG, Rosanowski F. Androglottia in a young female adolescent with congenital adrenal hyperplasia and 21-hydroxylase deficiency. *J Pediatr Endocrinol Metab.* 2000; 13: 959–962.

129. Heinemann M. Laryngeal and voice findings in congenital syndrome with adrenocortical hyperplasia. *Folia Phoniatrica.* 1974; 26: 450–460.

130. Nygren U, Södersten M, Falhammar H, Thoren M, Hagenfeldt K, Nordenskjöld A. Voice characteristics in women with congenital adrenal hyperplasia due to 21-hydroxylase deficiency. *Clin Endocrinol.* 2009; 70(1):18–25.

131. Nygren U, Nyström HF, Falhammar H, Hagenfeldt K, Nordenskjöld A, Soedersten M. Voice problems due to virilization in adult women with congenital adrenal hyperplasia due to 21-hydroxylase deficiency. *Clin Endocrinol.* 2013;79(6):859–866.

132. Nygren U, Isberg B, Arver S, Hertegård S, Södersten M, Nordenskjöld A. Magnetic resonance imaging of the vocal folds in women with congenital adrenal hyperplasia and virilized voices. *J Speech Lang Hear Res.* 2016;59(4):713–721.

133. Huang G, Pencina KM, Coady JA, Beleva YM, Bhasin S, Basaria S. Functional voice testing detects early changes in vocal pitch in women during testosterone administration. *J Clin Endocrinol Metab.* 2015; 100(6):2254–2260.

134. Huang G, Basaria S, Travison TG, et al. Testosterone dose-response relationships in hysterectomized women with and without oophorectomy: effects on sexual function, body composition, muscle performance and physical function in a randomized trial. *Menopause.* 2014;21(6):612.

135. Nordenskjöld F, Fex S. Vocal effects of danazol therapy. *Acta Obstetric Gynecolog Scand.* 1984;63(S123):131–132.

136. Glaser R, York A, Dimitrakakis C. Effect of testosterone therapy on the female voice. *Climacteric.* 2016; 19(2):198–203.

137. Damrose EJ. Quantifying the impact of androgen therapy on the female larynx. *Auris Nasus Larynx.* 2009;36:110–112.

138. Van Borsel J, De Cuypere G, Rubens R, Destaerke B. Voice problems in female-to-male transsexuals. *Int J Lang Commun Disord.* 2000;35:427–442.

139. Talaat M, Angelo A, Talaat AM, Elwany S, Kelada I, Thabet H. Histologic and histochemical study of effects of anabolic steroids on the female larynx. *Ann Otol Rhinol Laryngol.* 1987;96:468–471.

140. Achilli C, Pundir J, Ramanathan P, Sabatini L, Hamoda H, Panay N. Efficacy and safety of transdermal testosterone in postmenopausal women with hypoactive sexual desire disorder: a systematic review and meta-analysis. *Fertil Steril.* 2017;107(2):475–482.

141. Pope HG, Kanayama G, Athey A, Ryan E, Hudson JI, Baggish A. The lifetime prevalence of anabolic-androgenic steroid use and dependence in Americans: current best estimates. *Am J Addictions.* 2014; 23(4):371–377.

142. Nieschlag E, Vorona E. Mechanisms in endocrinology: medical consequences of doping with anabolic androgenic steroids: effects on reproductive functions. *Euro J Endocrinol.* 2015;173(2):R47–58.

143. Huang G, Basaria S. Do anabolic-androgenic steroids have performance-enhancing effects in female athletes? *Molec Cell Endocrinol.* In press.

144. Strauss RH, Liggett MT, Lanese RR. Anabolic steroid use and perceived effects in ten weight-trained women athletes. *JAMA.* 1985;253(19):2871–2813.

145. Matin FG. Drugs and vocal function. *J Voice.* 1988;2: 338–344.

146. Wardle PG, Whitehead MI. Nonreversible and wide ranging voice changes after treatment with danazol. *Br Med J.* 1983; 287:946.

147. Mercaitis PA, Peaper RE, Schwartz PA. Effects of danazol on vocal pitch: a case study. *Obstet Gynecol.* 1985;65:13 I–135.

148. Boothroyd CV, Lepre F. Permanent voice change resulting from danazol therapy. *Aust NZ J Obstet Gynaecol.* 1990; 30:275–276.

149. Barbieri RL. Endometriosis. *Drugs.* 1990;39(4):502–510.

150. Barbieri RL, Evans S, Kistner RW. Danazol in the treatment of endometriosis: analysis of 100 cases with a 4-year follow-up. *Fertil Steril.* 1982;37(6):737–746.

151. Verkauf BS. Effects of danazol treatment. Collected letters of the international correspondence society of obstetricians and gynaecologists. *Gynakol Prax.* 1978;19:120–122.

152. Damste PH. Voice change in adult women caused by virilizing agents. *J Speech Hear Dis.* 1967;32:126–132.

153. Gerritsma EJ, Brocaar MP, Hakkesteegt MM, Birkenhäger JC. Virilization of the voice in post-menopausal women due to the anabolic steroid nandrolone decanoate (decadurabolin). The effects of medication for one year. *Clin Otolaryngol.* 1994;19(1):79–84.

154. Baker J. A report on alterations to the speaking and singing voices of four women following hormonal therapy with virilizing agents. *J Voice.* 1999;13(4):496–507.

155. Damrose EJ. Quantifying the impact of androgen therapy on the female larynx. *Auris Nasus Larynx.* 2009;36(1):110–112.

156. Van Borsel, G. De Cuypere, R. Rubens, B. Destaerke J. Voice problems in female-to-male transsexuals. *Int J Lang Comm Dis.* 2000;35(3):427–442.

157. Brodnitz FS. The age of the castrato voice. *J Speech Hear Dis.* 1975;40(3):291–295.

158. Bermon S, Vilain E, Fenichel P, Ritzen M. Women with hyperandrogenism in elite sports: scientific and ethical rationales for regulating. *J Clin Endocrinol Metab.* 2015;100(3):828–830.

159. van Durme CM, Kisters JM, van Paassen P, van Etten RW, Tervaert JW. Multiple endocrine abnormalities. *Lancet.* 2011;378(9790):540.

160. Beckford NS, Schaid D, Rood SR, Schanbacher B. Androgen stimulation and laryngeal development. *Ann Otology Rhinol Laryngol.* 1985;94(6):634–640.

161. Kahane JC. Growth of the human prepubertal and pubertal larynx. *J Speech Hear Res.* 1982;25(3):446–455.

162. Hirano M, Kurita S, Nakashima T. The structure of the vocal folds. *Vocal Fold Physiol.* 1981:33–41.

163. 163.Evans S, Neave N, Wakelin D, Hamilton C. The relationship between testosterone and vocal frequencies in human males. *Physiol Behav.* 2008;93(4):783–788.

164. Dabbs JM, Mallinger A. High testosterone levels predict low voice pitch among men. *Personality Indiv Differ.* 1999;27(4):801–804.

165. Bruckert L, Lienard J-S, Lacroix A, Kreutzer M, Leboucher G. Women use voice parameters to assess men's characteristics. *Proc Biol Sci.* 2006;273: 83–98.

166. Meuser W, Nieschlag. Sex hormones and depth of voice in the male (Author transl). *Deutsche medizinische Wochenschrift* (1946). 1977;102(8):261–264.

167. Griggs RC, Kingston WI, Jozefowicz RF, Herr BE, Forbes GI, Halliday DA. Effect of testosterone on muscle mass and muscle protein synthesis. *J Appl Physiol.* 1989;66(1):498–503.

168 Sassoon D, Segil N, Kelley D. Androgen-induced myogenesis and chondrogenesis in the larynx of Xenopus laevis. *Devel Biol.* 1986;113(1):135–140.

169. Akcam T, Bolu E, Merati AL, Durmus C, Gerek M, Ozkaptan Y. Voice changes after androgen therapy for hypogonadotrophic hypogonadism. *Laryngoscope.* 2004;114(9):1587–1591.

170. Hamdan AL, Jabbour J, Saadeh R, Kazan I, Nassar J, Bulbul M. Vocal changes in patients with prostate cancer following androgen ablation. *J Voice.* 2012; 26(6):812- e11.

171. Gugatschka M, Kiesler K, Obermayer-Pietsch B, et al. Sex hormones and the elderly male voice. *J Voice.* 2010;24(3):369–373.

172. Altman KW, Haines GK, Vakkalanka SK, Keni SP, Kopp PA, Radosevich JA. Identification of thyroid hormone receptors in the human larynx. *Laryngoscope.* 2003;113(11):1931–1934.

173. Vanderpump M, Tunbrldge W, French J, et al. The incidence of thyroid disorders in the community: a twenty-year follow-up of the Whickham Survey. *Clin Endocrinol,* 1995;43(1):55–68.

174. Hollowell JG, Staehling NW, Flanders WD, et al. "Serum TSH, T4, and thyroid antibodies in the United States population (1988 to 1994): National Health and Nutrition Examination Survey (NHANES III). *J Clin Endocrinol Metab.* 2002;87(2):489–499.

175. Ritter F, "The effect of hypothyroidism on the larynx of the rat. An explanation for hoarseness associated with hypothyroidism in the human. *Ann Otol Rhinol Laryngol.* 1964;73:404.

176. Werner S. *The Thyroid: A Fundamental and Clinical Text.* 1962.

177. Ingbar SH, Woeber KE. The thyroid gland. In: *Textbook of Endocrinology.* 1974:198–199.

178. Chhetri M, Guha S. Clinical and metabolic study in hypothyroidism. *J Ind Med Assn.* 1970; 54(8):351–357.

179. Bicknell PG. Mild hypothyroidism and its effects on the larynx. *J Laryngol Otol.* 1973;87(2):123–127.

180. Gupta O, Bhatia P, Agarwal M, Mehrotra M, Mishr S. Nasal, pharyngeal, and laryngeal manifestations of hypothyroidism. *Ear Nose Throat J.* 1977;56(9): 349.

181. Mohammadzadeh A, Heydari E, Azizi F. Speech impairment in primary hypothyroidism. *J Endocrinol Investi.* 2011;34(6):431–433.

182. Hamdan AL, Jabbour J, Nassar J, Kasti M, Azar S. Acoustic analysis and perceptual evaluation of patients with non-myxedematous hypothyroidism. *Adv Life Sci Health.* 2014;16.

183. Stöllberger C, Finsterer J, Brand E, Tschabitscher D. Dysarthria as the leading symptom of hypothyroidism. *Am J Otolaryngol.* 2001, 22: 70–72.

184. Ficarra B J. Myxedemic hoarseness. *Arch Otolaryngol.* 1960: 72:75–76.

185. Barton, RT. Pharyngeal and laryngeal symptoms of thyroid origin. *New Engl J Med.* 1951:244:398–399.

186. Hilger JA. Otolaryngologic aspects of hypometabolism. *Ann Otol Rhinol Laryngol.* 1956: 65:395–413.

187. Hamdan AL, Dowli A, Jabbour J, Sabri A, Azar ST. Phonatory symptoms and impact on quality of life in female patients with goiter. *Ear Nose Throat J.* 2016;95(7):248–249.

188. Holl-Allen R. Laryngeal nerve paralysis and benign thyroid disease. *Arch Otolaryngol.* 1967;85(3):335–337.

189. Rueger RG. Benign disease of the thyroid gland and vocal cord paralysis. *Laryngoscope.* 1974;84(6):897–907.

190. McCall A, Ott R, Jarosz H, Lawrence A, Paloyan E. Improvement of vocal cord paresis after thyroidectomy. *Am Surgeon.* 1987;53(7):377–379.

191. Rowe-Jones J, Rosswick R, Leighton S. Benign thyroid disease and vocal cord palsy. *Ann Roy Coll Surg Engl.* 1993;75(4):241.

192. Fiorentino E, Cipolla C, Graceffa G, et al. Local neck symptoms before and after thyroidectomy: a possible correlation with reflux laryngopharyngitis, *Euro Arch OtoRhino-Laryngol.* 2011;268(5):715–720.

193. Hamdan AL, Jabbour J, Al Zaghal Z, Azar ST. Goiter and laryngopharyngeal reflux. *ISRN Endocrinol.* 2012.

194. Momex R, Orgiazzi J. Hyperthyroidism. In: DeVisscher, ed. Comparative *Endocrinology*. New York, NY: Raven Press; 1985:284–285.

195. Mcgaffee J, Uppmann S. Psychiatric presentations of hyperthyroidism. *Am Fam Physician*. 1983; 27:257–262.

196. Tsudana T, Mochinaga N, Eto T, et al. Hashimoto's thyroiditis presenting with severe pressure symptoms. *Jap J Surg*. 1991; 21:450–453.

197. Lindem MC Jr, Clark JH. Indications for surgery in thyroiditis. *Am J Surg*. 1969; 118: 829–831.

198. Tripp W, Rao V, Creary LB. Various manifestations of hyperthyroidism in an ambulatory clinic: case studies. *J Nati Medi Assn*. 1987;79(11):1167.

199. Heman-Ackah YD, Joglekar SS, Caroline M, et al. The prevalence of undiagnosed thyroid disease in patients with symptomatic vocal fold paresis. *J Voice*. 2011;25(4):496–500.

200. Azar S, Jabour J, Dowli A, Kasti M, Ziade G, Hamdan AL. Prevalence of phonatory symptoms and impact on quality of life in patients with subacute thyroiditis. *Austin J Otolaryngol*. 2014; 1(4):4.

201. Hamdan AL, Nassar J, El-Dahouk I, Al Zaghal Z, Jabbour J, Azar ST. Vocal characteristics in patients with thyroiditis. *Am J Otolaryngol*. 2012;33(5):600–603.

202. Lucarotti ME, Holl-Allen RT. Recurrent laryngeal nerve palsy associated with thyroiditis. *Br J Surg*. 1988; 75: 1041–1042.

203. Langevitz P, Cabili S. Persistent vocal cord paralysis in subacute thyroiditis. *Postgrad Med J*. 1983; 59: 726–727.

204. Dedivitis RA, Coelbo LS. Vocal cord paralysis in subacute thyroiditis. *Rev Bras Otorhinolaringol*. 2007; 73: 138.

205. Kuan EC, Peng KA, Kita AE, Bergsneider M, Wang MB. Acromegaly: otolaryngic manifestations following pituitary surgery. *American J Otolaryngol*. 2015;36(4):521–525.

206. Barreto VM, D'Ávila JS, Sales NJ, et al. Laryngeal and vocal evaluation in untreated growth hormone deficient adults. *Otolaryngol Head Neck Surg*. 2009;140(1):37–42.

207. Valença EH, Souza AH, Oliveira AH, et al. Voice quality in short stature with and without GH deficiency. *J Voice*. 2012;26(5):673–e13.

208. Moore C, Shalet S, Manickam K, Willard T, Maheshwari H, Baumann G. Voice abnormality in adults with congenital and adult-acquired growth hormone deficiency. *J Clini Endocrinol Metab*. 2005;90(7):4128–4132.

209. Valença EH, Salvatori R, Souza AH, et al. Voice formants in individuals with congenital, isolated, lifetime growth hormone deficiency. *J Voice*. 2016;30(3):281–286.

210. Williams RG, Richards SH, Mills RG, Eccles R. Voice changes in acromegaly. *Laryngoscope*. 1994;104(4):484–487.

211. Bogazzi F, Nacci A, Campomori A, et al. Analysis of voice in patients with untreated active acromegaly. *J Endocrinol Investi*. 2010;33(3):178–185.

212. Aydin K, Turkyilmaz D, Ozturk B, et al. Voice characteristics of acromegaly. *Euro Archi Oto-Rhino-Laryngol*. 2013;270(4):1391–1396.

213. Cooper T, Dziegielewski PT, Singh P, Seemann R. Acromegaly presenting with bilateral vocal fold immobility: case report and review of the literature. *J Voice*. 2016;30(6):758–e13.

214. Boden G. Fatty acids and insulin resistance. *Diab Care*. 1996; 19(4):394–395.

215. Gat-Yablonski G, Shalitin S, Phillip M. Maturity onset diabetes of the young—review. *Pediatr Endocrinol Rev*. 3(suppl 3) 2006: 514–520.

216. Holmkvist J, Almgren P, Lyssenko V, et al. Common variants in maturity onset diabetes of the young genes and future risk of type 2 diabetes. *Diabetes*. 2008: 57(6):1738–1744.

217. National Institute of Diabetes and Digestive and Kidney Diseases. National Diabetes Statistics, 2007. National Diabetes Information Clearinghouse. Retrieved March 30, 2009, from http://diabetes.niddk.nih.gov/DM/PUBS/statistics/.

218. National Eye Institute. Diabetic eye disease FAQ: prevention & treatment. National Eye Institute. Retrived April 6, 2009, from http://www.nei.nih.gov/diabetes/content/english/faq2.asp.

219. Hamdan AL, Kurban Z, Azar ST. Prevalence of phonatory symptoms in patients with type 2 diabetes mellitus. *Acta Diabetolog*. 2013;50(5):731–736.

220. Krishnan JA, Glick S, Smith LJ. Systematic review of the association between lung function and type 2 diabetes mellitus. *Diabetes Med*. 2010: 27(9):977–987.

221. Hamdan AL, Jabbour J, Nassar J, Dahouk I, Azar ST. Vocal characteristics in patients with type 2 diabetes mellitus. *Eur Arch Oto-Rhino-Laryngol*. 2012;269(5):1489–1495.

222. Huang BK, Monu JU, Doumanian J. Diabetic myopathy: MRI patterns and current trends. *AJR Am J Roentgenol*. 2010: 195(1): 198–204.

223. Tajiri Y, Kato T, Nakayama H, Yamada K. Reduction of skeletal muscle, especially in lower limbs, in Japanese type 2 diabetic patients with insulin resistance and cardiovascular risk factors. *Metab Syndr Relat Disord*. 2010: 8(2):137–142.

224. Wong AD, Best JA, Shapiro RD. Diabetic polyneuropathy involving the maxillofacial region: a case report. *J Oral Maxillofac Surg*. 2002;60:935–938.

225. Lee B, Woo P. Chronic cough as a sign of laryngeal sensory neuropathy: diagnosis and treatment. *Ann Otol Rhinol Laryngol*. 2005;114:253–257.

226. Aviv JE, Kim T, Thomson JE, Sunshine S, Kaplan S, Close LG. Fiberoptic endoscopic evaluation of swallowing with sensory testing (FEESST) in healthy controls. *Dysphagia*. 1998;13: 87–92.

227. Bock JM, Blumin JH, Toohill RJ, Merati AL, Prieto TE, Jaradeh SS. A new noninvasive method for determination of laryngeal sensory function. *Laryngoscope*. 2011;121:158–163.

228. Hamdan AL, Dowli A, Barazi R, Jabbour J, Azar S. Laryngeal sensory neuropathy in patients with diabetes mellitus. *J Laryngol Otol*. 2014;128(08):725–729.

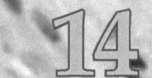

# Bodily Injuries and Their Effects on the Voice

*Robert Thayer Sataloff*

The ill effects of laryngitis, respiratory infections, direct trauma to the larynx, and other abnormalities in the head and neck are recognized routinely. However, the relevance of injuries elsewhere in the body is not always so obvious. Such maladies may affect the voice by altering abdominal support, introducing excess tension, distracting the singer through pain, or by other means that throw the vocal mechanism out of balance. Recognizing the potential hazard of injuries throughout the body often allows a singer or actor to compensate for them safely, preventing vocal stress and injury.

The anatomy of the singing voice involves the entire body. The larynx is inseparably interdependent with virtually all other body systems. The functions of the vocal folds (oscillator), supraglottic vocal tract (resonator), and abdomen and thorax (power source) were discussed in Chapter 1. The lower extremities and pelvis maintain a stable, balanced skeleton to optimize contraction of the abdominal and back musculature. Although the arms are less intimately involved with voice production under normal, relaxed circumstances, their direct association with neck and shoulder muscles and their location adjacent to the chest allow them, in abnormal use, to introduce undesirable neck tension or constriction of respiration. The brain is responsible for fine motor control, expression of emotion and stress, control of secretions (including those on the vocal folds), and coordination of all bodily functions. Injury to any part of the body may impair optimal vocal function.

## Anterior Neck Trauma

Injury to the front of the neck or to the larynx itself can be devastating. Usually, such injuries result from motor vehicle accidents in which the neck strikes the steering wheel or during altercations or playing sports. Direct trauma to the larynx can produce hemorrhage into the vocal folds, dislocation of the arytenoid cartilages, and fracture of the other laryngeal cartilages. Depending on the severity of the injury and other factors, the outlook ranges from complete recovery to permanent ruination of the voice.[1] Such injuries also have the life-threatening potential of airway obstruction. They can be avoided in many cases by proper use of seat belts with shoulder restraints. However, when anterior neck trauma occurs, immediate visualization of the larynx by a skilled laryngologist is essential. Laryngeal injuries are frequently worse than they appear to be at first.

## Posterior Neck Trauma

The most common form of posterior neck trauma is "whiplash," although a direct blow to the back of the neck may produce similar effects. Whiplash frequently is much more troublesome for singers and actors than it is for nonprofessional voice users. This injury can result in neck muscle spasms, hyperfunctional vocal technique, and abnormal neck posturing secondary to pain. The injury is especially problematic in singers who have already had to overcome a

341

tendency toward hyperfunctional voice abuse (eg, singing with tight jaw or neck muscles or with the tongue pulled back). In such people, whiplash will often result in decompensation and return to previous "bad habits." If the whiplash is associated with jaw trauma or temporomandibular joint injury, these problems may be aggravated. Temporomandibular joint dysfunction and pain may produce effects similar to those seen in whiplash.

## Head Trauma

Serious injuries to the head producing unconsciousness may be fatal. However, even when people recover from skull fractures or closed-head injury, subtle brain dysfunction may persist for many months, or even permanently.[2] This usually includes slight personality change, emotional liability, impaired memory, sometimes difficulty reading or speaking, and often nonspecific loss of "sharpness." Such impairments may be serious impediments to healthy singing.

Head trauma also may be associated with hearing loss.[3] This is most likely to occur if there is a blow directly to the ear or one severe enough to cause unconsciousness. Hearing should be checked after any serious head injury. If a hearing loss is found, counseling and rehabilitation usually avert vocal problems. However, if hearing loss goes unrecognized, the singer may "oversing" to compensate for the hearing impairment (especially if it is sensorineural hearing impairment (especially if it is sensorineural hearing loss or "nerve deafness"). Similar problems occur in actors or other professional speakers.

## Injury to the Supraglottic Vocal Tract

Injury to the nose such as nasal fracture can produce nasal obstruction. This alters the production of certain sounds (especially nasal consonants) and forces the singer to breathe unfiltered, unhumidified cold air through his or her mouth. This may result in voice irritation, especially in dusty or dry environments. Injury to the oral cavity, including surgical injury during tonsillectomy, changes a singer's sound. The shape and pliability of the tongue, palate, and pharyngeal muscles are important. They are trained during vocal studies, just as laryngeal muscles are. Although voice alterations caused by minor swelling or scarring in these areas are often more obvious to the singer or actor than they are to listeners,

they are hazardous, because performers (especially singers) tend to try to compensate for them. As these injuries produce structural changes in the anatomy of the vocal tract, there is no way to return the sound to "normal" while they are present. Many singers develop hyperfunctional technique in vain attempts to overcome them. The close supervision of a teacher and learning to "sing by feel" rather than "by ear" usually avoid these problems.

## Injury to the Upper Extremities

A broken arm, dislocated shoulder, or other upper extremity injury usually produces pain and muscle tension. This tension is often reflected in excess, asymmetric neck muscle tension and alterations of posture. Under most circumstances, awareness and special attention to these potential problems may avoid the hyperfunctional voice abuse that often supervenes.

## Chest and Abdominal Injuries

Chest and abdominal injuries may occur through vehicle accidents, surgery, or other trauma. Usually, they result in temporary muscle dysfunction. In general, singing should be avoided until support mechanisms are functional. A good rule of thumb is to require that the singer be able to do 10 sit-ups before resuming singing following chest or abdominal injury. This assumes reasonably good restoration of support muscle strength. It is generally safer not to sing at all than to sing without "support." Some less demanding vocal pursuits may be resumed sooner, with caution, such as gentle scales in the middle of a singer's range to maintain muscle tone. However, some injuries leave residual problems. If all or part of one lung is lost, voice technique may need to be modified. Similar problems may occur if lung function is impaired by inhalation injury. The greatest tendencies to voice abuse often come when a singer is nearly out of breath. Such singers must be careful to alter their phrasing to permit extra breaths, rather than attempt to sing extended phrases as they had prior to the injury. In addition, a vigorous program of aerobic rehabilitation is advisable. Following abdominal injuries, weaknesses in the abdominal muscle wall such as ventral hernias may persist. These may interfere with the support mechanism and require surgical repair.

## Injury to the Back

Back muscles are integral to voice support. Some of the consequences of cervical spine injury are discussed above in the section on posterior neck trauma. Thoracic, lumbar, and sacral injury also can interfere with voice performance. For example, such injuries may cause nerve dysfunction and consequent weakness in muscles used for respiration and support. Thoracic back pain may limit inspiration, and lumbosacral back pain may impede firm contraction of the abdominal and back muscles for support and may alter the balance of muscle function so essential to efficient phonation for singing or projected speech. These problems result commonly in unconscious attempts at compensation that often lead to hyperfunctional phonatory technique. This is not only counterproductive in terms of quality and endurance, but also may lead to structural injuries of the vocal folds. These problems can be avoided in many cases by expert voice therapy and training, which should be instituted as soon as possible after injury. They may be helped by physical therapy, skeletal manipulation, massage therapy, and other intervention.

## Injury to the Lower Extremities

Although singers do not regularly consider a sprained ankle or a broken leg as reason for a voice complaint, vocal dysfunction frequently follows such injuries, especially in singers and actors. It is extremely difficult to maintain good abdominal-thoracic and back muscle support while balancing awkwardly on one foot. It is common for singers to present with voice fatigue and hoarseness while on crutches or limping. Damage from the undesirable posture is aggravated by the distractions of trying to keep one's balance and pain associated with the injury. Usually, awareness of this potential hazard and the need for conscious attention to support will avert this problem in singers, actors, and other voice professionals.

## Conclusion

The voice mechanism is extremely sensitive to minor alterations anywhere in the body. Physicians must be alert for problems created not only by injuries to the larynx, but also by injuries elsewhere in the body. Helping the professional voice user to become aware of the problem, and to practice meticulous technique and good judgment, usually is sufficient to avoid serious or prolonged vocal disability from injuries with temporary effects. However, injuries that produce chronic pain or impairment frequently have chronic vocal consequences.

## References

1. Spiegel JR, Sataloff RT. Surgery for laryngeal trauma. In: Gould WJ, Sataloff RT, Spiegel JR, eds. *Voice Surgery.* St. Louis, MO: Mosby-Year Book; 1993:291–306.
2. Mandel S, Sataloff RT, Schapiro S. *Minor Head Trauma: Assessment, Management and Rehabilitation.* New York, NY: Springer-Verlag; 1993.
3. Sataloff RT, Sataloff J. *Hearing Loss.* 3rd ed. New York, NY: Marcel Dekker; 1993.

# Medications and the Voice

*Robert Thayer Sataloff, Mary J. Hawkshaw, Joseph Anticaglia,*
*Michelle White, Kirsten Meenan, and Jonathan J. Romak*

Medications are used to treat many problems encountered commonly in professional voice users. Some are used to treat illnesses affecting the head and neck, others involve other organs and systems in the body and can potentially affect the larynx and voice production. Many medications that potentially affect the voice are discussed in the first two editions of this book and in other literature.[1,2] In many cases, the effects are minor and not clinically significant. However, physicians, nurses, and others caring for professional voice users should be familiar with drug-induced phenomena that may affect the voice.

In addition to the recognized effects and side effects of medications, when trying to predict or recognize the potential vocal consequences of pharmacologic agents, it is important also to consider biological variability in individuals. An individual's response to medications is influenced also by gender, age, body size, metabolic status, and concurrent use of other medications or recreational drugs. "Recommended doses" are the amount of a drug generally required to achieve the desired balance between an effect or side effect. However, they are merely guidelines based on average responses in test populations. Optimizing the relationship between desired effects and undesirable side effects requires individualization, especially in professional voice users for whom even "minor" side effects may be vocally disabling.

## Antihistamines

Antihistamines are used commonly to treat allergies. However, virtually all antihistamines can have a drying effect on upper respiratory tract secretions, although severity varies widely with different drugs and from person to person. In addition, antihistamines are often combined with sympathomimetic or parasympatholytic agents, which further reduce and thicken mucosal secretions and may reduce lubrication to the point of producing a dry cough. This may be more harmful to phonation than the allergic condition itself. Normal mucosal secretions are extremely important for free movement of the vibratory margin of the vocal folds. If vocal tract lubrication is suboptimal as a result of dehydration, or by shifting the normal balance of serous and mucinous secretions, alterations in phonation occur. Laryngologists frequently discover that a patient has self-medicated with an over-the-counter (OTC) antihistamine preparation, thus making it imperative to seek this information when taking a patient's medical history. When professional voice users develop thick, viscous vocal fold secretions during performance, results can be disastrous.

The majority of antihistamine agents are acetylcholine antagonists that have parasympatholytic activity, which probably accounts for the increased viscosity of secretions by directly affecting the salivary glands and mucus-secreting membranes of the respiratory tract. They may also have a sedative effect that can impair sensorium and disturb performance. Milder, newer antihistamines such as fexofenadine (Allegra, Chattem, Inc., Chattanooga, Tennessee) and loratadine (Claritin, MSD Consumer Care, Inc., Memphis, Tennessee) produce less drowsiness and often less dryness; but in many people, they are often less effective in treating symptoms than drugs with more disturbing side effects. Mild antihistamines in small doses may be helpful for performers with intermittent allergic symptoms, but the medications should be tried between or before performances, not immediately prior to professional engagements. When medication is needed to treat an acute allergic response shortly before performance, oral or injected corticosteroids rather than antihistamines usually accomplish the desired result without causing significant side effects. Antihistamines used to treat allergies are different from the antihistamines (H2 blockers) used to treat other conditions such as reflux. H2 blockers (ranitidine, Zantac, Barbados, W.I.) are used to block the stimulant effects of histamine on gastric acid secretions.

The antihistamines most commonly used are those belonging to the alkylamine or chlorpheniramine family. Because they have been deregulated by the US Food and Drug Administration (FDA) and are now available over the counter (OTC), these agents are being used with increasing frequency. Diphenhydramine (Benadryl, McNeil-PPC, Inc. Fort Washington, Pennsylvania) and scopolamine (Transderm, Novartis Consumer Health, Inc., Parsippany, New Jersey), which have a significant drying effect, are present in some OTC sleep aids, presumably for their sedative effect. Promethazine (Phenergan, Baxter Healthcare Corp., Cherry Hill, New Jersey) is contained in several antitussive mixtures and can dry laryngeal secretions. Meclizine (Antivert, Pfizer Inc., Collegeville, Pennsylvania), another OTC antihistamine used to treat dizziness and motion sickness, is also encountered commonly. All antihistamines provide some degree of relief from motion sickness; and to a greater or lesser degree, all cause drying of the mucous membranes, especially of the nose and oropharynx.

## Mucolytic Agents

The lubricant viscosity of respiratory tract and vocal fold surface tension are essential to normal phonation. Dehydration and/or thickening of secretions may be caused by medications such as antihistamines, as discussed above, anticholinergics, generalized dehydration, and/or other factors. Dehydration may occur as the result of exercising, performing athletic or recreational activities, or from exposure to environmental factors such as the dry air on airplanes and the low humidity at high altitudes. Dehydration can also occur with febrile illness and/or prolonged vomiting or diarrhea. It must be remembered that the viscosity of respiratory secretions is directly related to available body water, assuming the absence of metabolic or pharmacologic interference. No medications, including mucolytic agents, are substitutes

for adequate hydration. However, mucolytics may be helpful in counteracting the effects of antihistamines and in ameliorating the mucosal consequences of dehydration quickly. Guaifenesin is a useful wetting agent, expectorant, and vasoconstrictor that increases and thins mucosal secretions. Guaifenesin (Mucinex, Reckitt Benckiser Inc., Parsippany, New Jersey) is currently among the most convenient preparations available. Mucolytics are relatively harmless and may be helpful in singers who complain of thick secretions, frequent throat clearing, or postnasal drip, which is often caused by secretions that are too thick rather than too plentiful.

## Corticosteroids

Corticosteroids are potent antiinflammatory agents that can be helpful in managing an acute allergy attack and acute laryngitis. Many laryngologists recommend using steroids in low doses, such as methylprednisolone 10 mg. However, the author (RTS) has found higher doses for short periods of time to be more effective. Depending on the indication, the steroid dosage may be methyl prednisolone 60 mg (Medrol, Upjohn) orally or dexamethasone 6 mg (Decadron, Merck & Co. Inc., Kenilworth, New Jersey) intramuscularly followed by a short course of a high-dose oral steroid tapered over 3 to 6 days. Regimens of oral steroid therapy, such as a dexamethasone (Decadron, Merck & Co. Inc., Kenilworth, New Jersey) or methylprednisolone (Depo-Medrol, Medrol, or Medrol Dosepak, Pfizer, Inc., Collegeville, Pennsylvania) may also be used. Physicians should be familiar with the dose relationship among steroids (Table 15–1).

Adrenocorticotropic hormone (ACTH) may also be used to increase endogenous cortisone output, thus decreasing inflammation and mobilizing water from an edematous larynx,[3] although the author (RTS) has found traditional steroid therapy entirely satisfactory. Care must be taken not to prescribe steroids excessively, and they should not be used habitually (or in females for monthly dysphonia premenstrualis). They should be used only when there is a pressing professional commitment that is being hampered by vocal fold inflammation. If there is any question that the inflammation may be of infectious origin, antibiotic coverage is recommended. Steroids, whether administered short term or long term, must be used with extreme caution in diabetics. Steroids elevate serum glucose; and in the diabetic patient, they can cause blood sugars to become uncontrolled. Laryngologists should have their patients consult

| Table 15–1. Steroid Equivalency | | | |
|---|---|---|---|
| Adrenocorticosteroids | Common Trade Name | Glucocorticoid (Anti-Inflammatory Potency) Equivalent Dose (mg) | Mineralocorticoid (Sodium Retention) Relative Potency |
| Betamethasone | Celestone (Schering) | 0.06 | 0 |
| Cortisone | Cortone (M-S-D) | 25 | 0.8 |
| Dexamethasone | Decadron (M-S-D) Deronil (Schering) Dexameth (Major) Gammacorten (CIBA) Hexadrol (Organon) | 0.75 | 0 |
| Fludrocortisone | Florinef (Squibb) | 0.1 | 100 |
| Fluprednisolone | Alphadrol (Upjohn) | 2 | 0 |
| Hydrocortisone | Cort-Dome (Dome) Cortef (Upjohn) Cortenema (Rowell) Cortril (Pfizer) Hydrocortone (M-S-D) | 20 | 1 |
| Methylprednisolone | Depo-Medrol (Upjohn) Medrol (Upjohn) Solu-Medrol (Upjohn) | 4 | 4 |
| Paramethasone | Haldrone (Lilly) Stemex (Syntex) | 2 | 0 |
| Prednisolone | Delta-Cortef (Upjohn) Hydeltra T.B.A. (M-S-D) Hydeltrasol (M-S-D) Meticortelone (Schering) Nisolone (Ascher) Sterane (Pfizer) | 5 | 0.8 |
| Prednisone | Delta Dome (Dome) Deltasone (Upjohn) Deltra (M-S-D) Meticorten (Schering) Paracort (Parke-Davis) Servisone (Lederle) | 5 | 0.8 |
| Triamcinolone | Aristocort (Lederle) Aristospan (Lederle) Kenacort (Squibb) Kenalog (Squibb) | 4 | 0 |

*Note.* Abbreviation: M-S-D = Merck, Sharp & Dohme.

their endocrinologist before starting steroids so that a schedule for monitoring blood glucose can be established while a patient is on steroid therapy.

Corticosteroids may have additional significant adverse effects; although they are not generally seen following short-term steroid use, they may occur in any patient. The side effects encountered most frequently include gastric irritation with possible ulceration and hemorrhage, increased appetite, increased energy, insomnia, mild mucosal drying, blurred vision, mood change (euphoria, occasionally psychosis), irritability, and fluid retention. These side effects can range from mild to severe depending on the dosage given and the patient's metabolism and response to the medication.

The author (RTS) routinely prescribes ranitidine (Zantac, Concordia Pharmaceuticals, Barbados, W.I.) when treating patients with steroids, as prophylaxis against gastric irritation. Patients that are already taking H2 blockers and/or proton pump inhibitors (PPIs) might require increased dosages of their medication while on steroids. Long-term effects such as muscle wasting and fat redistribution are generally not encountered with appropriate short-term use of steroids.

Another potential problem peculiar to professional voice users is steroid abuse. Because the side effects of steroids generally are uncommon and because steroids work extremely well, there is a tendency (especially among singers) to overuse or abuse them and to share their medication with other performers. This practice must be avoided.

## Diuretics and Other Medications for Edema

Diuretics are potent medications that help the body eliminate excess fluid and should be taken only with a physician's prescription and supervision. Like steroids, they should be taken only by the individual for whom they were prescribed. Diuretics are indicated and used to treat certain illnesses, such as heart or kidney failure, when the body is unable to excrete fluids at a rate needed to maintain its fluid and electrolyte balance. Diuretics also are used in conjunction with antihypertensive agents for the treatment of high blood pressure.

The premenstrual period is a temporary physiological condition in which women retain fluid as a result of decreased estrogen and progesterone levels associated with altered pituitary activity. An increase in circulating antidiuretic hormone results in fluid retention in Reinke's space as well as in other tissues. The fluid retained in the vocal fold during inflammation and hormonal fluid shifts is protein bound, not free water.[4] Diuretics do not remobilize this fluid effectively and can dehydrate the performer, resulting in decreased lubrication and thickened secretions and persistently edematous vocal folds, and thus should not be used for vocal fold symptoms related to these conditions. If diuretics must be used for other medical purposes, the voice should be monitored closely.

Topical and systemic decongestants such as oxymetazoline hydrochloride (Afrin, Bayer HealthCare LLC, Tarrytown, New York) and pseudoephedrine (Sudafed, McNeil-PPC, Inc. Fort Washington, Pennsylvania) have also been used to treat edema/congestion in the upper respiratory tract. Oxymetazoline hydrochloride (Afrin) applied by a large particle mist to the larynx is particularly helpful in treating severe edema immediately prior to performance, but it should be used only under emergent and extreme circumstances. Afrin is more commonly used as a nasal spray to treat nasal congestion. Its primary action involves reduction in the diameter and volume of vascular structures in the submucosal area; however, it may also produce "rebound" phenomena and thus requires use with caution.

## Sprays, Mists, and Inhalants

Diphenhydramine hydrochloride 0.5% (Benadryl, McNeil-PPC Inc., Fort Washington, Pennsylvania) in distilled water, delivered to the larynx as a mist may be helpful for its vasoconstrictive properties, but it is also dangerous because of its topical anesthetic effect and is not recommended by the author (RTS). However, Punt advocated this mixture and several modifications of it.[5]

Five percent propylene glycol in a physiologically balanced salt solution may be delivered by large particle mist and can provide lubrication, particularly helpful in cases of laryngitis sicca after air travel or as associated with dry climates. Such treatment is harmless and may also provide a beneficial placebo effect. Water, saline, or other physiologically balanced solutions delivered via a vaporizer or steam generator are frequently effective and sufficient. This therapy should be augmented by oral hydration, which is the mainstay of treatment for dehydration.

Nasal steroid sprays such as beclomethasone dipropionate (Beconase AQ, GlaxoSmithKline, Brentford, United Kingdom, and Qnasl, Teva Pharmaceuticals USA, Inc., North Wales, Pennsylvania), budesonide (Rhinocort Aqua, AstraZeneca Pharmaceuticals, LP, Wilmington, Delaware), triamcinolone (Nasacort, Chattem, Inc., Chattanooga, Tennessee), and mometasone (Nasonex, Merck & Co., Inc., Kenilworth, New Jersey) do not appear to harm the voice. The steroid in the nasal spray works topically on the nasal mucosa and is not absorbed systemically. However, certain propellants in these nasal sprays may cause mucosal drying. For this reason, the author (RTS) generally prescribes steroid nasal sprays that have an aqueous medium, such as budesonide (Rhinocort Aqua).

Most oral steroid inhalers, such as triamcinolone acetonide (Azmacort, Abbott Laboratories, Chicago,

Illinois) used to treat asthma are not recommended for use in professional voice users.[6,7] Dysphonia caused by contact inflammation from oral steroid inhalers occurs in up to 50% of patients and is related to the aerosolized steroid itself and not to the Freon propellant. Steroid inhalers used for prolonged periods may result in *Candida* laryngitis; and as is common in asthmatics, prolonged use of steroid inhalers can cause atrophy of the vocalis muscle.[7,8]

## Antibiotics

When antibiotics are used in professional voice users, high doses are recommended to achieve therapeutic blood levels rapidly, especially if important performances are imminent. When there is little time between initial treatment and performance, starting treatment with an intramuscular injection may be helpful. Selecting oral antibiotics that are absorbed rapidly and achieve optimal blood levels faster may also be helpful.

When patients have no pressing engagements, antibiotic use should be based on cultures whenever appropriate (eg, throat culture for streptococcus infection). However, in the common situation in which a performance must proceed and when there is clinical evidence of bacterial infection, antibiotics should be instituted after cultures are taken, without waiting for the results. The potential damage of delayed treatment in an active performer is greater than the potential harm of antibiotic use for an unproven organism.

## Antiviral Agents

A limited number of antiviral agents are available commercially. Acyclovir (Zovirax, GlaxoSmithKline, Brentford, United Kingdom) is used specifically for treating the herpes simplex virus (HSV) types I and II and may be appropriate in patients with recurrent herpetic superior laryngeal nerve paresis or paralysis. Oseltamivir (Tamiflu, Genentech Inc., San Franscisco, California) is a relatively new antiviral drug that can be effective in the treatment of acute influenza and for prophylaxis of influenza in adults and children, 13 years and older. It is not a substitute for a flu vaccination. Voice problems have not been reported with Tamiflu; however, rash and swelling of the face and tongue have been reported, which could have a negative impact on vocal performance. Zanamivir (Relenza, GlaxoSmithKline, Brentford, United Kingdom) is another antiviral medication administered

by oral inhalation, which delivers the medication directly to the respiratory tract. Relenza is indicated for treatment of influenza A and B in patients who have been symptomatic for no more than 2 days, and in adults and children 7 years or older. However, it is generally not recommended for patients with underlying airway disease; bronchospasm and decreased lung function have been reported with use of this drug. Recently, a new medication to reduce the length and degree of symptoms of the common cold has been introduced and should be available in less than 1 year pending FDA approval. Pleconaril (Picovir, Schering-Plough, Kenilworth, New Jersey) specifically attacks the rhinovirus, which is the most common cause of the common cold. Pending FDA approval of this medication, it will be available by prescription only and its brand name will be Picovir.

Vistide (cidofovir, Gilead Sciences, Foster City, California) is now being used as an intralesional injection in treating human papilloma virus (HPV) involving the larynx. An in-depth discussion of its use can be found in Chapter 55. Patients with human immunodeficiency virus (HIV) are also treated with antivirals such as zidovudine (Retrovir, ViiV Healthcare, Brentford, United Kingdom), which was previously called azidothymidine (AZT). This drug has the potential to cause very severe side effects; however, it is often difficult to determine what is a side effect of a medication, because many of the side effects can be manifestations of the HIV disease process itself. Zidovudine can cause hoarseness, cough, pharyngitis, nervousness, muscle spasm, tremor, and many other systemic side effects, all of which can have a negative impact on vocal performance.

Amantadine (Symmetrel, Endo Health Solutions Inc., Malvern, Pennsylvania) used in the treatment of Parkinson's disease, also has been found to be effective against influenza[9-12] and other viruses. If a performer must work in an area in which there is a flu epidemic, it may be reasonable to use this drug. However, agitation, tachycardia, and extreme xerostomia and xerophonia may occur. When these side effects occur, they are generally severe enough to require cancellation of a performance.

## Antitussive Medications

Cough suppressants (antitussives) often contain an antihistamine and codeine, a narcotic, that can have a secondary drying effect on vocal tract secretions.[13,14] Benzonatate (Tessalon, Pfizer Inc., New York, New York) is a non-narcotic antitussive that acts peripherally by anesthetizing stretch receptors in the upper respiratory tract, thereby suppressing the cough reflex. However, severe hypersensitivity reactions including laryngospasm and bronchospasm have been reported. Dextromethorphan is a non-narcotic, antitussive agent found in most cough syrups and has pharmacologic actions similar to those of codeine. Generally, the over-the-counter preparations that contain dextromethorphan and guaifenesin (Robitussin DM, Pfizer Inc., Richmond, Virginia) work well for voice professionals. All patients, including singers, should be instructed to read the labels on all OTC medications. If there is any question regarding safety or ingredients of a product, it should be discussed with their primary physician and/or laryngologist.

## Antihypertensive Agents

Almost all of the antihypertensive agents used currently have a parasympathomimetic action of varying degrees and thus dry mucous membranes of the respiratory tract. Often, they are used in combination with a diuretic that promotes dehydration. The authors have frequently noted dryness with reserpines and agents of the methyldopa group, and occasionally a dry cough with some of the newer medications used to treat hypertension. When mucosal drying and a dry, nonproductive cough are thought to be a side effect of an antihypertensive medication, the laryngologist may recommend that the patient's internist prescribe another antihypertensive agent. Beta-blockers such as propranolol (Inderal, Akrimax Pharmaceuticals, Cranford, New Jersey) are also used in the treatment of hypertension but are not recommended treatment for preperformance anxiety.[15]

## Gastroenterologic Medications

Medical management of gastroesophageal reflux disease (GERD) generally includes neutralization of gastric acid with antacids; suppression of acid secretion with histamine receptor antagonists (H2 blockers), such as ranitidine (Zantac, Concordia Pharmaceuticals, Inc., Oakville, Ontario); blocking of the gastric proton pump enzyme (H+/K+ATPase) with antagonists such as omeprazole (Prilosec, AstraZeneca Pharmaceuticals, LP, London, United Kingdom); and modifications in lifestyle and diet. In the laryngologist's (RTS) practice, the authors frequently encounter patients who misunderstand their medical treatment for laryngopharyngeal reflux despite receiving oral and written explanations and instruc-

tions by the authors and being reinforced by other members of our voice team involved in a patient's care. The most common misconception is that H2 blockers and/or proton pump inhibitors (PPIs) eliminate the need for antacids and other lifestyle modifications. It is especially important for singers and all patients to understand the correct rationale for use of their medications, because inadequately treated reflux laryngitis can have deleterious effects on the voice over time including cancer of the larynx or esophagus. A more in-depth discussion of reflux management can be found in Chapter 59. Laryngeal cancer and its treatment can be found in Chapter 103.

Antacids can cause constipation, diarrhea, or bloating in some people, which may affect performance by impairing the support mechanism vital to singers and other musicians. Occasionally, they also have a drying effect. However, it is usually possible to find an antacid that can be tolerated by any individual. It is also possible to select antacids that do not contain chemicals (eg, aluminum) that some people wish to avoid (Tables 15–2 and 15–3).

H2 receptor antagonists have revolutionized the treatment of gastroesophageal reflux disease and proved beneficial for the treatment of reflux laryngitis (RL) and are now used widely by most laryngologists who treat a large number of professional voice users.

H2 receptor antagonists inhibit the stimulation of gastric acid secretion and are generally effective in reducing acid output from gastric parietal cells, although they have little affect on the basal rate of acid production. The H2 blockers most commonly used include ranitidine (Zantac, Concordia Pharmaceuticals, Inc., Oakville, Ontario), famotidine (Pepcid, Merck & Co., Inc., Kenilworth, New Jersey), cimetidine (Tagamet, Prestige Brands Holdings, Inc., Greenburgh, New York), and nizatidine (Axid, Braintree Laboratories, Inc., Braintree, Massachusetts) have been deregulated by the FDA and are now available OTC, but in much lower doses than prescription doses. Patients should be made aware of this. Although drying of the laryngeal mucosa (from its antihistamine action) is not a major side effect of the H2 blockers, it does occur and must be considered. Occasionally, the drying effects of H2 blockers can be severe enough to cause not only dry mouth, but also dry and irritated eyes. This condition makes it difficult to read scores and causes excessive blinking, especially under spotlights, which can be misinterpreted by an audience as nervousness.

Gastric proton pump (H+/K+ATPase) inhibitors (PPIs) suppress gastric acid production and are generally highly effective in the management of GERD

| Table 15–2. Contents of Liquid Antacids (in mg/tsp) | | | | | | | |
|---|---|---|---|---|---|---|---|
| | Aluminum Hydroxide | Magnesium Hydroxide | Calcium Carbonate | Magnesium Carbonate | Magaldrate | Simethicone | Sodium |
| Alternagel | 600 | | | | | | <2.5 |
| Aludrox | 307 | 103 | | | | | |
| Amphojel | 320 | | | | | | |
| Camalox | 225 | 200 | 250 | | | | |
| Delcid | 600 | 665 | | | | | <15 |
| Di-Gel | 200 | 200 | | | | 20 | |
| Gaviscon (mg/tbsp) | 95 | | | 412 | | | |
| Gelusil | 200 | 200 | | | | 25 | |
| Gelusil II | 400 | 400 | | | | 30 | |
| Kolantyl | 150 | 150 | | | | | |
| Maalox | 225 | 200 | | | | | |
| Maalox Plus | 225 | 200 | | | | | |
| Mag-Ox | | 400 | | | | 25 | |
| Mylanta | 200 | 200 | | | | 20 | |
| Mylanta II | 400 | 400 | | | | 40 | |
| Riopan | | | | | 540 | | 0.1 |
| Riopan Plus | | | | | 540 | 20 | 0.1 |
| Riopan Plus E-S | | | | | 1,080 | 30 | 0.3 |
| Uro-Mag | | 140 | | | | | |

and RL. Medications such as omeprazole (Prilosec, AstraZeneca Pharmaceuticals, LP, London, United Kingdom), lansoprazole (Prevacid, Takeda Pharmaceuticals, Osaka, Japan), rabeprazole (Aciphex, Janssen Pharmaceuticals, Horsham, Pennsylvania), pantoprazole (Protonix, Pfizer Inc., New York, New York), and esomeprazole (Nexium, AstraZeneca Pharmaceuticals, LP, London, United Kingdom) inhibit the H+/K+ATPase system, which is virtually unique to the gastric parietal cell. H+/K+ATPase competitive inhibitors cause inactivation of the H+/K+ATPase enzyme, suppressing both basal and stimulated gastric acid secretion for prolonged periods of time. In most patients, once or twice daily dosing usually provides excellent control of acid production. Proton pump inhibitors do not adversely affect the lower esophageal sphincter or esophageal motility, but they do slow the linear emptying rate of solids

from the stomach.[16] Although the incidence of side effects of PPIs is low, they can cause diarrhea, abdominal pain, and nausea and elevation of liver enzymes (this is also true of most H2 blockers). Dry mouth, esophageal candidiasis, muscle cramps, depression, tremors, dizziness, fatigue, and headaches have also been reported. Resistance to omeprazole has also been reported.[17]

Hyperkinetic agents improve motility and help prevent reflux by increasing the rate of gastric emptying. For several years, metoclopramide (Reglan, ANI Pharmaceuticals, Inc., Baudette, Minnesota) was the only such agent available. Because of troublesome side effects, particularly neurological abnormalities in approximately 10% of patients, the drug was never used extensively in professional singers; and it has now been largely replaced by newer agents. At present, the most commonly prescribed medication

**Table 15–3.** Contents of Antacids: Tablets-Chewables-Gums (in mg)

| | Aluminum Hydroxide | Magnesium Hydroxide | Calcium Carbonate | Simethicone | Dihydroxy-Aluminum Na$^+$ Carbonate | Magnesium Carbonate |
|---|---|---|---|---|---|---|
| Alka-Mints | | | 850 | | | |
| Algicon | 360 | | | | | 320 |
| Alu-cap | | | 194 | | | |
| Alu-tab | | | 585 | | | |
| Bisodol | | 178 | | | | |
| Calcitrel | | 120 | 585 | | | |
| Chooz | | 500 | | | | |
| Remegel | Mg carbonate codried gel 476.4 | | | | | |
| Rolaids (cherry) | | | 550 | | 334 | |
| Rolaids (plain) | | 64 | 317 | | | |
| Tempo | 133 | 81 | 414 | 20 | | |
| Titralac | | | 420 | | | |
| Tums | | | 500 | | | |
| Tums E-X | | | 750 | | | |

in this drug class is cisapride (Propulsid, Janssen Pharmaceuticals, Inc., Horsham, Pennsylvania). Cisapride increases lower esophageal sphincter pressure and lower esophageal peristalsis, which significantly accelerates gastric emptying of liquids and solids. The most common side effects are headache, abdominal pain, nausea, diarrhea, constipation, dizziness, pharyngitis, depression, dehydration, and rhinitis. Dry mouth, tremor, and somnolence have been reported in less than 1% of patients, and numerous other adverse reactions are seen uncommonly.

Other medications used to treat disorders of the gastrointestinal tract include phenobarbital (many manufacturers), prochlorperazine (Compazine, GlaxoSmithKline, Brentford, United Kingdom), isopropamide (many manufacturers), and propantheline bromide (many manufacturers). Members of the belladonna alkaloid group, including scopolamine (Scopace, Hope Pharmaceuticals, Scottsdale, Arizona) and atropine (AtroPen, Meridian Medical Technologies, Columbia, Maryland), are widely used and prescribed for their antispasmodic effects. All of these agents have a significant drying effect on secretions in the vocal tract.

Not infrequently the laryngologist may encounter a patient who consumes large amounts of vitamin C (ascorbic acid) in an effort to maintain health or to prevent the common cold. However, large amounts of ascorbic acid can irritate the stomach lining and consequently aggravate gastroesophageal reflux laryngitis. In some patients, a drying effect may occur when vitamin C is taken in large doses, probably due to a mild diuretic effect.[18] Additionally, in patients with impaired renal function, high doses of vitamin C may produce acidic urine and possibly renal calculi.

## Sleeping Pills

Sleeping pills generally should not be necessary for healthy people. Occasionally, the stresses of a tour and the aggravations of travel, along with frequent changes in time zones, can disturb sleep patterns. For this reason it is appropriate to take a small supply of a mild sleeping medication when traveling and to use it with great caution. These should be prescribed with instructions regarding rebound insomnia and the risk of habituation and physical dependence. Performers should avoid using diphenhydramine (Benadryl, McNeil-PPC, Inc. Fort Washington, Pennsylvania), an antihistamine that is a common ingredient in many OTC sleep aids. It is a safe drug and works well, but it produces excessive drying of mucosal membranes.

## Analgesics

Aspirin and other analgesics such as ibuprofen (many manufacturers) are prescribed frequently for relief of minor to moderate pain. The platelet dysfunction caused by aspirin (many manufacturers) predisposes an individual to bleeding and even hemorrhage, especially in vocal folds traumatized by excessive voice use in the face of vocal dysfunction. A vocal fold hemorrhage can be devastating to a professional voice user; and for this reason, the laryngologist (RTS) prohibits aspirin use and recommends minimal use of NSAIDs in his singers and all voice patients. However, the author (RTS) has one exception to the aspirin rule for singers and other professional voice users. A low daily dose of aspirin, generally one children's aspirin (81 mg), is used commonly in the treatment of patients with known coronary artery disease and for the prevention of heart disease in others. Because this dosage of aspirin is so small, its potential for jeopardizing the voice is low; and treatment of heart disease always takes precedence over maintenance of a healthy voice. Acetaminophen (Tylenol, McNeil-PPC, Inc., Fort Washington, Pennsylvania) is the recommended analgesic for mild to moderate pain. The nonsteroidal antiinflammatory drugs (NSAIDs) such as ibuprofen (Motrin, McNeil-PPC, Inc., Fort Washington, Pennsylvania) and ketoprofen (Oruvail, Sanofi, Malvern, Pennsylvania similar to ibuprofen, but taken only once daily) may interfere with the clotting mechanism, and their use is also discouraged in professional voice users.

A new class of analgesics, selective COX-2 inhibitors, is now being used to treat acute and chronic pain. These medications do not interfere with the COX-1 pathway and, do not cause bleeding dyscrasias or gastrointestinal side effects as seen with traditional NSAIDs.

Caruso used a spray of ether and iodoform on his vocal folds when he had to sing with laryngitis. However, such use of analgesics is extremely dangerous and should be avoided. Pain has an important protective physiologic function. Masking it risks incurring significant vocal damage that may not be recognized until after the analgesic wears off. If a singer requires analgesics taken orally or topical anesthetics to alleviate laryngeal discomfort, the laryngitis is severe enough to warrant canceling a performance. If the analgesic is used for headache or some other discomfort not directly associated with voice production, symptomatic treatment should be discouraged until singing commitments have been completed or cancelled.

Narcotic analgesics should not be used for any reason shortly before performance, especially if the medications are being used for laryngeal discomfort. Even when the pain is outside the head and neck, narcotics may cause sufficient change in sensorium to impair performance and risk vocal fold injury through unconscious technical voice abuse. As Damsté reported, sedatives and narcotics, in addition to impairing intellectual function, may cause an uninhabited drive to speak and symptoms of dysarthria.[19] Occasional exceptions can be made. For example, if a low dose of codeine early on a performance day is sufficient to control moderate menstrual cramping, its use is certainly not unreasonable. However, if menstrual cramps are so severe that high doses of codeine (in the 60 mg range) are required within a few hours of performance, cancellation may be more appropriate.

## Hormones

The most significant group of drugs that can adversely affect the voice are hormones such as androgens and anabolic steroids.[20–25] These drugs cause changes in voice quality by alterations in fluid content and structural changes. Structural alterations in laryngeal architecture seldom occur as the result of pharmacologic influences, but androgens are an exception. They may produce irreversible lowering of fundamental frequencies and coarsening of the voice, especially in females.[22–30] Androgenic agents such as Danocrine (danazol, Sanofi, Malvern, Pennsylvania) are used in the treatment of endometriosis, as part of chemotherapy regimens for some breast cancers, and to treat postmenopausal sexual dysfunction and other problems.[31–40] Birth control pills with relatively high progesterone content are most likely to produce androgen-like changes in the voice.[41–48] Most oral contraceptives marketed in the United States now have an appropriate estrogen-progesterone ratio, and voice changes are seen in only about 5% of women who use birth control pills (C. Carroll, MD, and H. von Leden, MD personal communication, September 1992). These changes generally are temporary, abating when oral contraceptive use is discontinued.

Estrogen replacement is helpful in forestalling the typical voice changes that follow menopause. The conjugated estrogen preparation used most frequently in the United States is Premarin (Prempro, Pfizer Inc.,

New York, New York). Until recently, the conjugated estrogens were thought to be preferable to estradiol; however, it now appears that there is no real difference with regard to the effect on the voice (J. Abitbol, personal communication, 2001). The progesterone, Provera (Pfizer Inc., New York, New York) is often prescribed in combination with Premarin (Prempro). In low doses, natural progesterones usually do not cause significant voice problems. However, some of the synthetic progesterone substitutes have androgenic effects and the potential for permanent virilization of the voice. Unless medical contraindications are present, professional voice users should be offered hormone replacement under appropriate medical supervision at the time of menopause.

Other hormone replacement medications may also affect the voice, often beneficially. Thyroid replacement may restore vocal efficiency and "ring" lost with even a mild degree of hypothyroidism. Agents used to treat maladies in any part of the diencephalic pituitary axis should be presumed to have laryngeal effects and warrant close monitoring of voice function.

## Bronchoactive Medications

Phonation depends on the availability of a powerfully supported airstream passing between the vocal folds. Impairment of pulmonary function can cause severe problems for professional voice users. Pulmonary function is affected deleteriously by bronchoconstriction, which occurs in allergic reactions and asthma. These conditions may hamper or prevent vocal performance unless recognized and treated promptly. Bronchodilators can be used to counteract the bronchoconstrictive effects of such environmental factors as house dust, pollen, other inhalant allergens, and common air pollutants produced by our increasingly industrialized society. Bronchodilators often are used to treat patients with reactive airway disease, although inhaled bronchodilators may produce chronic laryngitis, as discussed previously. Clinically, inhaled cromolyn sodium (Intal, Pfizer, Inc., New York, New York) appears to cause fewer problems than most of the other inhalant bronchodilators commonly used in the treatment of asthma. The bronchodilator used most often is epinephrine and its related compounds, including xanthines (aminophylline is an example). In professional voice users, the author (RTS) favors asthma management primarily with oral medications and minimal inhaler use, as discussed in Chapter 46 in greater detail.

Cystic fibrosis is an autosomal recessive disorder in which systemic dysfunction of the exocrine glands causes excessive mucus production in the airways and reduced pulmonary function. Dornase alfa (Pulmozyme, Genenctech, Inc., San Franscisco, California), an enzyme used in the treatment of cystic fibrosis, has been reported to cause sore throat, hoarseness and other voice alterations, laryngitis, and chest pain.[49] However, these side effects are not severe and generally will subside without adjustment of dosage.

## Beta-Blockers

Propranolol (Inderal, Akrimax Pharmaceuticals, Cranford, New Jersey) and other beta-blockers have been used successfully in the treatment of hypertension, cardiac tachyarrhythmias, and migraine headaches. Beta-blockers also have been used to treat stage fright. British investigators[50] found that instrumental musicians given propranolol did, in fact, exhibit less anxiety during performance; however, a significant response was not seen in voice professionals or musicians.

A subsequent study reported that propranolol, given for preperformance anxiety, lessened anxiety and also produced an increase in salivation.[51] This investigation was conducted by measuring the weight increase in saliva-saturated dental rolls of cotton placed in the mouth during performance. This indicated that the problem of upper respiratory tract secretion dryness had been avoided and that some of the parasympathomimetic effects of performance anxiety had been negated.

Today, laryngologists generally agree that these drugs should not be used by singers or other voice professionals. Beta-blockers are potentially dangerous because they can slow the heart rate, decrease blood pressure, and cause bronchospasm that can trigger asthma attacks in susceptible patients. In addition, when given in doses sufficient to ameliorate stage fright, they produce a lackluster performance.[15] Any professional voice user who requires an ingested substance to perform the daily activities of his or her chosen profession is manifesting a more significant psychological problem and should be referred for appropriate counseling and treatment and not merely medicated.

## Neurologic Medications

Professional voice users may be diagnosed with a neurologic disease during evaluation of their voice complaint or have a coexisting illness. A number of highly potent medications are used in the medical management of neurologic disorders. The side effects of some of these medications and/or the course of the illness itself may ultimately force the end of a performance career or, at the very least, require significant modifications. Some of the most common neurologic diseases and the medications used to treat them are discussed. Parkinson's disease is treated with medications having anticholinergic properties such as L-dopa (and L-dopa in combination with other agents), dopamine receptor agonists, and monamine oxidase inhibitors (MAOIs). Parkinsonian syndrome, not secondary to Parkinson's disease, may also be a focus of treatment with these drugs.

The MAOIs are also used in the treatment of depression. However, many other drugs used in the treatment of depression also have anticholinergic properties and have been associated with speech disorders, hoarseness, and aphonia.[52,53] Side effects are related to a drug's mechanism of action on the central nervous system and peripheral target organs.[54] Anticholinergic side effects include blurred vision, dryness, impaired urination, constipation, nervousness, dizziness, and drowsiness, as well as confusion, memory loss, headache, hallucinations, and delusions.[55] Side effects most commonly associated with L-dopa are gastrointestinal disturbance, orthostatic hypotension, syncope, oral dryness, blurred vision, and cardiac arrhythmia. Dyskinesias, nightmares, confusion, agitation, psychosis, depression, increased libido, and end-of-dose akinesia have been reported.[55] L-dopa in combination with other agents is used to decrease peripheral and systemic side effects. Amantadine (Symmetrel, Endo Health Solutions, Inc., Malvern, Pennsylvania) used in the treatment of Parkinson's disease is also used as an antiviral drug to treat influenza.

Dopamine receptor agonists can cause gastrointestinal (GI) disturbance, postural hypotension, and fatigue as well as skin rash, headache, involuntary movements, depression, and sometimes confusion or hallucinations.[49]

Myasthenia gravis is an autoimmune disease in which serum antibodies impair synaptic transmission at the neuromuscular junction by disturbance of the neurotransmitter acetylcholine.[56] Pyridostigmine bromide (Mestinon, Valeant Pharmaceuticals International, Inc., Bridgewater, New Jersey) is used to treat myasthenia. Mestinon enhances the action of acetylcholine by inhibiting the enzyme acetylcholinesterase. Excessive salivation and gastrointestinal disturbances are common side effects of acetylcholinesterase inhibitors. Skin rash, nervousness, confusion, or weakness is also reported. Attention deficit disorder (ADD) is a commonly diagnosed medical problem that affects children and adults. Once the diagnosis is confirmed and symptoms persist, medication is indicated. The medication prescribed most often is methylphenidate hydrochloride (Ritalin, Novartis Pharmaceuticals, Inc., Philadelphia, Pennsylvania). Most of the time, Ritalin, in appropriate doses, does not cause significant voice problems even in singers. However, it may produce a slight tremor that could, theoretically, be audible in singing.

Multiple sclerosis (MS) involves the progressive loss of myelin in white matter adjacent to the ventricles of the brain, optic nerves, brainstem, cerebellum, and spinal cord.[56] Drug therapy aims at reducing the frequency of exacerbations and/or reducing the degree of myelin loss during an attack. Medications are also used to treat associated symptoms such as spasticity, cerebellar dysfunction, and depression.[55] These medications include immunosuppressants such as corticosteroids, adrenocorticotrophic hormone, azothioprine, and cyclophosphamide. Corticosteroid side effects have been previously discussed. Other immunosuppressants may also be used in patients with an inability to tolerate corticosteroids, but these side effects are potentially extremely serious. Beta-interferon (Avonex, Biogen, Weston, Massachusetts) is a potent immunosuppressant given by injection; its side effects include local inflammation, flu-like syndrome, fever, chills, muscle aches, and asthenia. The incidence of these side effects will diminish with continued treatment. The side effects of medications used to treat MS, along with symptoms of the disease, can affect performance but are reported to rarely cause speech disturbance.

## Herbs and Supplements

Over the past decade or so, more and more individuals, including singers, are seeking alternatives to medications in the form of herbs and dietary supplements. Many common herbs have potential side effects for voice users; additionally, some herbs should never be taken by anyone because of potentially severe consequences. Some are highlighted in Table 15–4, and selected substances are summarized in greater detail in Table 15–5. In addition, it is helpful to be familiar with some of the most common dietary supplements and their intended usage (Table 15–6).

These dietary supplements are not to be considered prevention, treatment, or cure for any medical problem. Some supplements are dangerous. For example, glucosamine, which is extracted from shellfish, should not be taken by individuals with shellfish allergy. The ingredients of all supplements must be studied carefully, and patients should be encouraged to discuss the use of dietary supplements with their physician before using them. Nevertheless, their use is ubiquitous.

**Table 15–4.** Herbal Medications and Their Common Risks

| Herbal Medications | Risks Associated With Use |
| --- | --- |
| Chaparral, Coltsfoot, Comfrey | Potential for hepatotoxicity |
| Cowslip | Anticoagulation activity (salicylates) |
| Dong quai | Anticoagulation activity (Coumadin), and alteration in hormonal activity |
| Dandelion | Diuretic, dehydration |
| Echinacea | Can be immunosuppressive if used >8 weeks continuously; also may induce allergic response |
| Elder | Diuretic activity, dehydration |
| Ephedra (Ma Huang) | Stimulant, potential for seizures, HTN (hypertension), death |
| Fennel | Anticoagulation activity (Coumadin) |
| Feverfew | Anticoagulation activity, diuretic activity |
| Garlic, Ginger, and Ginkgo | Anticoagulation activity (inhibition of platelet aggregation) |
| Goldenseal | May elevate blood pressure, and cause allergic responses |
| Jack-in-the-pulpit | Anticoagulation activity |
| Licorice root | Hormonal activity (estrogen/progesterone); also a steroid and antidiuretic, capable of inducing a cushingoid syndrome/hypertension |
| Melatonin | Used by many as a sleep aid; it has hormonal activity and can also cause immune dysregulation |
| Nettles | Diuretic activity |
| Primrose | Anticoagulation activity (salicylates), hormonal activity |
| Red Root | Anticoagulation activity |
| Vitamin E | Taken in megadoses (4000 IU or greater), it has anticoagulation activity (antiplatelet) |
| Willow bark | Anticoagulation activity (salicylates) |
| Yam | Hormonal activity (potent progesterone) |
| Yohimbe | Hormonal activity (androgen/testosterone) |

**Table 15–5.** Herbal Products

| Common Name | Scientific Name | Uses | Adverse Reactions | Comments |
|---|---|---|---|---|
| **Ginkgo**, Maidenhair tree | *Ginkgo, Ginkgo biloba* | Memory, and concentration, intermittent claudication, Alzheimer's, altitude sickness | Bleeding, GI upset, headache, palpations, restlessness, nausea, vomiting | Avoid using it with blood thinning medication (eg, Coumadin, aspirin), insulin, thiazide diuretics, antidepressants, antipsychotics |
| **Echinacea**, Purple coneflower, Black Sampson | *Echinacea purpura, E. pallida, E. angustifolia* | Common cold, upper respiratory infections (flu) | Liver damage; initially, it stimulates the immune system; after 8 weeks may be immunosuppressive | Avoid using it with liver toxic drugs (methotrexate), calcium channel blockers, (verapamil), anti-anxiety drugs (valium), steroids (prednisone), patients with autoimmune disease (eg, HIV/AIDS); cross-allergenicity (eg, daisies, ragweed, marigolds) |
| **St John's Wort**, SJW, Amber, Goatweed, Klamath weed | *Hypericum perforatum* | Antidepressant, seasonal affective disorder (SAD), anxiety | Insomnia, anxiety, GI upset, vivid dreams, fatigue, photosensitivity, intermenstrual bleeding | Avoid using SJW with herbal or prescription products until you are aware of the adverse reactions and interactions of these medications (refer to text) |
| **Ephedra**, Ma Huang | *Ephedra sinica* | Reduce weight, enhance physical performance | Heart attacks, strokes, seizures, hypertension, death | Avoid its use; Ephedra may be fatal |
| **Valerian**, Phu, Garden heliotrope | Valeriana officinalis | Sedative-hypnotic, anxiolytic[81] | Morning drowsiness[82] | Can cause additive effects with alcohol, and other medications that have sedative properties |
| **Ginseng**, Korean and American ginseng | *Panax ginseng* (Korean); *Panax quinque-folium* (American) | Improves cognitive function[83]; lowers fasting blood glucose[84] | Agitation, insomnia nervousness; estrogenic effects may cause vaginal bleeding | Avoid using with caffeine, blood thinning, and antidiabetic medications |
| **Saw Palmetto**, Dwarf palm tree | Serenoa repens | Benign prostatic hypertrophy (BPH) | Infrequently, GI upset, an instance of intraoperative hemorrhage | Improves urinary symptoms of BPH with fewer side effects[85] compared to the drug finasteride (Proscar); use cautiously if at all with blood thinning medication |
| **Horse Chestnut** (seed) | *Aesculus hippocastanum* | Chronic venous insufficiency (CVI), varicose veins | GI upset, kidney toxicity[86] | Useful for CVI[87]; avoid use with blood thinning medication; monitor glucose levels in diabetic patients |

*continues*

**Table 15–5.** *continued*

| Common Name | Scientific Name | Uses | Adverse Reactions | Comments |
|---|---|---|---|---|
| **Pycnogenol**, Pine bark extract | *Pinus maritime, P. pinaster* | CVI, varicose veins,[88] diabetic and other retinopathies | None reported | Reduces edema by decreasing capillary permeability |
| **Milk Thistle** | *Silybum marianum* | Cirrhosis of the liver, hepatitis, jaundice, liver poisoning (eg, mushroom poisoning) | Occasional laxative effects | A member of the daisy family, the German E Commission (comparable to FDA in the United States) has approved its use for liver disorders as noted here under "use" |
| Garlic | *Allium sativum* | Lowers LDH (low density lipoprotein) and cholesterol[89] | Halitosis, GI upset | Can increase the risk of bleeding; therapeutic effect is modest compared to other cholesterol-lowering drugs |
| **Kava**, Kava-Kava | *Piper methysticum* | Stress, anxiety disorders[90] | Liver toxicity, gastrointestinal (GI) upset, headache, dizziness | Avoid using it; several European governments have banned its use; especially harmful in combination with liver toxic drugs, sedatives, sleeping pills, alcohol, levodopa (Parkinson's disease) |

## Complementary, Alternative, and Integrative Medicine

Millions of Americans spend billions of dollars annually on complementary alternative medicine (CAM), and many of these are herbal products. Some CAM herbal preparations are useful, others have no proven efficacy. Some are safe, others are potentially harmful. The quality of the product may vary from one manufacturing company to another. Occasionally, the ingredients listed on the label do not correspond to the product in the bottle. The recommended dosage is not uniformly agreed on, and the manufacturers of herbal products are not regulated sufficiently at this time. Some singers and other voice patients use CAM indiscriminately; and it behooves them, their teachers, and their health care providers to become familiar with the potential benefits and risks of taking complementary and alternative remedies.

*Complementary* medicine uses therapies "along with" conventional medicine (eg, the use of massage for low back pain "along with" muscle relaxants). *Alternative* medicine uses therapies "in place"

of conventional medicine (eg, homeopathy to treat rheumatoid arthritis or the unsuccessful attempt to treat cancer with laetrile). *Integrative* medicine incorporates proven effective outcomes of CAM with conventional medicine.

CAM is not limited to herbal products. Homeopathy uses principles of similars and dilutions. Similars work on the concept that if a specific substance causes symptoms in a healthy person similar to that of an ill patient, that substance can be used to cure the sick individual ("like cures like"). Dilutions use the principle that small doses "stimulate" a beneficial immune response or "vital force" in the body.

Traditional Chinese medicine incorporates acupuncture and herbal remedies. Chiropractors and osteopaths use manipulation techniques. Some CAM practitioners utilize massage, hypnosis, biofeedback, or meditation; others use prayer and spirituality, energy, or naturopathy as well as a host of other modalities.

The field of alternative and complementary medicine is vast. As of December 2016, the online research resource PubMed of the National Library of Medi-

**Table 15–6.** Other Natural Products

| Other Natural Products | What They Are Used For |
|---|---|
| Supplements<br>Glucosamine<br>Chondroitin<br>Calcium<br>Vitamin D<br>Sam-e<br>Ipriflavone | Bones and joints |
| Herbals<br>Ginkgo biloba<br>Ginseng<br>Niacin<br>Folic acid<br>Riboflavin<br>Zinc<br>Copper<br>Vitamin $B_6$ and $B_{12}$ | Memory and mental acuity |
| Stanol Esters<br>Garlic<br>Vitamin B complex<br>Folic acid, E, D, and K<br>Calcium | Control cholesterol and healthy heart |
| Isoflavones<br>Black cohosh (botanical) | Supplements menopause symptoms |
| For men: Herbals<br>Jujube dates, Ginseng, Ginkgo biloba;<br>Amino acids—Arginine Alanine, Lysine,<br>Glutamic acid, Vitamins, B-Vitamins | Sex drive and function |
| For Women: Herbals<br>Wild Yam, Chaste Berry, Avena Sativa,<br>Vitamin E | Sex drive and function |

cine (https://www.ncbi.nlm.nih.gov/pubmed/) cites more than 26 million publications, abstracts, or full articles. The challenge is to weed out the useful from the useless and the safe from the dangerous.

Herbal products come from plants that have been investigated for their biochemical composition and potential use as medication. The distinction between herbal products and conventional drugs is gradually being obliterated. All biochemical products are potential poisons. The side effects of medications, although usually minor, may at times be disabling, devastating, or even fatal, whether it is an herbal product or conventional drug. When one introduces a foreign substance into the body, there is the potential for an adverse reaction. Singers take herbal products for a variety of reasons, and many erroneously equate "natural" with safe and effective.

## Quality Control and Product Regulation

Pharmaceutical companies must go through several phases before their drugs can be sold to the public. The safety, effectiveness, and side effects of the product must meet premarket standards of the FDA.

In contrast, when Congress passed the 1994 Dietary Supplement Health and Education Act (DSHEA), CAM manufacturers were allowed to put their products on the market without quality control standards. This "free ride" is now being challenged by the FDA, which proposed regulations regarding the purity, quality, and strength of the products (recommended daily doses).[57]

The FDA has documented cases of supplements that have been contaminated with lead, instances in which the declared amount of an ingredient (isoflavone) was lacking by 50%, probiotics, lacking by 99%, and an instance in which the strength of a product (niacin) had been increased by a factor of 10, resulting in nausea, vomiting, heart attack, and liver damage before the manufacturer recalled the product.[57] Contamination of herbal products has occurred with microorganisms (eg, *Staphylococcus aureus*), heavy metals (ie, lead, mercury, arsenic), radioactive agents (I-131), pesticides (DDT), microbial toxins (bacterial endotoxins), other plants (digitalis, belladonna), and fumigation agents (ethylene oxide) and adulterated with analgesics, diuretics, nonsteroidal antiinflammatory medication, and steroids.[58]

Until better labeling and manufacturing controls are put in place, one must be especially diligent about purchasing supplements and herbal products from reputable companies with standardized formulations. The FDA has proposed rules regarding the labeling and manufacturing of supplements and herbal products; it has not addressed the question of safety and efficacy of these preparations, yet.

## Herbal Products

Hundreds of herbal products (alone or in combination) are marketed in the United States. CAM manufacturers are not allowed legally to claim their product cures or prevents disease, but they can and have claimed that products boost the immune system, burn fat, enhance stamina and energy, stimulate mental function, fight fatigue, improve memory, elevate mood, fight osteoporosis, and many other assertions. Below (and in Table 15–6) are selective considerations of herbal products.

### Kava

Kava, also known as Kava-Kava, is derived from the plant *Piper methysticum,* and is a member of the piper family, a plant native to the South Pacific islands. People use kava to treat restlessness, and to reduce stress and anxiety. Studies support the effectiveness of kava for short-term use (1–8 weeks) for anxiety disorders.[59,60] Kava's ingredients, known as kavalactones, have an anxiolytic (calming) and sedative effect.

One of the problems with kava is that it can cause unpredictable, severe liver damage, which has required liver transplants in several patients.[61,62] Hepatitis, cirrhosis, and liver failure have been reported, as well as adverse effects including jaundice (yellowing of the skin), gastrointestinal upset,

and impaired motor reflexes. Of paramount concern, the use of kava has been implicated in deaths due to liver toxicity.

Some countries have limited its distribution or banned its use (Switzerland, Germany, Canada). If one cannot ascertain a set dosage for kava or the mechanism by which it is broken down in the body, the consumption of products containing kava poses an unacceptable health risk, and it should be avoided. Certainly, the health risk is heightened in patients with liver problems or those who use drugs, herbs, or products with effects or side effects similar to kava. For example, antihistamines, sedatives, alcohol, sleeping pills, St. John's wort, ginseng, and chamomile are among the substances that can heighten drowsiness, as well as place one more at risk for liver damage.

### Ginkgo Biloba

The ginkgo tree, which comes from China, Korea, and Japan, has been around for more than two hundred million years, can live more than one thousand years, and is considered by some to be one of the wonders of the world, a "living fossil."[63] Extracts of the gingko leaves contain active ingredients such as flavonoids, terpenoids that have antioxidant and anticoagulant (blood thinning) properties. The majority of studies indicate that gingko is likely to be effective in helping concentration and memory and can help circulation for "intermittent claudication" (pain in the lower legs after walking due to vascular insufficiency).

The usual dose of ginkgo can cause palpations, gastrointestinal episodes, headache, and other side effects. Large doses can cause nausea, vomiting, and restlessness. One of the most worrisome, potential side effects of gingko is excessive spontaneous bleeding. There have been reports of spontaneous brain hemorrhage, and excessive postoperative bleeding associated with gingko use.[64–66] These are rare occurrences, but potentially devastating.

It is conceivable that inappropriate use of ginkgo in singers could be a contributing factor in vocal fold hemorrhage, particularly in combination with anticlotting products such as aspirin, nonsteroidal antiinflammatory drugs (NSAIDs), Coumadin, or other herbs such as garlic, ginger, or ginseng. Ginkgo extract can alter blood glucose levels. Therefore, in diabetic patients using insulin, glucose monitoring should be done more frequently.[67] Ginkgo may reduce the effectiveness of seizure medications and should be used cautiously or avoided totally in patients prone to seizures disorders.[68] Ginkgo might interfere with fertility and generally should not be used by couples who are trying to conceive.[69] People taking thiazide, a diuretic, should avoid using gingko leaves because it can increase blood pressure.[70]

## Echinacea

Echinacea is a perennial herb that is native to the United States. *Echinacea purpura* is the plant most frequently used for research and herbal treatment. People use this American purple coneflower to treat upper respiratory infections, influenza, and the common cold, as well as a myriad of other conditions.[71] Echinacea seems to be most effective in reducing the duration and severity of certain symptoms of the common cold or influenza if it is taken when symptoms first appear and continued for 7 to 10 days. Certain allergic patients should avoid taking echinacea, particularly if they are allergic to ragweed, marigolds, daisies, chrysanthemums, or chamomile.

Echinacea, in the short term, can have a stimulating effect on the immune system. However, if it is used for more than 8 weeks, it may suppress the immune system and may cause liver damage.[72] Because echinacea might stimulate the autoimmune system, it should be avoided in individuals with autoimmune disorders such as multiple sclerosis, rheumatoid arthritis, and perhaps patients with HIV/AIDS.[73] If a patient has liver problems or is taking medications that potentially can cause liver toxicity such as methotrexate (a chemotherapeutic agent that is sometimes used for rheumatoid arthritis and autoimmune ear disease), he or she should avoid taking echinacea.

## St John's Wort

St John's wort is an herb with yellow flowers derived from *Hypericun perforatum*, which is cultivated in the United States, Africa, Asia, and Europe. In the Middle Ages, people used St John's wort to cast out evil spirits for afflictions such as mental illness. Wort, not to be confused with "wart," comes from the old English *wyrt*, meaning plant. One explanation for the plant's common name is that its flowers typically blossom around June 24, the birthday of St John the Baptist. However, there are other folklore explanations for its name.

St John's wort is as effective as traditional antidepressant medication with fewer side effects for mild to moderate depression[74] and for seasonal affective disorder (SAD), a depression peaking in the fall/winter and declining during the spring/summer when there is more sunlight.

The side effects of St John's wort, although uncommon, include insomnia, dry mouth, upset stomach, fatigue, dizziness, photosensitivity (hypersensitivity to light), and headache. This herb should be used cautiously with other antidepressants such as nefazodone (Serzone, Bristol-Myers Squibb Co., Philadelphia, Pennsylvania), sertraline (Zoloft, Pfizer Inc., New York, New York), or paroxetine (Paxil, Apotex Corp., Toronto, Ontario), because it might cause serotonin syndrome, a serious complication resulting in an increase in serotonin levels that may result in hypertension, extreme anxiety, tachycardia (increase in heart rate), confusion, and coma.[75] The herb may reduce the therapeutic effect of digitalis, decrease the concentration of oral contraceptives causing breakthrough bleeding and possibly pregnancy, and decrease the concentration of protease inhibitors and medications used for HIV/AIDS patients. It should be avoided with tetracycline, sulfa, and quinolones (eg, Cipro); because in combination with these drugs, it can contribute to an increased sensitivity to sunlight with resultant dermatitis, inflamed mucous membranes, and oral blistering. The interaction of St John's wort with certain amino acids, for example, tyramine-containing foods (red wine, chocolate, cheese, eggs) and tryptophan (cottage cheese, beef liver, fish, peanuts), might cause a hypertensive crisis.[76] People with hypertension should be especially alert to these interactions of St John's wort.

## Ephedra, Ma Huang

Ephedra, also called Ma Huang, comes principally from *Ephedra sinica*, a shrub-like plant that is native to China. It should be distinguished from the alkaloid-free American ephedra or Mormon tea, which does not have either the toxicity or therapeutic effects of ephedra.

For thousands of years, the Chinese have used ephedra in pill or tea form for asthma, cough, and the common cold. Today, ephedra is used most commonly to lose weight and to improve physical performance. It is clinically related to amphetamine (speed) and is found in a variety of products. Aspiring singers may use it to lose weight. A milder form of ephedra, pseudoephedrine, is found in many decongestants, cold, and cough medicines.

Side effects from ephedra are not infrequent and can be life threatening. It has been linked to heart attacks, hypertension, stroke, and seizures; and some such incidents have occurred in young professional athletes. Ephedra can constrict blood vessels, increase heart rate, and cause thermogenesis (elevation of the body temperature) and heat stroke. It has been associated with personality changes and dependency after long-term use.[77,78]

The interaction of ephedra with caffeinated drinks can increase the side effects of nervousness, insomnia, and dizziness. It can make some steroids less effective, elevate blood glucose, and should be avoided in patients with conditions such as angina, anxiety, heart disease, hypothyroidism, hypertension, and urinary retention (eg, patients with enlarged prostates).

The FDA has received hundreds of reports linking ephedra or ephedrine use to serious side effects including deaths. Until better guidelines are formulated, it is best to avoid ephedra products.

## Common Vocal Remedies—What Are They and Do They Really Work?

Other common vocal remedies used commonly by singers have been reviewed by the authors elsewhere.[79] The information is included here, with permission.

Herbal medicine, or botanical medicine, has a rich and ancient history, featured prominently in the healing arts of numerous civilizations over thousands of years. Seeds, berries, flowers, leaves, roots, and bark have been used traditionally in the treatment of many common and uncommon health conditions, including asthma, allergy, migraine, irritable bowel syndrome, menstrual disorders, cancer, and the common cold, among others. In 2008, the World Health Organization reported that the annual market for herbal medicines is nearly $60 billion.[80] As more and more is invested into development and marketing of these products, more and more people are trying them. Among these are professional and avocational singers.

The voice is a delicate instrument, sensitive to dryness and inflammation from the environment, allergens, irritants, reflux, and infection. A number of herbal products are marketed to singers to help prevent and reduce hoarseness, dryness, laryngitis, inflammation, and cough, while providing lubrication of the mucosa and improved voice quality. This chapter reviews the efficacy and safety of 7 of the most popular herbal products marketed to singers (Throat Coat, Entertainer's Secret Spray, Vocal Eze Throat Spray, Thayer's Cherry Lozenges, Vocal Zone Pastilles, Vitavocal Throat and Voice Enhancer, Sprout's Voice Remedy) and 2 home voice remedies (singer's tea recipe and singer's gargle).

The effects of herbal remedies have not been researched adequately and are thus poorly understood.

The FDA, which is responsible for ensuring that all drugs brought to market are both safe and effective, does not endorse or regulate the sale of herbal preparations. Many of the claimed effects of herbal remedies have not faced the same rigorous scrutiny that prescription medications have, including extensive preclinical and clinical trials prior to approval. Although many herbal products contain agents that provide health benefits and alleviate symptoms, they cannot be marketed as medicines. Therefore, all herbal preparations must be marketed as "dietary supplements," and it is not acceptable to make specific health claims about these supplements.[81]

In Germany, different requirements and standards exist for the regulation and control of herbal supplements. The German government's Commission E evaluated and approved hundreds of herbal products found to be reasonably safe and effective. Products that have been approved by Commission E provide information about potential treatment options for a wide array of illnesses. In the United States, the National Institutes of Health is carrying out an increasing number of well-controlled clinical trials evaluating herbal medications and supplements. Until a more substantial body of evidence develops focusing on herbal preparations, it is important to be cautious when interpreting claims that herbal remedy companies may make about their products.[82,83]

### Throat Coat

Throat Coat, marketed by the company Traditional Medicinals (Sebastopol, California), is an herbal tea containing 4 main ingredients: licorice root (760 mg), slippery elm bark (60 mg), marshmallow root (60 mg), and licorice root dry aqueous extract (60 mg). It also contains a proprietary blend (1040 mg) of wild cherry bark, bitter fennel fruit, Saigon cinnamon bark, and sweet orange peel. A proprietary blend is a mix of ingredients listed together in decreasing quantities. As such, consumers do not know the actual amount of each of these individual ingredients.[84]

Licorice root (*Glycyrrhiza glabra*) is a demulcent. In Germany, it is prescribed to relieve inflammation of the airway mucus membranes. It is used in China for treatment of bronchitis, pharyngitis, laryngitis, peptic ulcers, asthma, malaria, abdominal pain, insomnia, and infections.[85,86] It has been shown to have estrogenic, aldosterone-like, cortisol-like (anti-inflammatory), antiallergic, antibacterial, antiviral, antihepatotoxic, anticancer, expectorant, and antitussive properties.[86-88] The FDA recognizes licorice and its derivatives, such as glycyrrhizin, to be safe for use in foods. Many different numbers have been quoted as the safest maximum dose based on small clinical trials. Caution should be advised to people who ingest more than 60 to 70 grams per day of licorice root or more than 2 mg/kg per day (150 mg for a 75 kg person) of the extracted active compound, glycyrrhizinic acid.[89] Because of the aldosterone-like effects, high doses for extended periods of time can cause elevated blood pressure and low potassium. Licorice should be avoided or used with caution in people with hypertension, kidney failure, digitalis use, diuretic use, or antihypertensive use. People on oral hypoglycemic drugs or insulin should monitor blood glucose levels carefully.[86]

Slippery elm bark (*Ulmus rubra* or *Ulmus fulva*) is another demulcent often used to relieve symptoms of pharyngitis.[85] To the best of our knowledge, there have been no clinical trials evaluating the efficacy of slippery elm in the treatment of upper respiratory tract pathology. The most remarkable trials of slippery elm have been in patients with breast cancer. However, oncologists have recommended against using slippery elm bark, in the form of Essiac (Essiac Canada International, Fredericton, New Brunswick, Canada), because it lacks efficacy and may delay beneficial medical treatment if patients rely on it to the exclusion of proven allopathic treatments.[90,91]

Marshmallow root (*Althaea officinalis*) is another demulcent used often for dry cough and pharyngitis symptoms.[85] The main antitussive and emollient effects are attributed to the root's polysaccharide component, which forms a protective coating over the mucosa, decreasing irritation and the cough reflex.[92] Commission E approved its use in cough and bronchitis. Average daily doses of 6 grams of root, 5 grams of leaf, and 10 grams of syrup are believed to be safe.[93]

To date, there has been one clinical trial comparing Throat Coat to a placebo tea for symptomatic relief of pharyngitis. The trial included a total of sixty subjects. Thirty patients used Throat Coat 4 to 6 times per day, while the other 30 used placebo tea. Throat Coat use led to a statistically significant decrease in pain on swallowing and total pain compared to placebo. The pain relief was immediate and lasted at least 30 minutes. There were no serious adverse effects from drinking 4 to 6 cups of Throat Coat each day. Overall, Throat Coat, taken as recommended on the label, is safe and effective in transiently alleviating symptoms of pharyngitis.[85] This trial did not attempt to address whether Throat Coat shortens the duration of pharyngitis. Throat Coat is unlikely to shorten the duration of viral or bacterial pharyngitis, and if bacterial pharyngitis is confirmed, one should still be treated with an antibiotic to prevent sequelae

of a Group A Streptococcal infection (eg, rheumatic fever/heart disease and poststreptococcal glomerulonephritis), as well as other potential complications of bacterial infection.

**Entertainer's Secret Spray**

Entertainer's Secret Spray (Entertainer's Secret, Carmel, Indiana) is a combination of carboxymethycellulose, aloe vera gel, and glycerin in a mixture of dibasic sodium phosphate and potassium chloride. The first three of these ingredients act as lubricants to moisten, clean, and coat the mucosa on which it is sprayed. The latter 2 ingredients generate the hypertonicity of the spray, for which it is marketed.[94] Hypertonicity refers to a solution that has a higher concentration of solutes than a reference solution. Water will flow from a region of low tonicity (hypotonicity) to a region of high tonicity (hypertonicity). Hypertonic spray is therefore presumed to be beneficial in moistening any area of the mouth, throat, or vocal folds that the spray contacts.

To the authors' knowledge, there has been one clinical trial evaluating the effects of Entertainer's Secret on the voice. The trial compared the effects of mannitol, sterile water, and Entertainer's Secret on lowering the phonation threshold pressure (PTP) in 18 healthy women who were nonsingers. The PTP is the minimum pressure needed to initiate vocal fold oscillation, and it has been used in a number of studies to assess the respiratory effort needed to produce sound. At one point, it was assumed that a decrease in PTP correlates with decreased phonatory effort and more efficient phonation. It was also assumed that dryness of the larynx secondary to decreased water content increases the viscosity of mucus and resistance to airflow, thus increasing PTP. However, numerous studies in the past 10 years have shown varying effects of desiccation on the PTP. In this trial, subjects were given 1 of the 3 treatment options each week through a nebulizer, which allows the medication to be delivered to the respiratory system as a mist. The PTP was measured 15 minutes prior to treatment, immediately before treatment, and 5, 20, 35, and 50 minutes following treatment. The results of this study showed that only mannitol decreased the PTP at 5 minutes, but the PTP returned to baseline by 20 minutes. Water was shown to lower the PTP at 5 minutes, but this was not deemed statically significant. Water also showed a rebound increase in PTP for the remainder of the study. Entertainer's Secret showed an oscillating pattern of increasing and decreasing PTP at the recorded times, but the PTP was never significantly reduced from baseline.[95]

Mannitol, is an osmotic agent, and the proposed mechanism of action is that it pulls water into the larynx for lubrication. Sterile water, through the nebulizer, may either have no effect on an already healthy voice, or it may be absorbed rapidly because it is hypo-osmolar (less concentrated) relative to the tissue, causing dryness.[95] Entertainer's Secret has both lubricating properties and potential osmotic properties. However, the actual measured osmolality of Entertainer's Secret is not shared on their website, so it is unclear if it would be hyper- or hypo-osmotic relative to the tissue in the body.

Although this study showed that only mannitol transiently but significantly decreases the PTP, there are many weakness of the study. First, it did not assess the participant's perceived phonatory effort, which may be more relevant than simply measuring the PTP. Furthermore, it was performed only in a handful of healthy, young women. The results from this study may vary in a larger population including men, varying ages, and people with pathology. Also, Entertainer's Secret is taken normally as an oral spray, not as a nebulized treatment. The assumption of Roy et al was that a nebulizer would be more effective in delivering medicine to the larynx than an oral spray.[95] However, the product may still be beneficial to singers by lubricating the mouth and pharynx.

**Vocal Eze Throat Spray**

Vocal Eze Throat Spray (multiple manufacturers), like many other similar products, is endorsed by famous vocalists and is a proprietary blend of many herbal products. As a proprietary blend, it is not required to document the amount of each active ingredient. It includes marshmallow root, Osha root, licorice root, Echinacea purpurea root, propolis, Echinacea purpurea flower, ginger root, *Echinacea angustifolia* root, and *Echinacea purpurea* seed. It also contains Aloe vera gel, vegetable glycerin, wildflower honey, natural flavors, and spring water.[96] While there has been a substantial amount of research on Echinacea and licorice root, some of its other ingredients are discussed less thoroughly in the literature. There are no studies known to the authors evaluating the efficacy of Vocal Eze.

Native American populations commonly use Osha root for the treatment of respiratory illnesses. It has been shown to have antimicrobial, antiviral, antiinflammatory, sedative, spasmolytic, and vasodilatory properties.[97,98] It is used as a remedy for cough, sore throat, indigestion, headache, sinusitis, wounds, arthritis, cancer, and angina.[98] However, clinical evidence supporting its use is lacking.

Ginger root (multiple manufacturers) has been studied in numerous in vitro, animal, and human studies. Ginger has been shown to have antiemetic, antiinflammatory, antiplatelet aggregation, antidiabetic, and analgesic effects.[99–101] Interestingly, ginger root also has been found to have antiviral properties against human respiratory syncytial virus in human respiratory tract cells.[102] However, human trials are lacking, and results have been inconsistent.[101,103] While there is some evidence of these effects in humans, there is not enough evidence to fully support ginger as a treatment for any disease from the medical perspective. Commission E approved the use of ginger for loss of appetite, travel sickness, and dyspepsia. Chinese and Indian medicine use ginger to treat colds and pharyngitis.[99] The lethal dose in mice is extremely high, which can be extrapolated to also be very high in humans. Thus, while ginger's clinical efficacy is questionable, it is considered safe when taken at the recommended doses.

Echinacea (multiple manufacturers) is used widely for the treatment of the common cold and is discussed elsewhere in this chapter. It is the second top-selling herbal product in the United States. Echinacea may work by modulating the immune system or through antiinflammatory and antiviral effects. In 2014, a Cochrane review was published analyzing Echinacea verses placebo for the prevention and treatment of the common cold. The preparations used in different trials varied and were therefore not comparable. Also, the methods for assessing outcomes varied greatly from trial to trial. With this in mind, the Cochrane review concluded that a variety of Echinacea products might be able to reduce healthy people's risk of catching a cold. However, the overall evidence supporting Echinacea for the treatment of cold is clinically weak.[104]

Propolis (multiple manufacturers) is a waxy mixture of substances from plants, buds, and exudates made by honeybees to seal their hives. Historically, it has been used to embalm cadavers, seal violin cracks, heal wounds, treat sore throat, and disinfect the mouth. Today, it is a remedy used for the treatment of upper respiratory tract infections, wounds, burns, acne, herpes simplex, and neurodermatitis. It also is utilized in dental hygiene to prevent caries and to treat gingivitis and stomatitis. It is composed of resins, waxes, oils, pollen, and organic compounds. Hundreds of different compounds are identified in different samples. It has been reported to have antioxidant, antibacterial, antiinflammatory, and immunomodulatory effects.[105] While there are multiple clinical trials evaluating its effects on the treatment of dental pathologies,[106] there is limited evidence supporting its use in the treatment of cold symptoms. To our knowledge there are no trials evaluating its use as a demulcent or its effects on the voice.

### Thayers Cherry Slippery Elm Lozenges

Vocalists have used Thayers lozenges (Thayers Natural Remedies, Westport, Connecticut) for over 136 years to relieve symptoms of vocal irritation and hoarseness. Each lozenge contains 150 mg of slippery elm bark, contributing to its demulcent effect. Thayers prides itself on having menthol-free products.[107] This is especially important to singers when using remedies to treat a sore throat. Pain is a protective physiologic function. Analgesics like menthol dampen the pain but do not fix the cause. Masking pain permits more stress to be added to an already damaged mucosal surface, which can lead to further and more serious damage. If pain and discomfort are great enough to require an analgesic, serious consideration should be given to cancelling the performance.

### Vocal Zone Pastilles

Marketed by Kestrel Medical Ltd. in Broadstone, United Kingdom, as a formulation for singers, actors, and voice professionals, Vocal Zone Pastilles are a popular option among many celebrities for relieving dry or irritated throats from excessive singing, speaking, or smoking. This product also has a rich and interesting history. In 1907, an otolaryngologist named William Floyd produced a treatment he called "Vocalzone" as a voice remedy for the great Italian opera singer Enrico Caruso. His product gained such popularity that it is (supposedly) still being sold in its original formulation today.[108]

Ingredients in Vocal Zone Pastilles include Levomenthol 1.07%, Peppermint oil 0.54%, and Myrrh Tincture 1.39%, as well as sucrose, glucose, Crystal Tex 85, vegetable oil, liquorice extract, beeswax, and purified water.[108] Peppermint leaves yield a volatile oil that is composed primarily of menthol and menthone. Evidence-based medicine has demonstrated peppermint oil to be beneficial in preventing and relieving intestinal gas, indigestion, and irritable bowel syndrome–related intestinal spasms. This physiologic mechanism is due to smooth muscle relaxation in the gastrointestinal (GI) tract, and thus peppermint oil is contraindicated in conditions such as hiatal hernias, severe gastroesophageal reflux, and gallbladder disorders.[109,110] Further, peppermint oil may cause symptoms of heartburn.[110]

Additionally, peppermint oil has been shown to be effective topically for analgesia and muscle relax-

ation, and in mouthwash to relieve gum inflammation.[111] Commission E approved peppermint oil for relief of the common cold, cough, bronchitis, and inflammation of the mouth and pharynx.[112]

Interestingly, an animal study has shown that peppermint oil has an antispasmodic effect on tracheal smooth muscle in rats. The study found that the mechanism likely involves 2 well-studied chemical mediators that promote bronchial relaxation, nitric oxide and prostaglandin $E_2$, possibly explaining the popular use of peppermint oil in respiratory diseases.[113] Use of peppermint oil should be avoided in children due to potential for asthma-like attacks and possible respiratory failure[112]; however, the dosage used in Vocal Zone is likely too minimal for this to occur.

Myrrh's use in analgesia and wound cleaning dates back over 2000 years, prior to the discovery of morphine.[114] A number of studies have explored the antiinflammatory and analgesic activities of myrrh. Thus, there is support for using myrrh to treat various diseases associated with inflammatory pain, such as rheumatoid arthritis.[115,116] Commission E has also approved myrrh for treatment of conditions involving inflammation of the mouth and pharynx. Unproven uses for myrrh include topical treatment of mild infections of the oral and pharyngeal mucosa and as an expectorant for cough. Myrrh is contraindicated during pregnancy, although there are no known hazardous side effects associated with therapeutic dosages.[117] Those who choose to use this product should do so with caution, as it may mask the protective physiologic response of pain.

### Vita Vocal Throat and Voice Enhancer

Vita Vocal Health (New York, New York) markets their Throat and Voice Enhancer to singers, promising to "assist" in strengthening the voice, enhancing vocal clarity, soothing the throat, minimizing dryness, and preventing vocal fold inflammation. They also claim that it "may help with laryngitis." Like many of the other products discussed in this review, the marketers use words like "assist" and *may* help" to avoid making "guarantees" to their consumers because there are no substantial clinical trials evaluating the efficacy of the product. Throat and Voice Enhancer is taken as 2 capsules, each 400 mg of a proprietary blend of herbs and natural flavors.[118] Many of the herbs in this product have been discussed already, such as Osha root, Echinacea, slippery elm bark, licorice root, and marshmallow root. Additionally, this product contains vitamin $B_{12}$. This is a vitamin that is rarely deficient in an average, healthy, person because the body stores it for very long periods of time. The product label does not provide the consumer with the specific amount of vitamin $B_{12}$. Throat and Voice Enhancer also contains Chamomile, Eucalyptus, and Wild cherry bark for flavoring and its desired soothing effect. However, Eucalyptus can be a laryngeal irritant.

The first ingredient listed on the bottle in Throat and Voice Enhancer is American ginseng root. Many clinical trials have assessed the safety and efficacy of ginseng in preventing cold symptoms. Commission E approved its use for lack of stamina, fatigue, and decreased concentration.[119] In a 227 person trial, Scaglione et al[120] demonstrated that 100 mg of the ginseng extract G15 used daily decreased the incidence and duration of cold symptoms in influenza-vaccinated adults compared to adults who received the vaccine alone. It also increased the amount of antibodies, natural killer cells, and phagocytes in the blood, which are all involved in the immune system. Two similar studies were done in geriatric populations evaluating the extract CVT-E002.[121,122] Influenza-vaccinated volunteers older than 65 years who took 400 mg per day of CVT-E002 for 4 months had decreased incidence and duration of acute respiratory symptoms during November and December.[122] Additionally, doses up to 600 mg 3 times per day of ginseng extract were shown to be safe and well tolerated in children when used for a short period of time.[123]

It is important to point out that these studies evaluating the efficacy of ginseng have used specific doses of specific ginseng *extracts*. The product in question, Throat and Voice Enhancer, contains a total of 400 mg of all its ingredients. As far as the authors of this paper are aware, the ginseng included in Throat and Voice Enhancer is not a specific extract, and the dosage or mechanism of extraction is not known.

### Sprout's Voice Remedy

Sprout's Voice Remedy, manufactured by Kosher Vitamins in Brooklyn, New York, contains slippery elm bark, fennel seed, horseradish root, thyme herb, and celery seed in a proprietary herbal blend. It is advertised as an effective treatment for hoarseness, congestion, and inflammation. It is recommended for use 3 to 4 hours prior to performing or speaking. The product is administered by a dropper that dispels 25 mL in water once to twice per day, or as needed.[124] To our knowledge, no clinical trials investigating the effectiveness of Sprout's in comparison to other voice remedies or placebo have been published. We will therefore focus on uses that have been supported by Commission E.

Slippery elm bark, discussed as an ingredient in other remedies aforementioned, acts as a demulcent and an emollient that is soothing to the alimentary canal.[125]

Fennel seed promotes gastrointestinal motility and is antispasmodic. Two ingredients in fennel seed have been shown to suppress secretions in the respiratory tracts of frogs. Fennel extracts also have been shown to enhance mucociliary clearance, facilitating removal of mucus and preventing pathogen invasion into respiratory epithelium. Commission E approved fennel oil for treatment of cough and bronchitis. Its use is contraindicated in pregnant women and small children.[126]

Horseradish root has antimicrobial, hyperemic, and carcinostatic properties, and is approved by Commission E for cough and bronchitis. Unproven uses for horseradish root include treatment of respiratory tract inflammation and as supportive therapy for respiratory tract infections.[127]

Thyme is a bronchial antispasmodic, expectorant, and antibacterial agent. Commission E approved its use for cough and bronchitis. Though its effectiveness has not been proven, the herb was used initially for thinning upper respiratory tract secretions, asthma, laryngitis, and whooping cough. Externally, it has been used as a mouthwash to treat inflammation of the mouth and throat, although its effectiveness in doing so has not been proven.[128]

Use of celery seed as a cough treatment has been reported, but its effectiveness has not been validated.[129]

### Home Remedies

Many singers use recipes for voice remedies that combine several easy-to-obtain ingredients in the comfort of their own homes. One particular recipe, "Singer's Tea," contains 1 fresh ginger root, 6 ounces of apple juice concentrate, juice from 1 fresh lemon, one-third cup of honey, and one-quarter teaspoon of cayenne pepper. Vocalists may choose to drink Singer's Tea during a rehearsal or recording session. The warm liquid is said to humidify, lubricate, and thin mucosal secretions.

Honey is more than just a sweet spreadable substance produced by bees. Its clinical effectiveness in promoting wound healing has been well established.[130] Honey also has immunomodulatory, antioxidant, and antimicrobial capacities.[131–133] Studies have shown that single-dose treatment with honey was superior to over-the-counter cough medication for treatment of nocturnal childhood cough.[134,135] Another study showed that treatment of persistent postinfectious cough with honey and caffeine was more effective than systemic steroid treatment.[136]

Interestingly, intraoperative administration and post-op consumption of honey after adenotonsillectomy and tonsillectomy in children led to improved healing and decreased use of pain killers.[137] This finding may suggest that swallowing honey may have beneficial effects on inflammation and healing in the upper aerodigestive tract.

Cayenne pepper contains capsaicin, a substance that has vasodilatory, analgesic, and antimicrobial properties. Clinical trials have demonstrated its positive effects on pain modulation as well as its gastroprotective effects. Commission E approved capsaicin for muscular tension and rheumatism. Unproven uses include gargling to treat hoarseness and pharyngitis.[138] Cayenne pepper may relieve symptoms of laryngitis by lessening the pain associated with inflammation and promoting healing by dilating surrounding blood vessels, which enhances diffusion of oxygen and nutrients.

Singer's gargle is another home remedy that contains one-half teaspoon of baking soda, one-half teaspoon of salt, 1 tablespoon of honey, and 8 ounces of warm water. Instructions state to "gargle quietly and gently for two long, boring minutes. Do not rinse and use as often as necessary to help your dry, irritated throat." Of note, gargling has been found to have little proven efficacy, and loud, forceful gargling may be phonotraumatic. Any beneficial effects that a gargle solution contains last only briefly after spitting out the solution. However, if the process does not involve loud and aggressive vocalization, gargling is not likely to be harmful.

Baking soda is sodium bicarbonate, a basic substance that can be used as an antacid. It may buffer and soothe acidic tissues that are present during a cold or due to acid reflux. As an added bonus, baking soda has a teeth whitening effect. However, it is important to exercise caution when using baking soda. Misuse has been reported to cause significant electrolyte and acid-base abnormalities, abdominal pain, vomiting, drowsiness, and lethargy.[139]

## Discussion

Herbal teas, sprays, lozenges, and capsules are extremely popular among singers and performers. Many of the active ingredients in these herbal remedies have been shown to have valuable properties in vitro, in animal studies, and in some human clinical trials. However, the actual amount, potency, and rheological characteristics of the active components in each product are affected by extraction conditions (temperature, time, pH, ratio of water to solid), extraction techniques,[103] and genus type.[140] Without well-controlled clinical trials, it is difficult to assess whether these singing products objectively or subjectively improve the singing voice. At least, according to the current, limited amount of literature, it appears that none of the discussed remedies cause significant harm if used as recommended. Products with possible analgesic effects, such as Vocal Zone pastilles, should be used with caution in vocalists as they can mask pain, possibly leading to injury. Products that may irritate laryngeal mucosa, relax the lower esophageal sphincter, or increase ingested acidity require caution and further study.

While marketed by different companies under different names, the products discussed in this chapter share many of the same ingredients, many of which act in some way as a demulcent. Therefore, a relevant question is whether one form (spray, lozenge, pill, or tea) has an advantage over the others in delivering the active ingredients. Limb et al[141] explored this question using a technique called scintigraphy. In scintigraphy, a radioisotope, such as Technetium-99m, is ingested. The radioisotope emits radiation, which is captured by a camera to assess its location in the body. In the study, lozenges, tablets, spray, and gargle were labeled with Technetium-99m and administered to volunteers. Images were then obtained to localize the radioisotope distribution immediately after lozenge/tablet placement in the mouth, spray followed by swallow, or gargle followed by spit. Images also were obtained at time intervals up to 2 hours post-administration. Limb et al found that a significantly larger percentage of the metered dose was deposited initially in the mouth using a lozenge or tablet. Only 5% of the spray and less of the other formulations was deposited initially in the throat. After 20 minutes, significantly more Technetium-99m from the lozenge remained in the mouth and throat than any other formulation. Over the 2-hour span, the lozenge delivered the most Technetium-99m to the mouth and throat combined. However, the spray delivered more to the throat alone. Both the lozenge and spray showed low, but detectable, levels of Technetium-99m for up to 2 hours postadministration in the mouth and throat. The gargle was by far the least effective in delivering the radioisotope; its presence in the mouth and throat was lost soon after spitting out the solution. Based on this study, a lozenge or spray form of a demulcent would be more effective than a tablet or gargle. The effect of tea would likely be similar to that of a lozenge, but evidence to confirm that speculation is lacking.

The supraglottic larynx, pharynx, palate, oral cavity, nasal cavity, tongue, lips, and sinuses are all part of the conduction system for the voice. Therefore, appropriate moisture and decreased irritation in these regions may make singing more comfortable and improve the quality of the sound. Nasal breathing filters, warms, and humidifies air and therefore should be used whenever possible. The lubricating remedies discussed in this paper may be beneficial in rapidly relieving mucosal dryness that occurs after being exposed to dry air on airplanes, smoke-filled rooms, and artificial fog.

Just as dry mucosa can cause changes in voice quality, copious and viscous mucosal secretions also can cause detrimental changes in the voice. This effect can be caused by foods like milk and chocolate. Spicy foods can irritate the mouth and throat and increase symptoms of reflux laryngitis. Singers should avoid these foods if they experience any of these effects. Vocalists should also remain hydrated to ensure proper lubrication of the laryngeal mucosa. Diuretics, alcohol, caffeine, and fluid loss from vomiting and diarrhea can cause systemic dehydration, which can alter the moisture of the larynx and voice conduction system. None of the products discussed is a substitute for adequate hydration.

It is believed that proper oscillation of the vocal folds requires both adequate systemic hydration and adequate flux of fluid and electrolytes across the laryngeal mucosa to provide a thin, liquid layer of lubricant over the vocal folds. Numerous studies have been published evaluating the vocal effects of hypertonic, hypotonic, and isotonic steam delivered via a nebulizer to healthy, nonsingers.[95,142–146] A nebulizer is a device used to deliver a mist to the larynx and lungs. It is a common method used to deliver asthma medication. These previous small studies showed that inhaled dry air increased the phonatory threshold pressure (PTP) and self-perceived phonatory effort (PPE).[95,142] We have already discussed one study investigating Entertainer's Secret Spray,[95] and here we look at the results of 2 similar studies evaluating the effects in classically trained singers.

The first study assessed the PTP and PPE in 34 classically trained female sopranos. Participants inhaled dry air through the mouth for 15 minutes, followed by nebulized isotonic saline, sterile water (hypotonic), or no treatment. Singers received a different therapy each week. The PTP and PPE were then recorded at time intervals up to 2 hours while singing in the upper passaggio. It was presumed that the upper passaggio is the range most susceptible to surface tissue dehydration. The results showed that PTP did not change significantly following laryngeal desiccation. However, the PPE did increase signifi-

cantly. In the isotonic saline group, the PPE values were near baseline by 5 minutes posttreatment and did return to baseline by 110 minutes. In the sterile water group, the PPE did not return to baseline in the 2-hour period. These results indicate that isotonic saline promotes immediate relief for perceived laryngeal dryness. It appears to act as a lubricant, and because it has the same tonicity, or concentration, of the tissue it does not affect the flow of electrolytes or water. Sterile water is hypotonic relative to the tissue; therefore, water is more likely to move into the tissue causing thickening and drying of the surface fluid. The absence of change in PTP suggests that singers, unlike nonsingers, may be able to compensate for the physiologic changes of laryngeal desiccation. This may have led to the significant increase in the perceived vocal effort (PPE).[147]

The second important study by Tanner et al[148] evaluated the effects of nebulized isotonic saline in young, healthy male singers compared to nonsingers. In both groups, the PTP, a measure of the physiologic response to desiccation, remained unchanged following laryngeal desiccation. Additionally, both groups perceived an increase in vocal effort, mouth dryness, and throat dryness postdesiccation and a decrease postnebulization. However, the self-perceived effects were greater in nonsingers but had shorter duration, whereas the singers reported a smaller increase in vocal effort and dryness, but the effects lasted longer. This suggests that trained vocalists may possess an advantage over nonsingers that allows them to adapt to dry conditions. It is also possible that the expectation of drying effects influenced the rating of self-perceived measures. Finally, the gender difference in self-perceived measures is worth noting. Classically trained female sopranos reported twice the increase in vocal effort post-desiccation, even though the men received dry air for twice the amount of time. This suggests that males may be less susceptible to laryngeal dehydration. It has been postulated that a deeper position of the male larynx in the neck facilitates humidification and warming of the air.[149] Nonetheless, both studies in singers provide evidence that isotonic saline inhalation is beneficial to singers.

All of the products discussed in this review have the potential to provide relief of symptoms. The authors of this paper do not recommend any specific product over another. If desired, performers should experiment with these products and choose the one that provides the desired effect. Above all, singers must listen to their bodies, heed warning signs, avoid masking symptoms, and seek the care and guidance of a laryngologist when vocal health is in question.

## Surgery and Herbal Products

One should avoid herbal medications for at least 14 days prior to surgery according to the American Society of Anesthesiologists.[150] Ginkgo, ginger, ginseng, and garlic can contribute to excessive bleeding. Valerian and kava can potentiate (increase) the sedative effects of anesthetics. Ephedra can provoke hypertension, cardiac irregularities, and temperature elevation. Ginseng can lower blood sugar.[151] Kava and echinacea can cause liver damage, particularly in conjunction with certain anesthetic agents that may also be toxic to the liver. Preoperatively, patients should let their surgeon and anesthesiologist know about "all" of the medications they are taking including all herbal and other CAM products.

## Conclusion

It is essential for laryngologists, nurses, speech-language pathologists, singing voice teachers, vocal coaches, and others involved in caring for professional voice users to be familiar with the potential vocal effects of all ingested substances, including medications. This chapter reviewed only a small number of the pharmacological agents that may affect voice adversely. It is also incumbent on health care providers to educate voice professionals about the action of medications and the potential consequences of drugs (prescription and nonprescription) on the voice, thus enabling individuals to make an informed consent for recommended treatment.

In general, herbal therapies and conventional drugs are safe. Legally, herbs are foods that do not treat or cure disease. However, in the medical world, they are drugs that can help or hurt one's well-being.

Even if the FDA imposes premarket safety and efficacy standards, singers and other voice professionals should take herbal products for the right reasons, at the right time, and from reputable manufacturers who have standardized the formulations of their products. They should let responsible people know what medications they are taking and recognize that at certain times they will be at greater risks compared to others because of the use of these substances.

The side effects, interactions, lack of quality control, and proven effectiveness of some herbal preparations have serious ramifications for professional voice users and the risks may seriously outweigh the benefits. What is on the label may neither work nor be in the bottle. Until more randomized control trials are done to substantiate the safety and usefulness of herbal products, one should use caution in buying supplements.

Singing and acting teachers and laryngologists are in a unique position to influence the behavior of their clients. The examples given above highlight several of the great many herbal products available, and they emphasize the need for all of us who interact with voice performers to be aware of the strengths and limitations of CAM and to educate the singers and other voice professionals under our care.

## References

1. Sataloff RT, Lawrence VL, Hawkshaw M, Rosen DC. Medications and their effects on the voice. In: Benninger MS, Jacobson BH, Johnson AF, eds. *Vocal Arts Medicine: The Care and Prevention of Professional Voice Disorders.* New York, NY: Thieme Medical Publishers; 1994:216–225.

2. Lawrence VL. Common medications with laryngeal effects. *Ear Nose Throat J.* 1987;66(8):318–322.

3. Schiff M. Medical management of acute laryngitis. In: Lawrence VL, ed. *Transcripts of the Sixth Symposium: Care of the Professional Voice.* New York, NY: The Voice Foundation; 1977:99–102.

4. Schiff M. *Comment at the Seventh Symposium: Care of the Professional Voice.* New York, NY: The Juilliard School; 1978.

5. Punt NA. Vocal disabilities of singers. Applied laryngology—singers and actors. *Proc R Soc Med.* 1968;61:1152–1156.

6. Williams AJ, Baghat MS, Stableforth DE, et al. Dysphonia caused by inhaled steroids: recognition of a characteristic laryngeal abnormality. *Thorax.* 1983;38:813–821.

7. Watkin KL, Ewanowski SJ. Effects of aerosol corticosteroids on the voice: triamcinolone acetonide and beclomethasone dipropionate. *J Speech Hear Res.* 1985;28:301–304.

8. Toogood JH, Jennings B, Greenway RW, Chuang L. Candidiasis and dysphonia complicating beclomethasone treatment of asthma. *J Allergy Clin Immunol.* 1980;65(2):145–153.

9. Davies WL, Grunert RR, Haff RF, et al. Antiviral activity of 1-amantanamine (amantadine). *Science.* 1964;144:862–863.

10. McGahen JW, Hoffman CE. Influenza infections of mice. Curative activity of amantadine HCl. *Proc Soc Exp Biol Med.* 1968;129:678–681.

11. Wingfield WL, Pollack D, Grunert RR. Therapeutic efficacy of amantadine-HCl and rumantidine-HCl in naturally occurring influenza A2 respiratory illness in man. *N Engl J Med.* 1969;281:579–584.

12. Council on Drugs. The amantadine controversy. *JAMA.* 1967;201:372–373.

13. Martin FG. Drugs and vocal function. *J Voice*. 1988;2(4): 338–344.

14. *Nursing '89 Drug Handbook*. Springhouse, PA: Springhouse Corporation; 1989:236.

15. Gates GA, Saegert J, Wilson N, et al. Effect of beta-blockade on singing performance. *Ann Otol Rhinol Laryngol*. 1985;94:570–574.

16. Rasmussen L, Oster-Jorgensen E, Qvist N, et al. Short report: a double-blind placebo-controlled trial of omeprazole on characteristics of gastric emptying in healthy subjects. *Aliment Pharmacol Ther*. 1991;5:85–89.

17. Bough ID Jr, Sataloff RT, Castell DO, et al. Gastroesophageal reflux laryngitis resistant to omeprazole therapy. *J Voice*. 1995;9(2):205–211.

18. Lawrence VL. Medical care for professional voice. [Panel.] In: Lawrence VL, ed. *Transcripts from the Annual Symposium: Care of the Professional Voice*. New York, NY: The Voice Foundation; 1978:3:17–18.

19. Damsté PH. Changes in the voice caused by drugs. In: Meyer L, Pach HM, eds. *Drug Induced Diseases*. Amsterdam, The Netherlands: Excerpta Medica; 1978:543–548.

20. Damsté PH. [Virilization of the voice due to anabolic steroids.] *Ned Tijdschr Geneeskd*. 1963;107:891–892.

21. Damsté PH. Voice change in adult women caused by virilizing agents. *J Speech Hear Disord*. 1967;32:126–132.

22. Derman RJ. Effects of sex steroids on women's health: implication for practitioners. *Am J Med*. 1995;98(1A): 137S–143S.

23. Pinsky L, Kaufman M, Killinger DW. Impaired spermatogenesis is not an obligate expression of receptor defective androgen resistance. *Am J Med Genet*. 1989; 32(1):100–104.

24. Rolf C, Nieschlag E. Potential adverse effects on long-term testosterone therapy. *Baillieres Clin Endocrinol Metab*. 1998;12(3):521–534.

25. Pedersen MF, Moller S, Krabbe S, et al. Fundamental voice frequency in female puberty measured with electroglottography during continuous speech as a secondary sex characteristic. A comparison between voice, pubertal stages, oestrogens and androgens. *Int J Pediatr Otorhinolaryngol*. 1990;20(1):17–24.

26. Saez S, Francoise S. Recepteurs dandrogenes: mise en evidence dans la fraction cytosolique de muqueuse normale et d'epitheliomas pharyngolaryngés humains. *CR Acad Sci (Paris)*. 1975;280:935–938.

27. Vuorenkoski V, Lenko HL, Tjernlund P, et al. Fundamental voice frequency during normal and abnormal growth, and after androgen treatment. *Arch Dis Child*. 1978;53:201–209.

28. Arndt HJ. Stimmstörungen nach Behandlung mit androgenen und anabolen hormonen. *Munch Med Wochenschr*. 1974;116:1715–1720.

29. Bourdial J. Les troubles de la voix provoques par la therapeutique hormonale androgene. *Ann Otolaryngol Chir Cervicofac*. 1970;87:725–734.

30. Joura EA, Zeisler H, Brancher-Todesca D, et al. Short-term effects of topical testosterone in vulvar lichen sclerosus. *Obstet Gynecol*. 1997;89(2):297–299.

31. Hansen J, Eckert L, Mlytz H. Sex hormones and carcinoma of the larynx in women. *Arch Klin Exp Ohren Nasen Kehlkopfheilkd*. 1969;193(3):277–286.

32. Slayden SM. Risks of menopausal androgen supplementation. *Semin Reprod Endocrinol*. 1998;16(2): 145–152.

33. Need AG, Durbridge TC, Nordin BE. Anabolic steroids in postmenopausal osteoporosis. *Wien Med Wochenschr*. 1993;143(14–15):392–395.

34. Petit JC, Klein T, Rodier D. Hormone therapy for advanced breast cancer with drostanolone propionate. *Bull Cancer*. 1971;58(4):511–522.

35. Wardle PG, Whitehead MI. Non reversible and wide ranging voice changes after treatment with danazol. *Brit Med J*. 1983;287:540.

36. Gelfand MM, Witta B. Androgen and estrogen-androgen hormone replacement therapy: a review of the safety literature, 1941–1996. *Clin Ther*. 1997;19(3):383–404; discussion 367–368.

37. Abitbol J, Abitbol B. [The voice and menopause: the twilight of the divas.] *Contracep Fertil Sex*. 1998;26(9): 649–655.

38. Mercaitis PA, Peaper RE, Schwartz PA. Effect of danazol on vocal pitch: a case study. *Obstet Gynecol*. 1985;65:131–135.

39. Sorgo W, Zachmann M. [Virilization caused by methandrostenoline-containing cream in prepubertal girls.] *Helv Paediatric Acta*. 1982;37(4):401–406.

40. Abitbol J, Abitbol P, Abitbol B. Sex hormones and the female voice. *J Voice*. 1999;13(3):424–446.

41. Dordain M. Étude statistique de l'influence des contraceptifs hormonaux sur la voix. *Folia Phoniatr*. 1972; 24:86–96.

42. Pahn V, Goretzlehner G. Stimmstörungen durch hormonale Kontrazeptiva. *Zentralb Gynakol*. 1978;100: 341–346.

43. Schiff M. The "pill" in otolaryngology. *Trans Am Acad Ophthalmol Otolaryngol*. 1968;72:76–84.

44. Brodnitz F. Medical care preventive therapy. In Lawrence V, ed. *Transcripts of the Seventh Annual Symposium: Care of the Professional Voice*. New York, NY: The Voice Foundation; 1978:3:86.

45. Bausch J. Effects and side-effects of hormonal contraceptives in the region of the nose, throat and ear. [In German]. *HNO*. 1983;31(12):409–414.

46. Could contraceptives with progestational effect cause voice change? [In Dutch]. *Ned Tijdschr Geneeskd*. 1975; 119(44):1726–1727.

47. Krahulec I, Urbanova O, Simko S. [Voice changes during hormonal contraception.] [In Czech]. *Cesk Otolaryngol*. 1977;26(4):234–237.

48. Wendler J. Cyclicly dependent variations in efficiency of the voice and its influencing by ovulation inhibitors. [In German]. *Folia Phoniatr* (Basel).1972;24(4):259–277.

49. Ramsey BW, Astley SJ, Aitken ML, et al. Efficacy and safety of short-term administration of aerolized recombinant human deoxyribonuclease in patients with cystic fibrosis. *Am Rev Respir Dis*. 1993;148:145–151.

50. James IM, Griffith DN, Pearson RM, Newbury P. Effect of oxprenolol on stage-fright in musicians. *Lancet*. 1977;2:952–954.

51. Brantigan CO, Brantigan TA, Joseph N. Effect of beta blockade and beta stimulation on stage fright. *Am J Med*. 1982;72(1):88–94.

52. Lyskowski JC, Dunner FJ. Hoarseness and tricyclic antidepressants. *Am J Psychiatry*. 1980;137:636.

53. Rhoads JH, Lowell SH, Hedgepeth EM. Hoarseness and aphonia as a side effect of tricyclic antidepressants. *Am J Psychiatry*. 1979;136:1599.

54. Vogel D, Carter J. *The Effects of Drugs on Communication Disorders*. San Diego, CA: Singular Publishing Group; 1995:29–135.

55. Schatzberg A, Cole J. *Manual of Clinical Psychopharmacology*. 2nd ed. Washington, DC: APA Press; 1991:40, 50, 55, 58, 66, 68, 69, 72, 73–77, 110–125, 158–165, 169–177, 185–227, 313–348.

56. Sataloff RT, Mandel S, Caputo Rosen D. Neurological disorders affecting the voice in performance. In: Sataloff RT, ed. *Professional Voice: The Science and Art of Clinical Care*. 2nd ed. San Diego, CA: Singular Publishing Group; 1997:479–498.

57. US Food and Drug Administration. FDA proposes labeling and manufacturing standards for all dietary supplements. *FDA News*. March 7, 2003. http://www.fda.gov/bbs/topics/NEWS/2003/NEW 00876.html.

58. Ernst E, Pittler MH. Herbal medicine. *Med Clin North Am*. 2002;86(1):149–161.

59. Pittler MH, Ernst E. Efficacy of kava extract for treating anxiety: systemic review and meta-analysis. *J Clin Psychopharmacol*. 2000;20(1):84–89.

60. Volz HP, Kieser N. Kava-kava extract. WS 1490 vs. placebo in anxiety disorders—a randomized placebo controlled 25-week outpatient trial. *Pharmacopsychiatry*. 1997;30(1):1–5.

61. Escher N, Desmeules J, Giostra E, Gilles M. Hepatitis associated with Kava, an herbal remedy for anxiety. *Br Med J*. 2001;322:139.

62. Shaver K. Liver toxicity with Kava. *Pharm Lett/Prescrib Lett*. 2001;18:180115. http://www.pharmacistsletter.com; http://www.prescribersletter.com.

63. Murray MT. *The Healing Power of Herbs*. Rocklin, CA: Prima Publishing; 1995.

64. Gilbert J. Ginkgo biloba. *Neurology*. 1997;48:1137.

65. Rowin J, Lewis SL. Spontaneous bilateral subdural hematomas with chronic Ginkgo biloba ingestion. *Neurology*. 1996;46:1775–1776.

66. Fesseden JN, Wittenborn WW, Clarke L. Ginkgo biloba: a case report of herbal medicine and bleeding postoperatively from a laparoscopic cholecystectomy. *Am Surg*. 2001:67:33–35.

67. Kudolo GB. The effect of 3-month ingestion of Ginkgo biloba extract on pancreatic beta-cell function in response to glucose loading in normal glucose tolerant individuals. *J Clin Pharmacol*. 2000;40(6):647–654.

68. Gregory BJ. A seizure associated with Ginkgo biloba? *Ann Intern Med*. 2001;134(4):324.

69. Ondrizek RR, Chan PJ, Patton WC, King A. Inhibition of human sperm motility by specific herbs used in alternative medicines. *J Assist Reprod Genet*. 1999;16:87–91.

70. Jellin MJ, Gregory BJ, Patz S, et al. *Natural Medicine Comprehensive Data Base*. 4th ed. Stockton, CA: Therapeutic Research Factory; 2002:589.

71. Brinkeborn RN, Shah DV, Degenring FH. Echinaforce and other Echinacea fresh plant preparations in the treatment of the common cold. A randomized, placebo controlled, double-blind clinical trial. *Phytomedicine*. 1999;6:1–6.

72. Giles JT, Palat CT III, Chien SH, et al. Evaluation of echinacea for the treatment of the common cold. *Pharmacotherapy*. 2000;20(6):690–697.

73. Bruss K, ed. *The American Cancer Society Guide to Complementary and Alternative Cancer Methods Handbook*. Atlanta, GA: American Cancer Society; 2000:273.

74. Kim HL, Streltzer J, Goebert D. St. John's wort for depression: a meta-analysis of well-defined clinical trials. *J Nerv Ment Dis*. 1999;187:532–538.

75. Brown TM. Acute St. John's wort toxicity. *Am J Emerg Med*. 2000;18:231–232.

76. Miller LG. Herbal medicinals: selective clinical considerations focusing on known or potential drug-herb interactions. *Arch Int Med*. 1998;158:2200–2201.

77. Doyle H, Kargin N. Herbal stimulant containing ephedrine has also caused psychosis. *Br J Med*. 1996;313(7059):756.

78. Haller CA, Benowitz ML. Adverse cardiovascular and central nervous system events associated with dietary supplements containing ephedra alkaloids. *N Eng J Med*. 2000;343(25):1833–1838.

79. Meenan KD, White MK, Romak J, Sataloff RT. Common vocal remedies: What are they and do they really work? *J Singing*. 2016;73(2).

80. Tilburt J, Kaptchuk T. Herbal medicine research and global health: an ethical analysis. *Bull World Health Org*. 2008;86(8):594–599.

81. Angell M, Kassirer JP. Alternative medicine: the risks of untested and unregulated remedies. *N Eng J Med*. 1998;339(12):839–841.

82. Cirigliano M, Sun A. Advising patients about herbal therapies. *JAMA*. 1998;18:1565–1566.

83. Fong HS. Integration of herbal medicine into modern medical practices: issues and prospects. *Integr Cancer Ther*. 2002;3:287–293.

84. Traditionalmedicinals.com [Internet]. Sebastopol, CA: Traditional Medicinals; 2013. http://www.traditionalmedicinals.com/products/throat-coat/. Accessed November 12, 2015.

85. Brinckmann J, Sigwart H, van Houten Taylor L. Safety and efficacy of a traditional herbal medicine (Throat Coat) in symptomatic temporary relief of pain in patients with acute pharyngitis: a multicenter, prospective, randomized, double-blinded, placebo-controlled study. *J Altern Complement Med*. 2003;9(2):285–298.

86. Murray M. *Glycyrrhiza globra* (Licorice). In: Pizzorno JE, Murray MT, eds. *Textbook of Natural Medicine.* 4th ed. St. Louis: Elsevier/Churchill Livingstone; 2013: 804–812.

87. Izzo A, Di Carlo G, Borrelli F, Ernst E. Cardiovascular pharmacotherapy and herbal medicines: the risk of drug interaction. *Int J Cardiol.* 2005;98:1–14.

88. Kamei J, Nakamura R, Ichiki H, Kubo M. Antitussive principles of *Glycyrrhizae radix*, a main component of the Kampo preparations Bakumondo-to (Mai-men-dong-tang). *Eur J Pharmacol.* 2003;469(1–3):159–163.

89. Omar HR, Komarova I, El-Ghonemi M, et al. Licorice abuse: time to send a warning message. *Ther Adv Endocrinol Metab.* 2012;3(4):125–138.

90. Zick SM, Sen A, Feng Y, Green J, Olatunde S, Boon H. Trial of Essiac to ascertain its effect in women with breast cancer (TEA-BC). *J Altern Complement Med.* 2006;12(10):971–980.

91. Cassileth B. Essiac. *Oncology (Williston Park).* 2011; 25(11):1098–1099.

92. Benbassat N, Kostova B, Nikolova I, Rachev D. Development and evaluation of novel lozenges containing marshmallow root extract. *Pak J Pharm Sci.* 2013; 26(6):1103–1107.

93. Marshmallow: *Althaea officinalis*. In: Fleming T, ed. *PDR for Herbal Medicine.* 4th ed. Montvale, NJ: Medical Economics Company; 2000:505–506.

94. Entertainers-secret.com [Internet]. Carmel, IN: Entertainer's Secret; 2014. http://www.entertainers-secret.com/. Accessed November 12, 2015.

95. Roy N, Tanner K, Gray SD, Blomgren M, Fisher KV. An evaluation of the effects of three laryngeal lubricants on phonation threshold pressure (PTP). *J Voice.* 2003;17(3):331–342.

96. Vocaleze.com [Internet]. Colorado Springs, CO: Vocaleze; 2014. http://vocaleze.com/index.php/. Accessed November 12, 2015.

97. Terrell B, Fennell A. Oshá (Bear Root): *Ligusticum porteri* J.M. Coult. & Rose var. porteri. *NPJ.* 2009;10(2): 110–117.

98. Leon A, Toscano RA, Tortoriello, J, Delgado G. Phthalides and other constituents from *Ligusticum porteri*; sedative and spasmolytic activities of some natural products and derivatives. *Nat Prod Res.* 2011; 25(13):1234–1242.

99. Ginger: *Zingiber officinale*. In: Fleming T, ed. *PDR for Herbal Medicine.* 4th ed. Montvale, NJ: Medical Economics Company; 2000:334–341.

100. Ojewole JA. Analgesic, anti-inflammatory and hypoglycaemic effects of ethanol extracts of *Zingiber officinale* (Roscoe) rhizomes (Zingiberaceae) in mice and rats. *Phytother Res.* 2006;20(9):764–772.

101. Terry R, Posadzki P, Watson LK, Ernst E. The use of ginger (*Zingiber officinale*) for the treatment of pain: a systematic review of clinical trials. *Pain Med.* 2011; 12(12):1808–1818.

102. Chang JS, Wang KC, Yeh CF, Shieh DE, Chiang LC. Fresh ginger (*Zingiber officinale*) has anti-viral activity against human respiratory syncytial virus in human respiratory tract cell lines. *J Ethnopharmacol.* 2013; 145(1):145–151.

103. Malu SP, Obochi GO, Tawo EN, Nyong BE. Antibacterial activity and medicinal properites of ginger (*Zingiber officinale*). *Global J Pure Appl Sci.* 2009;15(3): 365–368.

104. Karsch-Völk M, Barrett B, Kiefer D, Bauer R, Ardjoman-Woelkart K, Linde K. Echinacea for preventing and treating the common cold. *Cochrane Acute Respiratory Infections Group.* 2014. doi:10.1002/14651858. CD000530.pub3

105. Wagh VD. Propolis: A wonder bees product and its pharmacologic potentials. *Adv Pharmacol Sci.* 2013. doi:10.1155/2013/308249

106. Hwu YJ, Lin FY. Effectiveness of propolis on oral health: a systematic review. *JBI Database System Rev Implement Rep.* 2013;11(5):28–61.

107. Thayers.com [Internet]. Westport, CT: Thayers Natural Remedies; 2014. http://www.thayers.com/. Accessed November 12, 2015.

108. Vocalzone.com [Internet]. Broadstone, England: Kestrel Medical Ltd. http://www.vocalzone.com/. Accessed November 12, 2015.

109. Pimentel M, Bonorris GG, Chow EJ, Lin HC. Peppermint oil improves the manometric findings in Diffuse Esophageal Spasm. *J Clin Gastroenterol.* 2001;1:27–31.

110. Klinger B, Chaudhary S. Peppermint Oil. *Am Fam Physician.* 2007;7:1027–1030.

111. Wells LK. Evidence-based herbal medicine. *Dental Abstracts.* 2012;57(6):305–307.

112. Peppermint: *Mentha piperita*. In: Fleming, T, ed. *PDR for Herbal Medicine.* 4th ed. Montvale, NJ: Medical Economics Company; 2000:580–583.

113. de Sousa AAS, Soares PMG, de Almeida ANS, Maia AR, de Souza EP, Assreuy AMS. Antispasmodic effect of *Mentha piperita* essential oil on tracheal smooth muscle of rats. *J Ethnopharmacol.* 2010;130(2):433–436.

114. Su S, Duan J, Chen T, et al. Frankincense and myrrh suppress inflammation via regulation of the metabolic profiling and the MAPK signaling pathway. *Sci Rep.* 2015;13668. doi:10.1038/srep13668.

115. Cheng YW, Cheah KP, Lin CW, et al. Myrrh mediates haem oxygenase-1 expression to suppress the lipopolysaccharide-induced inflammatory response in RAW264.7 macrophages. *J Pharm Pharmacol.* 2011; 63(9):1211–1218.

116. Su S, Wang T, Duan JA, et al. Anti-inflammatory and analgesic activity of different extracts of *Commiphora myrrha*. *J Ethnopharmacol.* 2011;134(2):251–258.

117. Myrrh: *Commiphora molmol*. In: Fleming, T, ed. *PDR for Herbal Medicine.* 4th ed. Montvale, NJ: Medical Economics Company; 2000:534–536.

118. Vitavocalhealth.com [Internet]. VitaVocal Health. http://www.vitavocalhealth.com/product/vitavocal-throat-voice-enhancer/. Accessed November 12, 2015.

119. Ginseng: *Panax ginseng*. In: Fleming, T, ed. *PDR for Herbal Medicine.* 4th ed. Montvale, NJ: Medical Economics Company; 2000:346–349.

120. Scaglione F, Cattaneo G, Alessandria M, Cogo R. Efficacy and safety of the standardized Ginseng extract G115 for potentiating vaccination against the influenza syndrome and protection against the common cold [corrected]. *Drugs Exp Clin Res.* 1996;22(2):65–72.

121. McElhaney JE, Gravenstein S, Cole SK, et al. A placebo-controlled trial of a proprietary extract of North American ginseng (CVT-E002) to prevent acute respiratory illness in institutionalized older adults. *J Am Geriatr Soc.* 2004;52(1):13–19.

122. McElhaney JE, Goel V, Toane B, Hooten J, Shan JJ. Efficacy of COLD-fX in the prevention of respiratory symptoms in community-dwelling adults: a randomized, double-blinded, placebo-controlled trial. *J Altern Complement Med.* 2006;12(2):153–157.

123. Vohra S, Johnston BC, Laycock KL, et al. Safety and tolerability of North American ginseng extract in the treatment of pediatric upper respiratory tract infection: a phase II randomized, controlled trial of 2 dosing schedules. *Pediatrics.* 2008;122(2):e402–410.

124. Saveritemedical.com [Internet]. Brooklyn, NY: Save Rite Medical. http://www.saveritemedical.com/product/sprouts-voice-formula-for-singers-a-voice-remedy-for-hoarsness-laryngitis-and-expectorant.html. Accessed November 12, 2015.

125. Slippery elm: *Ulmus rubra.* In: Fleming T, ed. *PDR for Herbal Medicine.* 4th ed. Montvale, NJ: Medical Economics Company; 2000:697.

126. Fennel: *Foeniculum vulgare.* In: Fleming T, ed. *PDR for Herbal Medicine.* 4th ed. Montvale, NJ: Medical Economics Company; 2000:302–304.

127. Horseradish: *Armor acta rusticana.* In: Fleming T, ed. *PDR for Herbal Medicine.* 4th ed. Montvale, NJ: Medical Economics Company; 2000:408–409.

128. Thyme: *Thymus vulgaris.* In: Fleming T, ed. *PDR for Herbal Medicine.* 4th ed. Montvale, NJ: Medical Economics Company; 2000:761–762.

129. Celery: *Apium graveolens.* In: Fleming T, ed. *PDR for Herbal Medicine.* 4th ed. Montvale, NJ: Medical Economics Company; 2000:172–174.

130. Molan PP, Rhodes T. Honey: A biologic wound dressing. *Wounds.* 2015;27(6):141–151.

131. Al-Waili NS, Boni BS. Natural honey lowers plasma prostaglandin concentrations in normal individuals. *J Med Food.* 2004;6(2):129–133.

132. Al-Waili NS. Effects of honey on the urinary total nitrite and prostaglandin concentration. *Int Urol Nephrol.* 2005;37(1):107–111.

133. Timm M, Bartlet S, Hansen EW. Immunomodulatory effects of honey cannot be distinguished from endotoxin. *Cytokine.* 2008;42(1):113–120.

134. Paul IM, Beiler J, McMonagle A, Shaffer ML, Duda L, Berlin CM. Effect of honey, dextromethorphan, and no treatment on nocturnal cough and sleep quality for coughing children and their parents. *JAMA Pediatr.* 2007;161(12):1140–1146.

135. Shadkam MN, Mozaffari-Khosravi H, Mozayan MR. A comparison of the effect of honey, dextromethorphan, and diphenhydramine on nightly cough and sleep quality in children and their parents. *J Altern Complement Med.* 2010;16(7):787–793.

136. Raeessi MA, Aslani J, Raeessi N, Gharaie H, Zarchi AAK, Raeessi F. Honey plus coffee versus systemic steroid in the treatment of post-infectious cough: a randomized controlled trial. *Prim Care Respir J.* 2013; 22:325-330.

137. Henatsch D, Wesseling F, Kross KW, Stokroos RJ. Honey and beehive products in otorhinolaryngology: a narrative review. *Clin Otolaryngol.* 2016;41(5):519–531.

138. Cayenne: Capsicum species. In: Fleming T, ed. *PDR for Herbal Medicine.* 4th ed. Montvale, NJ: Medical Economics Company; 2000:165–168.

139. Al-Abri SA, Kearney T. Baking soda misuse as a home remedy: case experience of the California Poison Control System. *J Clin Pharm Ther.* 2014;39(1):73–77.

140. Pakrokh GP. The extraction process optimization of antioxidant polysaccharides from Marshmallow (*Althaea officinalis L.*) roots. *Int J Biol Macromol.* 2015; 75:51–57. doi:10.1016/j.ijbiomac.2014.11.047.

141. Limb M, Connor A, Pickford M, et al. Scintigraphy can be used to compare delivery of sore throat formulations. *Int J Clin Pract.* 2009;63(4):606–612.

142. Tanner K, Roy N, Merrill RM, Elstad M. The effects of three nebulized osmotic agents in the dry larynx. *J Speech Lang Hear Res.* 2007;50(3):635–646.

143. Verdolini K, Titze IR, Fennell A. Dependence of phonatory effort on hydration level. *J Speech Hear Res.* 1994;37(5):1001–1007.

144. Verdolini-Marston K, Titze IR, Druker DG. Changes in phonation threshold pressure with induced conditions of hydration. *J Voice.* 1990;4(2):142–151.

145. Solomon NP, Glaze LE, Arnold RR, van Mersbergen M. Effects of a vocally fatiguing task and systemic hydration on men's voices. *J Voice.* 2003;17(1):31–46.

146. Solomon NP, DiMattia MS. Effects of a vocally fatiguing task and systemic hydration on phonation threshold pressure. *J Voice.* 2000;14(3):341–362.

147. Tanner K, Roy N, Merrill RM, et al. Nebulized isotonic saline versus water following a laryngeal dessication challenge in classically trained sopranos. *J Speech Lang Hear Res.* 2010;53(6):1555–1566.

148. Tanner K, Fujiki RB, Dromey C, et al. Laryngeal desiccation challenge and nebulized isotonic saline in healthy male singers and nonsingers: effects on acoustic, aerodynamic, and self-perceived effort and dryness measures [published online September 26, 2015]. *J Voice.* 2016;30(6):670–676.

149. Hunter E, Tanner K, Smith M. Gender differences affecting vocal health of women in vocally demanding careers. *Logoped Phoniatr Vocol.* 2011;36(3):128–136.

150. Sabar R, Kaye AD, Frost, EA. Perioperative considerations for the patient taking herbal medicines. *Heart Dis.* 2001;3(2):87–96.

151. Surow JB, Lovetri J. "Alternative medical therapy" use among singers: prevalence and implications for the medical care of the singer. *J Voice.* 2000;14(3):398–409.

# Index

Note: Page numbers in italic reference non-text material.